Cha
from
co Mart
Minneapolis

MEDICAL REVOLUTION IN MINNESOTA

MEDICAL REVOLUTION IN MINNESOTA

A History of the University of Minnesota Medical School

Leonard G. Wilson

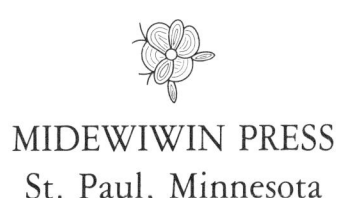

MIDEWIWIN PRESS
St. Paul, Minnesota

Copyright © 1989 by Leonard G. Wilson

All rights reserved. No part of this book may be reproduced or transmitted in any form or by any means, electronic or mechanical, including photocopying, recording or by any informational storage or retrieval system—except by a reviewer who may quote brief passages in a review for the public press—without permission in writing from the author. For information contact:

Midewiwin Press
797 Goodrich Avenue
St. Paul, Minnesota 55105

Printed in the United States of America

Library of Congress Cataloging-in-Publication Data
Wilson, Leonard G. (Leonard Gilchrist), 1928–
  Medical revolution in Minnesota : a history of the University of Minnesota Medical School / Leonard G. Wilson.
    p. cm.
  Bibliography: p.
  Includes index.
  1. University of Minnesota. Medical School—History. I. Title.
R747.U68344W55 1989
610'.7' 11776581—dc19   88-29563
ISBN 0-9620884-0-4   CIP

Designed by Lois Stanfield
Set in Garamond type by Stanton Publication Services, Inc., Minneapolis
Printed and bound by Bookcrafters, Chelsea, Michigan

To
the whole company of teachers and students,
past and present,
of medicine and surgery
at the University of Minnesota

Contents

Preface	ix
1. Introduction	3
2. The Origins of the Medical Profession and the Beginnings of Medical Teaching in Minnesota	6
3. The Department of Medicine, 1888–1892	32
4. The Early Years of the School on the University Campus, 1893–1897	60
5. The Medical School under Dean Parks Ritchie, 1897–1906	82
6. The Elliot Memorial Gift and the New Medical Campus	109
7. The College of Medicine and Surgery under Dean Wesbrook	124
8. The Convulsion of 1913 and the Appointment of Dean Lyon	141
9. Affiliation of the University with the Mayo Foundation, 1915–1917	159
10. The Medical School in the First World War, 1917–1919	213
11. Renewed Controversy and Continued Stagnation, 1919–1923	235
12. "Hope Resurgent:" Expansion of the University Hospitals, 1923–1929	251
13. The Development of a Full-time Clinical Faculty, 1925–1930	282
14. The Clinical Renaissance of the Medical School, 1930–1941	305
15. Research in the Basic Medical Sciences, 1913 to 1941	372
16. Developments in Biochemistry, the Laboratory of Physiological Hygiene, and the Identification of Risk Factors in Coronary Heart Disease	400

CONTENTS

17.	The Medical School in the Second World War, 1941–1945	416
18.	The Mayo Memorial Campaign and Campaigners	426
19.	The Fusion of Basic & Clinical Research at Minnesota, 1942–1960	463
20.	The Development of Cardiac Surgery at Minnesota, 1940–1960	481
21.	The Development of Organ Transplantation at Minnesota	529
22.	Change and Expansion after 1970	544
23.	New Developments in the 1980s	557
24.	The Medical School in Retrospect	564
	Appendix I: The First Faculty of the Department of Medicine	567
	Manuscript Sources	570
	Abbreviations of Journals Cited	573
	Bibliography	578
	Index	583

Preface

The life of such a large and complex institution as a university medical center is so diverse and so constantly active that it is difficult to grasp it at any one moment in time. The successive changes through which such an institution has evolved over the course of a century cannot, therefore, be described with any approach to completeness—certainly not in one volume. The history of a medical school must be limited to the discussion of a relatively few developments (few in proportion to the total life of the school) that may be used to portray the overall history. The result is nonetheless a large book that might easily have been larger. It was conceived and written so that its publication might coincide approximately with the centennial of the University of Minnesota Medical School in 1988, but it is written as history rather than as promotion for the medical school. Some of the school's history is sad, burdened with unrealized possibilities; part may be controversial, because truth is not always agreeable to everyone; but the history of the University of Minnesota Medical School is also a proud record of brilliant accomplishment, often in the face of adversity.

Late in 1983 former president of the University of Minnesota C. Peter Magrath and Vice-president for Health Sciences Neal A. Vanselow made funds available to support the research and writing of a history of the University of Minnesota Medical School. University funds were later supplemented by grants from the Minnesota Medical Foundation. The funds were used to support a research fellow to assist with the project and to pay the costs of photocopying and other expenses associated with historical research. In September 1984 Jane M. Hult (now Jane M. Tang, Ph.D.) was appointed as research fellow, and from then until June 1987 carried out extensive historical research for the book in various archives at the University of Minnesota, the Minnesota Historical Society, and the Minneapolis Public Library. Although I, too, spent long periods at work in archives, particularly the University of Minnesota Archives, Jane Tang's assistance enabled me to concentrate my attention primarily on the actual writing. I am deeply indebted to her for an immense amount of conscientious and thoroughly efficient work, and

PREFACE

for highly intelligent and scientifically informed advice on many aspects of the book.

At the University Archives Penelope S. Krosch, archivist, her assistant Lois G. Hendrickson, and their student assistants gave us invaluable assistance in our search for documents and photographs relating to the history of the medical school. Norma Peterson, director of the Office of Academic Personnel System, University of Minnesota, kindly made available to us the personnel files of deceased faculty members, which frequently contained otherwise unobtainable biographical information. The staff of the Bio-medical Library has been most helpful in locating books and journals and in answering reference questions.

The staff of the Minnesota Historical Society Archives were unfailingly helpful as were also the staffs of the Minneapolis Collection at the Minneapolis Public Library and the Stillwater Public Library. Laurenda Daniels, university archivist at the University of British Columbia Library, Vancouver, Canada, kindly provided me with photocopies of correspondence from the Wesbrook papers. During a visit to the Rockefeller Archive Center at Pocantico Hills, North Tarrytown, New York, in April 1987 I received courteous assistance from J. William Hess, associate director, and his staff in locating documents relating to the University of Minnesota among the papers of the General Education Board and the Rockefeller Foundation.

In addition to the staffs of archives and libraries various individuals assisted in various ways to enrich the book. Dr. Stuart Lane Arey allowed me to use his tape-recorded interview with the late Dr. Lawrence Richdorf. Dr. Jesse Barron most generously provided letters, papers, and photographs of his father, Dr. Moses Barron. Saul Benison, professor of history at the University of Cincinnati, informed me of correspondence among the Walter B. Cannon papers at Harvard University relating to the invitation in 1913 to Cannon to become dean of the University of Minnesota Medical School; and Richard J. Wolfe, curator of rare books and manuscripts at the Francis A. Countway Library of Medicine, Harvard University, kindly provided me with photocopies of the relevant letters. Professor Benison also drew my attention to the importance of the work of Sister Kenny in Minnesota. Over many years Dr. Howard Burchell has advised me on many aspects of medicine and medical history. His advice on questions of cardiology was particularly valuable in the chapter on cardiac surgery. Horace W. Davenport, William Beaumont Professor of Physiology, Emeritus, at the University of Michigan drew my attention to letters from Dr. Charles Lyman Greene to Victor Vaughan concerning the University of Minnesota Medical School among the Vaughan papers at the University of Michigan and generously sent me photocopies of them. Dr. Royal C. Gray spent an afternoon sharing with Jane Tang and me his memories of the medical school as he first knew it in the 1920s.

Sally E. Howard, director of Health Sciences Public Relations, University of Minnesota, provided photographs of the new medical buildings, including the new university hospital, and helped to locate photographs of certain faculty members. Doreen Bower provided a photograph of Lewis Wannamaker. Dr. Lyle O.

PREFACE

Johnson, chief surgeon at the Shriners Hospital for Crippled Children, Minneapolis, provided a photograph of Dr. Wallace Cole. Eleanor M. Larson of Richfield, Minnesota, provided me with a portrait photograph of Dr. Karl Wilhelm Stenstrom. Dr. C. Walton Lillehei provided photographs of his early open heart surgery patients. Mr. Perry H. Millard of Hazelcrest, Illinois, sent me letters, other papers, and photographs relating to his grandfather, Perry H. Millard, M.D., founder and first dean of the College of Medicine and Surgery at the University of Minnesota, and allowed me to make photocopies of them. Dr. Frederic J. Kottke provided photographs of Dr. Miland E. Knapp and of Sister Kenny. Sister Ann Thomasine Sampson, historian of St. Mary's Hospital, Minneapolis, provided photographs of St. Mary's Hospital and of the medical campus of the university from across the Mississippi River, both taken in 1920, and shared with me her experience of writing the history of St. Mary's. Sarah D. Wangensteen read a large portion of the manuscript and improved it greatly by numerous constructive criticisms and suggestions. From her deep knowledge of the history of Minnesota, Mrs. Wangensteen suggested various sources of information about the medical history of the state.

My wife, Adelia K. Wilson, has helped with the book in many ways. In a search for biographical information about the first dean, Perry H. Millard, she located Dr. Millard's will among the probate court records in St. Paul, and from the records of Fairview Cemetery at Stillwater, Minnesota, she obtained information that enabled us ultimately to locate Dr. Millard's grandson, Perry H. Millard, in Hazelcrest, Illinois. At the Stillwater Public Library she read microfilms of Stillwater newspapers of the 1870s for information about Dr. Millard's medical practice and other activities in Stillwater. She read critically the whole manuscript, copy-edited it for the press, and prepared the index.

For the preparation of the manuscript I am especially indebted to two secretaries. Kathryn Kosiak, who was my secretary from the beginning of the project until June 1987, typed the first draft of the whole work into our word processor. Her successor, Elizabeth Carveth, has guided the manuscript through the multitudinous changes required by several revisions of the original manuscript. Mrs. Carveth has also kept track of the photographs used as illustrations.

John Ervin, director of the University of Minnesota Press, obtained reviews of the manuscript, and the criticisms and suggestions of the three anonymous reviewers proved most helpful in the revision of the manuscript. Mr. Ervin encouraged us to publish the work and advised on publication.

For the help of all these persons I am deeply grateful. I remain responsible for all errors of fact or judgment and for historical interpretations in the book.

MEDICAL REVOLUTION IN MINNESOTA

CHAPTER 1

Introduction

Minnesota is unusually distinguished in medicine. The fame of its physicians and surgeons has drawn both medical students and patients to the state from all over the world. At the University of Minnesota in the 1930s, surgeons revolutionized the treatment of intestinal obstruction and introduced gastric suction, procedures that changed profoundly all abdominal surgery. During the 1950s the university pioneered in the introduction of open heart surgery, including the introduction of the heart pacemaker and artificial heart valves. In the 1960s and 1970s Minnesota played a leading role in bringing organ transplantation from the experimental laboratory to a successful surgical specialty. Minnesota has also made landmark contributions to knowledge of tuberculosis and brucellosis, and of children's diseases, especially immune deficiency diseases. The university's pioneering work in bone marrow transplantation in the 1980s is making that procedure safer and more successful. The role of diet in heart disease and of fluoride in the prevention of tooth decay were both revealed at the University of Minnesota. Its many contributions to medicine have given rise to great hospitals and clinics, and to a sophisticated technological industry that produces heart pacemakers, artificial heart valves, insulin pumps, and biological substances to heal the sick and prolong their lives.

The history of the University of Minnesota Medical School is part of the history of a revolution in medicine over the past century that has exerted profound effects on the lives and health not only of Americans, but of all the world's people. The medical school at the university has been the great engine that has powered the development of the health care industry in Minnesota, an industry that contributes greatly to the economy of the state, employing in an agricultural state more people than does agriculture. From its beginning the school pursued medical science and carried on research that has produced a rich harvest of medical discoveries. The school has trained successive generations of Minnesota physicians who collectively have given the hospitals and clinics of the state their far-reaching reputation.

INTRODUCTION

The introduction of antiseptic surgery to Minnesota in the 1880s was followed by the rapid development of surgery throughout the state. At St. Paul in 1886 Justus Ohage performed the first operation in America for the removal of a diseased gallbladder, and the following year another St. Paul surgeon, Anton Shimonek, performed the first appendectomy in Minnesota. In 1887 Minnesota passed a new medical practice act, creating a state board of medical examiners that established effective standards of qualification for medical practice. The act served both to exclude untrained practitioners from Minnesota and to attract to the state graduates of the better Eastern medical schools. The medical school, founded at the university in 1888, sought from the beginning to produce well-qualified physicians, trained thoroughly in scientific medicine to meet the standards of the state board of medical examiners. In cooperation with the state board of health, the school worked also to control such infectious diseases as rabies, diphtheria, and typhoid fever.

Soon after 1900 the Mayo Clinic, at Rochester, Minnesota, became world famous, and has continued to be preeminent as a center for the highest quality of medical care. The surgery of the Mayo brothers was a particularly brilliant reflection of the high quality of surgery practiced in Minnesota. The history of the University of Minnesota Medical School has been intertwined closely with that of the Mayo Clinic. Many graduates of the school have worked at the clinic, a number of them developing international reputations. Relations between the medical school and the Mayo Clinic have been marked both by warm cooperation and keen rivalry. For several decades the influence of the Mayo Clinic tended to inhibit the development of clinical teaching and research at the university, but the high quality of surgery and medicine practiced at the clinic also set a standard that the clinical faculty of the medical school was obliged to meet. Moreover, rivalry between the medical school and the Mayo Clinic was tempered by regular cooperation and a spirit of mutual helpfulness.

The medical school was born in the midst of rivalries—between regular and homeopathic physicians, between the physicians of Minneapolis and those of St. Paul, and between all educated physicians and untrained practitioners. The remarkable characteristic of medical rivalries in Minnesota was that although vigorous they were restrained. Usually contending groups sought accommodation with their opponents rather than their destruction. In the midst of quarrels kindliness kept breaking in.

What was true of rivalries among contending groups of Minnesota physicians was even more true of relations within local medical groups. Competition among physicians for patients was tempered by generosity and kindness. The doctors of St. Paul were known for their unusually good relations with each other. No one could quarrel with the genial Dr. Alexander Stone who was always willing to go out of his way to help a young doctor or a poor patient. Dr. Stone practiced obstetrics and gynecology. When one of his poor women patients died without any place in which to be buried, he provided a grave in his family plot. Dr. Stone acted in this generous manner so often that upon his death in 1910 there was no room left for him in the plot.

The character of the early Minnesota physicians is difficult to recapture, but it determined the character of the medical school that they created at the university. Their origins, their education, and their experience combined in the founding of the medical school and influenced its development.

CHAPTER 2

The Origins of the Medical Profession and the Beginnings of Medical Teaching in Minnesota

When in February 1851 the Minnesota territorial legislature enacted the bill establishing a university, their plan called for medicine to be one of the five constituent departments together with science, literature and the arts; law; elementary education; and agriculture.[1] The regents decided that a college of medicine was not practicable at that time, and more than thirty years were to pass before such a college was authorized. Meanwhile the University of Minnesota opened in the fall of 1851; by 1858, following problems over land acquisition, the financial crash of 1857, and lack of funds to complete the main building, the enterprise had approached extinction.[2] The precarious course of the university during its first thirty years delayed the opening of a medical college and consequently permitted private medical schools organized by the local medical profession to fill the need for medical instruction.

There were probably fewer than a dozen trained civilian physicians practicing in Minnesota Territory in 1851 when the legislators first contemplated a medical college. Dr. Christopher Carli, a graduate of the University of Heidelberg, who set up practice in 1841 in a house of tamarack logs on the bank of the St. Croix River on the site of what is now Stillwater, is often mentioned as the first trained physician to practice in the land that became Minnesota.[3] However, there had been several physicians among the early fur traders and missionaries at remote stations in the northern wilderness; United States Army surgeons had been posted at Fort Snelling since 1819; and a number of men had acted as both physician and recording scientist on government surveying expeditions into uncharted areas of the Northwest.[4]

In late 1847 Dr. John Jay Dewey, a recent graduate of Albany Medical College and brother of Wisconsin's first governor, came to the little village of St. Paul to set up practice and open the town's first drugstore (offering "tasteless castor oil" among other remedies).[5] When two years later St. Paul was incorporated as the capital of the new Minnesota Territory, the town's population was said to number between two hundred fifty and three hundred individuals, including "five physicians," one of whom was "a root and herb doctor."[6] The only qualified physicians besides Dr. Dewey were two new arrivals, Thomas Reid Potts and David Day, both medical graduates of the University of Pennsylvania. The same year, 1849, John Henry Murphy began practice at St. Anthony, but took a year off to complete his medical education at Rush Medical College at Chicago.[7] A fellow graduate, Dr. Alfred Elisha Ames, joined Murphy at St. Anthony in 1851, later moving across the Mississippi to the new settlement of Minneapolis on the west bank.

Throughout the 1850s additional physicians continued to come to St. Paul, which grew from a population of thirteen hundred in 1850 to more than ten thousand by 1860. Its growth was part of the expanding settlement of the Minnesota Territory where new towns and villages were springing up along the banks of the upper Mississippi and its navigable tributaries, the St. Croix and the Minnesota. In 1852 the United States government concluded treaties with the Sioux Indians by which the land west of the Mississippi in the lower valley of the Minnesota River became available for settlement, and in 1854 and 1855 federal treaties with the Chippewa opened to lumbering the great pine forests around the headwaters of the Mississippi and St. Louis rivers.

As more physicians came to the territory and its settlements, the desirability of a professional organization was discussed. On Saturday, 23 July 1853, eleven physicians met in the courthouse at St. Paul to found a medical society for the Minnesota Territory.[8] Among the eleven physicians present only nine, each of whom possessed a diploma from a medical college, participated in the organization of the society. Two young medical practitioners present, who were not allowed to participate in the organization, did not possess medical diplomas; their medical training had probably been received by apprenticeship. Five physicians, who could not attend but had expressed a desire to join, were elected members; all of them possessed medical diplomas.[9] Although the new medical society was intended to promote the professional interests of physicians, the founders also wished "to advance medical knowledge" and "to extend the bounds of medical science." They modeled their constitution and bylaws on those of the medical societies of Pennsylvania and Illinois.

In 1854 the Minnesota Medical Society sent a delegate to the seventh meeting of the American Medical Association held at St. Louis. Founded at Philadelphia in 1847 as a result of a convention of delegates from state medical societies and medical colleges from throughout the United States, the American Medical Association had as one of its primary purposes the advancement of the medical profession by the elevation of the standards of medical education.[10] In the 1850s the medical profession was unpopular in the United States and to a great extent had lost public confidence. Two forms of medical treatment commonly used by physicians, bloodletting and the administration of calomel (mercurous chloride), were widely recognized to be at least as dangerous as the diseases they were intended to cure. Bloodletting often so weakened patients as to hasten their deaths, while calomel might produce sores and deformities, or even serious nerve damage. Both treatments were used by doctors, and frequently to extremes. The public revulsion against such forms of treatment had caused most states to repeal their laws regulating medical practice. As a result anyone who wished might practice medicine.

As a group the regular American medical profession in the 1850s was composed mainly of young men, almost all of whom had received the same kind of medical training. Typically this training consisted of two to three years of apprenticeship in a doctor's office and attendance at two courses of lectures in a medical school, the second course being a repetition of the first. Because they had learned medicine for the most part as a body of authoritative doctrine taught in lectures, they were generally unfamiliar with modes of scientific inquiry. The medical theories on which their treatments were based were under attack, their motives impugned, and their incomes reduced by competition from various kinds of irregular practitioners. At the same time the number of doctors was great and growing as a result of large numbers of medical students graduating from the many new medical schools that had been founded in the United States and Canada during the nineteenth century.

In 1858 Minnesota was admitted to the union as a state. By 1860 its population had grown to one hundred seventy-two thousand, distributed mainly along the Mississippi River and its two important tributaries, the St. Croix and the Minnesota. In August 1860 an electric telegraph line was completed to St. Paul, placing the capital of the new state in instant communication with the rest of the country. During the 1860s Minnesota was deeply involved in two devastating conflicts—the Sioux Uprising of 1862 and the Civil War—in which Minnesota doctors bravely took part, using the skills and knowledge acquired in their early training and in later frontier experiences. They soon bitterly realized the shortcomings of their education and the failure of accepted techniques to contend with infected wounds and wartime epidemics. They returned with troubled memories to a burgeoning Minnesota. It was the great age of the lumber industry and wheat farming in the state; railroads were rapidly connecting remote towns; mills had sprung up along the rivers; and a concentration of flour mills at the Falls of St. Anthony foretold the future rapid growth of the city of Minneapolis. But the returning veterans could find little change in the status of their medical profession or answers to the health problems encountered by them in the war. The Civil War experience influenced profoundly the outlook of several men who were to lead the way in Minnesota toward establishment of a state medical college and public health measures.

Governor Alexander Ramsey was in Washington when the news came of the fall of Fort Sumter and was the first to offer state troops to the Union army. The First Minnesota was mustered at Fort Snelling 30 April 1861 with Dr. Jacob H. Stewart of St. Paul as surgeon and Dr. C. W. Le Boutellier of St. Anthony as assistant surgeon. Both were taken prisoner when they remained on the field to care for the wounded at the first battle of Bull Run. Their replacement was Dr. Daniel W. Hand of St. Paul, a native of New Jersey and a medical graduate in 1856 of the University of Pennsylvania. He was promoted rapidly and under General Gor-

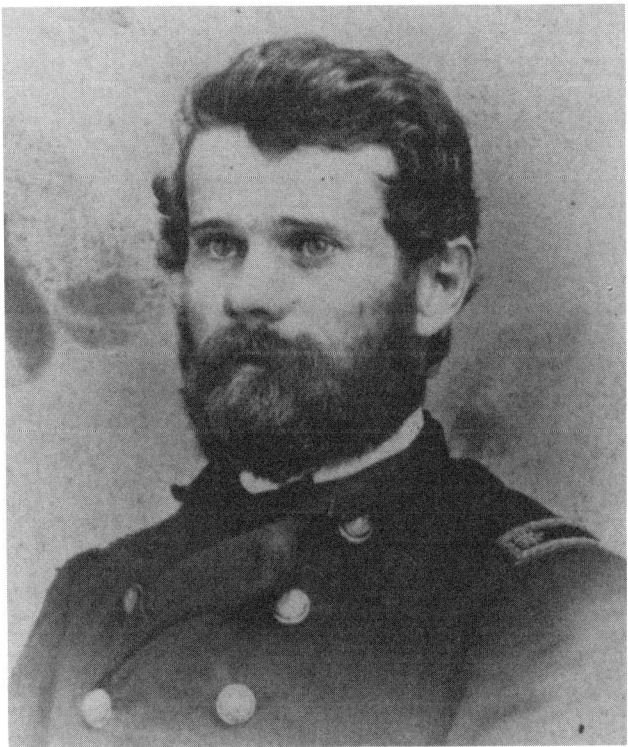

FIGURE 2:1   Daniel W. Hand in United States Army uniform. Courtesy National Library of Medicine.

man in the spring of 1862 was responsible for the care of large numbers of wounded men. As a lieutenant colonel he was in charge of the general hospital at Newport News which sometimes contained two thousand sick and wounded, many with a frequently fatal chronic diarrhea. As medical director for the army in North Carolina in the fall of 1863, faced with severe epidemics of intermittent and remittent fevers, Hand recommended sending inland regiments to the coast, where their health improved markedly. He also moved convalescing fever patients from inland hospitals to hospitals by the sea where they soon recovered. During the next two years Hand dealt with successive epidemics of malarial fevers, smallpox, yellow fever, and probably typhoid and typhus fevers. He learned the types of conditions in which epidemics arose, and devised means to limit their spread. His experience provided him with an intensive education in the conditions that tended to produce disease and the practical measures that might be taken to preserve public health.[11]

In June 1866 Daniel Hand resumed medical practice in St. Paul in association with Jacob Stewart, who after his capture at the first battle of Bull Run had been exchanged and paroled. The Confederates so respected Stewart's courage in re-

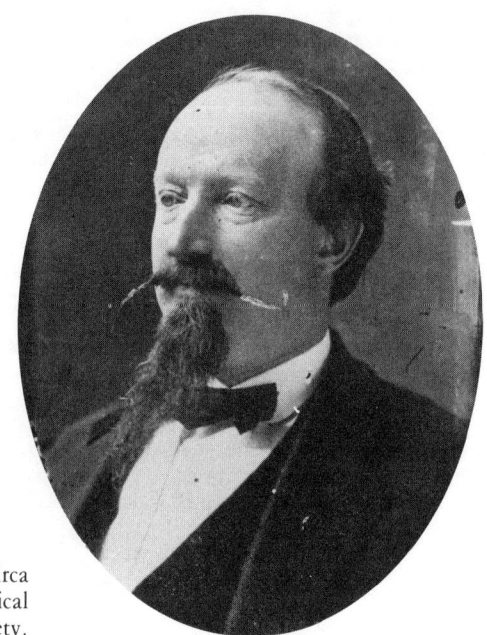

FIGURE 2:2 Jacob H. Stewart, circa 1865. Courtesy Minnesota Historical Society.

maining to care for the wounded on the battlefield that when he was exchanged at Richmond, General Pierre Beauregard returned his sword to him. Because of the great number and variety of operations performed during the war, surgeons like Hand and Stewart became very skillful. On their return to civilian life they were eager to improve upon the medical training that they had received. About 1868 Drs. Hand and Stewart began to give informal lessons in anatomy to a small group of students from various doctors' offices in St. Paul. They met on the second floor of a small stone dead house that stood beside St. Joseph's Hospital, and in a room containing only a table, a few chairs, and a skeleton, instructed students in the dissection of limbs amputated at the hospital.

Other physicians who had served as surgeons in the Union army likewise returned to Minnesota or came to settle after the war. Among the newcomers was Dr. Charles N. Hewitt, son of a Vermont physician, who in 1866 took over the practice of his old friend Dr. Augustine B. Hawley at Red Wing. Like Dr. Hand, Dr. Hewitt had extensive experience during the Civil War with surgery and with malarial fevers, typhoid fever, and scurvy among the troops; his insight through his war experience into disease prevention made him an active proponent of public health measures in Minnesota.

On 2 February 1869 the Minnesota Medical Society, which had been inactive since 1857, was reorganized as the Minnesota State Medical Society, and immediately urged the Minnesota legislature to enact laws to regulate the practice of medicine, or as the assembled doctors put it, "to protect the citizens of this State from quackery."[12] Two months later, on 4 March, the state of Minnesota enacted

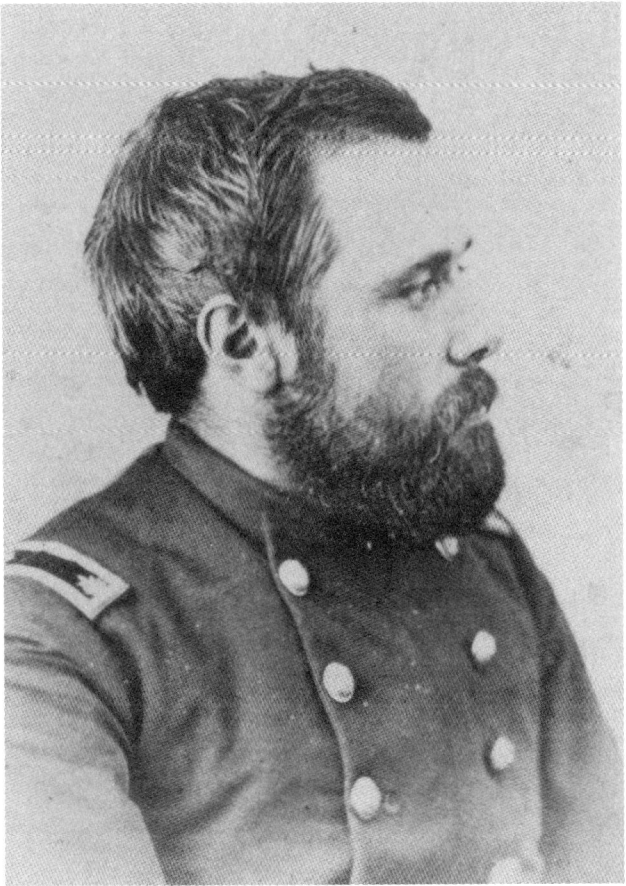

FIGURE 2:3   Charles N. Hewitt in United States Army uniform. Courtesy Minnesota Historical Society.

a law providing that no person might practice medicine or perform surgical operations "who has not attended at least two full courses of instruction, and graduated at some school of medicine within the United States, or of some foreign country, or who cannot produce a certificate of qualification from some State, district or county medical society . . . ."[13] The act also required every medical practitioner to file with the clerk of the district court in the county where he practiced a sworn copy of his medical diploma or certificate in order to sue for payment of fees. Nevertheless, the new law failed in its purpose because a medical diploma or certificate might easily be forged or stolen, and even when such a document was genuine, the level of medical qualification that it represented might vary enormously. Furthermore, the act included no provision for its enforcement.

In the spring of 1870, the young physician Dr. Alexander Stone moved to St. Paul from Stillwater where he had come the preceding summer from Boston at

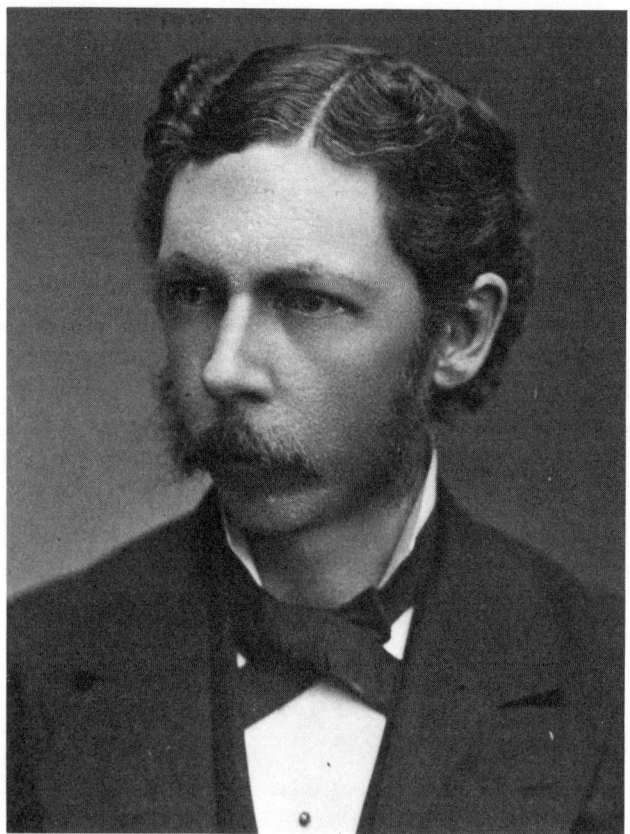

FIGURE 2:4   Alexander J. Stone, circa 1870. Courtesy Minnesota Historical Society.

the age of twenty-four with his bride. A native of Maine, Stone began his medical training in a simple preparatory school at Portland, and after periods of study at the Harvard Medical School and the Bowdoin College medical school, he received his M.D. degree from the Berkshire Medical Institution at Pittsfield, Massachusetts, in the last graduating class of that small but distinguished country medical school.[14] Following graduation Stone spent the year 1867–68 in Europe visiting clinics at Paris, London, and Edinburgh.[15] On his return to America he joined one of his former teachers at Pittsfield, Dr. Horatio R. Storer, in the practice of obstetrics and gynecology at Boston until coming to Minnesota in the summer of 1869.

On his arrival at St. Paul the energetic and ambitious Stone founded a medical journal, through which he came in contact with many physicians and learned their common concern to provide better instruction for the student apprentices reading medicine in their offices.[16] When he learned of the informal teaching carried on by Drs. Hand and Stewart at St. Joseph's Hospital, Dr. Stone undertook to organize their teaching into a preparatory medical school, similar to the one in which he had studied at Portland. The instruction was intended to be primarily clinical and to provide essentially a more organized form of apprenticeship training.[17] The school began in 1870 as the St. Paul School for Medical Instruction. It had a formal sixteen-week term that began in June, timed to allow attendance at the winter course in the medical colleges at Chicago. The faculty consisted of various St. Paul physicians, some of whom had already been teaching informally for several years. Daniel Hand taught surgery and Alexander Stone taught obstetrics and diseases of women. In 1871 the fees for the summer term were $30 and for the succeeding winter term of 1872, $25, or both terms together for $50. Initially the instruction was carried on in the offices of the various faculty members and in the second story of the dead house beside St. Joseph's Hospital.

In December 1872 a second preparatory medical school opened in Minnesota at Winona under the direction of Dr. Franklin Staples, who presided over a faculty of six physicians including himself. Like the St. Paul school, the Winona school conferred no degrees and did not pretend to offer complete medical training; it was simply a more organized form of apprenticeship instruction. The school closed in 1878, presumably because such preparatory training was less needed as the spread of railroads facilitated travel to cities with medical colleges.[18]

Although the Minnesota State Medical Society perhaps was concerned most urgently with efforts to obtain the regulation of medical practice by state law, the society also pursued other matters connected with medicine and public health. In 1871 the society sought and obtained passage of a state law for the registration of vital statistics. In 1872 Alexander Stone drew up for the consideration of the society a bill to be presented to the state legislature to legalize anatomical dissection. Dr. Stone also moved that the society establish a committee on medical education. Both motions were approved.[19]

In 1872, in his capacity as chairman of the Committee on Medical Education, Dr. Stone recommended to the society that they should establish a board of examiners to examine persons who wished to study medicine and that the qualifications required of beginning medical students should be as high as for students entering "literary institutions."[20] The committee also recommended that each medical college should adopt a progressive course of study to extend over four years, with examinations to be held at the end of each year, and a curriculum that would include anatomy, physical chemistry, and physiology as well as clinical subjects. The faculty should be nominated by a medical board, such nominations to be confirmed by the board of regents or trustees of the medical college. Dr. Stone's committee envisioned that the kind of medical college they desired would have to be part of a state university.

In 1872 the society also sought enactment of a bill to create a state board of health and vital statistics. The state board of health was, among other things, to "make sanitary investigations and inquiries respecting the causes of disease, especially of epidemics, the source of mortality and the effects of localities, employments, conditions, and circumstances on the public health . . . ."[21] The board was also to advise the state on all hygienic or medical matters. The bill, passed by the Minnesota legislature on 4 March 1872, provided that the State Board of Health would be composed of seven physicians, one from St. Paul and the other six from various sections of the state, and would elect from its members a president and secretary, of whom the latter would be the executive officer of the board. When the first board met, Dr. Charles N. Hewitt of Red Wing was elected secretary.[22]

In 1874 there were already sixty-one regular medical colleges in the United States, to which might be added eight homeopathic, six eclectic, and two botanic schools. The competition among schools for students was, therefore, more intense than ever and hindered efforts to raise the standards of medical education. In 1874 the Committee on Medical Education of the Minnesota State Medical Society recommended that the number of medical schools be reduced (by what means was unclear), the medical college course be made progressive through examinations for promotion from class to class, the course of study be lengthened to five years, and strict standards of preliminary education be established for admission to medical school. The custom of studying medicine in the office of a practitioner was generally unsatisfactory. The committee, therefore, recommended the establishment of private preparatory medical schools to take the place of the medical apprenticeship in the preparation of a student for entry into a medical college.

In the 1870s new ideas began to enter medicine. Anaesthesia, introduced thirty years before, was generally used in surgical operations, but surgery was performed only when absolutely necessary. The most common operation was amputation. The danger of surgical infection was great. Physicians were beginning to speak of the germ theory, then regarded as an interesting but unproven hypothesis, and some referred vaguely to Joseph Lister's antiseptic methods intended to exclude germs from wounds, but in Minnesota no one had yet attempted antisepsis.

During the 1870s medical education in Minnesota followed the same pattern as in other parts of the country. In an effort to improve upon the apprenticeship style of instruction, a physician or several physicians would organize a small school. After a very few years the school was likely to have combined with one or more other schools, changed its name at least once, or disbanded. The St. Paul School for Medical Instruction was no exception to this pattern. It was reorganized in 1878 as the St. Paul Medical College under Dr. Alexander J. Stone as dean. Instead of being a school to prepare students to enter a medical college, it was now intended to provide a complete medical education leading to a medical degree. In 1878 it offered a two-year course for the M.D. degree, but in 1880 extended the course to three years, the term each year being twenty-six weeks long. The school rented the upper two stories of a building on Third Street in St. Paul and enlarged its faculty by the addition of a young Minneapolis physician, Dr. Frederick Dunsmoor. A native of Richfield, Minnesota, Dunsmoor had begun the study of medicine in 1869 at the age of sixteen as an apprentice to two Minneapolis physicians.[23] After four years of apprenticeship Dunsmoor went to New York City to study at the Bellevue Hospital Medical College where he received his medical de —

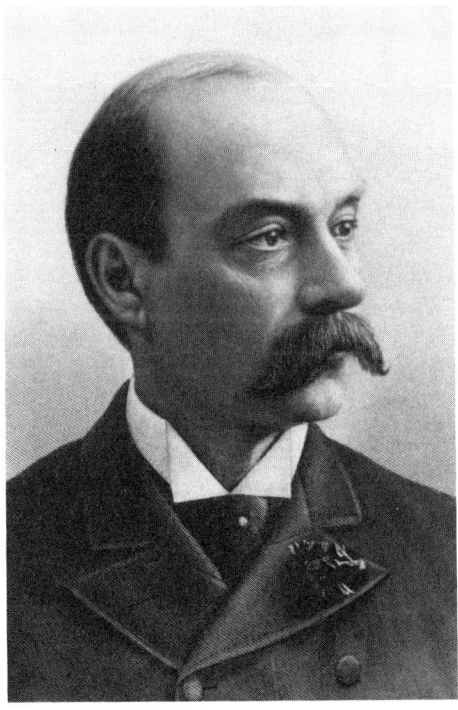

FIGURE 2:5 Frederick A. Dunsmoor, circa 1890. Courtesy Minnesota Historical Society.

gree in 1875. In 1878, at the age of twenty-five, Dr. Dunsmoor delivered his first course of lectures in the St. Paul Medical College on the subject of genitourinary surgery.[24] The following year he began to lecture on general surgery and Dr. Charles A. Wheaton began to teach anatomy. Dr. Wheaton, who had grown up at Northfield, Minnesota, had just returned to St. Paul from two years spent in the Massachusetts General Hospital and Boston City Hospital following his graduation from the Harvard Medical School in 1877.[25] In 1879, the St. Paul Medical College became affiliated with Hamline University in St. Paul, in order to be able to confer the M.D. degree on its students when they completed their medical course. The following year George F. French, who had recently come to Minneapolis from Portland, Maine, joined the faculty of the St. Paul Medical College, now called the Medical Department of Hamline University. Like Drs. Hand and Stewart, Dr. French was a former Union army surgeon. Immediately after graduation from the Harvard Medical School in 1862, he entered the army, and was assigned first to the staff of General Ulysses S. Grant at Vicksburg and then to the staff of General Sherman during his march to the sea. After leaving the army in 1865, Dr. French practiced medicine at Portland and taught in the Portland School for Medical Instruction until he moved to Minneapolis in 1879.[26]

Although affiliated with Hamline University, the medical college maintained its classrooms in downtown St. Paul. To perform their teaching duties, Dr. Duns-

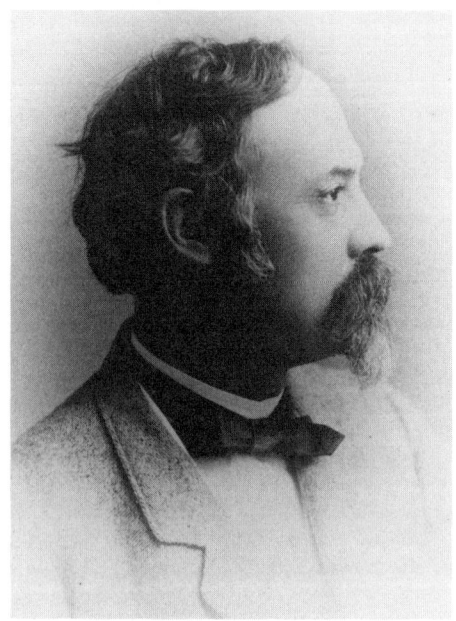

FIGURE 2:6 George F. French. Courtesy National Library of Medicine.

moor and Dr. French were accustomed to travel by train from Minneapolis to St. Paul on the Chicago, Milwaukee and St. Paul Railway which went by a roundabout route through Fort Snelling and Mendota, the trip taking an hour. In order to save time at the St. Paul end, they left the train at a small station on the Mississippi River front and climbed 150 steps up the cliff to the Third Street level. They then had an additional climb up an outside stairway to enter the rooms of the St. Paul Medical College.[27]

Classes began daily at three o'clock in the afternoon, so as to permit the professors to pursue their practices during the morning, and continued until ten o'clock at night. The class in anatomy met at 9 p.m. Such a course was strenuous for both students and faculty, especially so for Drs. French and Dunsmoor who had to make the time-consuming railway trip in addition to teaching. The St. Paul Medical College was also handicapped by the lack of facilities for clinical teaching.

In 1881 Dr. Dunsmoor sought to overcome both difficulties at once by purchasing the large building in St. Anthony (in 1881 part of East Minneapolis) belonging to Macalester College, but known formerly as the Winslow House. It had been built in 1857 by James M. Winslow as a hotel for the multitudes of rich Southerners who used to come on summer excursions up the Mississippi River by steamboat. With more than two hundred rooms the Winslow House possessed ample facilities for a combined hospital and medical school. The guest rooms could provide accommodation for patients and for medical students while the large public rooms could be adapted for lecture rooms and laboratories.[28]

The development of organized clinical instruction in hospitals at New York City and Brooklyn had made New York by 1880 the leading center of medical education in the United States, and Frederick Dunsmoor wished to create at Minneapolis a hospital-based medical school along the lines that had proven so successful there.[29] The rapid development of clinical medicine during the nineteenth century, the sorting out of many diseases and disease states, each identifiable by particular signs and symptoms, meant that there was a growing body of medical knowledge that could be learned effectively only at the bedside. Dunsmoor proposed to organize the Minnesota College Hospital along the lines of the Long Island College Hospital, which had opened at Brooklyn, New York, in 1858 as a combined hospital, outpatient dispensary, and medical school. Although the Long Island College Hospital was plagued by recurrent financial difficulties, it possessed from the beginning a distinguished faculty that included Austin Flint as professor of medicine and Frank Hamilton as professor of surgery. The term of its medical school extended through the spring and early summer when other medical schools were not in session so that it was able to draw both faculty and students from other schools.[30] When Frederick Dunsmoor was studying medicine at the Bellevue Hospital Medical College in New York City from 1873 to 1875, he supplemented the medical school instruction with private lessons from among others Frank Hamilton in surgery and Austin Flint on diseases of the chest. They may have impressed Dunsmoor with the desirability of including extensive clinical instruction as an integral part of medical education. The Long Island College had provided a model for the establishment of a medical school in connection with a hospital, a model that had been consciously followed in the establishment of the Bellevue Hospital Medical College in connection with Bellevue Hospital in New York City in 1861.[31] The founders of Bellevue Hospital Medical College also saw the medical schools of such London hospitals as Guy's and St. Thomas's as examples of the value of conducting medical teaching in connection with a hospital, with organized clinical instruction as an integral part of its curriculum.

In organizing the Minnesota College Hospital Frederick Dunsmoor enlisted the help of his fellow practitioner, George French, and also that of Amos Abbott, a physician who, shortly after his arrival at Minneapolis in 1876, had taught anatomy for a time in the St. Paul medical preparatory school. As a youth Amos Abbott had been taken prisoner while serving with the Union army in Louisiana. After escaping from a Confederate prison at New Orleans and hiding in a swamp, he came down with malaria so severely that he was discharged from the army and spent the remainder of the Civil War at Washington as a clerk in the army pay department. As a clerk he was sent frequently with messages to the White House where several times he saw and talked with President Lincoln—incidents which he cherished proudly in his memory.[32] At the age of thirty-seven in 1881 Amos Abbott was deeply interested in the possibilities of antiseptic surgery, and was emerging as an unusually capable surgeon. He was a strong ally in the development of the Minnesota College Hospital.

Although the Minnesota College Hospital was organized by Dr. Dunsmoor and his medical colleagues, they did not intend it to be a medical school operated by physicians for profit, and it was far from profitable. The incorporators included in addition to Frederick Dunsmoor and three other physicians, a justice of the Minnesota Supreme Court, Charles E. Vanderburgh, and the Minneapolis lawyer and businessman, Thomas Lowry. Thomas Lowry became president of the corporation while Frederick Dunsmoor was appointed dean of the medical school. Lowry also contributed financially to the Minnesota College Hospital and solicited a gift of $5,000 from his friend James J. Hill of St. Paul, president of the Great Northern Railroad. The faculty of the new medical school included the whole faculty of the former St. Paul Medical College, which obligingly closed in the spring of 1881 to permit the Minnesota College Hospital to open the following autumn. The plan for the new medical college was unusually complete with departments of dentistry, pharmacy, and veterinary medicine in addition to the college of medicine and surgery.[33] The faculty served without salary and the other expenses of the school were expected to be met from the annual tuition fees of fifty dollars paid by each student.

The opening exercises of the Minnesota College Hospital took place in "the large and elegant lecture room of the college" in the Winslow House on 31 October 1881, in the presence of a large crowd of the leading citizens of Minneapolis and St. Paul, including Governor John Sargent Pillsbury and other notables.[34] Thirty patients were already in the private rooms and wards of the hospital. The first session of the school began the next day, 1 November, and was intended to continue until mid-April, but for some reason, which may have been financial exigency or possibly faculty fatigue, the school cut short its term by several weeks to hold its first commencement on 24 March 1882 in the great ballroom. The first graduating class included four students, who must have received part of their medical education elsewhere, possibly at the St. Paul Medical College, and the valedictory address was given by the brightest student of the class, Edward C. Spencer. Many years later Dr. Dunsmoor recalled: "I well remember the great trepidation with which we waited to hear the opening sentences of the valedictory address . . . . That feeling was immediately dispelled by the speech with which Dr. Spencer, with almost matchless fire, electrified and captured his audience."[35]

The Minnesota College Hospital required entering students to take a preliminary examination for admission unless they possessed a high school education or its equivalent. It offered a graded course of three years. The medical teaching was by recitation, didactic lectures, and clinical lectures, and included clinical teaching at the bedside. In addition to patients who might be seen at the Minnesota College Hospital itself, the school had arranged for clinical teaching at four other hospitals and two outpatient dispensaries in Minneapolis and St. Paul. As a hospital the Minnesota College Hospital was successful in attracting patients and soon had as many as one hundred beds occupied but, because as in almost all nineteenth-century hospitals most of the patients were charity patients, the hospital regularly operated at a deficit.[36]

From 1881 to 1885 the Minnesota College Hospital was a brilliant gathering place for physicians form Minneapolis and St. Paul, and the scene of some of the earliest operations by antiseptic surgery performed in Minnesota. At the hospital

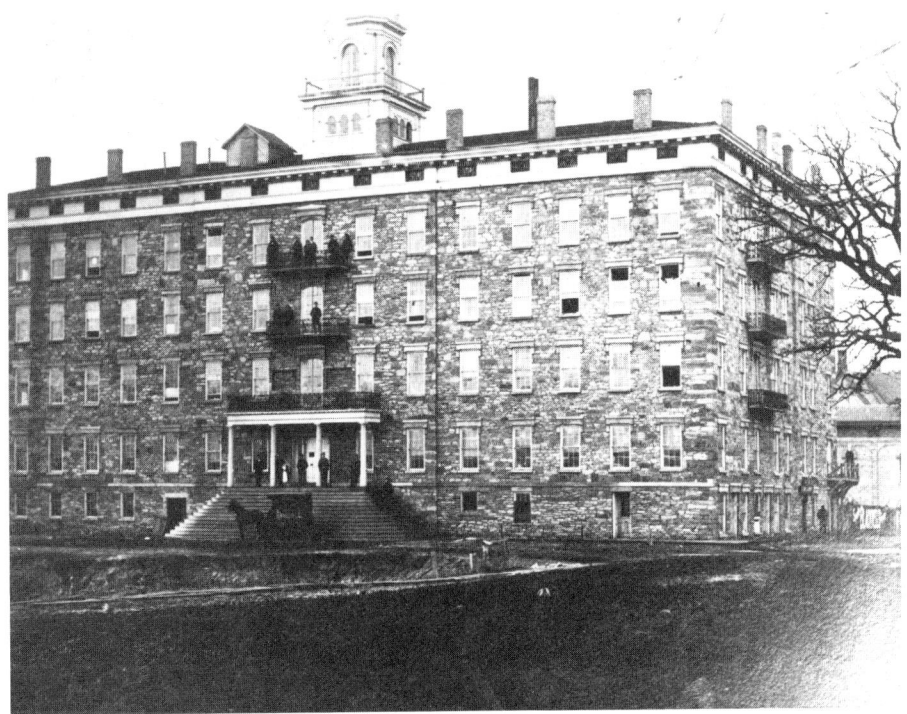

FIGURE 2:7 Minnesota College Hospital (Winslow House), circa 1881. Note the ambulance at entrance. Courtesy Minneapolis Public Library, Minneapolis Collection.

on 21 October 1882, with the assistance of Drs. Jay Owens and Charles Wheaton of St. Paul, Frederick Dunsmoor removed a large ovarian tumor, estimated to weigh sixty pounds, from a young married woman, the mother of two children. Dr. Dunsmoor performed the operation under a carbolic acid spray, and afterwards covered the wound with carbolic gauze and other dressings recommended by Joseph Lister. The patient recovered uneventfully and returned home on 4 December.[37] The operation may have been the first to be performed by strict Listerian antisepsis in the Twin Cities. During that same year, 1882, Charles H. Hunter settled in practice at Minneapolis after years of study and travel in Europe following his graduation from the College of Physicians and Surgeons in New York City. At London Dr. Hunter had spent some time on Lister's wards at King's College Hospital where he became thoroughly familiar with Lister's methods.[38] Soon after Hunter's arrival Dunsmoor added him to the faculty of the Minnesota College Hospital.

From the beginning the Minnesota College Hospital was also successful as a medical school whether measured by the quality of its faculty or the number and quality of its students. In 1884 Dr. John F. Fulton, an ophthalmologist who had come to St. Paul from Philadelphia two years earlier, joined the faculty and began a free weekly clinic on diseases of the eye and ear. During 1884–85 the school enrolled fifty-five students, including three women, and among the fifty-five, eighteen were college graduates and twenty-five were graduates of high schools or normal schools. A number of graduates later became eminent physicians in the Twin Cities; Dr. Arthur J. Gillette founded the Gillette Children's Hospital in St. Paul and Dr. George G. Eitel the Eitel Hospital in Minneapolis.[39]

Although the costs of running the medical school of the Minnesota College Hospital were small because the faculty were unpaid, the costs of operating the Winslow House as a hospital proved too great. Without any endowment, the hospital depended for income on its paying patients and they were too few to sustain it. That great building, containing so many rooms for patients and students, with its large ballroom so commodious for opening exercises and commencements, proved a nightmare to heat through the severe cold of a Minnesota winter. In a financial crisis during one winter, Thomas Lowry offered to pay the coal bill for one month and was astonished to learn that it was more than $700. As residents of houses with coal-burning boilers may remember, the coal all had to be shoveled into boilers and the ashes later removed. In the 1880s, $700 would have bought hundreds of tons of coal, and the Winslow House must have required several firemen to keep its boilers stoked through the winter months. By 1885 the directors decided that without endowment, or other continuing subsidy, they must close the Minnesota College Hospital. Nevertheless, they wished to continue to operate the medical school which, separated from the hospital, could operate by itself on the income from tuition fees.

On 13 July 1885 Frederick Dunsmoor and his colleagues created a new corporation to be called the Minnesota Hospital College. In separating the medical school from the hospital they wished to keep as close to the original name as possible so they simply changed the order of the words from "College Hospital" to "Hospital College."[40] The new Minnesota Hospital College bought land on the northeast corner of Ninth Avenue South and Sixth Street in Minneapolis, adjacent to St. Barnabas Hospital, a hospital first established in 1871 by members of the Protestant Episcopal Church as the Cottage Hospital of the Brotherhood of Gethsemane. On the new site the directors of the Minnesota Hospital College erected a building designed specifically for a medical school. The new building opened 20 September 1886 and contained a lecture amphitheater, dissecting rooms, chemical and pathological laboratories, and an outpatient dispensary. The school naturally wished to use St. Barnabas Hospital for clinical teaching, but St. Barnabas lacked a surgical operating room. To overcome that difficulty, Dr. Frederick Dunsmoor and Dr. Charles H. Hunter offered to build an operating room at St. Barnabas at their own expense if the hospital would permit clinical teaching in its wards. St. Barnabas Hospital accepted their offer, the operating room was built, and clinical teaching began in the hospital.

The board of directors of the Minnesota Hospital College included lay members who agreed to help manage the business affairs of the college on condition

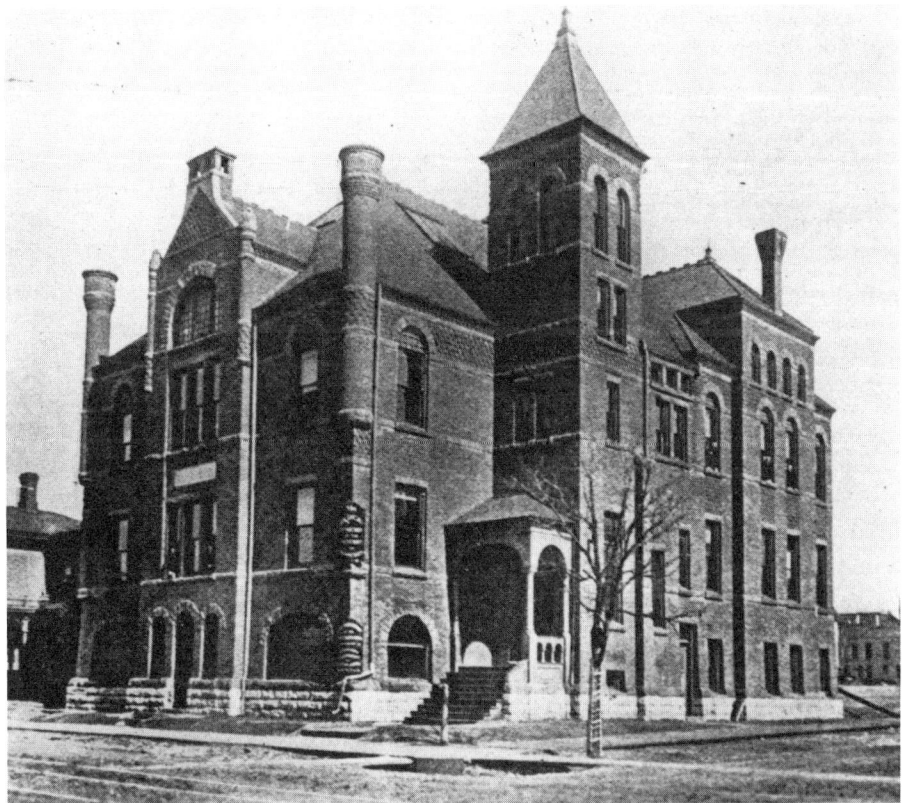

FIGURE 2:8   Minnesota Hospital College. Courtesy Mn U Archives.

that the college should incur no debt. As guarantors of that promise Drs. Dunsmoor and Hunter frequently had to advance funds to the college in exchange for stock in the corporation so that they presently came to be the majority stockholders.

The Minnesota College Hospital in the Winslow House had to face competition for students within two years of its opening. In October 1883 a second medical school opened in Minneapolis with the avowed purpose of offering a higher standard of medical education than that represented by the Minnesota College Hospital. The new school, called the Minneapolis College of Physicians and Surgeons, offered a three-year graded medical course, the session in each year to be six months in length. In order to be admitted students had to show evidence of adequate preliminary education, and at the conclusion of their medical course they were to be examined by the College of Medicine of the University of Minnesota, established by a legislative act in 1883 purely as an examining and licensing body. The practice of having the University of Minnesota examine students at the completion of their course continued until the third session of 1885–86 when the Minneapolis College began to invite leading physicians from various parts of Minnesota to examine their students. In 1887 the college began to conduct its own examinations and award diplomas to its own students who would in any case have to pass the examinations of the State Board of Medical Examiners created by the Minnesota state legislature in that year.[41]

At the time of the reorganization of the Minnesota College Hospital into the Minnesota Hospital College with its affiliation with St. Barnabas Hospital, the St. Paul physicians who had belonged to the faculty of the former Minnesota College Hospital resigned to organize themselves as a new St. Paul Medical College, of which Alexander Stone became president and Charles Wheaton vice president. The new St. Paul Medical College opened in the fall of 1885 and proceeded immediately to raise funds for the building that the college dedicated in 1886. Both the Minnesota Hospital College and the St. Paul Medical College were recognized by the University of Minnesota in 1885 as satisfactory medical schools so that graduates of either school could apply to the university for a medical degree. Thus after 1885 there were three medical colleges in the Twin Cities engaged in preparing students to be examined for the medical degrees of the University of Minnesota.

In October 1886 yet a fourth medical school appeared in the Twin Cities when the homeopathic physicians organized the Minnesota Homeopathic Medical College in Minneapolis. In 1867 sixteen homeopathic physicians met at the Globe Hotel in St. Paul to found the Minnesota State Homeopathic Institute that was empowered by its articles of incorporation to confer the degree of Doctor of Medicine after examination by a board of censors appointed by the institute. In 1884 a group of homeopathic physicians in Minneapolis established the Minneapolis Homeopathic Hospital on the corner of Fourth Avenue South and Twenty-fifth Street to enable them to provide homeopathic treatment to patients in hospital. Homeopathic physicians drew support from many prosperous and well-educated citizens because of the mild character of their treatments of disease. Homeopaths were particularly successful in the treatment of typhoid fever for which they could claim an unusually low fatality rate among their patients.[42] Two years after the opening of their hospital, a group of homeopathic physicians met in Minneapolis to incorporate themselves as the Minnesota Homeopathic Medical College, becoming the fourth medical school. The college opened 4 October 1886 in a building at Fourth Avenue and Twentieth Street with a faculty of sixteen professors under Dr. Philo L. Hatch as dean.[43] Dr. Hatch, who had come to Minnesota in 1858 at the age of thirty-five, was a graduate of the Homeopathic Hospital and College of Cleveland, Ohio. He had been one of the group of sixteen founders of the Minnesota State Homeopathic Institute.[44] The homeopathic college attempted to set a higher standard of medical education than other schools by offering a three-year graded course, of which they required a minimum of two years for the M.D. degree. Their terms were six months long. For clinical instruction the students had access to all the general hospitals in Minneapolis on the same terms as all medical students and they were especially welcome at the Minneapolis Homeopathic Hospital, only five blocks away. Seven students enrolled in the first class.

The College of Medicine at the University of Minnesota as a Medical Examining Board, 1883-1887

Early in 1882, Drs. Perry H. Millard of Stillwater and Charles N. Hewitt of Red Wing, acting together with Dr. William H. Leonard,[45] a St. Paul homeopathic physician, and William Watts Folwell, president of the University of Minnesota, moved to create a medical college at the university. At the meeting of the state medical society in June, Dr. Charles Hewitt, as its president, urged the University of Minnesota to establish a medical faculty whose sole function would be to examine candidates for medical degrees.[46] Meanwhile, Dr. Millard drew to the attention of state legislators a provision in the state constitution empowering the Board of Regents of the university to form a college of medicine intended to exercise no teaching function, but to exist solely as an examining body. The faculty of such a college could impose, in effect, a quarantine upon medical schools whose graduates could not pass muster. It was Millard's intention to establish a single state medical college at the university, but he recognized the wisdom of proceeding gradually toward that end. To force the closure of the several private medical schools currently in operation, or to create overnight a rival teaching institution at the university, would serve only to generate antagonism among physicians. The physicians associated with the active medical colleges of Minnesota were among the best educated and most influential in the state. Their cooperation was indispensable to the success of Millard's plan, and he believed that, after a few years of operation of the new college as an examining board, the leaders of the medical community would recognize that medical education in the state should be conducted by a single, central, state-operated institution.

Deficiencies inherent in the American system of medical education made difficult the establishment of uniform standards of competence for physicians. The often inadequate preliminary education of medical students, the absence of uniformity among medical colleges in the quality and quantity of academic and clinical instruction offered, and the failure of state and local laws to define reasonable requirements for the practice of the profession, all were factors contributing to great variations in competence among medical men. Physicians and laymen alike cited also the commercialism of medical education as a harmful influence. The precarious financial condition of many private medical colleges forced them to struggle competitively for students. Entrance requirements might be debased to attract students and performance requirements reduced to retain them. Even when high standards of achievement were enforced, the ability of medical faculties to confer degrees upon their own students created a clear conflict between their commercial and professional interests. By the establishment at the University of Minnesota of a single examining body, and by the vigorous enforcement of laws regulating qualifications for the practice of medicine, the influence of weaknesses, or even of corruption, in the training of young doctors could be eliminated.

After much discussion on the matter, the Board of Regents invited the drafting of a formal proposal for the creation of a college of medicine. On 29 June 1882 Dr. Charles N. Hewitt submitted such a document.[47] Six months later, on 28 December 1882, the Board of Regents entrusted a committee of four men to draw up a plan for the organization of the new college. Three physicians, Charles N. Hewitt, Perry H. Millard, and William H. Leonard, were appointed to the committee; the fourth member was William Watts Folwell, president of the university. In their report, the committee outlined four principles intended to provide a workable foundation for the functioning of the proposed college as an examining body. "Never before," the committee remarked in its introductory statement, "has there been such unanimity among medical men in demanding that examinations for degrees in medicine be separated entirely from the teaching of its theory and practice."[48] The statement went on to describe the struggle of reputable educational institutions, such as Harvard University, to maintain reasonable requirements for diplomas in competition with the vast number of inferior schools also legally empowered to teach medicine and grant diplomas. The establishment of the college of medicine at the University of Minnesota as an examining board would serve to distinguish the qualified from the unqualified regardless of their institutional affiliation.

The four principles for the organization of the new college of medicine were intended to establish a high standard. The first principle provided for a competent and independent faculty charged with examining all candidates for licenses and degrees in medicine in the state of Minnesota. Faculty members were to be in no way associated with the preparation of students for medical degrees or examinations. Secondly, the faculty was to demand of all applicants for examination preliminary literary and scientific education. Thirdly, professional examinations should be administered under strict but reasonable rules. Each candidate should be judged on the basis of his performance in written, oral, and clinical tests, and the results of those tests should be recorded and preserved. Finally, for the degree of doctor of medicine, in addition to satisfying the requirements for the bachelor of medicine degree, an original thesis upon a medical topic must be prepared and defended successfully before the faculty.

On 5 January 1883 the Board of Regents accepted the principles outlined above and the College of Medicine was officially organized.[49] At the same meeting the board adopted bylaws for the new college, also prepared by Hewitt, Leonard, Millard, and Folwell.[50] At their first formal meeting on 23 April 1883, the college faculty elected Perry Millard as their recording secretary.[51] At the same time, the chairman, Charles Hewitt, submitted to the faculty the constitution and bylaws for the college adopted by the Board of Regents on 5 January. The constitution contained three articles dealing, respectively, with terms and regulations for faculty appointments, with examinations and the degrees that the faculty could confer, and with the identification of approved schools of medical instruction.[52]

The College of Medicine was to consist of nine departments, including those of anatomy and physiology, pathology, materia medica and therapeutics, medical chemistry, preventive medicine (personal and public hygiene), practice of medicine, surgery, obstetrics and diseases of women and children, and, finally, diseases of the nervous system. The last department was to include also medical jurisprudence. In addition to nine faculty members, one for each department, the president of the university was to serve as a tenth faculty member, in an ex officio capacity. Because the Board of Regents was concerned to avoid any apparent conflicts of interest among the medical faculty, Article I of the bylaws specified that at *no* time might a faculty member be associated *in any way* with another college of medicine. The duties of the medical professors were to examine candidates for degrees in medicine and surgery, and to recommend them for graduation to the Board of Regents.[53]

Once appointed, the medical college faculty lost no time in preparing to execute their duties. On 30 April 1883, the five members who had been appointed met in the President's Room with William Folwell.[54] By the president's invitation, the general faculty of the university was also present to welcome the medical faculty to the university. During the business portion of the meeting, the medical faculty discussed its first application for a degree from B. J. Merrill, a Stillwater physician who had graduated in 1881 from the Bellevue College Hospital School in New York City. Individuals receiving the M.D. degree from approved schools were eligible for the same recognition from Minnesota upon their successful presentation and defense of an original thesis.[55] Minnesota M.B. graduates were eligible to do the same after three years of professional practice. An exception was granted to candidates who distinguished themselves during the examination for the M.B. degree by "evinc[ing] a high degree of proficiency in the literature, theory, and practice of medicine."[55] Such candidates were permitted to defend a thesis and, if successful, to receive the M.D. degree without delay. B. J. Merrill's credentials were in good order, and the faculty approved his request to submit a thesis for trial.

As a state examining board, the faculty of the College of Medicine had four functions:

1. To issue certificates to graduates of reputable medical colleges.

2. To issue licenses to practice to persons who had already practiced medicine continuously in Minnesota for more than five years.

3. To examine and license those who lacked a diploma from a recognized medical college, but who passed a satisfactory examination.

4. To withdraw a license to practice medicine from practitioners of medicine guilty of "unprofessional conduct."[57]

From 19 April 1883 until 10 May 1884 the faculty granted certificates to practice in Minnesota to 579 physicians who possessed diplomas from reputable medical colleges.[58] An additional 129 individuals who furnished affidavits to show that they had practiced medicine actively for five or more years in the state also received certificates allowing them to continue to practice without examination.[59]

Shortly after it was organized, the faculty began to conduct examinations primarily for the benefit of persons affected by a retroactive clause in the law that for a limited time allowed persons who were not graduates of approved medical colleges to qualify to practice in Minnesota if they could pass a formal examination. In 1883 and 1884 the faculty held three public examinations for such persons, and among forty-six persons examined, twenty-four received certification from the faculty.[60]

The faculty took their responsibilities as an examining body very seriously. No candidate was admitted to the examination whose preparation was deficient in any respect, and no examinee was passed whose performance during testing faltered in even one subject. The faculty was committed equally strongly to high standards for graduation in medicine. Initially they may have been a bit too rigid. At the examination on 15 April 1886 they were more flexible.[61] Seven applicants were approved for examination, and all were recommended to receive the M.B. degree. In framing their examination questions, each professor referred to specific criteria of competence.[62] In anatomy, in addition to knowledge of histology and regional anatomy, students were expected to show that they had performed autopsies and dissections, and had acquired practical skills in the use of the microscope. During the examination, candidates were required to identify anatomical specimens, both gross and microscopic. In the first examination in anatomy, Professor Millard asked candidates to give the chemical and microscopic structure of bone, to describe in detail the structure and anatomical relationships of the sterno-clavico mastoid muscle, the cornea of the eye, and the ovaries. They were asked also to name and locate the valves of the heart, to give the boundaries of the fourth ventricle of the brain, and to name the articulations of the sphenoid bone.[63] In physiology Millard questioned them on the composition and use of fats, sugars, bile, proteins, red blood cells, lymph, chyle, and epithelial cells. He asked additional questions about the fetal circulation and the development of a fertilized ovum. The professional examination was designed to test various skills as well as knowledge. In pathology, for example, in addition to the oral examination, candidates took a practical examination to demonstrate their skills in diagnostic pathology, using chemical tests, the microscope, or the dissection knife, as required.

In addition to the professional examination for the bachelor of medicine degree, the college also gave a preliminary examination for entrance to the study of medicine and a scientific examination. Both examinations were waived for students who were certified by the Minnesota State High School Board or had baccalaureate degrees from the university's colleges of Science, Literature, and Arts, Mechanical Arts, or Agriculture. In practice, the college seldom had occasion to administer the preliminary or scientific examinations.

The College of Medicine offered no instruction. Its faculty served as an examining body solely; but it published its requirements for the preliminary, scientific, and professional examinations, lists of recommended textbooks, and on occasion sample examination questions. The bulletin for the year 1886–87 differed sharply from those issued previously. Except for the names of two persons awarded the M.B. degree at the previous examination, it merely announced that the university was going to ask the legislature for an appropriation to establish a teaching school of medicine, and that the examining functions of the faculty had been transferred to a new state board.[64]

Thus ended the brief career of the College of Medicine of the university as a board of medical examiners. The experiment lasted only four years. During that interval fewer than three score individuals had applied and been approved to stand for the examination for the M.B. degree. Fewer than half of the approved candidates were successful. Meanwhile, the vast majority of physicians in the state of Minnesota had been granted a license to practice, in accordance with the law of 1883, either under the diploma clause or the five-year-practice clause. Although as an examining board the faculty prevented those who failed the examinations from practicing medicine, the high rate of failure and frequent low scores among the examinees demonstrated the urgent need for improved standards of medical education. The time was ripe for the University of Minnesota to open a teaching institution capable of delivering first-rate medical education.

NOTES

1. Minnesota. Laws, Statues, Etc., "An act to establish the University of Minnesota . . . ." Section 10, 13 February 1851.

2. James Gray, *The University of Minnesota 1851–1951*, pp. 18–24.

3. Robert Rosenthal, "Dr. Christopher Carli, pioneer physician of Minnesota," *Minn. Med.*, 1982, *65*, 765–768.

4. Theodore C. Blegen, "Frontier bookshelves," *Minn. Hist.*, 1941, *22*, 351–366, pp. 355–356; idem, *Grass roots history*, pp. 192–206. John M. Armstrong, "History of medicine in Ramsey County," *Minn. Med.*, 1938, *21*, 703–704.

5. John M. Armstrong, "History of medicine in Ramsey County," *Minn. Med.*, 1938, *21*, 698–703, 793–800, 850–855; 1939, *22*, 36–40, 109–115, 180–186, 251–257, 311–316, 409–416, 470–474, 543–547, 643–647, 709–714 [title varies]. Armstrong's account of Dr. Dewey is in *Minn. Med.*, 1938, *21*, 698–703, pp. 700–701.

6. Ibid., 1938, *21*, 698–703, pp. 702–703.

7. Ibid., 1938, *21*, 793–800, pp. 794–795.

8. Arthur S. Hamilton, "History of the Minnesota State Medical Society," *Minn. Med.*, 1942, *25*, 45–51. Their stated objectives were " . . . the advancement of medical knowledge, the elevation of professional character, the protection of the interests of its members, the extension of the bounds of medical sciences . . . and to improve the health and protect the lives of the community."

9. The medical colleges represented included the University of Pennsylvania Medical School, the College of Physicians and Surgeons of Columbia University, Harvard Medical School, Albany Medical College, and Rush Medical College at Chicago.

10. " . . . the great leading object of those who originated and carried into effect the [earlier] Convention of May 1846 was the improvement of our system of medical educa-

tion." Nathan S. Davis, *History of the American Medical Association from its organization up to January 1855.*

11. D. W. Hand, "Extracts from reports relative to the operations of the Medical Staff in the Department of North Carolina, from August 1863 to the close of the War," in U.S. Surgeon-general's Office, *The medical and surgical history of the War of the Rebellion (1861-65)*, I, 238-241, p. 238; [Obituary] "Daniel W. Hand, M.D.," *Trans. Minn. St. med. Soc.*, 1889, pp. 234-239.

12. "Historical account of organization and proceedings of first annual meeting of Minnesota State Medical Society," in *Trans. Minn. St. med. Soc.*, 1870, pp. 1-5, p. 4.

13. Samuel Willey, "State of Minnesota," *Med. Rec.*, 1869-70, *4*, 86.

14. Founded in 1823, the Berkshire Medical Institution continued for forty-five years during which it graduated 1,188 doctors of medicine. Primarily an educational institution, Berkshire was not organized for profit, and usually operated with a deficit. Although the faculty changed frequently, many distinguished men including Elisha Bartlett, who wrote on the fevers of the United States, and Willard Parker, who later became a leading New York surgeon, taught at Berkshire. See Peter D. Gibbons, "The Berkshire Medical Institution," *Bull. Hist. Med.*, 1964, *38*, 45-64.

15. Stone carried an introduction from Dr. Storer to Sir James Young Simpson, the discoverer of chloroform, who invited him to dinner. A highlight of Stone's stay in London was his visit to the clinic of Sir Thomas Spencer Wells, noted for his success as an ovariotomist.

16. Alexander J. Stone, "The St. Paul Medical College," *J. Minn. St. med. Ass. & Northwest. Lancet*, 1909, *29*, 42-43.

17. James Eckman, "Alexander J. Stone, M.D., LL.D., founder of Minnesota's first medical journal," *Ann. med. Hist.*, 1941, ser. 3, *3*, 306-325. On p. 318 Eckman reproduced the announcement of the St. Paul School for 1872 in which the members of the faculty are listed.

18. Richard Olding Beard, "The history of medical education in the state of Minnesota," *J. Minn. St. med. Ass. & Northwest. Lancet*, 1909, *29*, 24-42, pp. 28-29.

19. *Trans. Minn. St. med. Soc.*, 1872, p. 5.

20. Alex. J. Stone, "Report of committee on medical education," *Trans. Minn. St. med. Soc.*, 1872, pp. 96-99, p. 96.

21. "An act to establish a state board of health," *Trans. Minn. St. med. Soc.*, 1872, pp. 115-116.

22. The other members were Drs. Daniel W. Hand, St. Paul; Nathan B. Hill, Minneapolis; Asa W. Daniels, St. Peter; Vespasian Smith, Duluth; and George D. Winch, Blue Earth City.

23. Frederick A. Dunsmoor, "Medicine and surgery," in Isaac Atwater, ed., *History of Minneapolis, Minnesota*, II, 860-915, pp. 885-890. Dunsmoor's preceptors were Hannibal Hamlin Kimball and Calvin Gibson Goodrich. Dr. Kimball had come from Maine in 1867 when he was twenty-six years old to begin medical practice at Minneapolis. In 1869 Dr. Kimball was joined by Dr. Goodrich, a forty-nine-year-old physician who had been lured west the year before after twenty years in practice at Oxford, Ohio.

24. [Obituary] "Dr. Frederick A. Dunsmoor, 1853-1930," *Minn. Med.*, 1931, *14*, 89. Cf. Frederick A. Dunsmoor, "The Minnesota Hospital College," *J. Minn. St. med. Ass. & Northwest. Lancet*, 1909, *29*, 43-45.

25. John T. Rogers, "Charles A. Wheaton," *Surg. Gynec. Obstet.*, 1923, *37*, 699-700.

26. [Obituary] "George Franklin French," *J. Med. Sci., Portland, Maine*, 1896-97, *3*, 323-324. Dr. French, a native of Dover, New Hampshire, was educated at Harvard College and the Harvard Medical School where he received his M.D. degree in 1862.

27. Dunsmoor (n.24), p. 43. In terms of present-day St. Paul the railroad was located near the intersection of Chestnut Street and the railroad track adjacent to Shepard Road. The Civic Center Parking Ramp covers the site of the steps up the cliff to Third Street, renamed Kellogg Boulevard, and the site of the building that housed the medical school is now a parking area in front of the St. Paul Auditorium.

28. Dr. Dunsmoor paid $40,000 for the Winslow House, $10,000 in cash and a mortgage of $30,000 on the property. He then turned the property over to a corporation that he and his colleagues created, known as the Minnesota College Hospital, receiving voting stock for the $10,000 that he had paid. Dunsmoor (n.24), p. 44.

29. Dale Cary Smith, "The emergence of organized clinical instruction in the nineteenth-century American cities of Boston, New York, and Philadelphia," (Ph.D. diss., University of Minnesota, 1979), pp. 258–273.

30. James J. Walsh, *History of medicine in New York,* II, 506–527.

31. Ibid., p. 480.

32. Elizabeth Abbott, "Amos Wilson Abbott, Jan. 6, 1844 - Feb. 27, 1927," MHS Archives.

33. Dunsmoor (n.23), p. 866.

34. "A new medical college," *Northwest. Lancet,* 1881, *1,* 29.

35. Dunsmoor (n.24), p. 44.

36. David Rosner has traced the change of hospitals in Brooklyn and New York City from purely charitable institutions, dependent on endowments and gifts, to business enterprises supported by paying patients. See David Rosner, *A once charitable enterprise: Hospitals and health care in Brooklyn and New York, 1885–1915.*

37. F. A. Dunsmoor, "Report of a successful ovariotomy," *Trans. Minn. St. med. Soc.,* 1883, pp. 90–93.

38. Charles H. Hunter, "The treatment of wounds, with especial reference to the aseptic method of Mr. Lister," *Trans. Minn. St. med. Soc.,* 1883, pp. 93–103.

39. Dunsmoor (n. 24), p. 44.

40. Ibid.

41. In 1894 the Minneapolis College of Physicians and Surgeons moved to the Rand House on Seventh Street South in Minneapolis where it opened the Good Samaritan Dispensary. In 1897, while still remaining at its Minneapolis location, the college became the Department of Medicine of Hamline University in St. Paul, and agreed with the University of Minnesota on common standards of examination for entrance to medical school.

42. Out of fifty-three cases of typhoid fever cared for at the Minneapolis Homeopathic Hospital during the summer and fall of 1887, only four died, a mortality of less than 8 percent. "Minneapolis Homeopathic Hospital," *Minn. med. Mthly,* 1888, *3,* 9.

43. Eugene L. Mann, "College of Homeopathic Medicine and Surgery," in E. Bird Johnson, ed., *Forty years of the University of Minnesota,* pp. 165–170, p. 166. Cf. James Eckman, "Homeopathic and eclectic medicine in Minnesota," *Minn. Med.,* 1941, *24,* 474–479, 567–572, 667–674, 762–769, 863–873, 967–971, 1073–1077, pp. 670–672.

44. Eckman (n.43), pp. 766–767. At the same meeting on 23 February 1886 at which the Homeopathic Medical College was organized, the homeopathic physicians established a homeopathic medical journal, the *Minnesota Medical Monthly,* with Dr. William E. Leonard as editor.

45. Dr. William H. Leonard was born on 2 December 1826 in Mansfield, Tolland County, Connecticut. After teaching school for six years, Leonard entered the office of Orrin Witter, M.D., of Chaplin, Connecticut, to prepare himself for formal medical studies. He attended the winter session medical lectures at the University of New York in 1850 and 1851 and then matriculated at Yale Medical College, earning his M.D. in 1853. In 1855, Leonard came to Minneapolis to practice. Although trained in the regular school of medi-

cine, Leonard became interested in investigating the merits of homeopathy. In 1859, having become convinced of the superiority of homeopathic therapeutics, he announced his conversion to that school. Dr. Leonard served from 1862 to 1865 as assistant surgeon of the Fifth Minnesota Volunteer Infantry during the Civil War. Upon returning to his civilian practice, he became very active in state politics. As a member of the State Board of Health, Leonard introduced the collection of the vital statistics of the city and served as first commissioner of the State Insane Examining Board. Leonard was instrumental in the founding of the Hahnemann Medical Society of Hennepin County and served three times as president of the Homeopathic State Institute. He recognized early the need for the establishment of a department of medicine at the university to function as an examining board. In 1883 he was appointed to the first faculty of that department as professor of obstetrics. Atwater, ed. *History of Minneapolis* (n.23), II, 932–933.

46. C. N. Hewitt, "[Report of the] Committee on medical education," *Trans. Minn. St. med. Soc.*, 1883, pp. 238–246, p. 243.

47. "College of Medicine 1882; Plan for College as an Examining Body," unpaginated manuscript in the hand of Mrs. William Watts Folwell. Medical School papers [1878–1948]. Extract; Proceedings of the Board of Regents of the University of Minnesota, 28 December 1882.

48. Ibid., Extract; Proceedings of the Board of Regents . . . , Jan. 5, 1883.

49. Ibid.

50. At the meeting of the Board of Regents on 25 January 1883, regents Lucius F. Hubbard of Red Wing, Greenleaf Clark of St. Paul, and John S. Pillsbury of St. Anthony were selected to nominate persons to fill nine faculty chairs. By the close of the meeting that day, they had filled five of the chairs. Charles N. Hewitt became professor of preventive medicine, Perry H. Millard professor of anatomy and physiology, and William H. Leonard professor of obstetrics. Dr. Franklin Staples became professor of the practice of medicine and Dr. Daniel W. Hand professor of surgery. Each was a respected physician, and each had demonstrated, by previous membership on the State Board of Health, his ability at administrative tasks.

51. "College of Medicine 1882" (n. 47), Extract; Proceedings of the Board of Regents . . . 23 April 1883.

52. The constitution and bylaws for the medical department, extracted from the Proceedings of the Board of Regents dated 29 June 1882, appear in manuscript in the "Minutes, College of Medicine and Surgery. Executive Committee", vol. 2, 23 April 1883 - 15 April 1886, Medical School Papers. The minutes are in the hand of the faculty recording secretary, Dr. Perry Millard. The bylaws and regulations are printed in their final form in the *Special announcement: College of Medicine* (Minneapolis: University of Minnesota, 1884), 57 pp., pp. 21–25. All page references are to the printed document.

53. Ibid., Article I, Sec. 5, p. 22.

54. "Minutes" (n. 52), p. 15.

55. *Special announcement* (n. 52), Article II, Sec. 10, p. 23.

56. Ibid., Article II, Sec. 8, p. 23.

57. *Trans. Minn. St. med. Soc.*, 1883, p. 245.

58. *Special announcement* (n. 52), pp. 36–47. Those physicians holding diplomas and certified to practice in Minnesota are listed here alphabetically along with the name of their colleges and year of graduation.

59. Ibid., pp. 48–49.

60. Ibid., p. 48; "Minutes" (n. 52), pp. 18–19.

61. "Minutes" (n. 52), p. 48.

62. *Special announcement* (n. 52), pp. 11–14. In the discussion on the organization of the professional examination, the requirements of each of the nine departments of the

medical college are listed. Following those requirements is a list of textbooks recommended for use in preparation for the examinations (pp. 15–16).

63. The questions used in the M.B. examination given in October 1883 are printed in the *Special announcement* (n. 52), pp. 50–53. They were given to show prospective candidates the general range of information required to pass the examination, and to demonstrate the emphasis upon practical rather than theoretical knowledge. Two additional sets of examination questions, those used in the spring 1884 and in the spring 1885, are found in "Minutes" (n. 52), pp. 21–28, 33–44.

64. *University of Minnesota Bulletin, 1886–87,* "The College of Medicine," p. 85.

CHAPTER 3

The Department of Medicine 1888–1892

On 14 June 1886, the Board of Regents decided that the results of the medical college were unsatisfactory and that it should either be abandoned or modified.[1] The board did not indicate specific shortcomings of the medical college as an examining body. Indeed, it seems to have fulfilled its modest function efficiently. The decision to reorganize the college was instead the next step in a plan, conceived in broad outline by Perry Millard in 1882, to establish a teaching medical school at the university. In 1882 a medical school operating as part of the state university system, for various reasons, would have been unlikely to succeed. The founders recognized that the conditions of medical education and the laws regulating medical practice did not favor the survival of a state medical school with standards for entrance and graduation far above those of coexisting private institutions.

During the brief life of the College of Medicine as an examining body, the inadequacies of the existing system of medical education and regulation became increasingly apparent both to the members of the medical profession and politically active laymen. By 1887 Perry Millard, who had been biding his time, sensed that the climate of opinion in Minnesota would now support the adoption of his plan for the fundamental reform of medical education in Minnesota. Millard recognized further that if such reform were to be permanent, it must be enforced by statute. Efficient medical legislation, in Millard's view, was prerequisite to efficient medical education. With the help of Stillwater attorney Fayette Marsh, he drafted a new medical practice act that set an unprecedented standard for the control of quality in medical education, and then labored relentlessly for its passage.[2]

The medical practice act of 1883, which had empowered the College of Medicine to act as an examining board, had the unfortunate weakness of giving a legal interpretation to the medical diploma.[3] The "diploma law," as that statute came to be called, recognized the possession of a medical diploma as a test of fitness to practice medicine. The powers of the faculty as an examining board were limited accordingly to a determination of the medical colleges from which diplomas should be accepted as evidence of qualification to practice and, for students who lacked an acceptable diploma, the requirements for admittance to the examination for a medical license. The diploma law was weakened further by its lack of teeth. The faculty serving as a board of examiners was granted no power to enforce the provisions of the examination system, except by indirect means.[4]

In dramatic contrast to the statute of 1883, Dr. Millard's draft of a new medical practice act incorporated all the essentials of effective medical regulation and measures for enforcement.[5] The proposed law provided for a nine-member state board of medical examiners that included representatives from both the regular medical profession and the homeopaths. It differed from previous medical legislation in that it provided for:

1. The adoption of more rigid rules governing the admission of students to medical schools.

2. The determination of the applicants' fitness to practice by an examination upon all branches of medicine.

3. The right to refuse or revoke licenses for unprofessional or dishonorable conduct.

4. An adequate penalty for violation of the provisions of the law.

5. The boards of examiners to be appointed by the Governor, with proportionate representation from the various schools of practice.[6]

By requiring submission to a qualifying examination of *all* new applicants for a license to practice medicine in Minnesota, the act of 1887 no longer recognized the medical diploma as evidence of fitness to serve as a physician. Minnesota was the first state in the Union to enact such a measure and was, in this respect, one of the most progressive in promoting higher standards in medical education.[7]

The provisions of the medical practice act of 1887 reflected the dramatic changes taking place in medicine and in the sciences fundamental to medicine. "Medicine," Millard stated in one of his numerous pleas for more efficient medical legislation, "is now more nearly practiced from a scientific basis than at any time in its history."[8] Accordingly, he drafted the law to demand of all medical licensure candidates evidence of solid preparation in the appropriate sciences. Taking effect on 1 July 1887, the new law specified that the qualifying medical licensure examination be " . . . both scientific and practical, but of sufficient severity to test the candidate's fitness to practice medicine and surgery."[9] To ensure the maintenance of fairness and high standards, deans of any medical schools and presidents of state medical societies were to be admitted freely as observers of the examination sessions of the board. Successful candidates—those approved by at least seven of the nine-member board—would be licensed to practice medicine in the state of Minnesota. Violations of the statute constituted misdemeanors to be prosecuted by the respective county attorneys under the jurisdiction of the respective municipal courts. As in the law of 1883, the 1887 act included a grandfather clause protecting the professional security of established physicians. Persons licensed, either by diploma or by examination, under the statute of 1883 were exempted from further tests of qualification to practice medicine. Commissioned surgeons of the United States Army or Navy, physicians and surgeons called in from other states or territories for consultation, and medical students working under the direct supervision of a preceptor also were exempted from the operation of the law. The Minnesota medical practice act of 1887 represented the dawn of a new era in the setting and enforcement of uniformly high standards in medical education. By 1897 more than one-half of the states followed suit, passing legislation modeled closely upon the Minnesota statute.

Having established in law the standards to govern medical education in Minnesota, Millard and his associates set about to establish a medical college capable of meeting those standards. On 7 April 1887, Drs. Perry Millard, Charles N. Hewitt, and Daniel W. Hand presented to the Board of Regents their case for organizing a medical teaching department to replace the former examining faculty.[10] Their arguments were persuasive. At the close of the meeting, President Cyrus O. Northrop moved that application be made to the state legislature at its next session for appropriations sufficient to establish and maintain a medical teaching institution at the University of Minnesota.

For fully a decade, Drs. Perry Millard, Charles Hewitt, Daniel Hand, and William H. Leonard, along with many others, had worked toward a common goal, the establishment of a high quality medical teaching department at the university. Nevertheless, the decision of the Board of Regents to open such a school did not reflect unanimity of opinion among those advocates concerning the organization of that department. Drs. Millard and Hewitt, the dominant figures in the creation of the department, held opposite views about the proper modes of medical education. The decision of the regents signaled the beginning of a struggle from which only one plan could emerge victorious.

As executive secretary of the State Board of Health and Vital Statistics, chairman of the examining faculty of medicine at the University of Minnesota, past president and a dominating figure of the Minnesota State Medical Society, and, in 1888, as president of the American Public Health Association, Hewitt was a powerful individual. He approached his work and expressed his views with a zeal that shunned compromise. Hewitt's convictions concerning the premier importance of preventive medicine, shared and supported by his close friend, former President Folwell, were well known.[11] In his autocratic management of the State Board of Public Health, as well as in his courses, speeches, and correspondence, Hewitt expressed forcibly his belief that a medical teaching institution should function only as a branch of the State Board of Public Health, and that its curriculum should center upon preventive medicine. In 1886, in an effort to enlist the support of President Northrop, Hewitt urged that medical education should be based on a knowledge of public health, "which is more and more the admitted foundation of practical medicine."[12] Hewitt went on to explain that the education and work of not only the physician but also of the public health officer, sanitary engineer, plumber, pharmacist, water engineer, and others should center around preventive medicine. In a medical school conforming to his design, he told Northrop, facilities would include, in addition to lecture halls, library and recitation rooms, laboratories and a "sanitary museum." While the basic sciences, such as chemistry and biology, were not to be neglected, strong emphasis would be placed upon "laboratory instruction in original experimentation and research in sanitary science."[13]

Whatever may have been the merits of Hewitt's vision of medical education, President Northrop gave his support to Perry Millard's plan. Although the State Board of Public Health offices and laboratories were housed on the campus, and although Hewitt had been given a university appointment some years before, he did not participate in the reorganization of the medical school and none of his proposals were implemented. Clearly Hewitt had been ostracized, but not without provocation.

For Perry Millard, the organization and survival of a first-rate medical school represented the fulfillment of his life's purpose. His plan for the administration of medical education at the university, fully consistent with the current state of the art, was both progressive and realistic. Millard was keenly aware of the rapid development of clinical medicine, and especially of surgery, which held out the hope of effective treatment for many diseases and at the same time required much more rigorous training for its successful practice. By contrast, Hewitt's plan, although not without its attractive features, was impractical and, for its time, utopian. Certainly the success of Hewitt's scheme was hampered further by his personality. An opinionated, domineering, determined individual, Hewitt's inability to compromise or to admit the merits of other viewpoints made him an unpopular man in many circles. In order for the medical school to flourish, it required the cooperation and support of a broad base of medical educators and practitioners.[14] Hewitt's control of the State Board of Public Health, as well as of the other organizations in which he participated, was well known. Millard recognized that Hewitt would oppose his own design for medical education and led in the effort to exclude him. Hewitt's opposition to and continued criticism of the medical practice act of 1887 confirmed Millard's view that Hewitt must be regarded as a dangerous opponent. Millard's commitment to the medical practice act was absolute. "In medical legislation," he stated, "we have the *only* solution of the problem of higher medical education."[15] Millard admitted that he had "by force of circumstances been somewhat aggressive in urging [the] enactment" of this legislation. With victory at hand, he could not afford to be less aggressive in his treatment of Hewitt, who perhaps represented a threat to that victory.

Millard prevailed. Behind him rallied the prominent medical educators of Minnesota. On 18 January 1888, the Minnesota Hospital College and the St. Paul Medical College agreed to surrender their charters and offered the use of their buildings to the university for a period of five years.[16] In March, the Minnesota Homeopathic Medical College followed suit.[17] In exchange for the surrender of their charter and the temporary use of their property, the Board of Regents agreed to establish a college of homeopathic medicine and surgery within the new medical department. By the willingness of the three medical colleges to remove themselves voluntarily from competition with the university medical department, and by their willingness to provide temporary quarters for the new school, the medical educators of the state gave to Perry Millard and his plan a resounding vote of confidence.

On 26 April 1888 the Board of Regents established the Department of Medicine of the University of Minnesota. They intended it to be a high quality medical college offering a medical course three years in length, each year to include a term of six months. Students already enrolled in other medical schools in the state were granted admission to the new school without examination. The new school immediately enrolled 105 students, many of them from the Minnesota Hospital College or the St. Paul Medical College. Lecture and laboratory classes as well as an outpatient dispensary were housed at the former Minnesota Hospital College at Sixth Street and Ninth Avenue South in Minneapolis, while the building of the former St. Paul Medical College at Ninth and State Streets in St. Paul housed a dispensary and was used for clinical teaching.

The regents appointed Perry H. Millard dean of the medical faculty, thereby making him responsible for the Department of Medicine, and the three colleges it comprised: the College of Medicine and Surgery, the College of Homeopathic Medicine and Surgery, and the College of Dentistry. Dr. Millard was to serve both as dean of the Department of Medicine and dean of the College of Medicine and Surgery.

Perry Henry Millard was a native of New York State, born at Ogdensburg in 1848. After completing his work in chemistry at the University of Michigan at Ann Arbor, he attended Rush Medical College at Chicago where he received the M.D. degree in 1871. After graduation he set up a medical practice in Chicago, but almost immediately lost everything in the great Chicago fire. In April 1872 Dr. Millard arrived at Stillwater, Minnesota, where he established himself in practice and was soon successful. It was not unusual for him to be summoned at any hour to one of the lumber camps in eastern Minnesota to treat injuries caused by logging accidents that often resulted in amputation. He also saw many injuries associated with the railroads. In addition he treated the townspeople. In 1874, Perry Millard married Caroline E. Swain, the niece of his professional colleague and a senior Stillwater physician, Dr. Joel K. Reiner. They had two children, Lillian and John Jay. In the fall of 1881 Millard went to England where he spent about six months studying surgery at Guy's Hospital in London.

Shortly after his return from England, Millard, as president of the Minnesota State Medical Association in 1882, arranged hospitality for the members of the American Medical Association when they met that year in St. Paul. Several times he was a delegate to national medical meetings and actively promoted the American Association of Medical Colleges. His participation in Republican politics at the county level no doubt served him well when he worked to get the medical

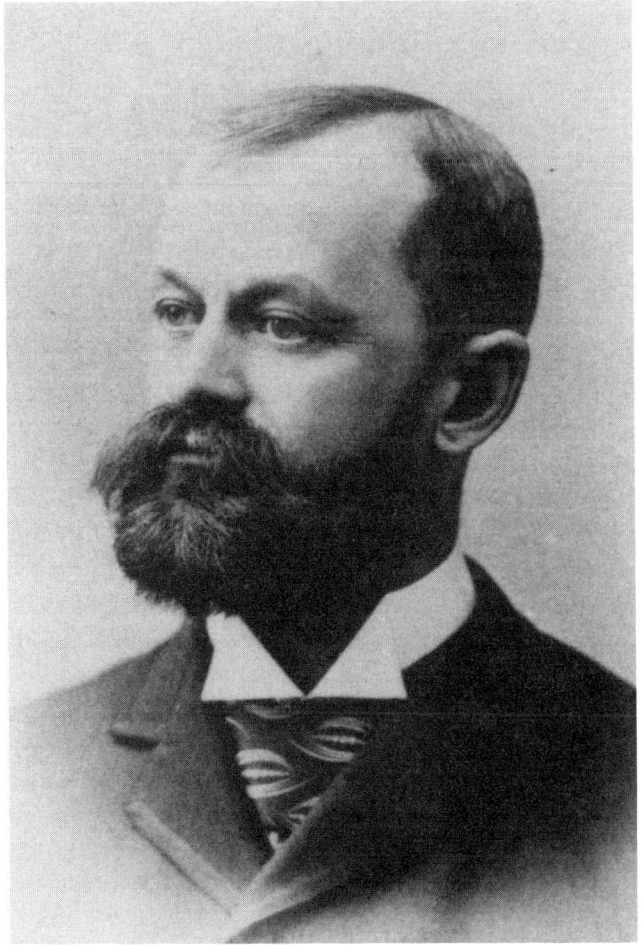

FIGURE 3:1   Perry H. Millard, circa 1887. Courtesy Mn U Archives.

practice acts of 1882 and 1887 through the legislature. In the fall of 1887 when he was actively engaged in negotiations for the establishment of a medical college at the university, Perry Millard moved from Stillwater to set up his surgical practice in St. Paul.[18]

After the regents' meeting of 26 April, Perry Millard had the authority as dean to proceed with organizing a Department of Medicine at the university, and within that department he had the framework of three colleges: medicine and surgery, homeopathic medicine and surgery, and dentistry. Furthermore, he had the mandate to create a high quality institution.[19] He lost no time getting down to the business at hand. In three months time he had his three faculties appointed, curricula established for a three-year course of study, faculty bylaws approved, student admissions standards and graduation requirements set, and a fee schedule.

Dean Millard must have worked night and day, but he had the cooperation and blessing of President Northrop and prominent Twin Cities physicians, many with appointments in the new medical school. The result of this intense activity appeared in the University of Minnesota Catalogue for 1887–88 where the Department of Medicine was listed with its three colleges and their courses of lectures, in place and ready to receive students.[20]

The faculty of the College of Medicine and Surgery was nominated by a committee consisting of President Northrop, Dean Millard, and the respective presidents of the State Medical Society, the State Board of Medical Examiners, and the State Board of Health. For more than a year before the regents formally established the Department of Medicine on 26 April 1888, the committee had held a succession of informal meetings in both Minneapolis and St. Paul. Their great difficulty was to select a medical faculty without offending professors of the two former schools. Not all could be included in the new school, and those who were omitted were bound to feel slighted. On 26 April the committee submitted a list of twenty-nine nominees for the medical faculty, and all of the nominees were appointed by the regents, each for a term of one year.[21] All were physicians in practice in Minneapolis or St. Paul, except Dr. Arthur Ritchie from Duluth. Twenty-five received the title of professor.[22] Two were appointed clinical professors, three as adjunct professors, and one as demonstrator in anatomy. Fourteen of the faculty were in medical practice in Minneapolis and fourteen in St. Paul; the university deliberately maintained an exact balance in the representation from the two cities. A need for balance may also have influenced clinical and adjunct appointments. Whereas Dr. John Fulton of St. Paul was professor of ophthalmology and otology, Dr. Frank Allport of Minneapolis was clinical professor of the same subjects; Dr. Alexander Stone of St. Paul was professor of diseases of women while Dr. Amos Abbott of Minneapolis was clinical professor. Although the exactness of the balance in appointments between Minneapolis and St. Paul suggests that it was influenced by rivalry between the two professional groups, the need to provide clinical instruction for students in the hospitals and dispensaries of both cities required clinical teachers in both places.

The teaching of the basic medical subjects posed other problems. The time required to provide a thorough course in anatomy for medical students was too great for the task to be performed in the spare hours of medical practice. The same was true for physiology, especially if the teaching were to include practical instruction in laboratory classes. Chemistry posed the further difficulty that in addition to the time required to set up a chemical laboratory and organize practical laboratory classes, the subject had advanced so rapidly during the nineteenth century that few physicians, most of whom remembered only a little of the meager chemical knowledge they had gained from lectures in medical school, were prepared to teach it. Consequently, although most of the medical professors were to receive no salaries, Dean Millard and President Northrop realized that an exception must be made for teachers of chemistry, anatomy, and physiology. At the 26 April meeting the regents cautiously decided that such professors and their assistants

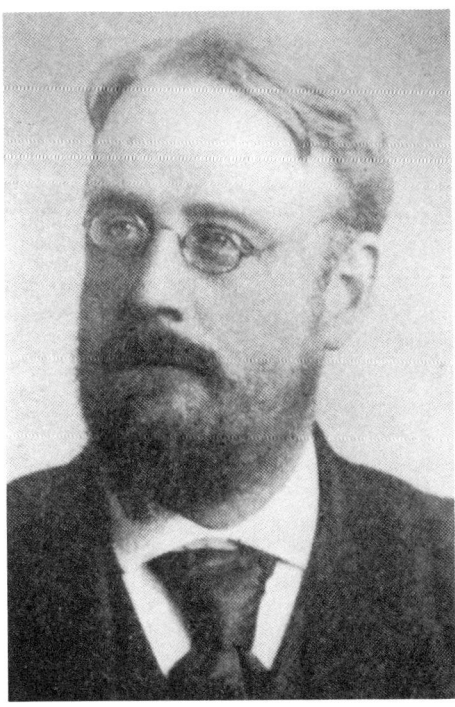

FIGURE 3:2 Charles J. Bell. Courtesy Mn U Archives.

might be paid salaries to the extent that the income from tuition fees would permit.[23] The tuition fees were to be thirty-five dollars per year for Minnesota residents, and sixty dollars for nonresidents, with additional fees to meet the cost of laboratory work and a graduation fee of ten dollars. Because Dean Millard knew the number of students who had been enrolled in the Minnesota Hospital College and the St. Paul Medical College, he could make a reasonably accurate estimate of the number of students who would enroll in the university medical college in the fall of 1888, which proved to be slightly over a hundred students. Thus he knew that he would have somewhat over $4,000 with which to pay the faculty during 1888–89. At their meeting on 14 May 1888 the regents appointed Charles J. Bell professor of chemistry in the Department of Medicine at a salary of $1,200 annually.[24] Charles Bell was a native of Massachusetts, receiving his education at Phillips Exeter Academy and Harvard College. After graduation from Harvard in 1876, Bell went to Germany where he spent six years studying chemistry at Munich with Adolf von Baeyer and at Berlin with August W. Hofmann. On his return to America, he taught chemistry for several years at Pennsylvania State College before becoming a fellow in chemistry at Johns Hopkins University, whence he came to Minnesota in 1888 at the age of thirty-five. Although the minutes of the regents meeting made no mention of other salary considerations, they also must have provided a salary for Dr. Arthur F. Ritchie, who came from Duluth for the six months of the medical school term to teach anatomy, for Dr. Burnside Foster

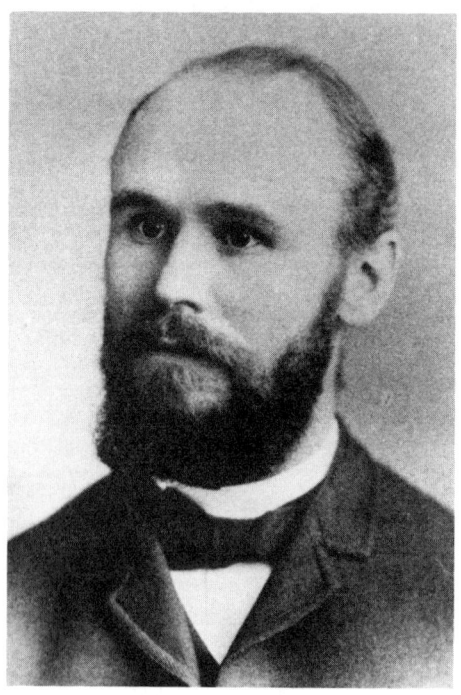

FIGURE 3:3   Richard Olding Beard, 1888. Courtesy Mn U Archives.

of Minneapolis, who acted as demonstrator in anatomy, and possibly for Dr. Richard O. Beard as professor of physiology.

The courses in the primary subjects of anatomy, physiology, and chemistry were taught also for the benefit of students in the College of Homeopathic Medicine and Surgery and the College of Dentistry. In the College of Homeopathic Medicine and Surgery the regents appointed fourteen professors.[25] The homeopathic faculty did not have equal representation from Minneapolis and St. Paul. There were eight professors from Minneapolis, four from St. Paul, one from Fergus Falls, and one from Duluth. Nevertheless, in other respects the homeopathic college was organized along lines very similar to those of the College of Medicine and Surgery.

On 14 May the committee on schedule of lectures, consisting of Dean Millard and representatives of the three colleges, met in the evening at Frederick Dunsmoor's home in Minneapolis. Professor Martindale of the College of Dentistry was elected chairman of the committee, and Dean Millard secretary. The committee decided that lectures in the basic subjects, that is, anatomy, physiology, and chemistry, should be given Monday through Friday mornings, the laboratory classes in chemistry and physiology in the afternoons from one until four o'clock, and anatomical dissection in the evenings.[26] They clearly intended to keep the first-year medical students from being over-burdened with leisure.

On 8 June 1888 the first meeting of the faculty of the Department of Medicine was held in President Northrop's office at ten o'clock in the morning. Twenty-six faculty members were present from the medical college, ten from the homeopathic college, and two from the dental college. President Northrop presided and agreed to give the inaugural address at the opening exercises of the department on 2 October. Members of the faculty reported progress in the organization of dispensaries in St. Paul and Minneapolis. A committee was appointed to obtain cadavers for dissection and another to seek clinical privileges for the medical students in the principal hospitals of the Twin Cities. The latter committee was also to seek the privilege of appointment of internes at the hospitals on the basis of a competitive examination to be taken by senior medical students at the time of graduation and to seek the construction at several of the hospitals of amphitheaters in which to conduct medical and surgical clinics. Drs. Charles Wheaton and Everton J. Abbott were deputed to seek the construction of such an amphitheater at St. Joseph's Hospital in St. Paul.[27]

Both the College of Medicine and Surgery and the College of Homeopathic Medicine offered a three-year graded course of study, a major departure from the long-standard two-year program in which the second year lectures simply repeated those of the first. The first year of study was nearly identical in the two colleges. The homeopathic college offered their own lectures on materia medica, which incorporated the principles of homeopathic therapeutics based on the writings of Samuel Hahnemann and other homeopathic authors, and the course in histology was omitted from their curriculum. By contrast the College of Medicine and Surgery offered both lectures and laboratory work in histology and suggested that each student should provide himself with a microscope.[28]

In the second year the same subjects were taught at a more advanced level, but each college also added a number of subjects. Only the regular college offered pathology, medical jurisprudence, and hygiene in addition to histology. The regular college laid considerable emphasis on pathology, which they said would include work in the dead house. Each student would be taught the techniques of autopsy in order to learn how to do a post-mortem examination properly. The catalogue stated that disease processes would be "illustrated by fresh and alcoholic specimens, that theories of disease may be as much matters of demonstration as the nature of the subjects will admit."[29]

The study of anatomy, physiology, chemistry, and materia medica was considered complete at the end of the second year in both colleges, but the other second year subjects were continued through the third-year with new courses added.[30] Both colleges emphasized the opportunities they offered for clinical experiences. The College of Medicine and Surgery promised access to the wards of the city hospitals of Minneapolis and St. Paul and to the principal private hospitals in both cities, in addition to a dispensary in each city where second and third-year students might attend clinics. The College of Homeopathic Medicine spoke enthusiastically of the hospitals devoted to homeopathic practice in Minneapolis and St. Paul, the latter ". . . situated in the natural center for accidents, within two blocks of

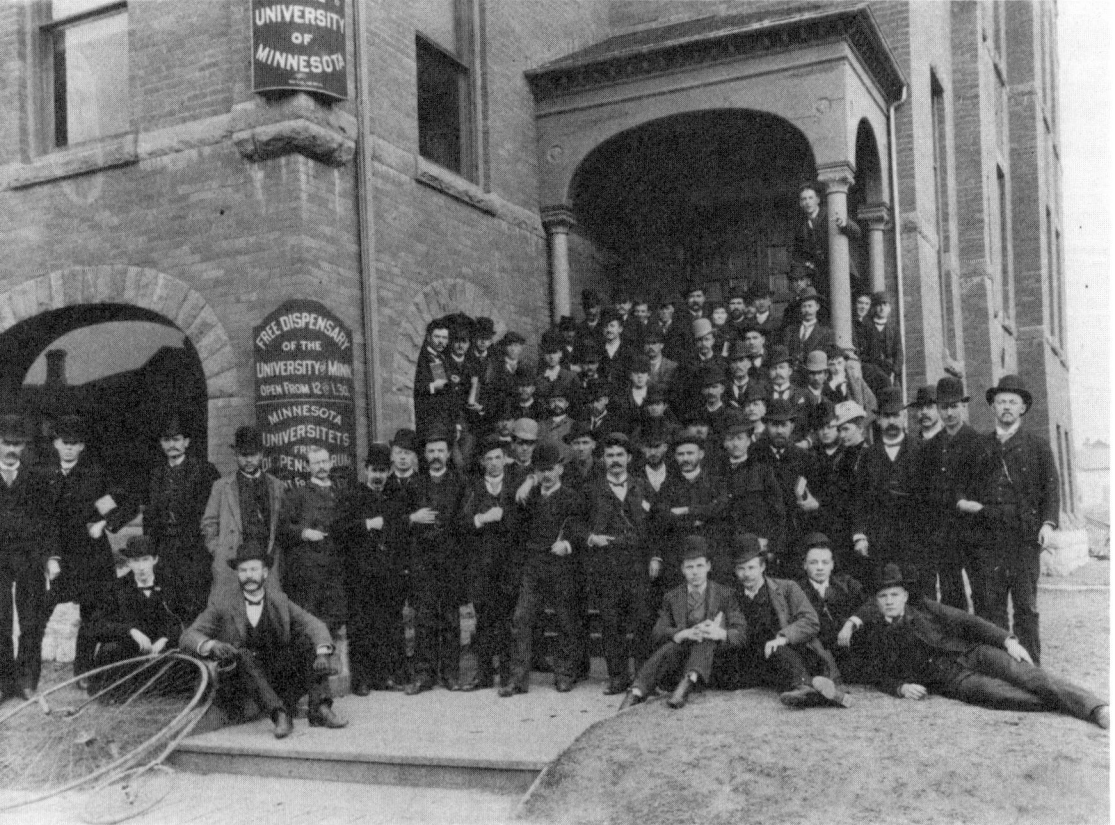

FIGURE 3:4 Medical students, College of Medicine and Surgery, circa 1889. Courtesy Mn U Archives.

most of the railroads that enter the city, and surrounded by car shops and manufacturing industries, secures a large share of surgical cases."[31] Students accompanied their homeopathic teachers to both hospitals where they visited patients at the bedside. Dean Millard made special arrangements with the railroads to carry the students from Minneapolis to St. Paul for the weekly clinic of both colleges held on Saturdays.

The first term opened on 1 October 1888 and continued until the end of March 1889. In addition an optional nine-week spring term beginning on 1 April offered special courses. Through the spring term the department also continued to provide opportunities for laboratory work and clinical instruction. A year later, at a meeting of the Department of Medicine on 18 April 1890, the faculty recommended that the annual session be extended from six to eight months, thereby making the spring term a required instead of optional part of the course. The change took effect with the academic year 1890–91.[32]

That the repeated mention of clinical opportunities in the university catalogue was not hollow rhetoric is suggested by the success of the department in obtaining amphitheaters for clinical instruction at several of the hospitals. The efforts of Drs. Wheaton and Abbott to obtain such an amphitheater at St. Joseph's Hospital in St. Paul were evidently successful. On 20 November 1888 the Board of Regents voted their thanks to Archbishop Ireland of the Archdioceses of St. Paul "for his generosity in providing an amphitheatre in connection with St. Joseph's Hospital for the benefit of the students in the medical department of the university and for his public exhibition of his appreciation of the importance of medical education."[33] The whole aim of the school in three months of strenuous creation in 1888 was summed up in the final paragraph of the announcement of the College of Medicine and Surgery, wherein Dean Millard wrote, " . . . the Faculty will spare no endeavor to put the College upon a plane with the foremost medical institutions of the country. . . ."[34] Brave words that Millard strove mightily to fulfill.

Whereas cooperation between the regular private medical schools of Minnesota and the Department of Medicine at the university made practical sense, such cooperation between the Minnesota Homeopathic Medical College and the university, from an historical perspective, was remarkable. Since the advent of homeopathy in the late eighteenth century, relations between physicians of the regular and homeopathic schools of medicine had deteriorated progressively until they were hardly on speaking terms. In the late 1840s and 1850s, one medical society after another adopted rules to exclude homeopathic doctors and to expel any of their own members caught consulting with, or even socializing with, homeopathic practitioners.[35]

The homeopathic system of medicine was developed in Germany in the 1780s by Dr. Samuel C. Hahnemann, a medical graduate of the University of Erlangen, during a period of great uncertainty in the treatment of disease. In the late eighteenth and early nineteenth centuries, physicians made unprecedented progress in the understanding of pathology and diagnosis, but achieved only minor advances in the field of treatment. Traditional treatment for most diseases included bloodletting and the administration of noxious, even toxic, emetics and purgatives. As knowledge of human physiology and pathology increased, physicians and their patients alike became less certain of the therapeutic benefits of standard treatments, and more certain of their adverse consequences. In the absence of a truly scientific basis for therapeutics, Samuel Hahnemann's system, when first introduced, attracted considerable interest and support.

In his book, *Organon of homeopathic medicine,* published in 1810, Samuel Hahnemann described two therapeutic "laws," the law of similars and the law of infinitesimals, upon which he based his system of medicine.[36] In about 1790 in an experiment conducted upon himself, Hahnemann discovered that when he took large doses of cinchona bark, he developed symptoms, such as fever, profuse sweating, and rapid pulse, similar to those experienced by patients ill with malaria. Since malaria could be cured by the administration of cinchona bark, Hahnemann theorized that the key to therapy was to administer a medicine that when given to a healthy person would produce symptoms similar to those of the disease to be treated. The experiment with cinchona bark, as well as subsequent self-experiments with other drugs, convinced Hahnemann of the correctness of his theory and led him to announce the first law of homeopathy, *similia similibus curantur,* or likes are cured by likes. The second law of homeopathy, the "law of infinitesimals," was based upon Hahnemann's belief that large doses of drugs served to aggravate illnesses and that small doses supported the "vital spirit" of the body in its effort to overcome disease.

While the chief tenets of homeopathic medicine were neither more absurd nor less amenable to scientific demonstration than the theories that governed regular therapeutics in the early nineteenth century, certain distinctly mystical features raised questions about the credibility of homeopathy. In Hahnemann's view, a "high potency" drug dose ought not to exceed 1/500,000 or 1/1,000,000 of a grain. But, Hahnemann explained, such an infinitesimal dose could not be effective unless prepared by a physician according to a prescribed ritual intended to potentize the medicine. Subsequently, Hahnemann elaborated further his system of medicine to include the claim that many chronic diseases, including dermatitis, insanity, asthma, and deafness, were consequences of medicines prescribed by regular physicians for the treatment of a condition he referred to as "the itch."[37]

During the nineteenth century a number of other nonorthodox systems of medicine, including hydropathy, electrotherapy, osteopathy, and new forms of herbalism, also came into vogue. In contrast to practitioners of such medical cults and fads, most homeopathic physicians were well-educated physicians who held M.D. degrees from respected medical schools and universities. They accepted the bulk of traditional medical ideas, differing from their orthodox colleagues only in matters of treatment. When homeopathic ideas were first introduced in the United States, their articulate spokesmen were received politely. In numerous published reports, homeopaths reported significantly better rates of survival than those reported by regular physicians when treating patients during epidemics of cholera and typhoid fever. Such results, together with the public's preference for more moderate treatments, moved many physicians to forsake the orthodox school of therapeutics and to offer instead homeopathic treatment. As the number of homeopathic practitioners increased, the regular medical profession began to feel threatened. Their initial policy of peaceful coexistence with the homeopaths gave way to mutual hostility between the two schools. In 1842, Dr. Oliver Wendell Holmes contributed his essay *Homeopathy and its kindred delusions* as part of the general offensive of orthodox physicians against homeopathy.[38] In his devastating analysis of homeopathic therapeutics, Holmes argued that the system had no rational or scientific basis and explained away its claims of therapeutic success by pointing out that, in nine cases out of ten, patients recovered with or without medical intervention. In the 10 percent of cases where the skills of a "true" physician made the difference between life and death, Holmes regarded homeopathy as both useless and dangerous.

For a number of reasons, homeopathy posed a serious threat to the sovereignty of the established medical profession. In contrast to other medical cults which attracted chiefly ignorant and poor patients, homeopathy achieved a broad base of public support that included many wealthy and prominent individuals. When, during the 1840s and 1850s, the regular medical profession launched a vigorous campaign to discredit homeopathy, the public and the medical profession divided into two hostile camps. Public sympathy for homeopathy was manifested by the repeated refusal of state legislatures to limit or prohibit homeopathic practice in their states. By its frequent and vituperative published attacks on homeopathy, and by its increasing tendency to punish by expulsion from medical societies members who consulted with homeopaths, the medical profession demonstrated its resolute animosity towards homeopathy.

In Minnesota, relations between regular and homeopathic physicians, although never perfectly cordial, showed more tolerance than in the East.[39] During Minnesota's years of territorial status and in the early years of its statehood, regular and homeopathic physicians labored side by side without closely scrutinizing one another's therapeutic ideas. Later, although sectarian rivalries prevented Minnesota homeopaths and regulars from regarding each other as equals, they were inclined to look upon members of the opposing school as misguided brethren of the same faith rather than, as the American Medical Association was claiming, heretics and charlatans.[40] At their professional meetings and in their respective journals, Minnesota homeopathic and orthodox physicians denounced each other regularly, but as a ritual performed without strong conviction. The opposing schools tended to recognize that their ideological similarities outweighed their differences. In 1883 in his presidential address before the Minnesota State Homeopathic Institute, Dr. George Hawes spoke for most homeopaths when he stated:

> I would not detract anything from the honors our friends of the opposing school have won in the collateral branches of medical science. We would accord them full credit for the reflected light we have absorbed from their researches in all departments, save that of therapeutics. In therapeutics, they stand where Hahnemann stood one hundred years ago.[41]

In the same year, the Minnesota State Homeopathic Institute and the Minnesota State Medical Society began the amicable gesture of exchanging copies of their respective *Transactions*.[42]

In 1888, when the Board of Regents of the University of Minnesota proposed a merger with the Minnesota Homeopathic Medical College, both parties recognized in such an arrangement advantages and disadvantages. The Board of Regents appreciated the prestige and influence homeopathic physicians enjoyed in Minnesota. A homeopath, Dr. William H. Leonard was a respected member of the State Board of Health.[43] During his tenure of office, he introduced the keeping of city vital statistics to the board, and became the first commissioner of the State Insane Examining Board. In Minneapolis, homeopathy and its institutions were supported by leading businessmen and political figures.[44] In St. Paul, the homeopaths enjoyed equally impressive patronage.[45]

During the planning stages of the new medical department at the university, the Board of Regents recognized that their success in this enterprise would depend, in large measure, upon public support. To include homeopathic instruction in the medical department would attract patronage that might have been alienated if the university were to compete with the Minnesota Homeopathic Medical College. Such considerations prompted the regents to offer, in exchange for the closing of the existing homeopathic college, the inclusion of homeopathic subjects in the curriculum of their medical department. Two chairs were proposed: *materia medica* and therapeutics.[46]

Leaders of Minnesota's homeopathic medical community rejected flatly the regents' offer to represent their school of medicine with two professorships in the regular medical department at the university. Under such an arrangement, the interests of homeopathy would be overshadowed quickly by those of the orthodox medical curriculum. The homeopaths were strong enough to bargain for more, but, they realized prudently, not strong enough to operate an independent school of the anticipated quality of the new university medical school. In exchange for the surrender of their charter, the trustees of the Minnesota Homeopathic Medical College demanded and obtained from the Board of Regents a separate homeopathic medical college, independent of the regular College of Medicine and Surgery, within the university's Department of Medicine. The homeopaths required a full faculty of homeopathic physicians authorized to offer a complete course leading to the doctorate of homeopathic medicine and surgery. Like the other private medical colleges, the trustees of the Minnesota Homeopathic Medical College offered the building occupied by their school as a temporary home for the university's new homeopathic college. Directly after the Board of Regents accepted their offer of accommodations, the regents appointed a special committee to nominate faculty for the homeopathic college of medicine and surgery.[47]

The standard of instruction in the homeopathic and regular medical colleges was remarkably similar. Except for the study of *materia medica* and therapeutics according to the principles of their founder, Samuel Hahnemann, homeopathic students mastered the same curriculum as their regular counterparts. During the twenty-one-year history of the homeopathic college at the university, every graduate *save one* passed the State Board Examinations. The regular college could boast no such record.[48]

In 1892 the homeopathic college gave up its building on the corner of Ninth Avenue South and Sixth Street to the new Asbury Hospital to move to the university campus. Henry W. Brazie, professor of pediatrics, was named dean of the college. In 1893, Dr. Brazie resigned as dean to be replaced by Alonzo P. Williamson, who held that office until 1903.[49]

During the deanship of Dr. Williamson significant changes were made both in the entrance requirements and the curriculum of the homeopathic college.[50] In addition to a faculty increase from thirteen to fifteen professors during the school's first twelve years, three lecturers were also employed to permit a broader division of subjects and a more detailed treatment of important topics in the curriculum. For instance, in 1900 four professors and two lecturers were responsible for teaching surgery, which in 1888 had been managed by only two professors.

Several hospitals participated in providing clinical experience for students of the homeopathic college, including the City Hospital of Minneapolis, and in St. Paul the City and County Hospital and St. Joseph's Hospital. Medical students of both the regular and homeopathic schools of medicine and surgery at the university acquired most of their early clinical training through dispensary work. For the homeopathic students, such work was accomplished at the Minneapolis Free Homeopathic Dispensary. Relocated in 1888 to the grounds of St. Barnabas Hospital, the clinic was reorganized and incorporated as the University Free Homeopathic Dispensary. The dispensary was administered as a charity and all medical services were free. Money for supplies was contributed by the faculty in amounts which varied, before 1900, between $400 and $600 per year. The faculty made a great effort to arrange the cases at the dispensary to provide systematic instruction for students. In 1892, over 2,000 patients were seen at the dispensary, including a large number of surgical cases. The dispensary staff served additional patients through house-call consultations. Over 8,000 prescriptions were prepared annually for patients calling at the dispensary. The high teacher-student ratio and low student-patient ratio, available in the homeopathic college from its beginning, combined to create conditions favorable for medical education. Between 1888 and 1900 an average of twenty-two students attended the college each year, with an annual graduation rate of five.

Growth and Change of the Department of Medicine

In 1889 the first changes in the medical faculty occurred when Dr. George A. Hendricks was appointed professor of anatomy to succeed Dr. Arthur F. Ritchie who had resigned, and Dr. J. Clark Stewart of Minneapolis succeeded Dr. Charles H. Hamilton as lecturer in pathology.[51] When Dr. George A. Hendricks came to the University of Minnesota in January 1889, he was at age thirty-eight considered an expert surgeon although he had been an instructor in anatomy at the University of Michigan since 1882. In order that he might devote the time required to teach anatomy properly, the university decided to pay Dr. Hendricks a salary of $1,800 per year, as they did Professor Charles Bell who taught chemistry. Dr. J. Clark Stewart's lectures on histology, pathology, and bacteriology constituted a burden sufficiently heavy that in 1889 the university provided him with a salary of $500. Similarly the professor of physiology, Dr. Richard O. Beard, received a salary of $400 for the lectures and laboratory classes in physiology. Dean Millard, whose

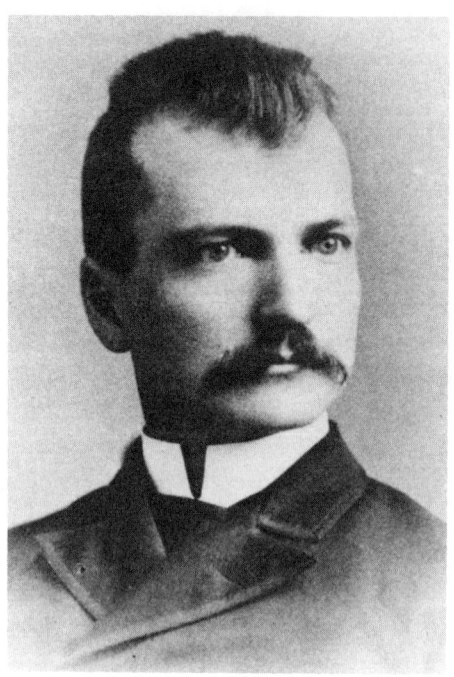

FIGURE 3:5 George A. Hendricks, circa 1889. Courtesy Mn U Archives.

duties in organizing and administering the three colleges of the Department of Medicine and as professor of surgery must have been quite heavy, received in 1889 a salary of $2,000.[52] The rest of the medical faculty remained unpaid.

In 1889 the Department of Medicine obtained additional apparatus, charts, and mannikins to be used in teaching. A new building was urgently needed because the greatly increased number of students in the three colleges was putting ever-greater pressure on the Minnesota Hospital College building. In October 1889 the department assigned the drug storeroom to Professor Charles Bell to use as a chemistry laboratory, Professor J. Clark Stewart took over the chemistry laboratory for his pathology courses, and the dental laboratory moved from the basement to the pathology laboratory—a sequence of changes that appear to have been desperate improvisations.[53] Even the inadequate building at Sixth Street and Ninth Avenue South was committed to the university only for five years, which meant the agreement terminated in 1893. On 1 November 1890 a newly constituted committee on buildings of the Department of Medicine met at the dean's office and decided that two buildings were needed: a laboratory building for teaching the basic subjects of anatomy, chemistry, physiology, and histology; and a clinical building containing a dispensary and infirmary for advanced clinical instruction.

In April 1891, when the Illinois State Board of Health announced their intention henceforth to recognize in Illinois only the diplomas of medical colleges that

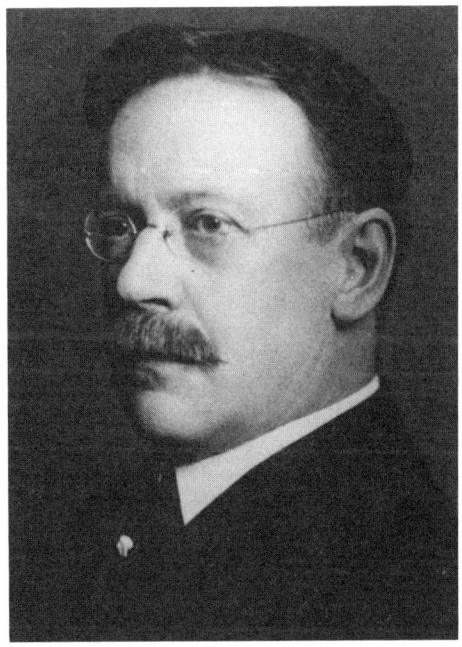

FIGURE 3:6 J. Clark Stewart, 1909. Courtesy Mn U Archives.

required four years of study for the M.D. degree, the faculty resolved that the medical course in both colleges should be increased from three to four years beginning with the class that would enter in the fall of 1891.[54] Their action was confirmed by the Board of Regents on 6 May.[55] Nevertheless, the decision to lengthen the medical course could not be implemented until a new building was obtained because the longer course would create four classes of students to teach instead of three, and more classrooms and laboratories would be needed to accommodate them. The four-year course did not take effect, therefore, until 1895.

On 19 August 1891 a special meeting of the faculty of the Department of Medicine convened in President Northrop's office at 8:30 in the morning. Thirteen members of the faculty were present together with President Northrop and two of the regents, John Sargent Pillsbury and William M. Liggett.[56] The purpose of the meeting was to select a site on the campus for the new medical building, and at the suggestion of the regents the faculty adjourned to the campus. The group walked across the campus that morning in late summer, the grass burnt brown, to select a site for the medical building on the bluff overlooking the gorge of the Mississippi River and the city of Minneapolis on the west bank. When they reconvened in President Northrop's office, the faculty recommended the site to the regents and then moved to have Dean Millard appoint a committee to select books for the library to be housed in the new building.[57]

On 15 September Perry Millard appeared before the regents to present the faculty's recommendation for the site of the new medical building and a set of plans prepared by the architect, Charles A. Reed of St. Paul.[58] Reed's plans called for a rectangular stone and brick building of three stories and a basement in an Italian Renaissance style with a handsome arched portico surrounded by richly ornamental stonework. The regents may have been slightly uneasy about the cost of the proposed building because they accepted Mr. Reed's plans provided that the building could be erected for $55,000. The university had not yet received from the state treasury the money appropriated by the legislature for university buildings so the regents were happy to accept Dr. Millard's offer of an interest-free loan of $20,000 until 1 April 1892 to allow work to begin on the foundation for the building that autumn.[59] Construction proceeded apace. On 2 November the faculty established a committee chaired by Dr. John F. Fulton to plan the dedicatory exercises for the new building. The following May Dr. Fulton announced that Dr. William Osler, professor of medicine at Johns Hopkins University, had agreed to give the dedicatory address, and recommended that the faculty give a reception in honor of the occasion.[60]

In 1891, after the Minnesota legislature appropriated $8,000 for the purpose, the Board of Regents created within the Department of Medicine a fourth college, the College of Pharmacy, to open for instruction in October 1892.[61] In May 1892 the regents appointed Frederick J. Wulling professor of the theory and practice of pharmacy and dean of the new college, which was to be housed initially in the new medical building then under construction.[62]

In 1892 Thomas G. Lee was appointed instructor in histology and bacteriology. Then thirty years old, Dr. Lee had studied medicine at the University of Pennsylvania where during his last two years he served as a student assistant to Professor Joseph Leidy in histology and embryology.[63] From 1888 to the spring of 1892 he taught histology and embryology in the Yale Medical School, and then spent the summer taking special courses at Munich before coming to Minnesota in the autumn. With the appointment of Dr. Lee, Dr. J. Clark Stewart gave up the teaching of histology and bacteriology, restricting himself to pathology.[64] In May 1892 Dr. Lee asked for an additional lecture hour per week throughout the session for the teaching of histology and bacteriology, and proposed that he also be entrusted with the teaching of embryology.[65] The fees for medical students were increased from $35 to $50, perhaps to reflect the more thorough training by a larger number of paid instructors that the students were to begin to receive in the new medical building that autumn.

With construction under way for a medical building on the campus, the owners of the buildings of the former Minnesota Hospital College and St. Paul Medical College decided to dispose of them. The Department of Medicine was then faced with relocating the two university dispensaries hitherto housed in these buildings. After considering tentatively a possible location in the basement of the Riverside Mission in Minneapolis, the faculty decided to locate the dispensary on the university campus in the new medical building.[66] Anxious to get a dispensary in operation, Dean Millard undertook personally to obtain the funds needed to

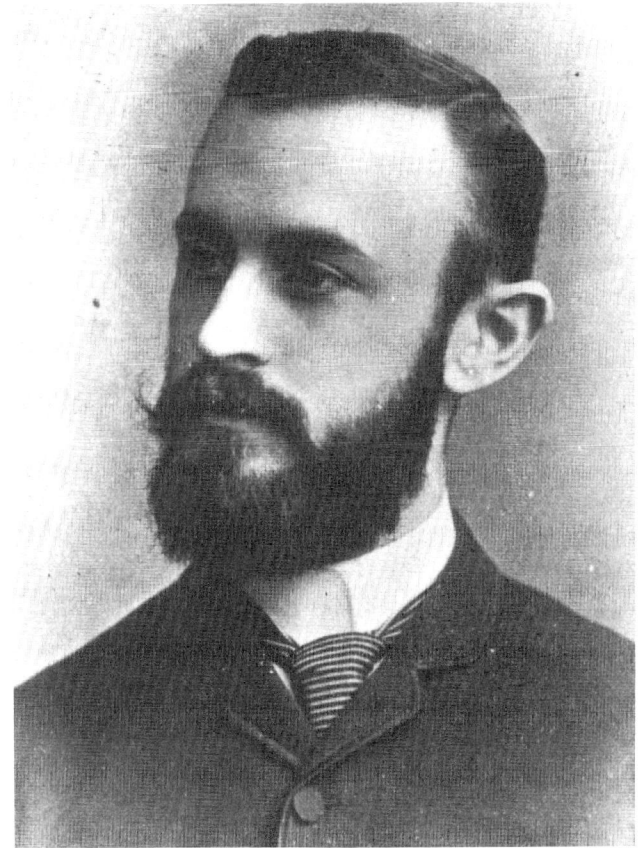

FIGURE 3:7   Thomas G. Lee, circa 1892. Courtesy Mn U Archives.

support the dispensary during its first year. The Board of Regents accepted his offer, but at the same time prohibited the dispensary from providing drugs to patients so that it could offer only outpatient medical and surgical services.[67] The facility would be open at specified hours from Monday to Friday, with days and times posted for clinics in the various specialties. A committee including representatives from both medical colleges of the Department of Medicine nominated a staff for the dispensary.[68]

On 4 October 1892 the new medical building on the university campus was dedicated. The ceremony was held at eight o'clock in the evening in the main lecture room of the medical building, which would accommodate only 500 of the 4,000 persons invited to attend. The room filled early and many were unable to gain entrance. The Reverend Wayland Hoyt, pastor of the First Baptist Church of Minneapolis, opened the proceedings with prayer. Governor William R. Merriam formally presented the building to the university and it was accepted on behalf of the Board of Regents by Regent John S. Pillsbury.[69] President Northrop introduced in succession the deans of the four colleges of the Department of Medicine and each spoke briefly. President Northrop then introduced Professor William Osler who spoke on the subject of medical education under the title "Teacher and Student."[70] Just the year before, Osler had completed the writing of his textbook, *The principles and practice of medicine*. For Osler this was a period of relative leisure at the Johns Hopkins Hospital before the Johns Hopkins medical school would open the following year. In May 1892 Osler married and for their wedding trip the Oslers traveled to Britain, where in July Osler attended the meeting of the British Medical Association at Nottingham. At that meeting Dr. George R. Murray described the successful treatment of patients suffering from myxedema, a condition shown only a few years before to result from thyroid deficiency. Dr. Murray's discovery of the effective use of thyroid gland extract suggested how the clinical and pathological data accumulated by successive generations of physicians might begin to offer effective modes of treatment for disease. It was a hint of the promise inherent in scientific medicine, a promise in which Osler believed deeply.

In his address Osler referred first to the great change that had occurred in medical education during the preceding twenty years, beginning with the reform of the Harvard medical school in 1876, to which he referred obliquely. He emphasized the importance to a medical school of its connection with a university, and said that the responsibility of the university's regents was to select the best possible teachers for the faculty of its medical school. The United States, he suggested, had hitherto neglected its teachers of science. A medical school should have well-equipped laboratories in anatomy, physiology, chemistry (both physiological and pharmacological chemistry), pathology, and hygiene, and such laboratories should be staffed with trained instructors who devoted their full time to teaching and research. In 1892, Osler said, no medical school in the United States possessed such a complement of scientific departments; the best medical schools might have two or three well-organized departments, but none had all.

The instructor in a scientific department must be an investigator as well as a teacher, and in order to be an effective investigator he must keep abreast of research in his field. "To avoid mistakes," Osler said, "he must know what is going on in the laboratories of England, France and Germany, as well as in those of his own country, and he must receive and read six or ten journals devoted to the subject."[71] Osler added with emphasis: "Thoroughly equipped laboratories, in charge of men thoroughly equipped as teachers and investigators, is the most pressing want to-day in the medical schools of this country."[72]

The clinical teachers too, Osler thought, had an obligation "to know and teach the best that is known and taught in the world . . . to teach to their students habits of reliance, and to be to them examples of gentleness, forbearance and courtesy in dealing with their suffering brethren."[73] As he went on, Osler's speech assumed more and more the tone and content of a sermon, embellished with Biblical allusions and moral reflections. The art of preaching came naturally to Osler, the son of a clergyman, and the note of a sermon probably struck a responsive chord in

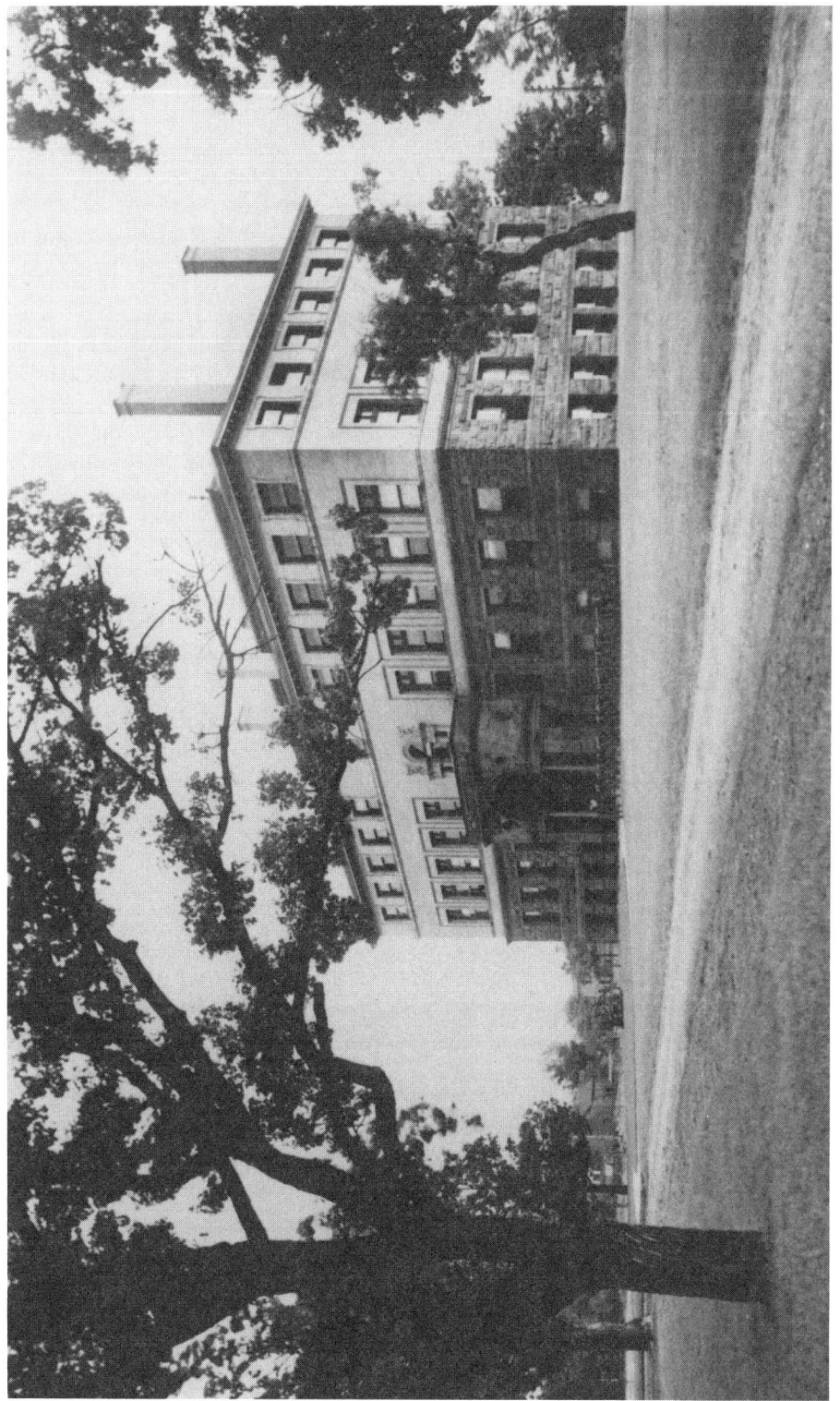

FIGURE 3:8 Medical Hall, 1890s. Courtesy Mn U Archives.

his audience. In 1892 undergraduates at the University of Minnesota attended daily chapel, Sabbath obervance was strict, and most of the students, professors, and ordinary citizens in the audience would be accustomed to attend church. To them it seemed only natural and fitting that Osler should urge the renunciation of pleasure in favor of regular study, and the cultivation of disciplined habits, thoroughness, and humility for the student to become a good physician. While in England during the preceding summer, Osler had attended service at the Norman-aged Gothic cathedral at Lincoln on Sunday, 31 July. That evening in October he recalled the experience:

> Sitting in Lincoln cathedral and gazing at one of the loveliest of human works — for such the angel Choir has been said to be — there arose within me, obliterating for the moment the thousand heraldries and twilight saints and dim emblazonings, a strong sense of reverence for the minds which had conceived and the hands which had executed such things of beauty. What manner of men were they who could in those (to us) dark days, build such transcendent monuments? What was the secret of their art? By what spirit were they moved? Absorbed in thought, I did not hear the beginning of the music and then, as a response to my reverie and arousing me from it, rang out the clear voice of the boy leading the antiphon, "That thy power, thy glory and mightiness of thy kingdom be known unto men." Here was the answer.[74]

Osler thus suggested that the study of medicine and its practice might be a high and holy endeavor. To his Minnesota audience, whose lives were passed amid the frame houses and muddy streets of raw prairie towns, Osler's evocation of the strange, rich beauties of European civilization may have been exhilarating. To the students as they sat in their new medical building of Renaissance design, with its elaborately wrought, decorative stonework, that building, through Osler's dedicatory address, became a symbol of the wealth and promise of the world of medical knowledge they were about to enter. The next day the *Minneapolis Tribune* commented:

> If old Esculapius, god of medicine, still lingers about looking after the welfare of humanity, he must needs have been pleased last night. For over on the State University campus there was being dedicated to him a new temple. In point of architecture and equipment, this new medical building is not to be surpassed, and its dedication marks another stride in the advance of Minnesota's university.[75]

As he returned by train to Baltimore and to the Johns Hopkins Hospital, where there was as yet no medical school, no building for anatomy or the other scientific departments, which he had asserted in Minneapolis were so necessary for medicine, and as yet no money to erect one, Osler may have been slightly envious of the splendid building he had just helped to dedicate. Nevertheless, there were two respects in which Osler was far more fortunate than his Minnesota colleagues, and he knew that he was. When the Johns Hopkins Medical School opened a year later, in October 1893, it was located next to the Johns Hopkins Hospital where Osler was chief of the medical staff and could use the wards fully for clinical teaching. By contrast the new medical building on the campus of the University of Minnesota was more than a mile and a half distant from the nearest hospitals across the Mississippi River in Minneapolis, and the university did not possess control over the wards of any hospital in the Twin Cities to guarantee their right of access for clinical teaching or clinical investigation.

In September 1892 the Board of Regents addressed a memorial to the mayor, Common Council, and Board of Charities of the city of Minneapolis to urge that the new public hospital then being planned for Minneapolis should be located in close proximity to the university so that the medical faculty could use it for clinical teaching.[76] Nevertheless, when a new Minneapolis City Hospital was built it was located on Sixth Street and Portland Avenue, close to the original site of the medical school and about two miles from the medical building on the university campus.

In 1892 at Johns Hopkins, graduate study and research were already well established, especially in pathology under William Henry Welch. Medical research and graduate study still lay in the future at the University of Minnesota.

NOTES

1. Board of Regents, Minutes, 1868–87 (14 June 1886), p. 282.

2. Perry Millard was regarded both as "the author and inspirer of the laws which have governed the practice of medicine in the State . . . " and as the man in whose " . . . brain . . . this institution, which has taken rank among the foremost professional schools of America, first took shape." *J. Am. med. Ass.*, 1897, *28*, 327.

3. "An act to regulate the practice of medicine in Minnesota," Ch. 125, Sec. 2, *Minnesota General Laws*, 1883, *23*, 167–169.

4. Ibid., Sec. 3. A license tax of one dollar was imposed upon those presenting genuine and approved diplomas. The board was entitled to exact a fine of twenty dollars from those submitting fraudulent diplomas, but the means of collection were unspecified. Penalties for violation of the 1883 act were rather stiff (Ibid., Sec. 12). A first offense could result in fines ranging from $50 to $500 or imprisonment from 30 to 365 days for each offense. Those submitting fraudulent diplomas were subject to prosecution for the felony of forgery.

5. "Board of Medical Examiners," Title 24, *Minnesota General Statutes*, 1, (St. Paul, 1891), 192–195.

6. Perry H. Millard, "A plea for efficient legislation regarding medical practice," *Bull. Am. Acad. Med.*, 1895, *2*, 100–110, p. 103. In the last decade of his life Millard lectured and wrote extensively on the reform of medical education by statute.

7. Richard H. Shryock, *Medical licensing in America, 1650–1965*, pp. 43–76.

8. Ibid., p. 104.

9. It was to encompass the disciplines of anatomy, physiology, chemistry, histology, materia medica, therapeutics, preventive medicine, practice of medicine, surgery, obstetrics, diseases of women and children, diseases of the nervous system, diseases of the eye and ear, medical jurisprudence and, in concert with the development of scientific medicine, " . . . such other branches as the board shall deem advisable." See "A bill to regulate the practice of medicine in the state of Minnesota, to license physicians and surgeons, and to punish persons violating the provisions of this Act," *Northwest. Lancet*, 1886–87, *6*, 201–203, p. 201.

10. At the meeting with the regents on 7 April 1887, Dr. Perry Millard submitted a written report pleading the present wisdom of establishing at the university a high grade medical teaching institution. A search for this document or a copy of it has been unsuccessful. University of Minnesota, *Catalogue, Academic year 1887-88*, pp. 93–111, p. 93.

11. Philip Jordan, *The people's health: a history of public health in Minnesota to 1948*, pp. 62–65.

12. Hewitt to Northrop, 22 May 1886. In his account of Hewitt's involvement in the plans for the reorganization of the medical school, Philip Jordan cites and quotes from letters in the Folwell papers held by the Minnesota State Historical Society. Those papers have since been reorganized and the cited letters are found neither in the boxes Jordan lists, nor in their proper places among the chronologically arranged correspondence.

13. Jordan, *People's health* (n. 11), p. 64.

14. Ibid., p. 65.

15. Millard (n. 6), p. 108.

16. Board of Regents, Minutes, 1888 - 1905 (28 January 1888), p. 303.

17. Ibid. (6 March 1888), p. 308.

18. The Millards lived first at 145 Nina and then at 530 Holly Avenue. Dr. Millard took office space at 326 Wabasha in downtown St. Paul on the site of the present Commerce Building, where he maintained a practice throughout the period of his deanship. Howard A. Kelly and Walter L. Burrage, eds., *American medical biographies* (1920), s.v. "Millard, Perry H.," by Burnside Foster; *Stillwater Gazette,* 1872-87, 1, 5 February 1897, 25 June 1926, 8 June 1936, 6 March 1961; *Stillwater Messenger,* 1872-87, 6 February 1897; *Minneapolis Journal,* 1 February 1897; *St. Paul Pioneer Press,* 2, 5, 8 February 1897; *Washington County Journal,* 5 February 1897; *St. Paul Dispatch,* 1 June 1936; Ramsey County (Minn.) Probate Court, No. 8706, "Millard, Perry H.," will and inventory of estate; Perry H. Millard (grandson), Hazelcrest, Illinois, telephone conversation and family papers.

19. Cyrus Northrop, "Reminiscences", *Minn. Alumni Wkly,* 1919, *19* (no. 13), 23–36, pp. 32–33.

20. *Catalogue* (n. 10), pp. 93–111.

21. Board of Regents, Minutes, 1888 - 1905 (26 April 1888), pp. 311–326.

22. Ibid., Appendix I. First Faculty of the Department of Medicine, University of Minnesota.

23. Ibid. (26 April 1888), p. 325.

24. Ibid. (14 May 1888), p. 328.

25. Ibid., Appendix I.

26. Department of Medicine, Record book, 1888-95 (14 May 1888), p.9

27. The hospitals included St. Joseph's Hospital, St. Luke's Hospital, the City Hospital and the Homeopathic Hospital in St. Paul, and St. Barnabas' Hospital, St. Mary's Hospital, the City Hospital and the Homeopathic Hospital in Minneapolis. College of Medicine and Surgery, Record book, 1888-96 (8 June 1888), pp. 31–38.

28. *Catalogue, 1887-88* (n. 10) pp. 93–111.

First Year Course

College of Medicine and Surgery	College of Homeopathic Medicine and Surgery
Anatomy	Anatomy
Physiology	Physiology
Chemistry	Chemistry
Materia Medica	Materia Medica (homeopathic)
Histology	
Laboratory Work	

29. Ibid., p. 102.
30. Ibid., pp. 93–111.

Second Year Course

College of Medicine and Surgery	College of Homeopathic Medicine and Surgery
Pathology	
Physical Diagnosis	Physical Diagnosis
Hygiene	
Theory and Practice	Theory and Practice
Surgery	Surgery
Clinical Medicine	Clinical Medicine
Obstetrics	Obstetrics
Gynecology	Gynecology
Diseases of Children	Paedology
Clinical Instruction	

Third Year Course

College of Medicine and Surgery	College of Homeopathic Medicine and Surgery
Neurology	
Electro Therapy	
Ophthalmmology	Ophthalmology
Otology	Otology
Dermatology	Dermatology and Venereal Diseases
Genito-Uriniary Diseases	
Laryngology	
Orthopaedia	
	Mental and Nervous Disorders
	Medical Jurisprudence
Clinical instruction in all branches	Opportunity to attend outdoor patients, to assist in surgical operations and to attend at least one obstetrical case.

31. Ibid., p. 106.
32. University of Minnesota, *Catalogue, Academic year 1889–90*, p. 116.
33. Board of Regents, Minutes, 1888 - 1905 (20 November 1888), p. 334.
34. Ibid.
35. For a comprehensive discussion of the relationship between homeopathic and regular physicians during the nineteenth century, see Martin Kaufman, *Homeopathy in America, the rise and fall of a medical heresy*. The so-called "consultation clause" of the American Medical Association is discussed in Chapter 4, pp. 48–62.
36. Samuel Hahnemann, *Organon of homeopathic medicine*.
37. Kaufman, *Homeopathy* (n.35), pp. 23–27.
38. Oliver Wendell Holmes, *Homeopathy and its kindred delusions*.
39. For a thorough treatment of the history of homeopathic physicians and their professional organizations in Minnesota, see James Eckman, "Homeopathic and eclectic medicine in Minnesota," *Minn. Med.*, 1931, *24,* 474–479, 567–572, 667–674, 762–769, 863–873, 967–971, 1073–1077.
40. Ibid., p. 567. "Proceedings of the twenty-seventh annual meeting of the Minnesota State Medical Society," *Trans. Minn. St. med. Soc.*, 1895.
41. George H. Hawes, "Annual address of the president," *Trans. Minn. St. homeo. Inst.*, 1882, 1883, 1884. The transactions of the Minnesota State Homeopathic Institute

for the years 1882, 1883, and 1884 were bound as a single volume without date or place of issuance, and consisted of reprints from the *Medical Counselor* of Chicago.

42. Eckman (n.39), p. 479.

43. Henry C. Aldrich, "Homeopathy in Minnesota," in Isaac Atwater, ed., *History of Minneapolis, Minnesota,* II, 916–934, p. 933.

44. William D. Washburn, president of the Minneapolis and St. Louis Railroad Company and a United States senator for Minnesota supported homeopathy and its institutions in Minneapolis. Washburn served as president of the board of trustees of the Minnesota Homeopathic College at it organization in 1886 and, together with Frederick C. Pillsbury, miller and president of the Minneapolis, Lyndale, and Minnetonka Railway Company, served on the board of directors of the Minneapolis Homeopathic Hospital Association. Thomas Lowry, founder of the Twin City Rapid Transit Company, and Charles M. Loring, long-time president of the Minneapolis Board of Park Commissioners, contributed financially toward the erection of an annex to the Minneapolis Homeopathic Hospital at Twenty-fifth Street South and Clinton Avenue. Eckman (n.39), p. 667.

45. When in the spring of 1887, a proposal was made to build a homeopathic hospital in St. Paul, former state Governor William R. Marshall was elected to the board of directors of the projected institution, as was future Governor William R. Merriam. Incorporators of the hospital included such prominent men as Senator Cushman K. Davis; former state governor, senator, and secretary of war, Alexander Ramsey; James J. Hill, creator of the Great Northern Railroad; Congressman Edmund Rice, president of the St. Paul and Pacific Railroad Company; and Charles E. Flandrau, former associate justice of the Supreme Court of Minnesota. Ibid., p. 667.

46. Ibid., p. 671 and Eugene L. Mann, "College of Homeopathic Medicine and Surgery," in E. Bird Johnson, ed., *Forty years of the University of Minnesota,* pp. 165–170.

47. Ibid., p. 167.

48. Statement by Dr. R. D. Matchan, Chairman, Legislative Committee, 1909, "Why the homeopathic people of Minnesota demand a college at the university," p. 5. Mann papers.

49. Eckman (n.39), p. 671.

50. In 1900 the faculty of the college submitted a report on their work to the Minnesota State Institute of Homeopathy. The report documented the college's efforts to keep pace both with the increasingly demanding standards for qualifications among regular practitioners and the steady increase in scientific knowlege. A. P. Williamson, *Report of the College of Homeopathic Medicine and Surgery of the University of Minnesota, 1900.* Mann papers.

51. Board of Regents, Minutes, 1888–1905 (3 May 1889), p. 345.

52. Ibid. (1 June 1889), p. 348.

53. Department of Medicine, Record book, 1888–95 (8 October 1889), p. 51.

54. College of Medicine and Surgery, Record book, 1888–96 (10 April 1891), p. 119.

55. Board of Regents, Minutes, 1888–1905 (6 May 1891), p. 373.

56. William M. Liggett (1846–1909), a native of Ohio, was dean of the State Agricultural School and Experiment School. He was a member of the Board of Regents from 1888 to 1905.

57. College of Medicine and Surgery, Record book, 1888–96 (19 August 1891), p. 147.

58. The St. Paul architectural firm of Charles A. Reed (1858–1911) and Allen H. Stem (1856–1931) later designed the Saint Paul Hotel, Saint Paul Auditorium, and Metropolitan Opera House in St. Paul, and the Grand Central Terminal in New York City.

59. Board of Regents, Minutes, 1888–1905 (15 September 1891), p. 379.

60. College of Medicine and Surgery, Record book, 1888–96 (28 May 1892), p. 161.

61. Board of Regents, Minutes, 1888–1905 (8 December 1891), p. 381.

62. Ibid. (3 May 1892), p. 388.
63. C. M. Jackson, "Thomas George Lee," *Anat. Anz.*, 1933, *76*, 348–349.
64. Board of Regents, Minutes, 1888–1905 (3 May 1892), pp. 384–385.
65. College of Medicine and Surgery, Record book, 1888–96 (28 May 1892), p. 162.
66. Department of Medicine, Record Book, 1888–95 (2 August 1892), p. 107.
67. Ibid. (23 August 1892), p. 109.
68. Ibid. (22 September 1892), pp. 115, 119.
69. The occasion is described in some detail in James Eckman, "Osler in Minnesota, his interest in medical education licensure," *Minn. Med.*, 1948, *31*, 776–787, p. 777.
70. William Osler, "Teacher and student," in Osler, *Aequanimitas with other addresses* . . . , pp. 21–43.
71. Ibid., p. 31.
72. Ibid., pp. 31–32.
73. Ibid., pp. 31–32.
74. Ibid., pp. 41–44.
75. *Minneapolis Tribune*, 5 October 1892, p. 5. The *Tribune* described Osler's speech as "a masterly address." Harvey Cushing regarded it as one of Osler's most effective addresses. See Harvey Cushing, *The life of Sir William Osler*, I, 366.
76. Board of Regents, Minutes, 1888–1905 (20 September 1892), p. 405.

CHAPTER 4

The Early Years of the School on the University Campus 1893–1897

The Department of Medicine was growing so vigorously that even while the new medical building existed only as a set of architect's plans, it was seen to provide insufficient space. At their meeting of 8 December 1891 after the plans for the new building had been approved and its foundation was being laid, the Board of Regents approved the erection of a second building to be used as a laboratory for teaching chemistry and histology. The construction of such a laboratory was to be "at a cost not to exceed $4,500," and although the Medical Chemistry Building that ultimately took shape alongside Medical Hall cost more than that amount, the original limit placed on its cost may have accounted for its peculiar plan and appearance. At the west end was a small two-story hip-roofed brick block, possibly all that was contemplated because of budget consideration. It contained on the first floor a room for preparing chemical reagents and distilled water and on the second floor an office and private laboratory for Charles Bell, the professor of chemistry, and a storeroom. Extending east from behind the two-story portion was a long, low one-story building, the first part of which formed the student chemistry laboratory while the further portion contained four rooms, three for histology and embryology and one for bacteriology, presided over by Professor Thomas G. Lee. The unusual shape and appearance of the building was reflected in its nickname, "the Bowling Alley." The east end, housing histology, embryology, and bacteriology, may have been an afterthought to provide accommodation for the laboratory work of Professor Lee after his arrival at the university in the fall of 1892. The building was ultimately completed at a cost of $6,500. The student laboratory for histology, embryology, and bacteriology was lighted by large windows on the north and east and was well adapted for microscopic work using natural light. The catalogue for 1893–94 enumerated its equipment proudly:

> The students' work tables are of oak and placed immediately beneath the windows. The laboratory is well equipped with Leitz and Bausch and Lomb microscopes, Thoma, Minot freezing and other microtomes, water baths, incubators, special forms of glass-

ware, apparatus for injection, the reconstruction from sections of models in wax and other materials . . . .[1]

No longer did medical students have to provide themselves with their own microscopes in order to examine smears or sections of tissues. Professor Lee had his own study and laboratory in which he kept "a large and comprehensive library" of works on histology and embryology, and "one of the richest and most extensive collections of serial sections and vertebrate embryos in the country."[2] Adjoining the general student laboratory were two rooms, one used as a research laboratory and preparation room for histology and embryology; the other equipped with sterilizers, special glassware, and various apparatus for bacteriological work.

In these bright rooms with their polished oak tables, gleaming brass microscopes, and sparkling glassware, Thomas G. Lee began in the fall of 1893 to initiate Minnesota students into the practical details of preparing sections of tissues and examining them under the microscope. Lee's own interest was in the placentation of the ovum in rodents, and that autumn he got one of the freshman medical students, Louis B. Wilson, to shoot gophers for him. Under Professor Lee's direction, Wilson studied the embryology of kidney tissues, thereby launching him on a career of research.[3] In February 1894 when Lee began to teach bacteriology to the junior class, the students reported that the course was "far more comprehensive than heretofore."[4] For the first time medical students were introduced to the techniques of staining and identifying pathogenic bacteria.

In contrast to Professor Lee, who could devote his full time to teaching and research, Professor Richard O. Beard lectured on physiology only as a part-time activity, earning most of his income by medical practice. He had set up a laboratory of sorts on the second floor of Medical Hall for the purpose of preparing physiological demonstrations to accompany his lectures in the adjoining amphitheater. Nevertheless, in the autumn of 1893, with new equipment and the additional facilities of the Medical Chemistry Building, Professor Beard gave the second-year medical students a three-hour laboratory class in physiological chemistry in the general chemical laboratory of the Medical Chemistry Building. On 17 February the *Ariel,* a student weekly, reported that the laboratory work in physiological chemistry provided analysis of the various constituents of the body, including the digestive fluids and their action on various food substances.[5]

Yet not all was work. Dean Millard gave the freshman class permission to hold a party in Medical Hall on Friday, 9 February. The North Star Quartette and the Criterion Mandolin Club provided music, and there was a literary and music program in addition to dancing. Every freshman was urged to attend with a lady, and a majority did. The North Star Quartette sang several songs, Professor Hendricks presented a humorous skit on the "Origin of Genus, Freshman Medic." Miss Nellie Lake sang a solo; Miss Zoa Hotchkiss provided a reading. Finally Mrs. August Hamilton played Chopin's Polonaise No. 8 on the piano, and the Criterion Mandolin Club played the "Sleigh Ride Polka." The party then moved to the dental operating room for dancing. During the dancing the lights went out, leaving the

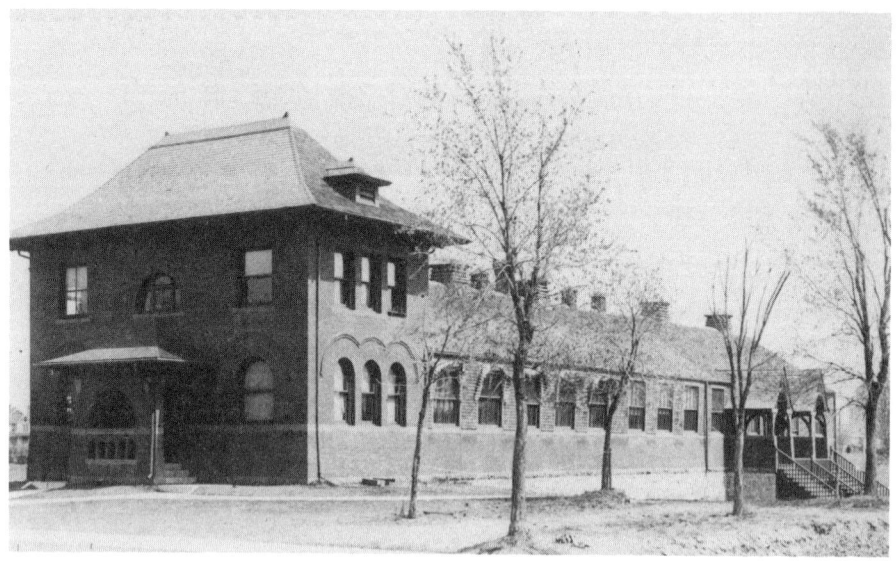

FIGURE 4:1 Medical Chemistry Building ("the Bowling Alley"), early 1890s. Courtesy Mn U Archives.

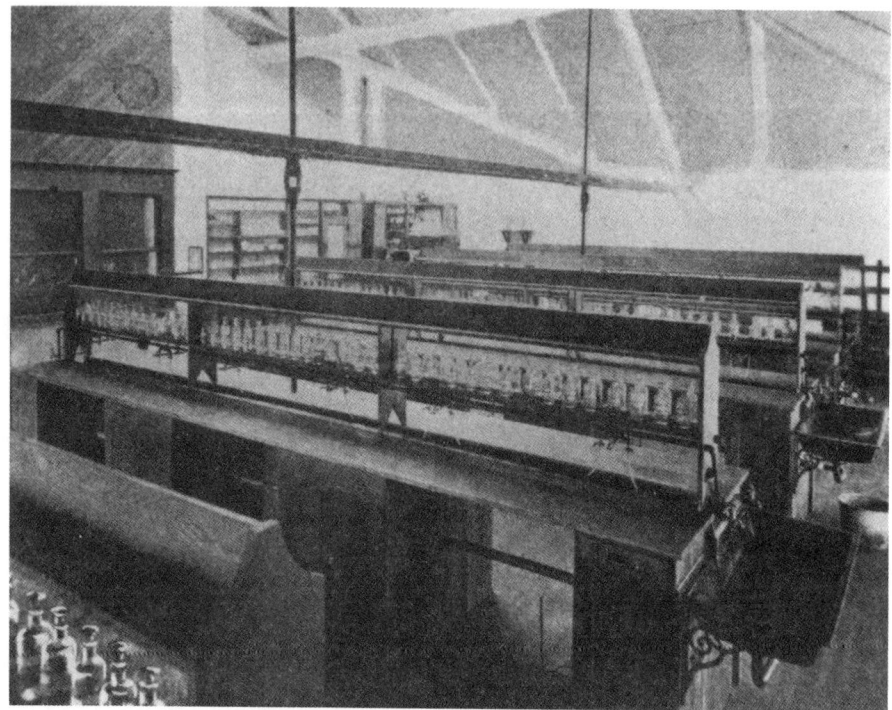

FIGURE 4:2 Chemistry laboratory, 1890s. Courtesy Mn U Archives.

party in complete darkness for thirty minutes—an emergency blamed on members of the junior class. The *Ariel* pronounced the party "a most decided success," and added, "Social gatherings of this nature should be more frequent in our department."[6] Diversions such as this party were most welcome during the latter months of a long Minnesota winter. A week later the *Ariel* reported that many medical students had attended a reception given by the university Y.W.C.A. and Y.M.C.A. "Just such gatherings as this," the reporter commented, "afford an opportunity for the students of the different departments to meet one another and break down any imaginary barrier which may exist between them."[7]

In December 1893 the faculty of the College of Medicine and Surgery recommended that the medical course be extended from three to four years and the Board of Regents approved the extension to four years, beginning with the class of 1895.[8] In June 1894 Dr. Charles A. Wheaton, deciding that he could no longer deliver the lectures on surgery, resigned from the didactic part of the chair and Perry Millard was appointed professor of the principles and practice of surgery.[9] Dr. Wheaton's resignation may have reflected the growing burdens imposed by the extension of the medical course from three to four years and the consequent need to teach larger numbers of students over longer periods of time. The increasing numbers of students and the longer course also placed increasing strain on the facilities of the new buildings.

At the ceremony opening the academic year of the Department of Medicine on Tuesday, 9 October 1894, Dr. J. Clark Stewart, professor of pathology, delivered the inaugural lecture on the history of pathology and its significance for modern medicine. He concluded by saying that he welcomed the extension of the medical course to four years because it would permit more time for the study of pathology, but he also noted that "our laboratory is too meager for the demands of all."[10] John Sargent Pillsbury, president of the Board of Regents and former governor of the state, followed Dr. Stewart on the podium. He remarked that when the medical building was designed, the regents had planned for 250 students. The enrollment had grown beyond the capacity of the building and the medical school needed to be enlarged in every respect. Mr. Pillsbury promised his aid and asked the alumni to use their influence to obtain the necessary medical appropriations from the state legislature.[11]

On 21 December 1894 a committee representing both the faculty of the Department of Medicine and the State Board of Health appeared before the Board of Regents to propose the construction of a new building to be known as the Laboratory of Hygiene to be used both for medical teaching and for the laboratories of the State Board of Health. In support of the proposal, the regents included $50,000 for the laboratory in their request to the Minnesota legislature. At the same meeting the regents decided to create a new position for a professor or instructor in bacteriology, and appointed a faculty search committee. J. Clark Stewart, who had delivered the lectures on bacteriology until Thomas Lee's arrival in 1892, appears to have acted as chairman of the committee, and corresponded with candidates for the position.

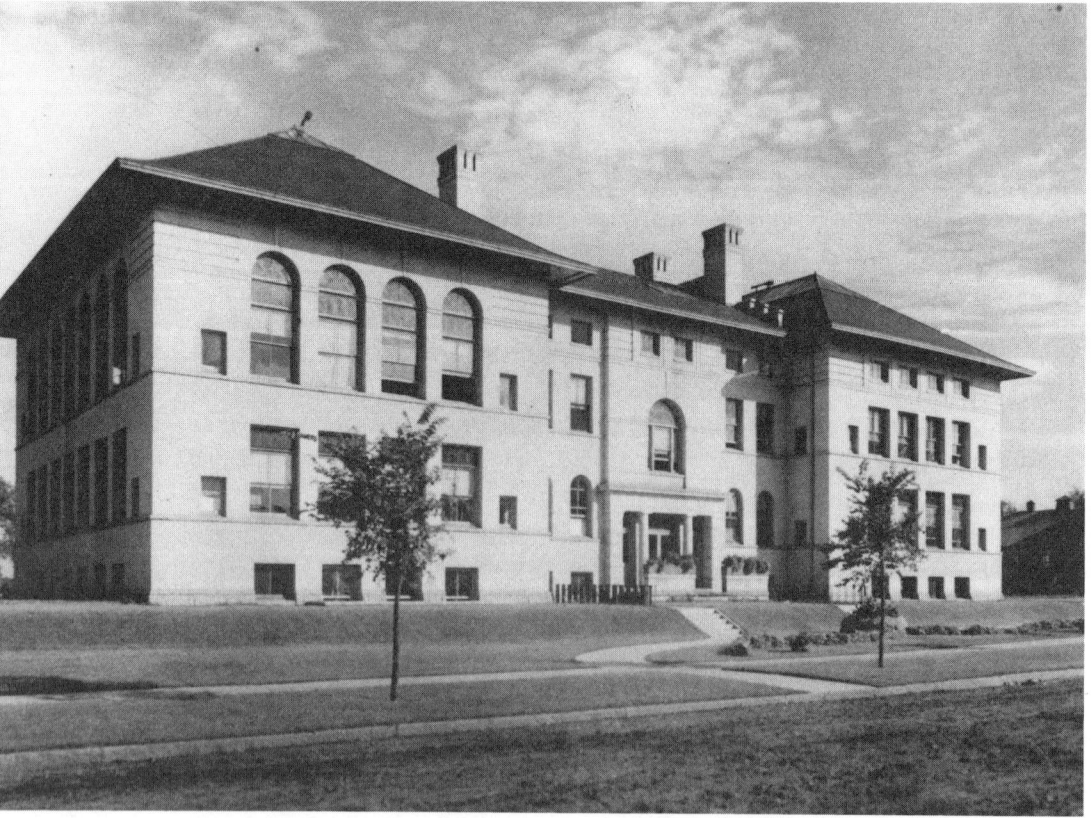

FIGURE 4:3 Laboratory of Medical Sciences, 1896. Medical Chemistry Building in background. Courtesy Mn U Archives.

In the spring of 1895 the Minnesota legislature appropriated $40,000 for the building of a new laboratory for pathology, bacteriology, histology, and embryology.[12] On 1 May the Board of Regents approved plans for the new building proposed by architect F. G. Corser.[13] Corser's plans called for an H-shaped approximately rectangular building of three stories set on a high basement. The outer walls would be of light, cream-colored brick, while the interior framework of heavy wood timbers was so designed as to be slow-burning in case of fire.[14] Half of the south pavilion, intended for the College of Pharmacy, possessed a separate entry and was separated by a fire wall from the rest of the building. The remainder of the building would contain a large amphitheater and laboratories for histology and embryology, pathology and bacteriology, and physiology. On the third floor were to be photographic laboratories and a pathological museum. On the second floor a large laboratory was intended for the bacteriological work of the State Board of Health. The basic plan as presented by the architect was accepted and construction began in June 1895. The building was finished and ready for use as the Laboratory of Medical Sciences by November 1895.[15]

Meanwhile, J. Clark Stewart's committee proceeded with its work to nominate an instructor in bacteriology. Toward the end of May 1895 Dr. Stewart received a letter of inquiry about the position from a young Canadian doctor, Frank F. Wesbrook, who was studying and doing research at Cambridge University in England.[16] As the recipient of the John Lucas Walker Studentship in pathology at Cambridge, Wesbrook was among a group of active young investigators working under Professor Charles S. Roy. The demonstrators in pathology included George Adami, Humphry Davy Rolleston, and Almroth Wright, all of whom later became famous. Charles Sherrington, the founder of modern neurophysiology, was also working in the laboratory. After initial collaboration with other investigators, Wesbrook in 1894 published a study of the toxins produced by the cholera bacillus using cultures of that organism obtained from Walldemar Haffkine at the Pasteur Institute in Paris.[17] At Cambridge in 1895 he studied the effects of sunlight on tetanus and cholera bacilli, showing that both kinds of bacilli were killed by sunlight only in the presence of oxygen.[18] He showed also that the cholera bacillus was much more virulent when grown under aerobic than under anaerobic conditions.[19] He also taught bacteriology to Cambridge undergraduates.

When in May 1895 Wesbrook learned of the opening for an instructor in bacteriology at the University of Minnesota, only a week remained until the deadline for receipt of applications. He wrote immediately, uncertain whether his application would arrive in time to be considered. The committee at Minnesota did consider his application together with some twenty others. Some of the applicants had strong credentials, such as an assistant to Harold Ernst at Harvard University, and an assistant to Alexander C. Abbott at the University of Pennsylvania. The committee's interest in Wesbrook was sufficient that they asked Dr. Henry M. Bracken, who was not a member of the committee, to write to London to make inquiries about him. In mid-June Bracken's letter was sent on by his London acquaintance to Arthur E. Shipley, Fellow of Christ's College, Cambridge and lecturer in invertebrate zoology in Cambridge University. Bracken stipulated that the man to be appointed must be "not only a scholar, but also a good teacher."[20] Shipley replied to Bracken's inquiry in glowing terms about Wesbrook's abilities as a teacher and investigator. Shipley's letter, together with the recommendations of Professor Roy and perhaps others, persuaded the committee that Wesbrook should be their choice. They may have recalled William Osler's exhortation in his dedicatory address in 1892 to appoint the best men wherever they might be found, and Perry Millard's eight months spent at London in Guy's Hospital and two months at Vienna in 1880–81 may have made him value Wesbrook's European scientific training. At Cambridge, Wesbrook was in the most active center of research in the medical and biological sciences in England. In July J. Clark Stewart wrote to Wesbrook to say that they had decided to offer him a full professorship of bacteriology with adjunct in pathology.[21]

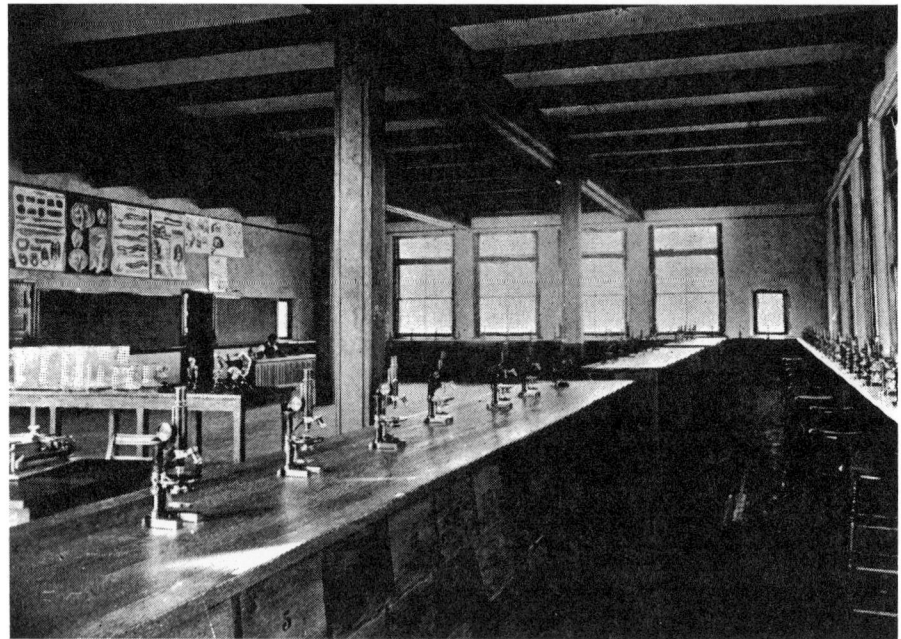

FIGURE 4:4 Histology and Embryology Laboratory in the Laboratory of Medical Sciences, 1896. Courtesy Mn U Archives.

In October 1895 Frank Wesbrook arrived in Minneapolis to find the new Laboratory of Medical Sciences with its splendid facilities for bacteriology, histology, pathology, and physiology, to be ready for occupancy within a few weeks. During the summer Professor Lee had spent the whole of his vacation in superintending the work, in overcoming delays, and in ordering and installing equipment. Despite his efforts the faculty was not able to hold classes in the new building until the beginning of the winter term on 1 January 1896. Professor Hendricks then took over Professor Beard's physiological laboratory in Medical Hall, and Professor Bell had the whole of "the Bowling Alley" for medical chemistry.

The freshman students entering the medical school in October 1895 were required to take a four-year course for the M.D. degree, which meant that they would study histology and embryology for two years instead of one and would also have a more thorough course in bacteriology with extensive laboratory work. The new building provided the room needed to accommodate all classes. The extension of the medical course to four years caused a slight drop in the number of entering students, but the faculty hoped that the school would attract better students.[22]

As the fall term of 1895 went on, the medical students at Minnesota began to realize that they possessed unusual advantages. In November the *Ariel* observed:

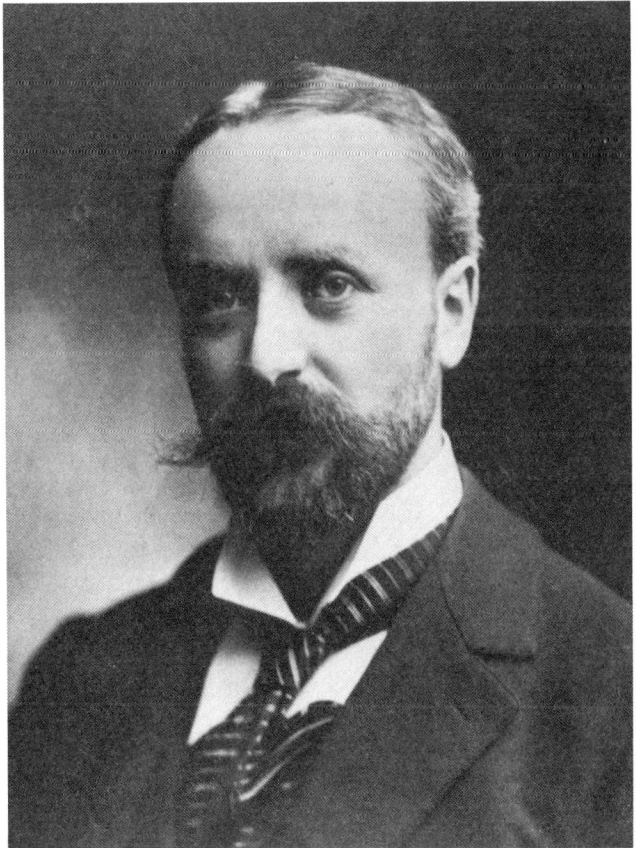

FIGURE 4:5   Frank F. Wesbrook, circa 1896. Courtesy Mn U Archives.

> The abundant and carefully planned demonstrations used by the primary chairs in illustrating their lectures make a visual and lasting impression on the student as nothing else can, and have incidentally raised our college in these branches abreast with the best in the land. In fact, after a careful examination of the different catalogues, we find that in anatomy and histology at least, we easily lead, both in amount and thoroughness of work required.[23]

Professor Lee began to use large charts, carefully prepared by his assistant, to illustrate the structure of typical animals and in particular the embryological development and structure of the human body. "Besides the large series of charts (constantly being increased)," the *Ariel* noted, "material in bulk and section will be used frequently as demonstrations during the lecture hour. Thus the student will get the full benefit of a large and valuable collection of Prof. Lee, which hitherto, on account of the cramped room, it has been impossible to use."[24]

Following his arrival at Minnesota in October 1895, Frank Wesbrook was occupied for several months in ordering equipment and setting up the bacteriology

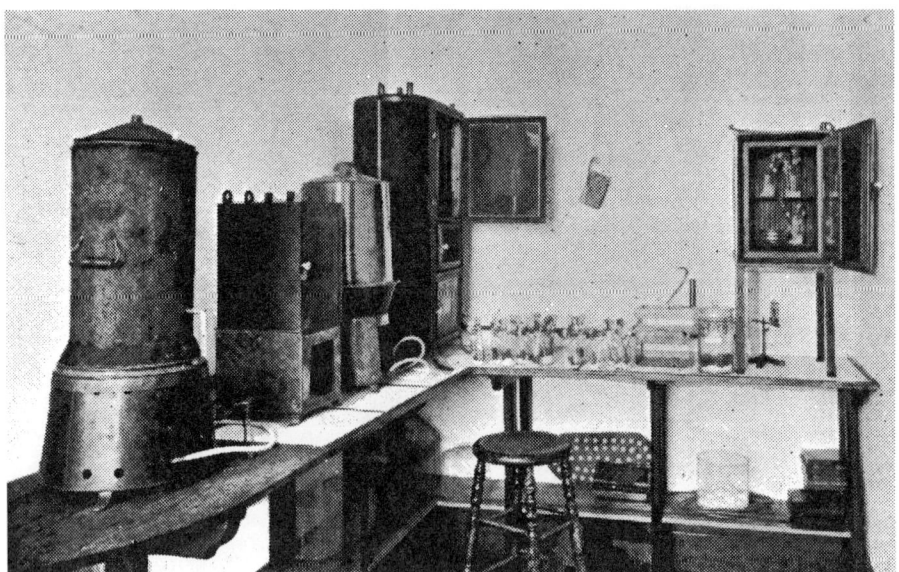

FIGURE 4:6 Bacteriology culture room in the Laboratory of Medical Sciences, 1896. Courtesy Mn U Archives.

laboratory. During the spring of 1896 he began to offer the medical students a much enlarged course in bacteriology. In January 1896 Frank Wesbrook assumed another responsibility in addition to his duties as professor of pathology and bacteriology in the medical school. The State Board of Health appointed him to be their bacteriologist and director of the bacteriological laboratory to begin in April at a salary of $100 per month.

From the time that Perry Millard was appointed to the State Board of Health in 1888, shortly after the founding of the medical school and his appointment as dean, he agitated to have the office of the board moved to St. Paul, the seat of state government. Dr. Charles N. Hewitt, as secretary of the State Board of Health, preferred his home town of Red Wing. After 1888 Dr. Hewitt was also professor of sanitary science at the university. He was given rooms on the top floor of the Mechanic Arts building for a laboratory and the State Board of Health provided two assistants, one in chemistry and one in bacteriology. After 1888 Hewitt was not a member of the medical faculty, and carried on his public health work quite separately from the medical school.[25] Over the years Dean Millard was both patient and persistent in recommending changes in the management of the State Board of Health. At a meeting of the board on 8 January 1895, speaking as dean of the medical school, Millard explained that the university wished to increase its facilities for laboratory teaching in medicine and asked the board to cooperate. The board agreed to support the university in its request.[26] When the Minnesota legislature passed an appropriation for the new laboratory building in the spring of 1895, the building was given entirely to the university, but the Board

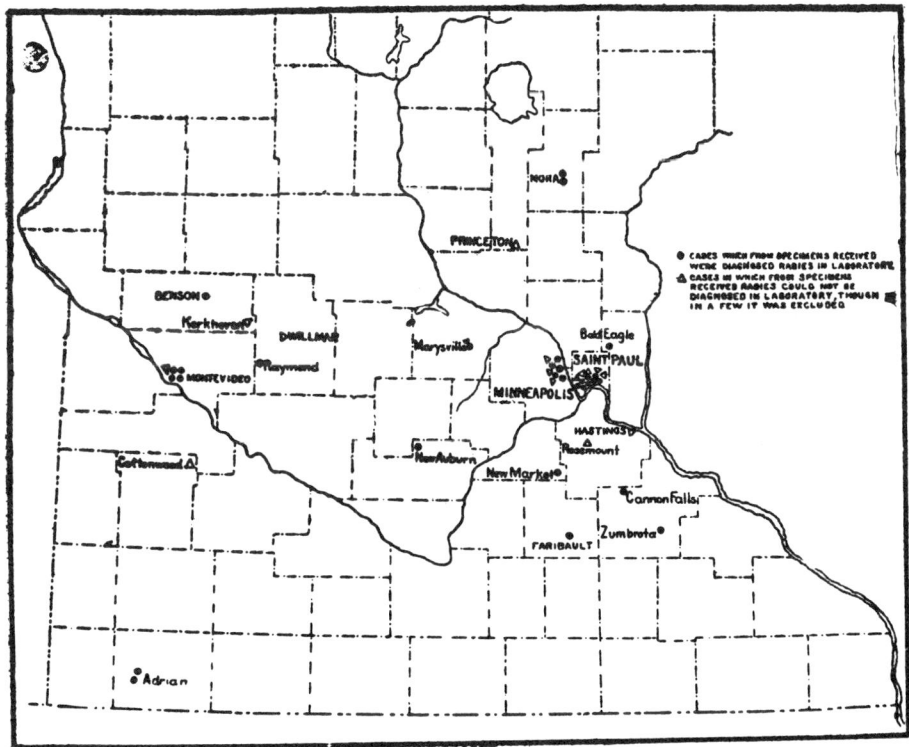

FIGURE 4:7 Distribution of Rabies in Minnesota, 1897–1900 (Wesbrook and Wilson, 1900).

of Regents set aside space within the new building for the laboratories of the State Board of Health. Dean Millard's patience was rewarded. With a minimum of dissension he had both acquired new laboratories for the medical school and had brought the laboratories of the State Board of Health in proximity to those of the medical school, a conjunction that over the years would prove very productive. Millard also obtained in the person of Frank Wesbrook an exceptional bacteriologist to direct the work of both laboratories.

Rabies

When Frank Wesbrook took over the laboratory of the State Board of Health in April 1896, the board offered him no guidance as to what the laboratory was supposed to do, so he decided to do whatever came to hand.[27] Anticipating that he would need assistants, Wesbrook hired Louis B. Wilson on Wilson's graduation in June from the medical school, and began to teach him the methods of bacteriology. He also hired Orianna McDaniel who had just received her M.D. degree from the University of Michigan where she studied bacteriology under Victor Vaughan. During the fall of 1896 the accurate diagnosis of rabies arose as an urgent public health problem because rabies appeared to be prevalent among dogs in St. Paul. During the previous two years six persons in St. Paul had died of rabies, contracted from the bites of stray dogs.[28] In a particularly terrible incident in a poor area of St. Paul in August 1896, a shepherd dog attacked three young children, two of whom died of rabies while the third child was sent to Chicago for Pasteur immunization.[29] Dr. John L. Rothrock, assistant health commissioner for St. Paul, asked Wesbrook to perform the laboratory diagnoses of rabies for the city. The heads of suspect dogs were sent to the laboratory where Wesbrook and Wilson prepared an emulsion from the brain or spinal cord in sterile saline solution for inoculation into the brains of rabbits under aseptic conditions. In the course of the first year they received brain or spinal cord material from twenty different sources. Sixteen proved positive for rabies. The high proportion of positive results was particularly striking because rabies had been thought to be a rare disease in the United States and especially in Minnesota. Wesbrook and Wilson found that the incubation period for rabies in the inoculated rabbits varied widely; they recorded incubation periods as short as 8 days and as long as 107 days.[30] For each case of suspected rabies examined, they inoculated from two to twenty-one rabbits, so that their report of twenty cases represented a large volume of work.[31]

In October 1897 Wesbrook and Wilson confirmed a diagnosis of rabies in a horse which had developed symptoms of the disease three or four months after it had been bitten by a stray dog.[32] From January to March 1898 they diagnosed rabies in two dogs, a cow, and a wolf, the heads of which were sent in from various parts of the state. The cumulative effect of their work was to show that rabies, far from being rare, was so prevalent among both domestic and wild animals in Minnesota as to be a serious health hazard. By June 1900 they had found rabies among dogs, cattle, horses, pigs, sheep, and wolves from various localities distributed in a band extending from east to west across southern Minnesota.[33]

Typhoid Fever

Concurrently with their work on rabies, Wesbrook and Wilson, together with Dr. Henry Bracken, were following exciting new developments in the diagnosis of typhoid fever. Although typhoid fever had been described early in the nineteenth century, its diagnosis, particularly in the early stages of the disease, was extremely difficult, because it could not be distinguished from fevers of other origin. Early in 1896 Richard Pfeiffer at Berlin and Max Gruber at Munich each observed independently that the blood serum of patients recovering from typhoid fever could be used to identify the typhoid fever bacillus (Eberth's bacillus) because, when the patient's serum was mixed with a broth culture of the typhoid bacillus, the bacilli, which previously had been swimming about rapidly, became motionless, clumped together, and settled to the bottom. The test was especially valuable because it distinguished the typhoid bacillus from the ordinary colon bacillus (Escherichia coli), which, although it otherwise looked very much like the typhoid bacillus, gave no reaction with the serum of typhoid fever patients. At Paris in June 1896 Fernand Widal announced that the reaction between blood serum and broth cultures of the typhoid bacillus could be used also as a diagnostic test for typhoid fever. If a known culture of typhoid bacillus were tested against the serum of various patients, only the serum of patients with typhoid fever would agglutinate and precipitate the typhoid bacilli.[34]

Widal's announcement of an exact and reliable test for typhoid fever attracted immediate attention among physicians throughout the world. At the meeting of the American Public Health Association at Buffalo, New York in September 1896, Wyatt Johnston of Montreal provided dramatic evidence for both the accuracy and value of the Widal test. Dr. Johnston found that the blood serum of typhoid fever patients retained its power to agglutinate typhoid bacilli even after it had been dried. When a sample of dried blood was moistened it would immobilize and agglutinate cultures of typhoid bacilli within fifteen minutes. Dr. Johnston arranged that the day after he left Montreal samples of blood were collected from six patients, dried, and sent to William E. Bissell, the city bacteriologist of Buffalo, together with a sealed envelope containing a key to their identity. At the meeting at Buffalo Dr. Johnston used the Widal test on the six blood samples, three of which were from typhoid fever patients and three not. After he identified each of the six samples as typhoid or nontyphoid, Dr. Bissell opened the sealed envelope and read the key to the anxious audience. Dr. Johnston's identifications corresponded exactly to those of clinical diagnosis given in the key.[35]

When Henry Bracken and Frank Wesbrook returned to Minneapolis from the Buffalo meeting, they began to study the feasibility of the Widal test for the routine diagnosis of typhoid fever. On 4 November Dr. Charles Lyman Greene reported to the Minnesota Academy of Medicine that at the City and County Hospital in St. Paul he and Dr. Harry P. Ritchie had used the Widal test on sixteen patients with typhoid fever all of whom showed the agglutination reaction, whereas ten other patients with fevers caused by septicaemia, erysipelas, pneumonia, tuberculosis or tubercular pleurisy failed to show the reaction.[36] At the State Board of Health Laboratory during November and December, Wesbrook and Wilson carried out the Widal test on samples of dried blood collected by Dr. Bracken from forty-seven patients according to Wyatt Johnston's method. In twenty-nine of the forty-seven patients the Widal test confirmed a clinical diagnosis of typhoid fever, while in other patients the Widal test showed that an initial diagnosis of typhoid fever was wrong, as was confirmed by the later clinical course of the illness. Dr. Bracken submitted the blood samples to Drs. Wesbrook and Wilson without any clinical history so that the diagnoses were made entirely on the basis of the test. Dr. Bracken reported the results of his study to the Minnesota Academy of Medicine at their meeting on 6 January 1897.[37]

About a month after Bracken's report, a typhoid fever epidemic broke out in Minneapolis and Wesbrook and Wilson were presented with an opportunity to study the value of the Widal test under the conditions of a large-scale epidemic. The clinical histories of patients suggested a common source of infection in the public water supply. Wesbrook and Wilson made cultures from samples of water taken from the laboratory tap and on 18 March 1897 isolated the typhoid bacillus from the water, using the reaction of the bacilli with the blood serum of a typhoid patient to distinguish the typhoid bacillus from ordinary colon bacilli. Later they used their culture of the typhoid bacillus from the Minneapolis water supply to perform the Widal test because it proved slightly more sensitive than stock laboratory cultures. Among 762 patients tested during the Minneapolis epidemic, 513 proved positive for typhoid fever.[38]

In September 1897 Louis B. Wilson devised a standard procedure for the collection and testing of blood samples by the Widal test. The State Board of Health Laboratory began to provide physicians with an envelope containing a piece of aluminum wire about three inches long with a small loop at one end for collecting a drop of blood, a piece of aluminum foil two inches square, a reporting form, and directions for collecting the blood sample. After pricking either the end of the patient's finger or the lobe of the ear, the physician transferred four or five loopfuls of blood to the surface of the aluminum foil, then carefully rolled up the foil without smearing the blood drops and allowed them to dry. When the blood was dry, the foil could be folded into a tight packet, placed in the envelope provided, and mailed to the laboratory. When the packets were opened in the laboratory, the dried blood easily flaked off from the foil. A measured quantity of dried blood was weighed out on a balance and dissolved in water. The diluted blood was then mixed with a suspension of typhoid bacilli in a hanging drop culture and observed under the microscope.

The advantages of this method of collecting standardized samples as devised by Louis B. Wilson were that the collecting outfit was light, inexpensive, and easy to distribute. It demanded little skill on the part of the physician, and the dried blood arrived at the laboratory perfectly preserved and unmixed with foreign matter so that it could be diluted accurately. By making the Widal test standard and quantitative, Wilson and Wesbrook ensured that it would be exact and reliable even when blood samples were collected by physicians of varying degrees of ability in all parts of the state. The results of the test were reported immediately to the attending physician with a request for information about the patient's subsequent clinical history. Among more than a thousand cases of suspected typhoid fever examined, Wesbrook and Wilson found that if the fever were actually typhoid, the Widal reaction appeared in most cases before the eighth day, and if delayed beyond the eighth day it appeared almost invariably at a later stage in the disease.[39]

Diphtheria

During the summer of 1896 the authorities at the Minnesota State Public Health School for Dependent and Neglected Children at Owatonna asked Frank Wesbrook to investigate the reasons for the unusual prevalence of diphtheria among children at the school. Ever since the school opened in 1887, cases of diphtheria had recurred repeatedly among the school's population of 220 to 275, despite great care taken to isolate those infected with the disease.

During the summer of 1896 there was a particularly severe diphtheria epidemic in the school with more than forty cases. The physician to the school, Dr. J. H. Adair, concerned at such a serious outbreak of diphtheria after nine years of efforts to control the disease, investigated every possible source of infection including the water supply and milk supply, but found nothing. It was then that he turned to the State Board of Health Laboratory and Dr. Wesbrook. In the course of the next two years, Wesbrook and his coworkers investigated the persistent occurrence of diphtheria at the Owatonna school. They made thousands of cultures from throat and nose, and for a period of time Dr. Orianna McDaniel, an assistant bacteriologist at the state laboratory, remained at Owatonna to run a bacteriological laboratory for this program. Although they never succeeded in identifying the reservoir of the diphtheria bacilli at the school, they learned a great deal from their research.

In examining the bacteria from large numbers of throat cultures, Wesbrook and his colleagues found both typical and atypical diphtheria bacilli in forms so various that they were compelled to question whether they were even observing diphtheria bacilli. So long as the patient was ill with clinical diphtheria, the presumption was that bacilli cultured from the throat were diphtheria bacilli causing the illness, but when the bacilli were cultured from the throat of a healthy child the presumption that they were diphtheria bacilli was lacking. The question became particularly acute in patients convalescing or recovered from diphtheria when the continuance or termination of quarantine was decided on the basis of the presence or absence of diphtheria bacilli in their throats. In the circumstances a bacteriologist needed definite criteria for deciding whether bacteria that appeared in a throat culture were diphtheria bacilli or not, but they lacked such criteria. As Wesbrook and his colleagues examined large numbers of cultures from the noses and throats of children in various schools and state institutions, they found that a large proportion of healthy children had diphtherialike bacilli, usually in their noses. They found that their original subdivision of diphtheria bacilli into *typical* and *atypical* forms was inadequate to describe the various forms of diphtheria bacilli that they encountered. It proved impossible to classify types of bacilli on a basis of the appearance of microscopic fields of presumed pure cultures, and they were forced to adopt a classification based on the morphology of individual bacilli. They made drawings of bacilli observed in twenty-four-hour cultures on solidified blood serum and stained with Löffler's methylene blue. They then classified the bacilli both according to their size and shape and according to whether they showed a granular, barred, or solid appearance as a result of staining with methylene blue. On the basis of size and shape they classified the bacilli into seven types A, B, C, D, E, F, and G, and each type might be granular, barred, or solid. Thus type A bacilli contained dark stained granules, type A_1 showed barred staining, type A_2 was stained solid blue, and so on for the other types. Both original and pure cultures usually showed a mixture of types. In the course of clinical diphtheria some types of diphtheria bacilli might disappear to be replaced by others. The granular forms, especially types C and D, were most frequently found to be the cause of clinical diphtheria.

From the numerous forms of the diphtheria bacillus, any one, or a mixture of which might occur either in patients with clinical diphtheria or in convalescent or healthy individuals, Wesbrook concluded that the presence or absence of diphtheria bacilli in the throat could not be used alone in deciding whether to impose or continue the quarantine of a patient. Clinical data had to be used together with bacteriological studies.[40]

Wesbrook did not consider that his types of diphtheria bacilli were necessarily distinct varieties. The purpose of his classification was to permit bacteriologists to describe diphtheria bacilli in precise terms. Nevertheless, in 1901 the classification proved of practical value in controlling a diphtheria epidemic at Park Rapids, Minnesota, a town of about a thousand persons in a lumbering area 200 miles from Minneapolis. During 1900 diphtheria had spread through the population of Park Rapids, attacking both children and adults in the town and extending to the surrounding lumber camps. The epidemic continued through the winter of 1900–1901, and persisted into the summer. In August 1901 the town authorities of Park Rapids, fearing an even worse diphtheria epidemic when the schools opened in September, appealed to the State Board of Health for help, and Henry Bracken and Frank Wesbrook went to investigate. After examining all cases of diphtheria that were then active, they met with the town council and school board in joint session and recommended that the opening of school be delayed in order to take throat cultures from all the children, their families, and their teachers. Any child or teacher who was infected with the large granular type of diphtheria bacilli would then be excluded from school until the child or teacher and all of his family were free of infection. Dr. Wesbrook then sent his assistant bacteriologist, E. H. Beckman, to Park Rapids where Dr. Beckman in two weeks took throat cultures from more than 350 school children and plotted the location, distribution, and dates of diphtheria infection on maps. All children who were infected with granular-staining diphtheria bacilli were excluded from school until the granular-staining forms could no longer be cultured from their throats. The campaign delayed the opening of school for a week, but when the school opened the diphtheria epidemic that had been greatly feared not only did not occur, but diphtheria disappeared from Park Rapids.[41]

The successful control of diphtheria at Park Rapids in 1901 was a tribute to Frank Wesbrook's ability to explain to ordinary people the scientific basis for the public health measures he proposed and to obtain their intelligent cooperation.

In 1903 Louis Wilson organized similar diphtheria control measures at Grand Rapids and in 1904 at Benson, Minnesota.

As a result of a study of diphtheria bacilli in healthy persons carried out by the Massachusetts Association of Boards of Health in 1902, to which Wesbrook and his colleagues contributed, the barred and solid-staining types of diphtheria bacilli were found more frequently in the nose than in the throat, and were, therefore, essentially nose bacteria when they were present in healthy persons.[42] At Providence, Rhode Island in 1901, Dr. Frederic P. Gorham extended Wesbrook's survey of the varieties of diphtheria bacilli to be found in the noses and throats of healthy persons. Gorham found Wesbrook's classification adequate for all types observed, and confirmed his observation that the granular types tended to predominate at the beginning of a diphtheria illness and that they tended to be replaced by barred and solid types shortly before diphtheria bacilli disappeared from the throat during convalescence.[43]

From 1892 when he worked on the anthrax bacillus with E. H. Hankin to the early years of the 1900s when diphtheria was being controlled, Frank Wesbrook had had ten years of exciting and productive research. His double appointment to the medical school faculty and as director of the State Board of Health Laboratory proved fortunate for all concerned. Wesbrook became known state-wide by physicians and lay people alike for the valuable research into rabies and diphtheria that he had directed and the common sense approach he had advocated for control of these public health problems. His work with the Minneapolis city officials during their typhoid epidemic also brought high praise.

X-rays

During the winter of 1896 the university was excited by the news of Roentgen's discovery of x-rays. In the physics laboratory at Minnesota, Professor Fred S. Jones repeated Roentgen's experiment of discharging high-voltage electricity through an evacuated glass tube and succeeded in taking "a number of excellent negatives, comparing favorably with the best obtained elsewhere."[44] On 25 March Professor Jones delivered a public lecture at the university on the new x-rays, during which he showed on a screen a number of the photographs he had taken with the x-ray apparatus. The *Ariel* reported that the best pictures were probably those of Professor Nachtrieb's frogs and fishes. "The bones in the frogs and the calcareous frame of the starfish were very clearly and distinctly outlined." The reporter added that a photograph of the hand of one of the laboratory assistants, known in the laboratory as the "Hand of Providence," was well worth a visit to the laboratory to see.[45] The potential value of x-rays to medical diagnoses was immediately apparent both to Professor Jones and his colleagues on the medical faculty. On 10 April Professor Jones lectured to the medical students on the use of x-rays for taking pictures of tubercular lesions in patients, and a week later he repeated his lecture in St. Paul.

On 16 October, shortly after the fall term began in 1896, the Department of Medicine held a special celebration for the semi-centennial of the discovery of anesthesia. Members of the medical profession from throughout the state were invited. During the morning a succession of speakers delivered lectures on various aspects of the history of anaesthesia and its influence upon surgery.[46] At noon the department provided a reception and luncheon for its guests in the Laboratory of Medical Sciences and after lunch the laboratories were opened for inspection by the visiting physicians. During the afternoon members of the faculty demonstrated in the clinic various modern methods used in anaesthesia, and at the end of the day Professor Jones of the physics department gave a demonstration of x-rays and a discussion of their uses. "The day was altogether one to stir the memories of the passing generation," said the *Northwestern Lancet,* "and to ensure the enthusiasm of the rising generation of physicians."[47]

One person most keenly interested in x-rays, because he saw their potential usefulness to surgery, was Perry Millard. During the week following the anesthesia celebration, at Dean Millard's request Professor Jones took his x-ray equipment to the City Hospital in St. Paul where he used x-ray photographs to locate bullets in the legs of two patients. Perry Millard then operated successfully to remove the bullets in the presence of several of his colleagues. The operations must have been one of the earliest effective uses of x-rays in surgery.[48] Millard and Jones planned to use x-rays for more such operations.

That fall some 220 students registered in the College of Medicine and Surgery. Some students had been expected to leave because of the introduction of the four-year course, but very few did. With the splendid new Laboratory of Medical Sciences in use and fully equipped for teaching and research, and in the afterglow of the anesthesia celebration, the faculty were proudly confident that they had one of the best medical schools in the United States. At his opening lecture in the course on surgical anatomy, Professor George A. Hendricks told his class that he was pleased to see so many of them back, and that it showed good judgment on their part to remain at Minnesota. During the preceding summer Professor Hendricks had made a study of medical colleges throughout the country and had concluded that the Department of Medicine at Minnesota was equal to the best. The reporter for the *Ariel* commented: "Dr. Hendricks is never inclined to be egotistical and his remarks consequently have a good deal of force."[49]

But in the midst of its new-found pride and confidence, Minnesota was to be struck a cruel blow. Early in November Dean Millard began to feel unwell. His initial symptoms may have been merely a sense of tiredness and weakness that suggested that he needed a rest. Certainly he had been working intensely during his eight years as dean. In addition to the appointment of a faculty and the organization of a curriculum that had grown from a medical course of two six-month terms to four eight-month terms, he had been responsible for bringing into being three new buildings on the university campus and the creation of dispensaries off-campus. And all the while that he was performing his administrative and teaching duties for the Department of Medicine in Minneapolis, Perry Millard was carrying on an active surgical practice in St. Paul. There was, therefore, reason for Dr. Millard to feel tired—reason, but not sufficient reason. During his years at Stillwater and later at St. Paul, Perry Millard had thrived on work. Ever active in a busy practice, he had served as secretary of the College of Medicine of the university when it was an examining body, had written the legislation creating a state board of medical examiners in Minnesota, and had conducted the negotiations that had brought together three medical schools into one Department of Medicine at the University of Minnesota. As dean of that department he had held the regular medical college and the homeopathic medical college together in uneasy, but on the whole effective, cooperation, creating a school of scientific medicine in the forefront of American medical schools. Dean Millard had also been active in the founding of the American Association of Medical Colleges. He enjoyed his work and did it well. It had never tired him before, or he could not have done so much. Now he was mysteriously and deeply weary.

On 14 November the *Ariel* announced that Dean Millard planned to leave the following Friday, 20 November, for a trip to the southwest on account of his health, and expected to be gone three weeks.[50] However, Dean Millard did not leave for the southwest as planned. A week later on 21 November the *Ariel* announced: "Dean Millard is seriously ill and will probably be gone several months."[51] Dr. Henry Bracken was to act as dean during Millard's absence. A few days later Perry Millard left his home in St. Paul, accompanied by his twenty-year-old daughter, Lillian, to go to Baltimore to become a patient of Dr. William Osler at the Johns Hopkins Hospital. Mrs. Millard could not accompany her husband to Baltimore because their seventeen-year-old son, John Jay Millard, was also ill.

Millard knew Osler from meetings of the American Association of Medical Colleges where they had served together on committees, and from meetings of the American Medical Association, as well as from Osler's visit to the University of Minnesota in 1892. It was, therefore, natural that, when he came down with a serious illness that puzzled his medical colleagues in Minnesota, Millard should travel to Baltimore to consult Osler. Before he left, Dean Millard met with President Northrop, presumably to discuss interim arrangements to carry on the Department of Medicine during Millard's absence.

On 4 December the *Ariel* reported that Dean Millard was at Baltimore under the care of Dr. Osler and added, "There is considerable doubt as to his recovery."[52] During the following week Perry Millard had some remission of his illness. On 10 December Dr. Osler sent a telegram to Dr. Bracken with the message, "Dr. Millard has passed the crisis. Symptoms point to recovery."[53] Nevertheless, on 30 December Perry Millard dictated his will to his nurse and it was put into its final form by the stenographer to Henry M. Hurd, the director of the hospital. On 9 January 1897 the *Ariel* reported cheerfully: "Dean Millard's condition is much improved, and he is expected back by February 1."[54] On 16 January the *Ariel* was less confident, "No marked change has been noted in Dean Millard's condition, but he writes hopefully."[55] A medical colleague, who visited Dr. Millard in hospital found him prematurely aged, like a man of eighty. Mrs. Millard was sum-

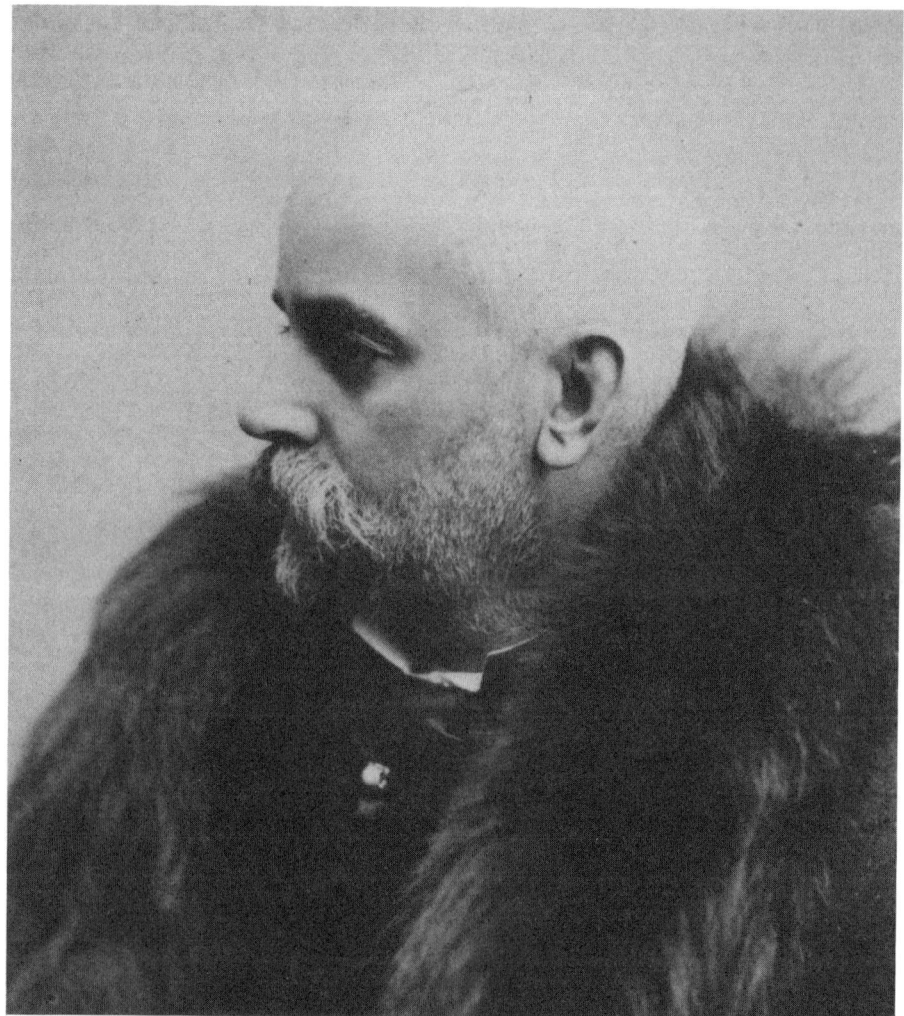

FIGURE 4:8   Perry H. Millard, circa 1896. Courtesy Mn U Archives.

moned to Baltimore. On Monday, 1 February, the day that he was expected back in St. Paul, Perry Millard died of what Osler diagnosed as anemia.[56] Mrs. Millard and her daughter, Lillian, returned to St. Paul with his body, arriving Thursday, 4 February.

At ten o'clock in the morning on Friday, 5 February, the funeral for Dr. Perry H. Millard was held at his house at 530 Holly Avenue. The Reverend S. G. Smith of the People's Church read the service. Over a hundred of his friends and colleagues attended. From the house they escorted his body to the railway station. A special train of three cars conveyed the funeral cortege over the line of the Omaha Railroad, which Perry Millard had served as chief surgeon, to Stillwater on the banks of the St. Croix where Perry Millard had practiced medicine for fourteen years. As the engine puffed slowly into Stillwater, where on one side of the track the frozen expanse of the St. Croix stretched over to the wooded hills of Wisconsin, and on the other rose the steep, tree-lined streets of the little town, some members of that train crew and many men from the sawmills waiting on the platform had been patients of Dr. Millard. From the station the procession went in carriages past Perry Millard's old office on the second floor at the corner of Chestnut and First Streets and past his former house on Third Street up the steep hills to Fairview Cemetery.

The following Sunday, 7 February, there was a memorial service for Dean Millard at the People's Church on Pleasant Avenue in St. Paul. In life Perry Millard had not been a particularly popular man, but now that he was dead his colleagues were suddenly aware of how much they owed to him. The faculty and the medical students attended the service en masse, together with many other physicians and friends. Both the Reverend Smith and President Northrop spoke, but Northrop dominated the occasion. Northrop said:

> I was associated closely with Dr. Millard for eight years . . . . It was his ambition to make the medical college of the university an institution that in its enduring life would show that he had lived and that in living he had been of use to the world. Dr. Millard is dead, but the medical college still lives, showing in every department the impress of his labor and his character. . . . Of Perry H. Millard may be said this . . . . He laid the foundation in this state for medical education and medical law, upon which his successors may build safely . . . .[57]

NOTES

1. University of Minnesota, *Catalogue, 1893-1894,* p. 199.
2. Ibid., pp. 199–200.
3. Louis B. Wilson, "Pioneers in research," *Minn. Alumni Wkly,* 1940, 39, 481–482.
4. "Medical Department," *Ariel,* 1893-94, 17, p. 179.
5. Ibid., p. 210.
6. Ibid., p. 195.
7. Ibid., p. 229.
8. Board of Regents, Minutes, 1888 -1905 (27 December 1893), p. 432.
9. Ibid. (4 June 1894), p. 439.
10. "Medical notes," *Ariel,* 13 October 1894, p. 11.
11. Ibid.
12. Ibid., 27 April 1895, pp. 13–14, p. 14.
13. Board of Regents, Minutes, 1888–1905 (1 May 1895), p. 451.
14. The building, now called Wesbrook Hall, has never burned, and is now used by the College of Education.
15. *Ariel,* 5 October 1895, p. 2.
16. Information obtained from the rough draft for the letter that Wesbrook sent to J. Clark Stewart, dated 15 May 1895, in the Wesbrook papers in the University of British Columbia Archives. The letter that Wesbrook actually sent to Stewart has not survived. For an account of Wesbrook's life, see William C. Gibson, *Wesbrook and his university.*

17. F. F. Wesbrook, "Contribution à l'étude des toxines du cholèra," *Annls Inst. Pasteur, Paris,* 1894, *8,* 318–337.

18. F. F. Wesbrook, "Some of the effects of sunlight on tetanus cultures," *J. Path. Bact.,* 1896, *3,* 70–79; idem, "The growth of cholera and other bacilli in direct sunlight," ibid., pp. 352–358.

19. F. F. Wesbrook, "The relative toxicity of aerobic and anaerobic cultures of the vibrio of Asiatic cholera," *J. Path. Bact.,* 1897, *4,* 1–7.

20. Walter S. Lazarus-Barlow to Wesbrook, 13 June 1895, Wesbrook papers.

21. Stewart to Wesbrook, 7 July 1895, Wesbrook papers.

22. "Medical notes," *Ariel,* 12 October 1895, pp. 9–10, p. 10.

23. Ibid., 2 November 1895, p. 12.

24. Ibid.

25. Henry M. Bracken, "Fifty years of public health work in Minnesota" (MS), p. 71, Bracken papers.

26. Ibid., pp. 20–27.

27. Ibid., p. 76.

28. Arthur Sweeney and C.F. Denny, "Rabies," *Northwest. Lancet,* 1896, *16,* 123–129.

29. "Mutilated by tramp cur," *St. Paul Pioneer Press,* 21 August 1896; "Death from hydrophobia . . . ," ibid., 3 October 1896, p. 8; "May escape hydrophobia. City sends Jennie Shaffer for Pasteur treatment," ibid, 4 October 1896, p. 7; Arthur Sweeney, "Rabies with reports of cases," *Northwest. Lancet,* 1897, *17,* 247–255.

30. F. F. Wesbrook and Louis B. Wilson, "Preliminary report on the laboratory diagnosis in twenty cases of suspected rabies," *Pub. Hlth Pap. Rep., N.Y.,* 1897, *23,* 219–235.

31. F. F. Wesbrook, "Quarterly reports of the bacteriological laboratory, 1897–1898," In Minnesota State Board Health, *Biennial report,* vol. 17 (1897–98), 123–182, p. 148.

32. Ibid., p. 153.

33. F. F. Wesbrook, "Rabies in Minnesota," *St. Paul med. J.,* 1900, *2,* 670–680.

34. Fernand Widal, "Sérodiagnostique de la fièvre typhoide," *Bull. Mém. Soc. méd. Hôp. Paris,* 1896, ser. 3, *13,* 561–566.

35. Wyatt Johnston, "On the application of the serum diagnosis of typhoid fever to the requirements of public health laboratories," *N. Y. med. J.,* 1896, *64,* 573–576, p. 574.

36. Chas. Lyman Greene, "Preliminary report upon the serum test for typhoid fever with demonstrations of method," *Northwest. Lancet,* 1896, *16,* 439–440.

37. Henry M. Bracken, "The practical application of the serum diagnosis of typhoid fever," *N. Y. med. J.,* 1897, *65,* 556–559.

38. Louis B. Wilson and F. F. Westbrook, "Preliminary report on the serum diagnosis of typhoid fever in an epidemic during which typhoid bacillus was isolated from the public water supply," *Br. med. J.,* 1897, *ii,* 1774–1775.

39. F. F. Wesbrook and Louis B. Wilson, "The serum diagnosis of typhoid fever from the public-health-laboratory point of view," *Phila. med. J.,* 1898, *1,* 549–553.

40. F. F. Westbrook, Louis B. Wilson, and O. McDaniel, "Varieties of Bacillus diphtheria," *Trans. Ass. Am. Phsns,* 1900, *15* 198–223, p. 223.

41. F. F. Wesbrook, "Diphtheria infection in Minnesota. — Recent experiences with the disease in school children and in institutional epidemics," *Pub. Hlth Pap. Rep. N.Y.,* 1905, *30,* 94–103, pp. 97–98.

42. F. F. Wesbrook, "Problems in the laboratory study of diphtheria," *Pub. Hlth Pap. Rep., N.Y.,* 1902, *28,* 381–387, p. 383.

43. Frederic P. Gorham, "Morphological varieties of Bacillus diphtheriae," *J. med. Res.,* 1901, *n.s. 1.,* 201–210.

44. Fred S. Jones, "Roentgen rays," *Ariel,* 19 March 1896, pp. 1–2.
45. "Prof. Jones' lecture on the X rays," *Ariel,* 28 March 1896, pp. 3–4.
46. The various papers were published in the *Northwest. Lancet,* 1896, *16,* 403–415. They included: Burnside Foster, "The history of the discovery of anaesthesia," pp. 403–405; Theodore F. Dewitt, "Fifty years of surgery under anaesthesia," pp. 406–409; B. H. Ogden, "Anaesthetics in obstetrics," pp. 409–412; Henry M. Bracken, "The therapeutics of anaesthesia," pp. 412–414; and Samuel Keith, "Preanaesthetic surgery," pp. 414–415.
47. "The semicentennial of the discovery of anaesthesia," *Northwest. Lancet,* 1896, *16,* 419–420, p. 420. Cf. "College of Medicine," *Ariel,* 24 October 1896, p. 15.
48. "X-ray operation," *Ariel,* 24 October 1896, p. 1.
49. "College of Medicine," *Ariel,* 24 October 1896, pp. 15–16.
50. Ibid., 14 November 1896, p. 14.
51. Ibid., 21 November 1896, p. 18.
52. Ibid., 4 October 1896, p. 15.
53. Ibid., 12 December 1896, p. 18.
54. Ibid., 9 January 1897, p. 16.
55. Ibid., 16 January 1897, p. 15.
56. *Minneapolis Journal,* 1 February 1897; *Saint Paul Pioneer Press,* 2 February 1897.
57. *St. Paul Pioneer Press,* 8 February 1897.

CHAPTER 5

The Medical School under Dean Parks Ritchie 1897–1906

On 25 May 1897 the Board of Regents appointed Dr. Parks Ritchie dean of the College of Medicine and Surgery. Then fifty-two years old, Parks Ritchie was a native of Indiana where he had received his early education. In 1864 at the age of nineteen he joined the 132nd regiment of Indiana volunteers, and served in the United States Army during the final year of the Civil War. Following the war, he studied medicine at the Medical College of Ohio in Cincinnati where he received the M.D. degree in 1870. In 1880 Dr. Ritchie came to St. Paul, where he specialized in obstetric practice and taught obstetrics at the St. Paul Medical College. With the founding of the medical school at the university in 1888 he became professor of obstetrics in the College of Medicine and Surgery. Now in 1897 he became dean, and with his new position he received his first salary in the sum of $1,800 from the university.[1]

At the regular meeting of the faculty of the College of Medicine and Surgery on May 28, three days after his appointment, Dean Ritchie made a short speech and assumed the chair. Conscious of the growth of the college, a faculty committee recommended that Roberts' rules of order be followed in faculty meetings, that faculty meetings should be held quarterly, and that a regular procedure should be followed for nominations to the faculty or changes in title, recommendations that the faculty adopted the following October.[2]

One of the first problems Dean Ritchie had to face was the inadequacy of the university dispensary and its funding. Dr. James Moore, professor of clinical surgery, presented his case to the executive committee in August 1897. He urged the college to develop its own hospital for clinical teaching, but in the meantime, the staff of the dispensary needed $1,500 immediately to improve its facilities and services. On recommendation of the committee, Dr. Moore addressed the regents along with a letter of support from Dean Ritchie. The regents voted $300 for clinical apparatus, far less than the sum Dr. Moore deemed necessary.

A year later, Dr. Moore again addressed the executive committee on the problem of a dispensary, but this time he had a plan. He suggested two possible solu-

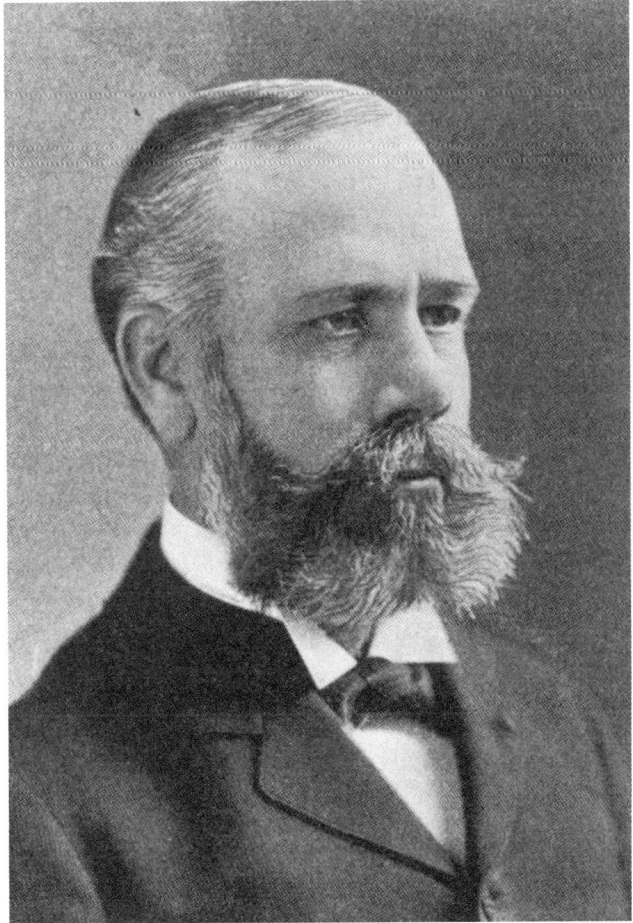

FIGURE 5:1 Parks Ritchie, 1897. Courtesy Mn U Archives.

tions. The university might buy land on the west side of the river and erect a building for a dispensary, or as a less expensive alternative, it might fit up a dispensary for about $2,000 in the Riverside Chapel in the same neighborhood on the west side of the river. The executive committee decided that both plans should be presented to the Board of Regents together with a request for $10,000 for a dispensary building, an indication that their own preference was for a new building specially adapted to dispensary needs.[3] At the same meeting Dr. Richard O. Beard, acting on behalf of the laboratory chairs, presented plans for an anatomy building to the west of Medical Hall to be connected to the existing anatomy laboratory in Medical Hall by a covered passageway for the transfer of bodies. The executive committee approved the plans and recommended them to the Board of Regents.

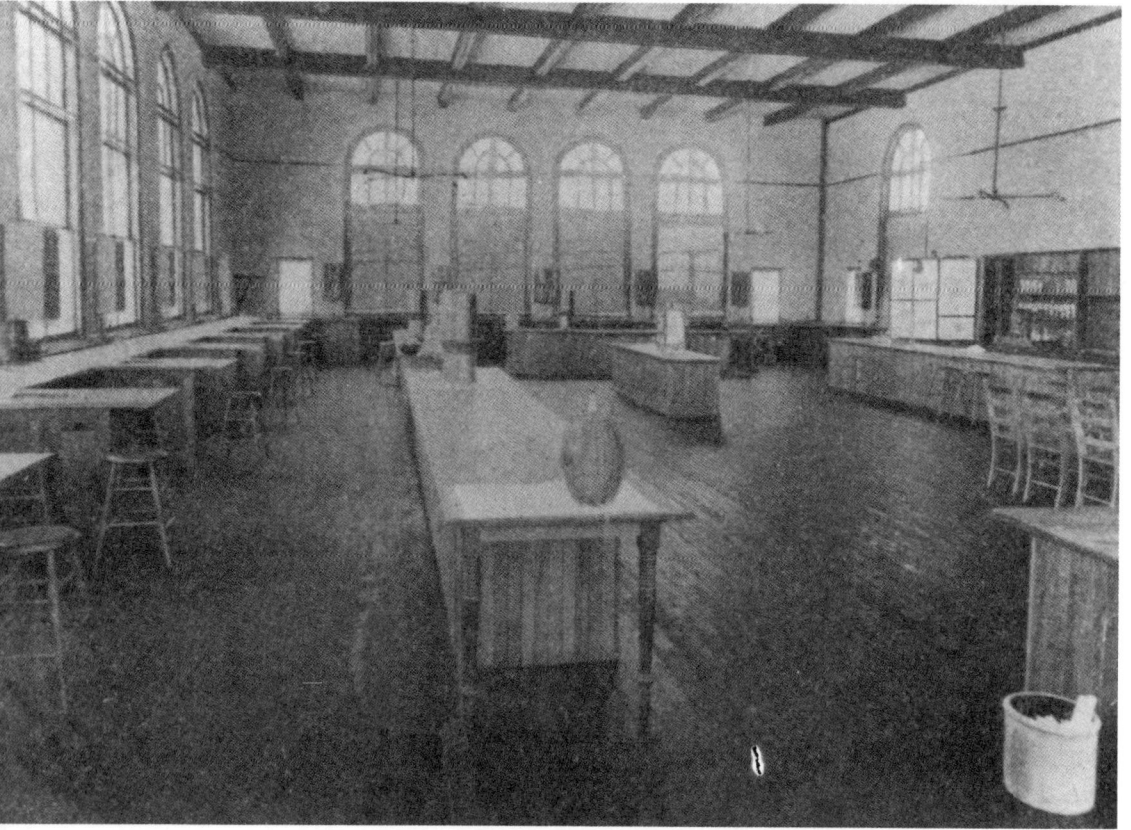

FIGURE 5:2 Bacteriology Laboratory, Laboratory of Medical Sciences. Courtesy Mn U Archives.

Dr. Beard also proposed and the executive committee approved the construction of an animal house to be built behind the Laboratory of Medical Sciences for rabbits, guinea pigs, and a small number of larger animals, together with aquaria for frogs and turtles. Altogether the executive committee recommended in 1898 that the university request $30,000 from the state legislature for additions to the medical buildings.[4]

In December 1898 the Board of Regents decided to request $12,000 from the legislature for a new anatomy building on the campus, and $15,000 to purchase land and erect a building for the dispensary.[5] They did not mention the animal house. In April 1899 the regents also approved substantial requisitions from Dr. Frank Wesbrook for supplies and new equipment for the laboratory of pathology and bacteriology.[6] The quality of the equipment and facilities in the Laboratory of Medical Sciences became evident the following October when the American Public Health Association met there. On that occasion William Henry Welch,

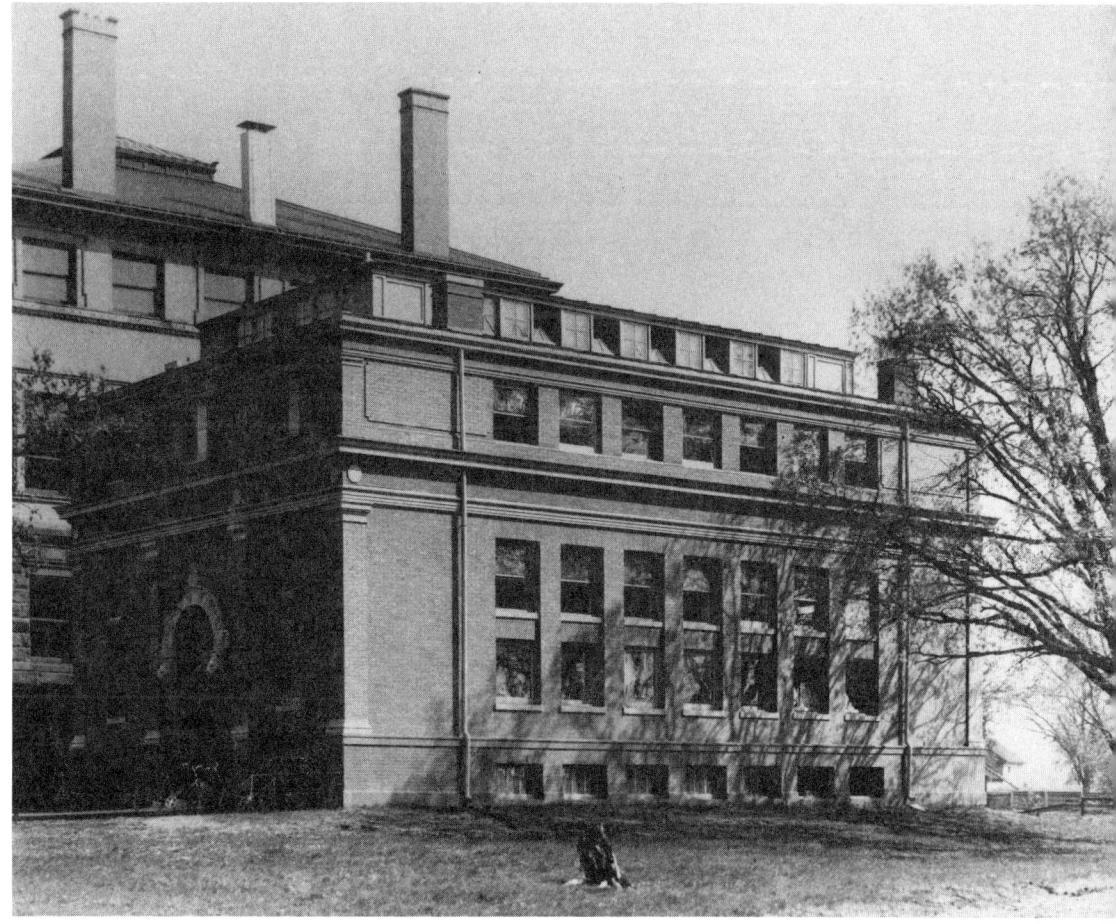

FIGURE 5:3   Anatomy Building, circa 1901. Courtesy Mn U Archives.

professor of pathology at Johns Hopkins University, remarked to Dr. Moore that the College of Medicine and Surgery was a great revelation to him. "We in the East," said Welch, "have no conception of the true status nor of the growth and progress of your college. The work done here by you is excelled by none and hereafter I shall advise students who desire to see good work to go West as well as East."[7] During the winter of 1899 the Minnesota legislature granted the university's requests for funds for an anatomy building and clinical building, and construction of both buildings began the following summer.

The new Anatomy Building built beside Medical Hall was a small, two-story structure containing a morgue, injecting room, cold storage vaults, and an engine to operate the refrigeration equipment. On the first floor was an amphitheater to seat 175 students, offices for professors and instructors, and a private dissecting

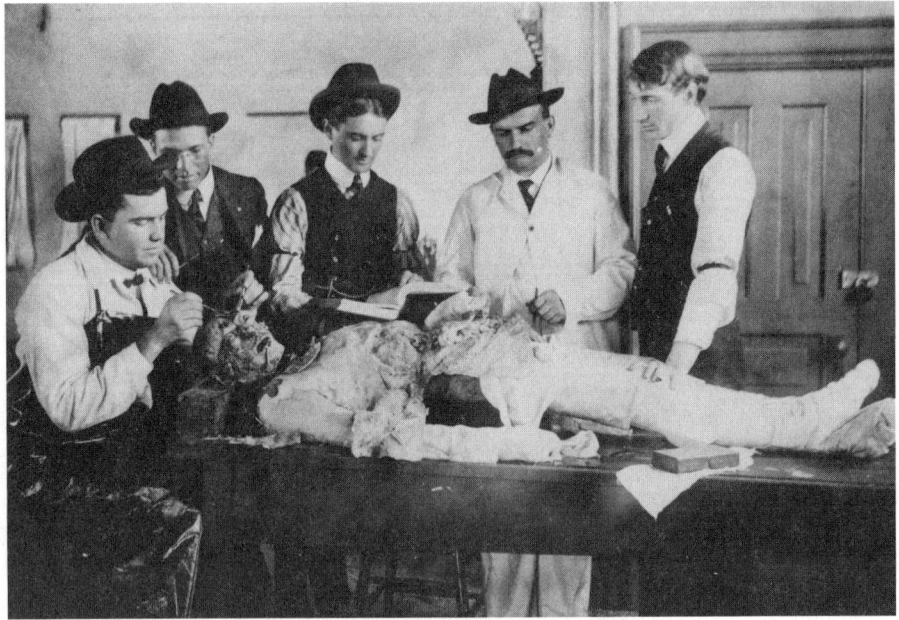
FIGURE 5:4 Anatomical dissection, early 1900s. Courtesy Mn U Archives.

room and research laboratory. The whole of the second floor was devoted to laboratories for practical anatomical dissection by the medical students.[8] The provision of cold storage vaults for cadavers enabled the anatomy department to acquire bodies whenever they might become available and store them until needed. The new building also permitted the complete removal of anatomical dissection from Medical Hall to relatively isolated and far more spacious quarters, thereby permitting students to learn anatomy by dissection much more thoroughly and completely than before. "This laboratory when completed," commented the *Ariel,* "will be the finest anatomical laboratory in the United States and will be fully equipped with the latest apparatus."[9]

A site for the clinical building was selected on Washington Avenue South in Minneapolis in the area known as Seven Corners. About a quarter of the space in the new building was to be allotted to the homeopathic college.[10] During the summer of 1899, in anticipation of the new clinical building then under construction, the dispensary was removed from the rooms it had occupied in the basement of Medical Hall, and the space thus vacated was given to the College of Dentistry.

Although its equipment and arrangements were not yet entirely finished, the university dispensary opened early in December 1899 at 1808–1810 Washington Avenue South on the west bank of the Mississippi. This was a modest, working-class neighborhood densely populated with Germans and Scandinavians, many of them recent immigrants, who were potential patients. The building was of two

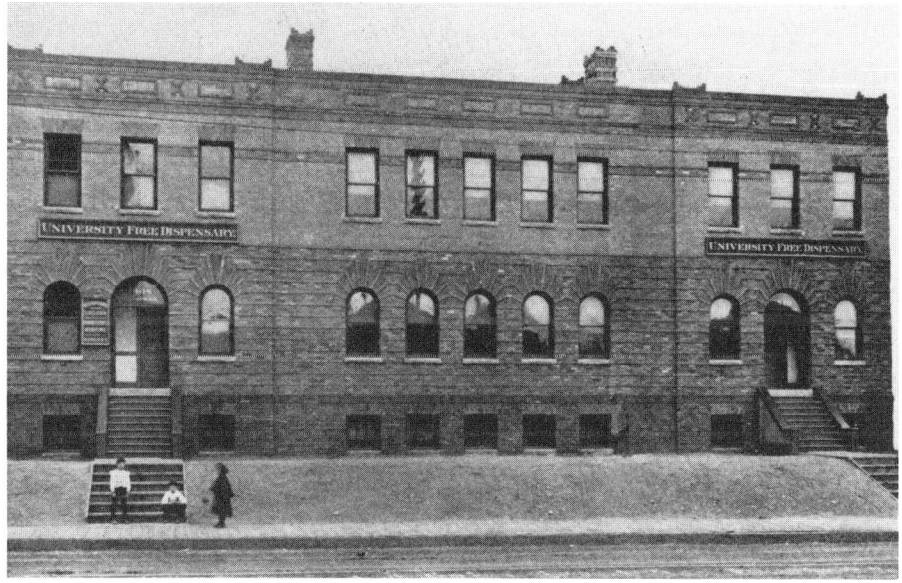

FIGURE 5:5 University Dispensary at Seven Corners, Minneapolis, 1900. Courtesy Mn U Archives.

stories, 40 by 150 feet, and contained amphitheaters, waiting rooms, a pharmacy, and class rooms for the various clinical specialties. There were also laboratories where the chemical and microscopic diagnostic tests, then being introduced to clinical medicine, might be performed. In May 1902 the Board of Regents also appropriated $1,000 for the physiology laboratory: half of the money was to be used to erect a building for laboratory animals on land belonging to a Mr. Greeley of Minnetonka Mills, and the other half was to be used for the care and feeding of the animals over a two-year period.

Disaster struck the night of 24 January 1902. The new Anatomy Building with its unrivaled facilities was gutted by fire. Although the stone walls survived, the whole interior burned. The loss of the Anatomy Building and its contents effectively halted the study of anatomy. In March the executive committee included among their requested appropriations an item for $500 to replace anatomical preparations that had been destroyed in the fire.[11]

Although the clinical building at 1810 Washington Avenue South had been open less than three years, it was already proving too small for the dispensary; the executive committee decided to ask the Board of Regents to request $20,000 from the legislature to enlarge and equip it. The committee also asked the regents to request $100,000 from the legislature for a new building for the pathology and bacteriology laboratories, part of which would be used by the State Board of Health.[12] On 2 October 1902 Drs. Richard O. Beard, Frank C. Todd, and Frank F. Wesbrook appeared before the regents to present the two requests.[13] After

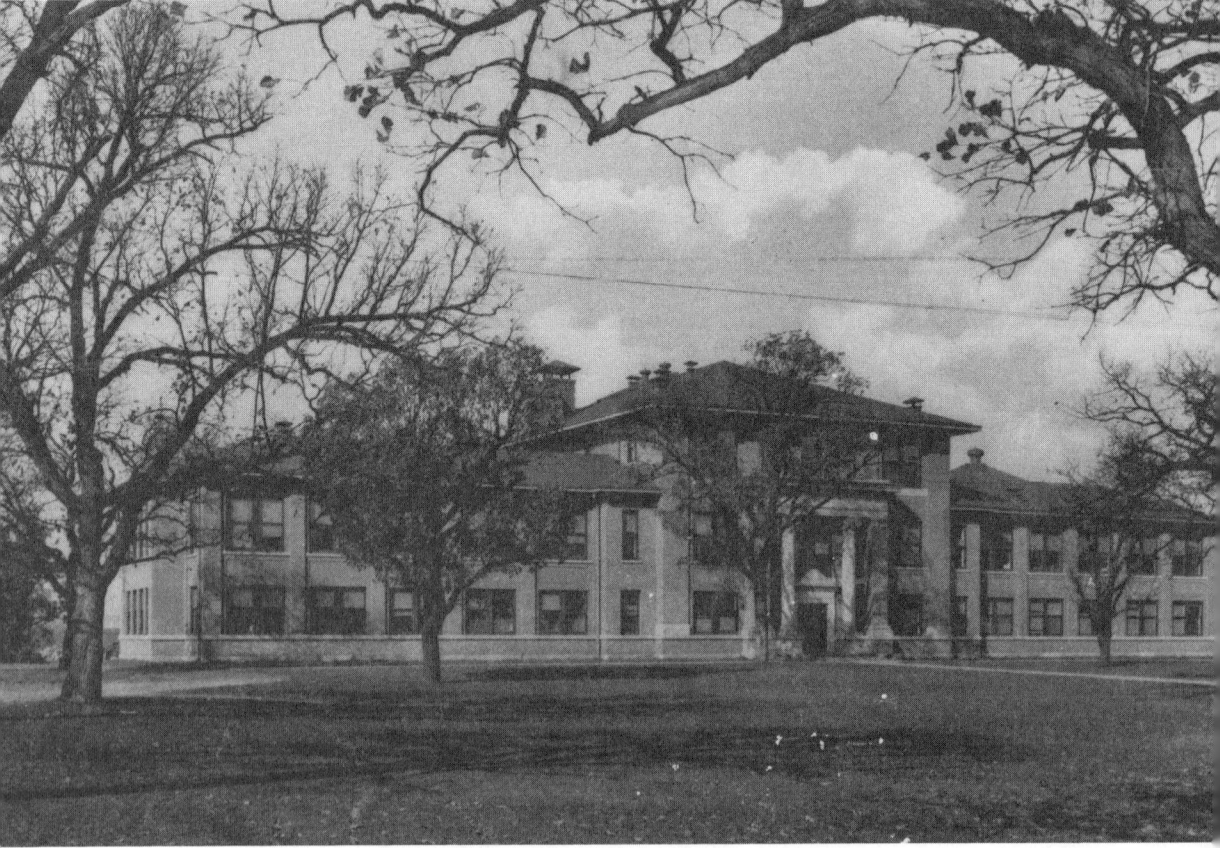

FIGURE 5:6 Institute of Public Health and Pathology, 1908. Courtesy Mn U Archives.

study the regents denied funds for an addition to the clinical building, but they forwarded to the legislature the request for $100,000 to build new laboratories for pathology and bacteriology. During their 1903 session the legislature appropriated the funds.

During the winter of 1904 Dr. Wesbrook traveled to Europe to visit laboratories in Great Britain, France, Germany, and Austria, including the Pasteur Institute at Paris and the Coke Institute for the Study of Tropical Diseases at Liverpool, all for the purpose of incorporating in the new building the best and most modern facilities for the study of bacteriology and infectious diseases.[14] Wesbrook returned to Minneapolis in April 1904, and during the remainder of the year he was deeply engaged in plans for the new building, to be known as the Institute of Public Health and Pathology. It was located overlooking the river, next to a small animal research laboratory built for the State Board of Health in 1902. It consisted of a large central block of three stories from which extended wings of two stories to the north and south. In addition to two large laboratories for teaching pathology, bacteriology, and public health, it contained a museum, a library, a large amphitheater and numerous offices and research laboratories.[15] To enable Minnesota residents to receive Pasteur treatment for the bites of rabid animals promptly and inexpensively, Dr. Wesbrook created a rabies prevention laboratory in the new building and placed it in the charge of Dr. Orianna McDaniel.

The new Pasteur Institute would meet an urgent need. Although relatively few people were bitten by rabid animals, when such bites occurred the victims had previously had to go out-of-the-state to receive Pasteur immunization treatment. Frequently, because they could not afford the journey, they did not go and hoped for the best. Often such bitten persons did not contract rabies, but some did. In April 1899 a fifteen-year-old St. Paul boy, Christian Bucka, was bitten on the left wrist while playing with his dog. The wound healed and he remained healthy until nearly a year later when, on 23 March 1900, he was vaccinated on the left arm. Three hours after vaccination the arm became severely painful at the site of the bite, the boy became feverish, began to show symptoms of rabies, and died on 30 March, a week after vaccination.[16] The tragic fate of Christian Bucka in 1900 was perhaps a factor in influencing the Minnesota legislature in 1903 to provide funds for the new Institute of Public Health and Pathology at the university. From January through July of 1906 there were reports of sixty-five persons bitten by rabid animals, including sixty-three bites by rabid dogs, one by a rabid cow, and one by a rabid cat. Forty-six of those bitten received Pasteur immunization treatment, but in order to obtain such treatment they had to travel either to Chicago or to Ann Arbor, Michigan. The other nineteen persons bitten received no treatment, but clearly they should have.[17]

The Hospital for Crippled Children

During the winter of 1897 Dr. Arthur J. Gillette of St. Paul caused to be introduced before the Minnesota legislature a bill which appropriated $5,000 per year for two years to the University of Minnesota to create a hospital for poor crippled children whose parents were unable to afford treatment for them. At that time many children were crippled and deformed as a result of tuberculous infection of the joints. They could often be treated effectively by draining the tuberculous abscesses and by orthopedic appliances to correct the deformity, but such treatments required continuous and prolonged periods in hospital. In 1897 there was no such thing as a state hospital for poor crippled children anywhere in the United States, and Dr. Gillette had to overcome the suspicions of legislators that his plan for the relief and cure of crippled children, who must eventually become in need of public charity if they were not so already, was merely a subtle scheme to enrich the medical profession. To their astonishment, Dr. Gillette assured the members of the legislative committee that the crippled children would be cared for by physicians and surgeons without charge, confident that the medical profession of Minnesota would fulfill the promise, and the legislature passed the bill.[18]

After examination of the various hospitals in Minneapolis and St. Paul the Board of Regents entered into a contract with the City and County Hospital of St. Paul whereby the hospital agreed to set aside a ward for the care of crippled children and the university agreed to pay the hospital for their care. The Hospital for Crippled Children opened in October 1897 as a hospital within a hospital; it was placed in charge of Dr. Gillette as chief surgeon and Dr. James E. Moore as consulting physician and surgeon.[19]

During the first two years, 1897–1899, Dr. Gillette examined eighty crippled children, among whom twenty-one were found incurable and were not treated. Five were treated as outpatients, but fifty-four received treatment in the hospital. The first case, admitted in October 1897, was a young boy from Pine County, Minnesota so severely crippled with tuberculous diseases of the vertebrae that he was bent at the hips nearly at a right angle and, thus bent over, could walk only with great difficulty so consequently he walked very little. He was suffering from double psoas abscesses and seven discharging sinuses, with the pains that usually accompanied such deep-seated tubercular disease. He was feverish, with a temperature of 100–102° F.

In the hospital the boy was placed in bed, flat on his back, with traction on his legs drawing along the line of the deformity, and the sinuses were dressed aseptically. "In a week," wrote Dr. Gillette, "he showed marked improvement, that is, he was relieved of all pain and the discharge from the abscesses immediately began to lessen. From day to day we found that we could gradually lower the inclined plane until the legs were perfectly straight thus completely overcoming the flexion due to psoas contractions."[20] His temperature became normal. Presently the sinuses had healed sufficiently that Dr. Gillette could apply a plaster of Paris cast around the body with a double spica about the thighs. By 30 September 1898, a year after admission, the boy was nearly cured, free from pain, and with all the sinuses healed. Somewhat later he was discharged from the hospital, healthy and free from pain, able to walk without any mechanical appliance and to attend school.

A critical factor in the achievement of such dramatic results was the complete rest which the tuberculous joints could be given in hospital as well as the orthopedic procedures which could there be applied. Dr. Gillette enjoyed similar successes in the treatment of clubbed feet (*talipes eqino varus*), which required surgical operation to correct. In April 1898 nine children were undergoing treatment in the Hospital for Crippled Children, and the regents of the University voted fifty dollars to provide an artificial limb for one Leon Filiatrault of Crookston, Minnesota, whose leg had been amputated. In July 1898 the hospital contained twelve children undergoing treatment. During its first year, expenditures for the hospital were some $1,500, including just over $100 for artificial limbs and braces. Dr. Gillette contributed his services without charge.

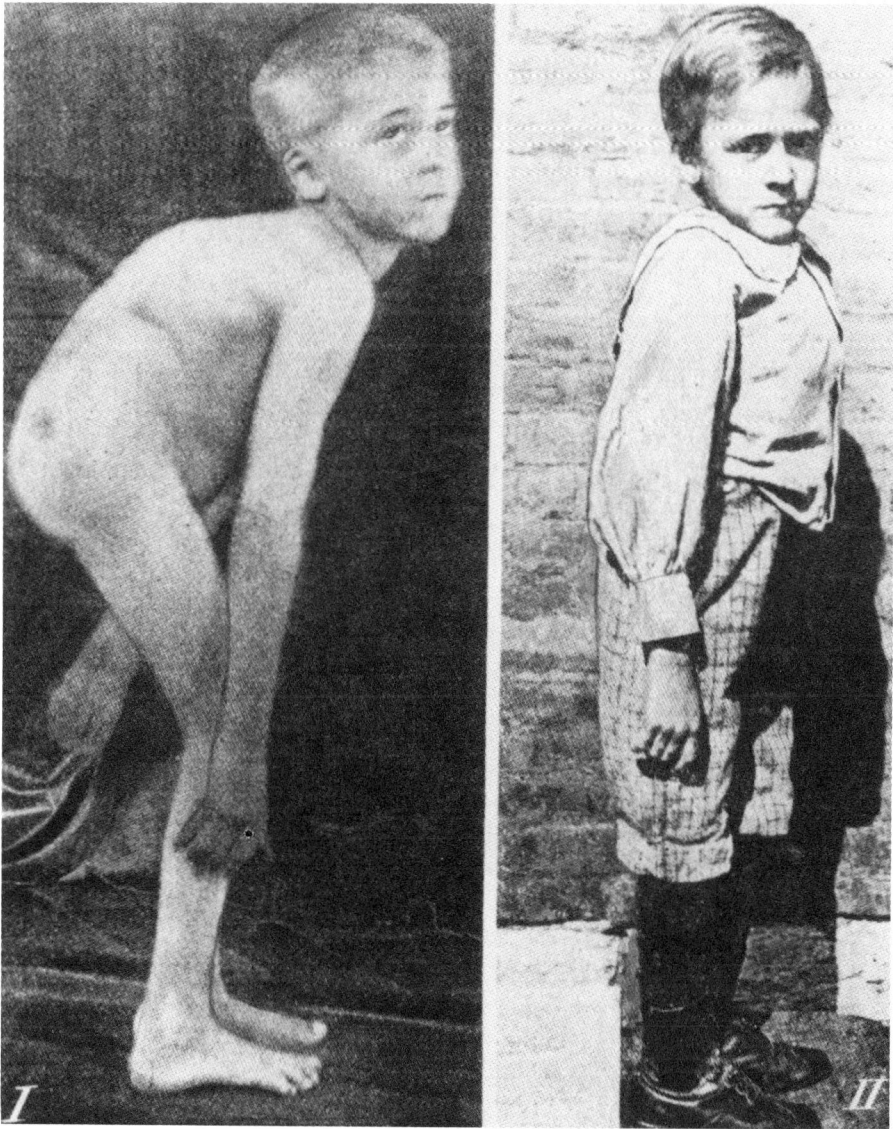

FIGURE 5:7 Arthur Gillette's first patient at the Hospital for Crippled Children. I. Before treatment. II. After treatment. *St. Paul Medical Journal,* 1900.

When in 1899 the members of the legislature visited the hospital they were "of one mind" that the hospital should be continued and should become a permanent institution of the state,[21] and the university renewed its contract with the City of St. Paul for another two years. The hospital continued to grow; in the four months December 1900 through March 1901 it cared for fifty-seven patients at a cost of $3,461.[22] By July 1901, near the end of its fourth year, the hospital had expended $11,513, and the university had received from the legislature a new appropriation to continue the cause.[23] In 1903 the University of Minnesota awarded an honorary M.D. degree to Arthur Gillette "in consideration of his valuable services and his eminence as a teacher of orthopaedic surgery . . . ."[24] Dr. Gillette and other members of the hospital staff were members of the medical faculty and the Hospital for Crippled Children was used to teach orthopedic surgery to medical students. To the glory of Minnesota, since 1897 no crippled child in the state has gone without treatment because of poverty.

The Medical Library

In May 1897 George S. Millard, brother of the late Dean Perry H. Millard and executor of his estate, wrote to the Board of Regents that before his death Dean Millard had told his family that he wanted to give his medical library to the medical department of the university, but in his will, written during his final illness in the Johns Hopkins Hospital at Baltimore, there was no mention of his library. His family, knowing Dean Millard's intentions, desired to fulfill his wishes by giving his medical library to the university, but they could not do so because the youngest heir, Dean Millard's seventeen-year-old son, John Jay Millard, was not of age. As a minor he could not give his consent to the gift, nor could the other heirs or the executor act for him. In the circumstances the family and executor had agreed to offer the library to the university to hold conditionally until John Jay Millard should come of age in four years' time when he would give his legal consent to the gift. The regents accepted the books on these conditions, and the university thus received the 700 volumes of Dean Millard's medical library including many old and rare medical books.[25]

Two years earlier, in December 1895, the executive committee of the College of Medicine and Surgery had established permanent subcommittees of which one was responsible for equipment and library.[26] In the spring Professor Thomas G. Lee was appointed chairman of the committee on equipment and library, and continued in that position for some years. The library was established in Medical Hall and shortly afterward Dr. Lee recommended that the Department of Medicine purchase an accession register, establish a card catalogue, and insert ownership labels in its books with special bookplates for the books given by the late Dean Millard.[27] The library collection benefited from gifts made by faculty members. Dr. James Moore and Dr. George Hendricks contributed runs of journals and Dr. Amos Abbott provided eighteen volumes of the *American Journal of Obstetrics* along with the promise to continue the subscription for the library at his own expense.[28] The library received 364 volumes from the Surgeon General's Office of the United States Army. In addition to gifts some purchases were made, such as copies of Gould's *Medical Dictionary* which was requested by the sophomore class.[29] Soon the library had received so many gifts of unbound journals that

Dr. Lee made a special request for $250 to bind them and provide additional bookcases.[30] With the students and faculty taking such an interest in the library, Dr. Lee asked for a list of leading books in the various branches of medicine to be considered for purchase and in November 1899 the executive committee appropriated $175 for the purchase of books.[31] In March 1900 the university librarian transferred to the medical library a number of medical dissertations from Kiel University in Germany.[32] A donation of 250 volumes of dental and homeopathic books and bound volumes of journals broadened the scope of the library's holdings, and the *Bulletin* for 1902-03 described the medical library as "containing some three thousand volumes and supplied with current periodicals."[33] By 1906 the medical library contained more than four thousand volumes.[34]

The medical library in Medical Hall was only part of the collection of books and journals in the Department of Medicine. The Colleges of Dentistry and Pharmacy each possessed their own libraries, and within the College of Medicine and Surgery many departments had organized departmental libraries. In 1907 Dr. Thomas G. Lee, in his capacity as librarian of the Department of Medicine, estimated that the various libraries within the department contained together nearly ten thousand bound volumes and fourteen thousand unbound volumes, including monographs, reprints of journal articles, and dissertations, and received about one hundred and seventy-five current periodicals. In 1905, through the generosity of Alfred F. Pillsbury, John S. Pillsbury, and Charles C. Pillsbury, the department of histology and embryology acquired a large part of the working library of the late Professor Wilhelm His of Leipzig, containing about eighty-five hundred titles by some twenty-five hundred authors.[35]

The libraries in the Department of Medicine were reinforced further by the general library of the University of Minnesota which in 1907 contained some one hundred and fifteen thousand volumes and received several hundred current periodicals.[36] The library of the department of animal biology in particular supplemented the libraries of the medical department. When in 1910 Hal Downey was working at Berlin, he found the library facilities there so poor that he had difficulty in consulting the scientific literature on blood cells. "If I could get aboard one of the dirigible balloons that we see flying over the city occasionally," Downey wrote to Henry Nachtrieb at Minnesota, "and have it take me to the U. of M. I could have my literature looked up in a short time."[37]

Changes in the Faculty

A striking feature of the life of the medical school at the turn of the century was the frequency of illness and death among both students and faculty. Students were frequently absent for periods of several weeks with typhoid fever, a disease which tended to occur among young adults who came to the city from small towns, villages, or farms, where they might have had no previous exposure to typhoid infection. Occasionally students came down with tuberculosis and had to leave the university without completing their medical course. It was all too easy for medical students to contract tuberculosis by exposure to tuberculous patients in clinics or from exposure to other students with tuberculosis.

The faculty, because older and more likely immune, were less liable to contract typhoid fever, and they may have possessed greater resistance to tuberculosis, but they, too, were frequently ill as well as being subject to grave hazards in their work. A prick of the finger or a minor cut while performing a post-mortem examination might lead to a serious infection if not to a fatal septicemia. Another common consequence of the performance of post-mortems was the development of tubercular infection, marked by the formation of tubercles on the fingers or hands. With alarming frequency members of the medical faculty died.

On 21 January 1898 Charles L. Wells of Minneapolis, who had been professor of diseases of children since the founding of the school, died suddenly and unexpectedly. To fill the immediate vacancy created by Dr. Wells's death, Albert Senkler of St. Paul, professor of clinical medicine, took over his lectures for the remainder of the academic year. The following June the Board of Regents appointed H. B. Sweetser clinical professor of diseases of children. In April they had already appointed James T. Christison a clinical instructor in pediatrics.[38] On 24 September 1899 the professor of anatomy, George Hendricks, died of an acute kidney infection (Bright's disease) after an illness of several months. The teaching of anatomy then fell entirely on the shoulders of the assistant professor, Charles A. Erdmann.[39]

On 10 December 1899 the beloved Albert Senkler died at his home in St. Paul at the age of fifty-seven after more than a year of illness from progressive heart failure.[40] At his death Dr. Senkler, like Dean Millard, left his medical library to the university. Among other books, Dr. Senkler's bound volumes of the *British Medical Journal* are now in the Biomedical Library of the University of Minnesota.

The death of Perry Millard in February 1897 had left vacant the chairs of the principles and practice of surgery and of medical jurisprudence as well as the deanship. For a time during the winter of 1897 no lectures were delivered in surgery, but on March 12 the professor of genito-urinary surgery, James Dunn, began lectures on general surgery.[41] In May 1897 Charles A. Wheaton of St. Paul was elected to succeed the late Dean Millard as professor of surgery, with a salary of $600 and responsibility for the delivery of some fifty lectures on surgery annually. The Board of Regents agreed that if Dr. Wheaton were not able to give all the lectures on surgery himself, he might ask the other surgical professors, Frederick A. Dunsmoor, James H. Dunn, and James E. Moore, to assist him and divide the $600 among them in proportion to the lectures given.[42]

Two years later, Dr. Wheaton resigned as professor of the practice of surgery because of ill health. James H. Dunn of Minneapolis, who had been professor of genito-urinary diseases and of clinical surgery, was appointed professor of the practice of surgery to succeed Dr. Wheaton. Then at the age of forty-six, James Henry Dunn was the leading surgeon in Minneapolis; he was greatly admired and

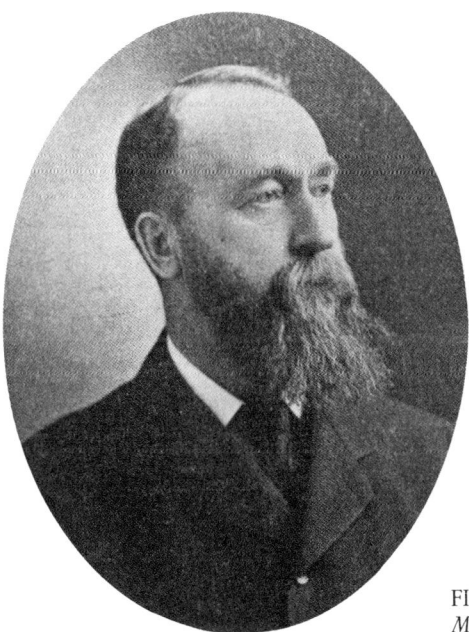

FIGURE 5:8 Albert Senkler. *St. Paul Medical Journal*, 1900.

loved by his professional colleagues, by his patients, and by the community at large. At age fifteen, James Dunn had been left to his own resources by the death of first his father and then a neighboring farmer who had given him a foster home. He decided to become a school teacher and completed his training in 1872 at the Winona Normal School. He became principal of public schools at Alexandria and Sauk Center, and during the summers taught in the Minnesota State Teachers Institute. While preparing to teach courses in hygiene, Dunn became interested in medicine and in 1875 entered Rush Medical College at Chicago. In 1876 he transferred to New York University where he was graduated M.D. in 1878. Dr. Dunn then began to practice medicine at Shakopee, Minnesota, where, because he was living in a community that included many German people, he acquired a working knowledge of the German language. His ability to speak German served Dr. Dunn very well when in 1883 he went abroad to Germany to visit and study in clinics at Berlin, Munich, Halle and Vienna. In Germany James Dunn was deeply impressed by the successful use of Lister's antiseptic methods by German surgeons, and by the complete absence of suppuration, pyemia, erysipelas, and septicemia from the surgical wards of the hospitals. Dr. Dunn returned to Minneapolis from Germany in 1885 an enthusiastic advocate of antiseptic surgery, and two years later he described sixty-one major operations that he had performed since his return without a single case of erysipelas, pyemia, septicemia, or excessive suppuration.[43]

James Dunn mastered the concepts and methods of antiseptic surgery by 1885, and, as he performed a greater number of operations, he became an increasingly

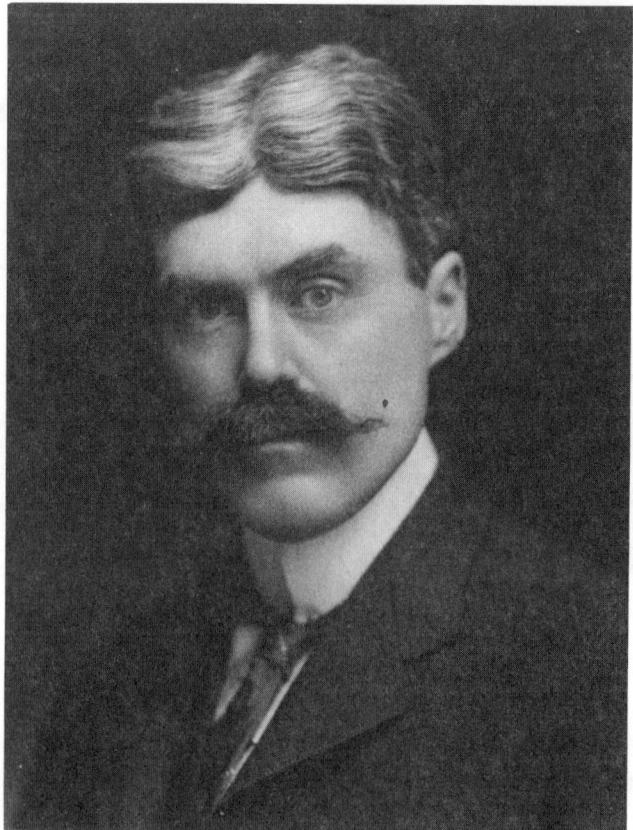

FIGURE 5:9   James Henry Dunn. Courtesy Mn U Archives.

skilled surgeon. As a surgeon he was also a devoted physician who gave his whole heart and mind to the care of his patients. Fluent in French and German, he read widely in the medical literature. So absorbed was he in things medical that in other matters he was extremely absent-minded. Shortly after his return to Minneapolis in 1885, Dr. Dunn married Miss Agnes Macdonald of St. Paul. Three months after his marriage he returned one day to the boardinghouse where he had lived as a bachelor, entered, and sat down at the dinner table. When one of his acquaintances asked whether Mrs. Dunn were out of the city, he said, "Oh—!", jumped up, took his hat, and went home.[44]

In 1887 Dr. Dunn became city physician of Minneapolis and organized the first city hospital for Minneapolis.[45] During the last three months of 1887 Dr. Dunn was responsible for the care of 164 patients who were received and treated at the Minneapolis City Hospital, many of them with typhoid fever.[46] He was also chief surgeon of St. Mary's Hospital and of Asbury Hospital in Minneapolis.

As a professor of surgery James Dunn was a brilliant lecturer who took great trouble to present the latest developments in surgery to his students. On 14

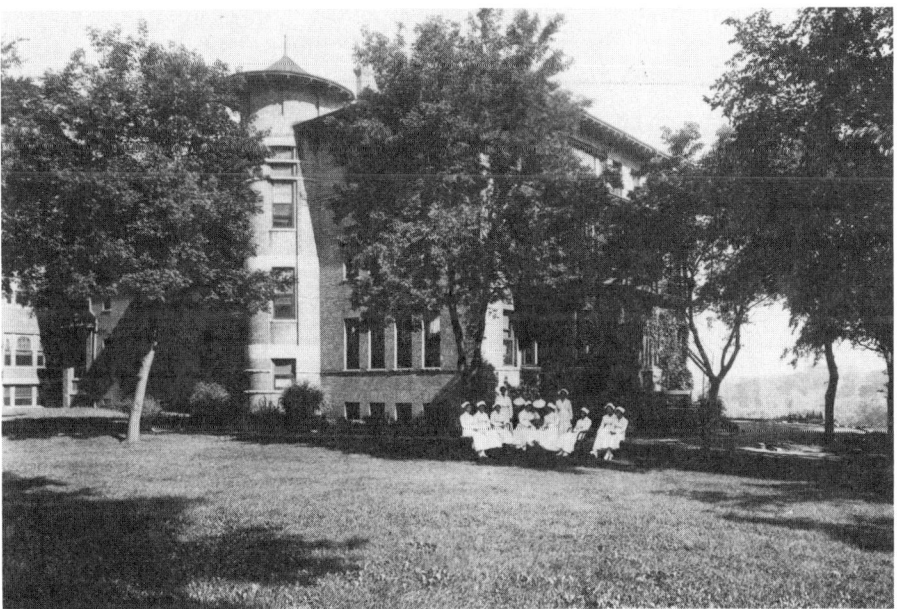

FIGURE 5:10   St. Mary's Hospital, Minneapolis, 1920. Courtesy St. Mary's Hospital.

November 1900, in the course of a clinical lecture at St. Mary's Hospital, Minneapolis, Dr. Dunn performed two operations, one for fistula in ano on a thirty-five-year-old man, and the other for tuberculous glands on the neck of a fifteen-year-old girl. He performed the operation for fistula in ano first because it could be completed quickly, wearing rubber gloves to do so. He then thoroughly cleaned his hands and operated on the neck of the girl without gloves because of the delicate nature of the surgery. In discussing the use of surgery on tuberculous glands, he presented the arguments for and against operation, and the factors essential to ensure that the surgery would benefit the patient. The second operation required so much time that Dr. Dunn did not complete it until after the class had left.[47]

Dr. Dunn urged his students to read the surgical literature extensively, especially in relation to the cases that they saw in clinics. In clinics Dunn warned his students not to regard the watching of major operations as the central feature of clinical education. They were not to assume that operating was the most essential thing in surgery.

> We have many operators in these days, but not so many surgeons. Most anybody can operate. In fact, some operate very beautifully who are very poor surgeons. Diagnosis, excellent surgical judgment, non-operative management, and many other things on the whole are certainly far more difficult to acquire, and not less necessary. Indeed, it is a curious fact that the greatest surgeons have rarely been brilliant operators. Understand me, I would not disparage beautiful technique. Acquire as much as possible

of it; only remember that it is to true surgery as polished manners are to character. The really difficult part of surgery is much deeper . . . . The whole object of surgery is to cure or relieve, not simply to operate.[48]

He advised students to master slight ailments and minor surgery as well as major operations.

Although Dr. Dunn said that his major duty was to deliver a course of thirty lectures on surgery, he acknowledged that lectures were of limited value in the teaching of surgery, but ". . . until we have a great University hospital, with material enough to illustrate at any time every phase of ordinary surgical practice, it will be desirable to cover systematically the more important and commoner surgical affections by didactic lectures. . . ."[49]

In June 1900 Dr. J. Clark Stewart, who since 1896 had held the title of professor of surgical and clinical pathology, requested that his title be changed to that of professor of the principles of surgery.[50] Initially Dr. Dunn objected to the change, but he later agreed on condition that his own title be changed to that of professor of surgery and that he be acknowledged as "Chief of the didactic surgical department, without whose cooperation changes in the various courses should not be made . . . ."[51] Dr. Dunn's letter of 25 February 1901 to Dr. J. Clark Stewart, in which he set forth the conditions of his agreement to Dr. Stewart's change of title, was also signed "Approved—C. A. Wheaton, F. A. Dunsmoor, J. E. Moore, J. Clark Stewart," so that the letter became a joint agreement among the surgical professors, establishing their relationship and acknowledging the authority of Dr. Dunn as professor of surgery to oversee surgical teaching. Thus several years before the College of Medicine and Surgery was organized into departments, the surgical professors were beginning to work together as a department of surgery. The forthright, vigorous, and generous character of James Dunn, and the high respect in which his colleagues held him, was undoubtedly essential to obtain such cooperation. The agreement among the surgeons was approved by the faculty and given effect by the Board of Regents.

During the autumn of 1897 Dr. Dunn suffered an illness that attacked his lungs resulting in an empyema from which he nearly lost his life. In January 1898 he went south for his health.[52] When he returned to Minneapolis at the beginning of April he was much improved, but the illness had left him with an impaired heart so that after 1898 he suffered to some degree from heart failure. On 17 June 1904, after delivering a paper on the surgical treatment of stricture of the oesophagus at a meeting of the American Surgical Association in St. Louis, James Dunn died of a heart attack in his hotel room.

In October 1904 the Board of Regents appointed James E. Moore as professor of surgery. Dr. Moore was one of the leading surgeons in Minnesota with a national reputation based upon his publications, especially upon his book on orthopedic surgery that had appeared in 1898.[53] The son of a Methodist minister, Moore was born at Clarkesville, Pennsylvania in 1852. He was educated at the Poland Union Seminary at Poland, Ohio and began to study medicine at the University of Michi-

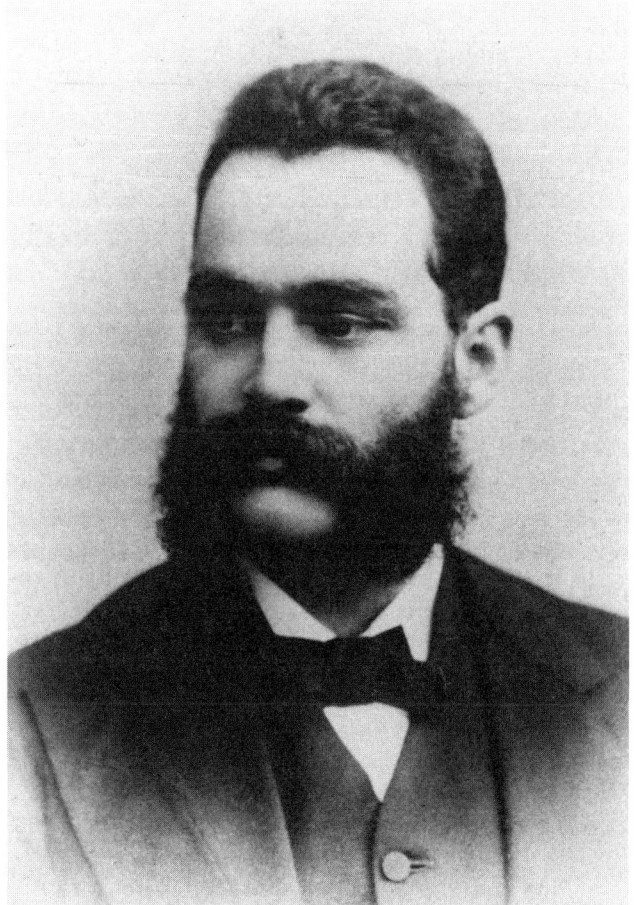

FIGURE 5:11 James E. Moore, 1888. Courtesy Mn U Archives.

gan. In 1872 he went to New York City to continue his medical studies at the Bellevue Hospital Medical College, where his interest was aroused in orthopedic surgery. Bellevue was then the only medical college in the United States to have a chair of orthopedic surgery, held by Lewis A. Sayre.[54] After graduating from Bellevue in 1873, and a year in practice at Fort Wayne, Indiana, Dr. Moore returned for two years of clinical study in hospitals at New York. He then spent six years in country medical practice at Emlenton, Pennsylvania where he made most of his calls on horseback, dispensing medicines from his saddlebags.

In 1882 Moore moved to Minnesota, but after three years in practice at Minneapolis went, like James Henry Dunn, to Europe for extended periods of study at Berlin, Paris, and London. On his return to Minneapolis in August 1887, Moore announced that he would restrict his practice to surgery—the first practitioner in the Northwest so to specialize. The following year he was appointed professor of orthopedic surgery in the newly founded medical college at the university. Like his fellow surgeons Millard, Wheaton, and Dunn, in the 1880s Moore practiced and advocated antiseptic surgery, and was prompt to adopt the techniques of aseptic surgery when they became practicable about 1890. After 1897 he gave his whole time to general surgery. As gentle and courteous as he was capable, and always moderate in his charges to patients, Moore was unfailing in his generosity in providing surgical care to poor patients. He was an unusually effective teacher who by his sincerity and charm drew students to himself and exerted a deep influence upon them.[55]

In March 1902 Dr. Rollin E. Cutts, a graduate of the medical school in 1893, died suddenly of a cerebral hemorrhage at the early age of thirty-five. Although a young man, Dr. Cutts was regarded very highly by his colleagues and the College of Medicine and Surgery was closed the afternoon of his funeral in respect for his memory. A year after his death his wife, Dr. Mary E. Smith Cutts, also a graduate of the medical school, gave as a memorial to her husband the sum of $500, the income from which was to provide a gold medal to be awarded annually for an essay on surgery by a senior medical student.

The Growth of the Curriculum

Early in 1898 the executive committee held meetings with the faculty to revise the teaching schedule for medicine and surgery and their related subjects. Changes were occurring rapidly, particularly in laboratory medicine, and such changes needed to be incorporated into the curriculum. At one meeting Frank Wesbrook presented a plan for the complete revision of the courses on bacteriology and pathology. He proposed that third-year students should have a lecture and laboratory course in which they would prepare their own cultures of pathogenic bacteria from diseased tissues, and would learn to distinguish pathogenic bacteria from other forms. Dr. Wesbrook would also teach general pathology at the beginning of the year and in the second semester the students would have lectures and laboratory work on the special pathology of various organs and tissues. Both the third and fourth-year students would have an opportunity to participate in autopsies at the various hospitals under the direction of the pathologist in charge.

When the third-year students began to take Wesbrook's laboratory course in the fall of 1898, they found that the preparation of culture media and the growing of bacterial cultures required long hours in the laboratory. "They seem to enjoy the work, however," *Ariel* reported, "and are much interested."[56] In October 1899 *Ariel* noted that bacteriology was keeping the third-year students in the laboratory until nearly six o'clock, but that they found the work very interesting.[57] A month later *Ariel* commented enthusiastically:

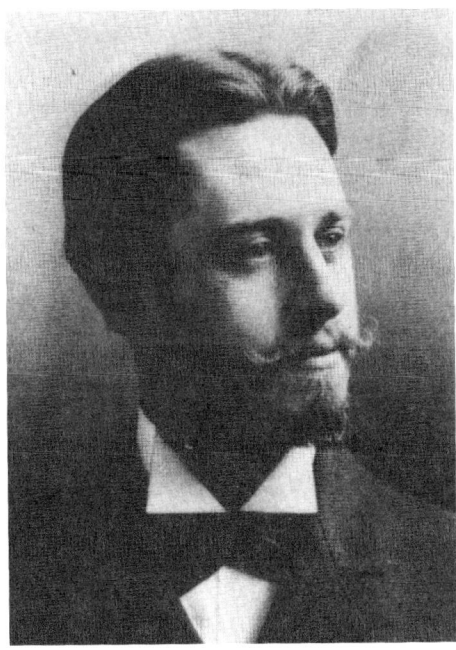

FIGURE 5:12 George Douglas Head, circa 1900. Courtesy Mn U Archives.

Dr. Wesbrook is giving the Juniors a very interesting and instructive course in Bacteriology. Medical students cannot too fully realize the important part in medicine played by this particular branch. Without it in many cases precision in diagnosis would be entirely lost . . . . We are very fortunate in having one of the most thoroughly equipped laboratories in America, and all should embrace the exceptional opportunities there offered. 'Twill pay an hundred fold, even though the hours are long and exacting.[58]

On 9 December *Ariel* again noted, "The work in Bacteriology goes merrily on."[59]

In January 1898 George Head included in a class on general microscopy an examination of the blood for diagnostic and clinical purposes. The students were greatly interested and on 22 January the *Ariel* suggested that such instruction be part of the regular required work.[60] In February the executive committee asked Dr. Wesbrook to prepare an outline for a course in clinical microscopy.[61] During the winter of 1900 such a course was taught as part (*b*) of Special Pathology to the third-year students in the second semester by Dr. Head. The course dealt with the microscopic and chemical study of blood, sputum, urine, and the contents of the alimentary canal. The students also examined animal parasites in tissues and studied the histology of various kinds of tumors, staining, mounting, and examining specimens for themselves.[62] On 7 April the *Ariel* noted that Dr. Head's "very interesting and practical course" had ended late in March. "It is to be hoped," *Ariel* added, "that in the near future the doctor may be able to extend this excellent course."[63]

Thus in 1900 George Head was able to introduce at Minnesota the latest refinements in microscopic methods of clinical diagnosis used at Johns Hopkins. The awareness of the existence of such techniques impressed the students deeply. At the end of the term in June 1900 a committee of the junior class wrote to Dean Ritchie to complain that much valuable clinical material was not being used and that they were "merely hearing of recent advances without receiving practical training and experience in modern clinical methods." They asked that a clinical laboratory be fitted up in the new dispensary building and placed in charge of a competent man such as Dr. Head.[64] The following October the executive committee granted Dr. Head money to equip a laboratory for clinical microscopy.[65] The laboratory proved useful; in March 1902, Dr. Head requested for clinical microscopy a longer, separate course and a larger budget.[66]

In addition to lengthening the medical course to four years and adding new courses and laboratory classes, the college in 1897 also proposed to raise its entrance requirements. As a result of a conference with Hamline University, which conducted the only other medical school in the state, the college decided that in 1898 its entrance examinations would cover English composition, elementary algebra, physics, Latin, United States history, and physiology, the last two subjects being new additions. The following year the requirements would increase to include more advanced examinations in Latin, consisting of examinations in Latin grammar and three books of Caesar's *Commentaries,* and plane geometry. By 1900 admission requirements would be the same as those for entrance to the academic departments of the University of Minnesota and Hamline University.[67] Medical students at Minnesota would no longer be of doubtful literacy.

Having raised their standards to the level of the university's academic departments, the medical school decided to require some college work before admittance. For admittance to the medical school in the fall of 1902, one year of college was required, and the number of students fell to only 40 from 136 the year before. The decline was so precipitous that the *Bulletin* for 1903 did not even include a list of the first-year class, as it had done the year before. Although by 1904 the second-year class had gained eight students, it was still little more than half the size of the third-year class. In the face of such a severe loss of students the college must not have thought it prudent to raise the admission requirements further in 1904. Nevertheless, the 1904 *Bulletin* announced that in 1905 two years' work in an accredited college or university would be required for admission to the medical college.[68]

In 1903 the university also established a six-year combined academic and medical course, leading at the end of four years to the degree of bachelor of science and at the end of six years to the M.D. degree. During the first two years students took courses in the college of science, literature, and the arts, and in their third year began courses in the college of medicine and surgery.

The question of admission requirements—one year of college work or two years—brought to light a "marked diversity of sentiment". The plummeting enrollment figures caused the executive committee to approve an expenditure of

$500 for advertising. The integrity of the six-year course of combined academic and medical studies was put in jeopardy. President Northrop intervened by asking the medical faculty to consider two questions: first, whether two years of college work were desirable "as a necessary preparation for medical study," and second, if the requirement were desirable, should it take effect in 1905.[69]

In accordance with President Northrop's request, Dean Ritchie called a meeting of the faculty for the evening of Friday, 14 April 1904, but only ten members of the faculty, including the dean, appeared, and three others were present by proxy. The professors of the basic medical sciences were all present, but very few of the professors of clinical subjects. Dean Ritchie stated that he favored a progressive raising of the standards for admission, but he thought that the announced requirement for 1905 should be postponed. After thorough discussion of the question, the faculty were unanimous in their answer to President Northrop's first question. They all believed that two years of college work were desirable as a preparation for medical study, but on the second question, whether the requirement should take effect in 1905, they were divided. Nine were for the maintenance of the announced requirement for 1905, while four, including Dean Ritchie, were against. All of the professors of the basic sciences (anatomy, histology and embryology, physiology, and pathology) were for the maintenance of the 1905 requirement, perhaps because they, more than the clinical faculty, had to deal with the educational deficiencies of the first and second-year students. Yet, standing up with Dean Ritchie in opposition was the professor of surgery, Dr. James Dunn, who with his quick wit and Irish eloquence was in debate a host in himself. Although the vote at the meeting was strongly for the maintenance of the 1905 requirement, so few of the medical faculty were present that the votes in favor may actually have represented a minority of faculty opinion.

Feelings evidently ran high over the question, whether because of the question itself or because it served to bring to light deep-seated tensions among the faculty. President Northrop, who was present at the meeting, informed the medical faculty that the Board of Regents had postponed indefinitely the 1905 requirement of two years of college preparation for admission to the medical course because of the lack of "any definite expression of the Faculty's views," and would rescind their action on the request of the faculty. The faculty voted unanimously to ask the Board of Regents to rescind its action at once.

On 17 June 1904 the *Minneapolis Journal* announced the death of Dr. Dunn of a heart attack, while attending the meeting of the American Surgical Association at St. Louis.[70] The next day the *Minneapolis Journal* contained another article describing opposition to Dean Ritchie among members of the medical faculty. The article stated that several members of the faculty had advised Dean Ritchie to resign. "Those who have so advised Dean Ritchie [the article continued] have told him frankly that they believed, for one thing, that his attitude toward the proposed raising of entrance requirements demonstrated that he did not share their desire to place the school on a higher plane, and to keep abreast of other colleges which are advancing rapidly."[71] The faculty members who spoke to Dean

Ritchie and who were interviewed by the reporter for the *Minneapolis Journal* were not identified. The newspaper article was clearly an effort to bring pressure on the dean to resign. The writer went on to say that Dean Ritchie had no intention of resigning and intended to do everything he could to maintain his position.

The admissions question was resolved when the Board of Regents decided in May 1906 to implement the requirement of two years of college education for admission to the medical college. Among the fifty-eight students of the first-year class, thirty-two, or 55 percent, could already satisfy the new requirement, and the proportion would be even higher if the students in the six-year course were included. The new building for the Institute of Public Health and Pathology was approaching completion. When it became available the college would possess much larger and better facilities for laboratory instruction, on a level comparable with the laboratories then existing at any medical school in the United States. The great deficiency of the college was the lack of a hospital in which to provide clinical education for the medical students, but by 1906 the college could hope presently to acquire a hospital. In 1905 Mary Ellen Hoar Elliot bequeathed to the university the residue of her estate with the instruction that the funds (amounting ultimately to $100,000) be used to build a hospital in memory of her husband, Dr. Adolphus F. Elliot, who died in 1901. Although there would be some delay before the funds became available, in 1906 the medical faculty could foresee that they would ultimately attain their dream of a university hospital.

In June 1906, in the midst of such pleasant prospects, Dean Ritchie resigned. During the nine years that Parks Ritchie had been dean, the College of Medicine and Surgery had added three substantial buildings, one of which, the Institute of Public Health and Pathology, was now the largest among the five medical buildings on the campus. The faculty had grown from forty-six instructors to eighty-seven, and the number of buildings from three to six, including the dispensary building at Seven Corners across the Mississippi River. During his deanship Parks Ritchie had continued his obstetric practice in St. Paul, spending only part of his time on the university campus. By 1906 the college required a dean who would be full time on the campus. Another consideration was the perennial tension between the physicians of Minneapolis and St. Paul. When the Board of Regents accepted Dr. Ritchie's resignation they appointed Frank F. Wesbrook as the new dean of the college. In selecting Dr. Wesbrook to succeed Dr. Ritchie, the Board of Regents found at once a man who was on the university campus full time, who had no links to either Minneapolis or St. Paul, and who was respected by the faculty of the whole college. Since his arrival at Minnesota in 1895, Wesbrook had built up his department of pathology and bacteriology from essentially nothing to make it recognized as one of the strongest in both teaching and research to be found in the United States. But more important than his personal achievements was Wesbrook's ability to gain the trust and enlist the cooperation not only of his faculty colleagues, but also of the community at large and most especially the members of the Minnesota legislature.

On 18 June, when the faculty of the College of Medicine and Surgery gave a testimonial banquet in honor of Dean Ritchie, President Northrop presented him with a silver loving cup to express the warm regard that his colleagues felt for him and their recognition of his long service to the university. At the banquet, Dean Wesbrook spoke also about the great contribution made by former Dean Perry H. Millard in establishing the State Board of Medical Examiners and the Department of Medicine in the university. Dr. Richard O. Beard then moved that Medical Hall, which had been built on the campus as a result of initiatives taken by Dean Millard and completed in 1892 under his supervision, should be named *Millard Hall*. Both retiring Dean Ritchie and Dean-elect Wesbrook supported the resolution, and President Northrop offered to present it to the Board of Regents for adoption at their next meeting.

Whatever may have been the disagreements among the faculty that led to Dean Ritchie's resignation, the faculty appreciated his work as dean and were united in their pride in the accomplishments of the medical school and their hopes for its future. To achieve that future Dean Wesbrook's immediate task was to bring into being a hospital directly under the control of the medical college.

NOTES

1. Board of Regents, Minutes, 1888–1905 (25 May 1897), p. 479.

2. College of Medicine and Surgery, Faculty, Minutes, 1895-1905(28 May 1897), pp. 35, 38.

3. College of Medicine and Surgery, Executive Committee, Minutes, 1895–1900 (16 September 1898), p. 93.

4. Ibid.

5. Board of Regents, Minutes, 1888–1905 (13 December 1898), p. 514.

6. Ibid. (6 April 1899), p. 515.

7. "College of Medicine and Surgery," *Ariel,* 1899–1900, *23,* 103.

8. University of Minnesota, *Bulletin, 1899,* vol. II, no. 9, "The College of Medicine and Surgery," p. 12.

9. "College of Medicine and Surgery," *Ariel,* 1899–1900, *23,* 53–54, p. 54.

10. College of Medicine and Surgery, Executive Committee, Minutes, 1895–1900 (26 May 1899), p. 111.

11. Ibid. (28 March 1902), p. 50.

12. Ibid. (26 September 1902), p. 77.

13. Board of Regents, Minutes, 1888–1905, (2 October 1902), p. 552.

14. "Dr. Wesbrook back from Europe with much interesting data," *Minn. Alumni Wkly,* 1904, *3,* no. 29, p. 6.

15. University of Minnesota, *Bulletin, 1905,* vol. IX, no. 9,"College of Medicine and Surgery," p. 14.

16. Arthur Sweeney, "A case of rabies," *St. Paul med. J.,* 1900, *2,* 550–554.

17. F. F. Wesbrook, "Extent of rabies" [letter to the editor, 7 August 1906], *J. Minn. St. med. Ass. & Northwest. Lancet,* 1906, *26,* 356.

18. Arthur J. Gillette, "State care of indigent crippled and deformed children," *St. Paul med. J.,* 1900, *2,* 76–86, pp. 77–78. A native of Rice County, Minnesota, where he was born in 1863, Arthur Gillette was educated in country schools and at Hamline Univer-

sity in St. Paul. He began the study of medicine at the Minnesota College Hospital but completed the medical course at the St. Paul Medical College where he was graduated in 1886. During 1886–87 he was a resident surgeon at the New York Orthopedic Dispensary and Hospital and then settled in practice at St. Paul. C. Eugene Riggs, Robert Earl, and Wallace H. Cole, "Memoriam to Dr. Gillette," *Minn. Med.*, 1921, *4*, 406–407.

19. In December 1897 Dr. Moore resigned the chair of orthopedics in the university, while retaining his title of professor of clinical surgery, and at the same time nominated Dr. Gillette to succeed him in the chair of orthopedics. Board of Regents, Minutes, 1888–1905 (25 August 1897), pp. 485–490. College of Medicine and Surgery, Executive Committee, Minutes, 1895–1900 (14 December 1897), p. 73.

20. Gillette (n.18).

21. Ibid.

22. Board of Regents, Minutes 1888–1905 (4 April 1901), p. 531.

23. Ibid. (3 October 1901), p. 539.

24. Ibid. The same year Dr. Moore resigned as consulting surgeon to the Hospital for Crippled Children.

25. Ibid. (25 May 1897), p. 476.

26. College of Medicine and Surgery, Executive Committee, Minutes, 1895–1900 (10 December 1895), p. 20; (28 February 1896) p. 29.

27. Ibid. (10 August 1897), p. 67.

28. Ibid. (8 March 1898), p. 82.

29. Ibid. (6 December 1898), p. 98

30. Ibid. (14 March 1899), p. 101.

31. Ibid. (10 October 1899), p. 117; (14 November 1899), p. 118.

32. Ibid. (20 March 1900), p. 135.

33. College of Medicine and Surgery, Executive Committee, Minutes, 1900–1905 (28 March 1902), p. 50; cf. College of Medicine and Surgery, *Bulletin*, 1902–03, p. 14.

34. College of Medicine and Surgery, *Bulletin, 1906–07*, p. 40.

35. Ibid., 1907–1908, vol. X, no. 13, p. 27.

36. Ibid.

37. Downey to Nachtrieb, 22 July 1910, quoted in Oliver P. Jones, "Hal Downey's hematological training in Germany, 1910–1911," *J. Hist. Med.*, 1972, *27*, 173–186, p. 176.

38. Board of Regents, Minutes, 1888–1905 (1 June 1898), p. 506; (12 April 1898), p. 497.

39. A native of Milwaukee, Wisconsin, Charles Erdmann was educated at the University of Wisconsin, but studied medicine at the University of Minnesota where he was graduated M.D. in 1893. After a year of postgraduate study at London and Vienna, he was appointed demonstrator of anatomy at Minnesota in 1894 and promoted to assistant professor in 1898. "Erdmann, Charles Andress," E. Bird Johnson, ed., *Forty years of the University of Minnesota,* p. 318. In April 1900 the Board of Regents appointed Dr. Erdmann acting professor of anatomy and a year later elected him professor of anatomy. Board of Regents. Minutes, 1888–1905 (5 April 1900), p. 522; (4 April 1901), p. 531.

40. Born in England, the son of a clergyman of the Church of England, Albert Senkler had come with his parents as a boy to Brockville, Ontario. Because he was a sickly child, he was educated at home by his father, a graduate of the University of Oxford, who gave his son a thorough classical education. Albert Senkler studied medicine at McGill University where he was graduated M.D. and Master of Surgery in 1863 at the age of twenty-one. In 1865 Dr. Senkler came to Minnesota where he practiced medicine first at St. Cloud, moving to St. Paul in 1880. His wide knowledge and extraordinary clinical judgment

caused Dr. Senkler to be held in unusually high esteem by his colleagues. "Obituary. Albert Edward Senkler, M.D., M.C.," *St. Paul med. J.*, 1900, *2*, 60–63.

41. "College of Medicine," *Ariel,* 27 February 1897, p. 14; 13 March 1897, p. 19.

42. Board of Regents, Minutes, 1888–1905 (25 May 1897), p. 478.

43. James H. Dunn, "A decade of observation and experience in antiseptic surgery," *Trans. Minn. St. med. Soc.,* 1887, pp. 56–81.

44. Robert Emmett Farr, "James Henry Dunn," *Surg. Gynec. Obstet.,* 1926, *43,* 396–398, p. 397.

45. "Obituary. Dr. James H. Dunn," *St. Paul med. J.,* 1904, *6,* 525–527.

46. Mary McNair McCune, "History of the Minneapolis General Hospital 1887–1930," (M.A. thesis, University of Minnesota, 1933), pp. 7, 10.

47. James H. Dunn, "Fistula in ano — tubercular glands of the neck," *Northwest. Lancet,* 1901, *21,* 5–8.

48. James H. Dunn, "Introductory lecture on surgery," *Northwest. Lancet,* 1902, *22,* 67–69, p. 68.

49. Ibid.

50. College of Medicine and Surgery, Executive Committee, Minutes, 1900–1905 (1 June 1900), p. 2.

51. James H. Dunn to J. Clark Stewart, 25 February 1901, College of Medicine and Surgery, Executive Committee, Minutes, 1900–1905 (8 March 1901), pp. 17–20.

52. "College of Medicine," *Ariel,* 1897, *21,* 205 ; p. 353.

53. James E. Moore, *Orthopedic surgery.*

54. Ibid., p. 18.

55. *Dictionary of American biography,* s.v. "Moore, James Edward" by Arthur T. Mann; *American medical biography,* s.v. "Moore, James Edward (1842–1918)" by A. A. Law; Ronald Dietzman, "James Edward Moore, M.D., educator and surgeon, his life and work," *J.-Lancet,* 1963, *83,* 157–160.

56. "College of Medicine. Medicine and Surgery," *Ariel,* 1898–99, *22,* 99.

57. Ibid., 1899–1900, *23,* p.67.

58. Ibid, pp. 127–128, p. 127.

59. Ibid., p. 150.

60. Ibid., 1897–98, *21,* 205.

61. College of Medicine and Surgery, Executive Committee, Minutes, 1895–1900 (7 February 1898), p. 79.

62. University of Minnesota, *Bulletin, The College of Medicine and Surgery, 1899,* vol. II, no. 9, p. 26.

63. "College of Medicine and Surgery," *Ariel,* 1899–1900, *23,* 330. George Douglas Head was born in Elgin, Minnesota in 1870, and was educated at the University of Minnesota where he was graduated B.A. in 1892 and then entered the College of Medicine and Surgery. After receiving the M.D. degree in 1895, Dr. Head began to practice medicine in Minneapolis. In 1897 he was appointed an instructor in pathology and in 1898 and again in 1900 went to the Johns Hopkins School of Medicine for postgraduate study, and in particular to learn more of the techniques of clinical microscopy. "Head, George Douglas," in Johnson, ed., *University of Minnesota* (n. 39), pp. 346–347.

64. College of Medicine and Surgery, Executive Committee, Minutes, 1900–1905 (1 June 1900), p. 2.

65. Ibid. (5 October 1900), p. 6.

66. Ibid. (28 March 1902), p. 51.

67. Ibid., 1895–1900 (13 April 1897), p. 59. Cf. University of Minnesota, *Bulletin, 1897–1898* (Department of Medicine) pp. 199–200.

68. *Bulletin* (n. 67), p. 18.
69. College of Medicine and Surgery, Faculty, Minutes, 1895–1905 (14 April 1904), pp. 115–116.
70. *Minneapolis Journal,* 17 June 1904, p. 6, col. 3.
71. *Minneapolis Journal,* 18 June 1904, p. 6, col. 2.

CHAPTER 6

The Elliot Memorial Gift and the New Medical Campus

In 1905 the death of Mary Ellen Hoar Elliot in California set in motion a train of events that led ultimately to the creation of a teaching hospital in conjunction with the medical school. Mary Elliot's husband, Dr. Adolphus F. Elliot, had practiced medicine in Minneapolis for about fifteen years until in 1883 his health forced him to leave Minnesota for the milder climate of California. During the Civil War, when Adolphus Elliot served as a junior officer with the Third Minnesota Regiment and was taken prisoner in Tennessee, he spent several months in a Confederate prison at Richmond, Virginia, an ordeal that had left his health permanently damaged. Dr. Elliot died in California in 1901, his wife surviving him by four years. In May 1905 Mr. Walter Trask, a close friend and attorney to the late Dr. Elliot, wrote to the university. As trustee under Mrs. Elliot's will, Mr. Trask stated that, after certain specific bequests, the residue of Mrs. Elliot's estate, estimated at more than one hundred thousand dollars, was available to the university for the building of a hospital in memory of her husband. The proposed hospital was to be operated in connection with the College of Medicine and Surgery. Dr. A. B. Cates of Minneapolis, professor of obstetrics, is said to have been instrumental in obtaining the Elliot gift.[1] The Board of Regents were hesitant to accept the gift, although one hundred thousand dollars in 1905 was a sum equal to more than twenty times that amount today and was even larger in proportion to the general level of wealth in Minnesota at that time. After months of inaction by the regents, on 15 November 1905 the executive committee recommended that at its next meeting the faculty of the College of Medicine and Surgery should urge the Board of Regents to accept the Elliot gift without further delay.[2] Through 1906 the matter of the Elliot gift remained unsettled, but as Dean Wesbrook reflected on the question of where to locate a hospital, whenever the Board of Regents might finally decide to accept the Elliot gift, he realized that there was no site on the existing university campus that would provide sufficient room for a hospital or allow for its future development together with the other buildings of the medical college that ought to be located in close relation to the hospital. In

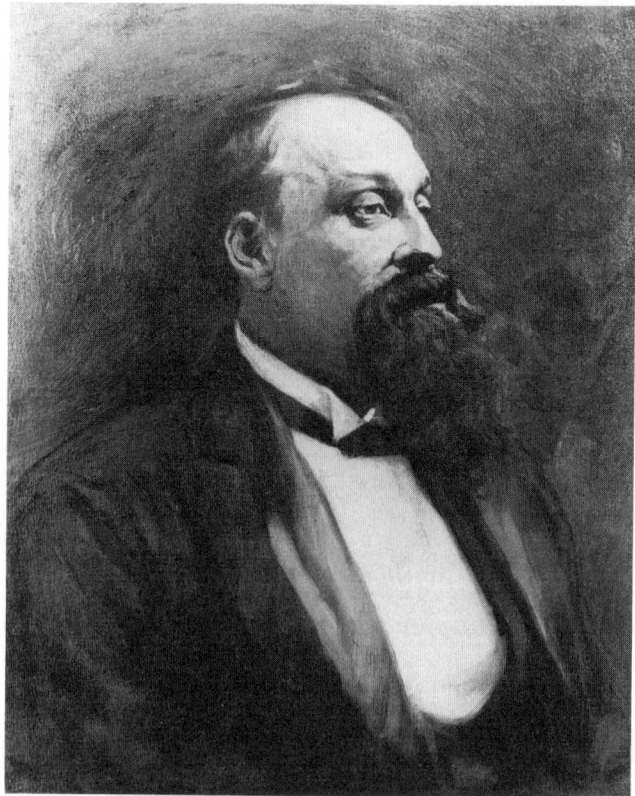

FIGURE 6:1   Adolphus F. Elliot. Courtesy Mn U Archives.

November 1906 Dean Wesbrook suggested to the executive committee that they should formulate plans for the most desirable arrangement of the laboratory departments then located in five separate buildings: Millard Hall, the Laboratory of Medical Sciences, the Chemistry Building, the Anatomy building and the Institute of Public Health and Pathology. Even though Dean Wesbrook recognized that several years would be required to accomplish the relocation of the basic science departments in new buildings on a new medical campus, such a rearrangement was much needed, and the college must be prepared to ask the legislature for the required funds.[3] Meanwhile, in 1906 the Board of Regents, which for several years had been chafing under the restrictions on their powers imposed by the state Board of Control, decided that they could not accept the Elliot bequest even though it could be used "to splendid advantage at the University."[4]

Confronted with the negative response of the regents to this generous gift and the possible unwillingness of the legislature to support a university hospital, in January 1907 a committee of eleven alumni of the medical college, led by Dr. George D. Head, addressed their fellow medical graduates in the following terms:

> The imperative need of the medical department of our state University is a clinical hospital entirely under its control in which clinical teaching can be done. Unless such a hospital is provided, and that speedily, the medical college of which you are now so justly proud will lose its high position among the first grade medical schools of the country and will graduate men inferior to the graduates of our best institutions. The condition of affairs exists not because our medical department has retrograded in the class of instruction which it gives, but because other medical schools with ample funds at their command have been able to provide themselves with hospital facilities entirely under their own control.[5]

Dr. Head's committee reminded their fellow alumni of how as medical students they had spent much time in traveling from one hospital to another in Minneapolis or St. Paul to attend clinics. Through the bequest of Mrs. Elliot, $115,000 had become available to build a university hospital, if the university could be enabled to accept it, and at its 1907 session the Minnesota legislature would be asked for appropriations to equip and maintain such a hospital. The hospital would be a charity hospital to which the counties of the state might send their sick poor, but for whom the counties would pay the state "a reasonable sum" per patient. Medical and surgical service would be provided by the medical faculty. To further the hospital project Dr. Head's committee said that a fund was being raised to purchase a site. They urged the medical alumni to " . . . do all in your power to instruct the state legislators of your district in this need of the medical department and place before them the reasons why a clinical hospital should be maintained by the state for its medical school."[6] In 1872 the Pennsylvania legislature had appropriated funds to build a hospital for the University of Pennsylvania medical school, and in 1875 the Michigan legislature had acted to create a hospital for the University of Michigan medical school at Ann Arbor. In 1900 the state of Missouri had built a hospital on the campus of the University of Missouri at Columbia. More recently the states of Massachusetts and New York had each provided state funds to create hospitals for medical teaching.[7] The *Minnesota Alumni Weekly* supported the committee's appeal editorially by contrasting the four and a half million dollars which had just been spent on the new state capitol building in St. Paul with the slightly more than two million that had been spent on buildings at the university throughout the whole history of the institution.[8]

On 2 April 1907 the Minnesota legislature responded to the urgings of Governor Johnson and the medical alumni by passing the "Elliot Memorial Hospital Bill" which provided that the Elliot Memorial Hospital would be part of the University of Minnesota, under the control of the Board of Regents. The hospital was to give free care and treatment to indigent sick persons who were residents of Minnesota. All medical or surgical care was to be given by members of the medical faculty, and the hospital was to be used for instruction in medicine and surgery.[9] The Board of Regents then acted to accept the Elliot gift.

During the winter of 1907, while the Elliot Hospital Bill was still pending in the legislature, Dean Wesbrook appointed a hospital committee composed of eleven members of the faculty, among whom seven were constituted a hospital site committee.[10] The first concern of the hospital site committee was to raise funds to purchase a site for the Elliot Memorial Hospital. The committee sought the help of Benjamin Gale of Minneapolis who proceeded to arrange a luncheon at which members of the site committee might explain their needs to a group of Minneapolis citizens. Among those whom Mr. Gale invited to the luncheon were various members of the family of the late Governor John Sargent Pillsbury, who until his death in 1901 had taken such a deep and generous interest in the university as to have been called its father. When Dr. James Moore and Dean Wesbrook described to the group assembled at the luncheon their need for money to buy land on which to build the hospital made possible by the Elliot gift, the various citizens present immediately subscribed $50,000. Afterward Dr. Moore remarked to Mr. Elbert L. Carpenter, one of the contributors, "Why it was all so easy. The people seemed glad to be asked to contribute." Later Mr. Carpenter explained why he and others gave so readily. They wished to honor the memory of Governor Pillsbury and to show their admiration and affection for President Northrop. "And finally," Carpenter added, they were moved by "a desire to uphold the hands of Dr. Wesbrook and the splendidly efficient Faculty of this medical school; for you may be sure our people know how this school is ranked in high places beyond the boundaries of Minnesota . . . ."[11]

In March 1907 the *Minnesota Alumni Weekly* announced that the money had been raised to purchase a site for the new hospital. The editor, noting that the medical faculty would provide free medical care to patients in the projected hospital, commented:

> Few people realize what the medical men are doing for the State at the present time. There are eighty-seven practicing physicians, who devote several hours each week to giving clinical instruction in the medical department, for which they receive no compensation. If these men were given anything like adequate pay for their service the expense to the State for the maintenance of that department would be about doubled.[12]

On 26 April 1907 the hospital committee and hospital site committee jointly recommended to the Board of Regents that the proposed hospital be located on four blocks of land between Washington Avenue and the Mississippi River in southeast Minneapolis, and that its precise location should be determined in relation to a general plan for a group of hospital buildings to be prepared by a committee of engineers, architects, and landscape gardeners. At that time the hospital committee thought that the Elliot Memorial building should be placed facing Washington Avenue on a site about midway between State Street and Riverside Parkway, slightly to the west of where the Coffman Memorial Union now stands. Various of the houses on the blocks to the south of Washington Avenue were to be used for a nurses' home, laundry, kitchen, and servants' quarters for the proposed hospital. The committee anticipated that the Elliot Memorial building would ultimately become an administration building for the university hospital surrounded by separate pavilions for medical patients, surgical patients, midwifery, diseases of children, isolation of contagious diseases, a pavilion for eye, ear,

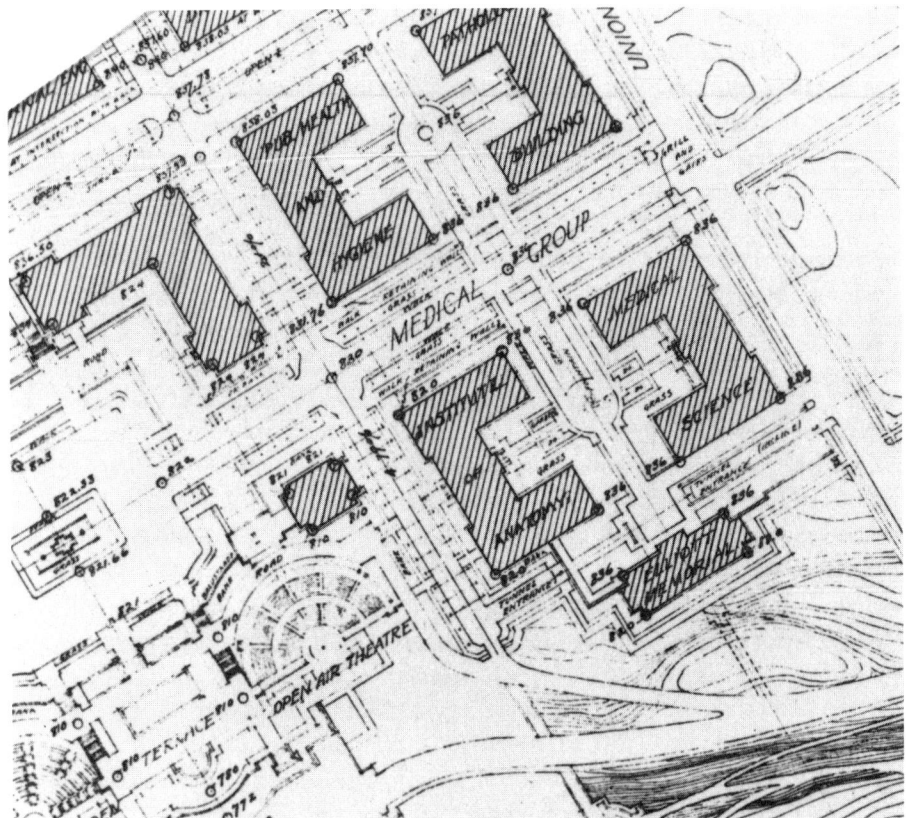

FIGURE 6:2 Cass Gilbert's original plan for the medical campus. Courtesy Mn U Archives.

nose, and throat patients, a tuberculosis pavilion, an outpatient building, and a residence for nurses. The Elliot Memorial building itself should be a fireproof structure of at least four storys, containing, in addition to medical and surgical wards, two amphitheaters, rooms for hospital offices and records, and clinical laboratories.[13]

By 1907, with a new hospital in prospect and in view of the growing needs of other colleges, the University of Minnesota was beginning to realize that it could no longer be contained within the narrow boundaries of the existing campus. At the meeting of the executive committee on 15 May 1907, to which the hospital committee presented its report, Dr. Frank Todd reported that two prominent alumni of Minneapolis, F. W. Clifford and Lewis S. Gillette, had become interested in the improvement of the university campus and had arranged to have the architects Cass Gilbert and F. W. Burnham prepare plans for the new campus, including the new university hospital.[14] In 1907 Cass Gilbert, then at the age of forty-eight, had recently acquired a national reputation as an architect through his design for the Minnesota State Capitol in St. Paul, completed in 1905, and his success in the competition to design the United States Customs House in New York City. He had recently received a commission to design the Woolworth Building in New York City and in 1908 would be elected president of the American Institute of Architects. Cass Gilbert now prepared a magnificent plan for the extension of the university campus along the axis of a central mall extending southward from the old campus to end in gardens and a park on the Mississippi River. Gilbert intended that Washington Avenue should be lowered and bridged over so as not to interrupt the continuity of the mall. The hospital and other medical buildings were to be arranged south of Washington Avenue to the east of the mall. Early in 1908 a Commission of Architects awarded Cass Gilbert a prize of $1,000 for the best plan for the extension of the university campus and in June of that year the Board of Regents placed Mr. Gilbert in charge of laying out the campus and of deciding the locations of the new buildings.[15]

During the summer and autumn of 1907 the medical faculty mulled over the various consequences that might follow from the location of the proposed hospital on a new part of the campus south of Washington Avenue, a half mile or more away from the existing group of medical buildings on the old campus. Meanwhile the College of Dentistry, extremely crowded in its quarters in Millard Hall, was clamoring for more space.[16] In December 1907 the executive committee recommended that block 10, north of Washington Avenue between Pleasant Street and the river, be reserved for a new anatomy building.[17] On 11 February 1908 the committee decided that the proposed anatomy building should house not only gross and microscopic anatomy, but also histology, embryology and neurology, activities then carried on in the Laboratory of Medical Sciences. They proposed to transfer physiology and pharmacology from the Laboratory of Medical Sciences to Millard Hall and to give the whole of the Laboratory of Medical Sciences to the College of Dentistry. The existing Anatomy Building was to be used for operative surgery and as a place to keep animals and to care for them following operations. It was also to be used by the departments of physiology and pharmacology for operative work on animals. With funds already available, the executive committee proposed to build an additional story on the Anatomy Building during the summer of 1908, the additional space to be used for the care of animals.

To implement their plans the executive committee recommended that the Board of Regents should request from the legislature $100,000 for a new anatomy building and $5,000 for its equipment. At the urging of the clinical members the committee also recommended a request for $150,000 for a hospital building to be an addition to the Elliot Memorial building, and $25,000 per year for maintenance of the proposed university hospital. Because such requests were so large the executive committee postponed final action on its recommendations to a second meeting to be held on 20 February 1908. This delay allowed Dean Wesbrook to confer with William J. Mayo, chairman of the medical committee of the Board of Regents, to obtain Dr. Mayo's opinion of the proposals. The minutes for the meeting of the executive committee on 20 February 1908 are missing. Dr. Mayo may have advised delay.

The following autumn the plans to use the existing Anatomy Building for operative surgery and the care of animals were shattered when on 6 October a fire destroyed it completely, leaving only the walls standing. Dr. Charles Erdmann lost his personal library and his papers together with many instruments and specimens.[18] The university was able to provide Dr. Erdmann with space for dissection and the teaching of gross anatomy in a house on Pleasant Street, but Dr. Moore had to postpone his dream of teaching operative surgery to senior medical students by actual operations on dogs.[19]

On 19 November 1908 the executive committee met for dinner at the Minneapolis Club with three members of the Board of Regents — John Lind, Benjamin F. Nelson, and Sidney M. Owen — to discuss the future development of the medical college. The regents present were favorable to a request for a new hospital building and in December the Board of Regents decided to ask the legislature for two buildings, an anatomy building and a medical science building, each to cost $200,000.[20] In the spring of 1909 the Minnesota legislature appropriated the funds requested, making the $200,000 for the anatomy building available 1 August 1909 and the same sum for a medical science building available two years later in August 1911. In 1909 the legislature also appropriated $350,000 for the purchase of land to implement the Gilbert plan for extension of the university.

On 10 February 1909 the executive committee received the report of a special committee that had conferred with Cass Gilbert about the general plans for new buildings for the college. The committee recommended that the college in its entirety be relocated south of Washington Avenue where there was some twenty-six acres in the area between Union Street and the Mississippi River. Even that area would probably within a few years become inadequate for the needs of the college. The committee noted that the buildings of the Harvard Medical School occupied fifteen acres and those of Johns Hopkins fourteen acres, with little space available for either on which to expand. Therefore, the committee recommended that nothing should be placed to the east of the proposed medical campus, that is, east of Union Street, that would prevent the ultimate extension of the medical buildings eastward.[21] The plan for the medical campus should provide for at least five large laboratory buildings in addition to the proposed university hospital. The Elliot Memorial building, for which the funds were already obtained, should in future become largely a hospital administration building. The university hospital should become a 1,000 bed hospital housed in ten separate pavilions each of 100 beds, with three pavilions each for medical and surgical cases, and individual pavilions for obstetrics, children's diseases, psychiatry, and infectious diseases. The hospital would also require buildings for a nurses' home, ambulances and storage, kitchens and service help, and laundry. After looking over the ground, Cass Gilbert had suggested that the western boundary of the medical campus should be State Street and that it should extend eastward as far as the needs of medical buildings might require. The executive committee approved the report and forwarded it to the Board of Regents.[22]

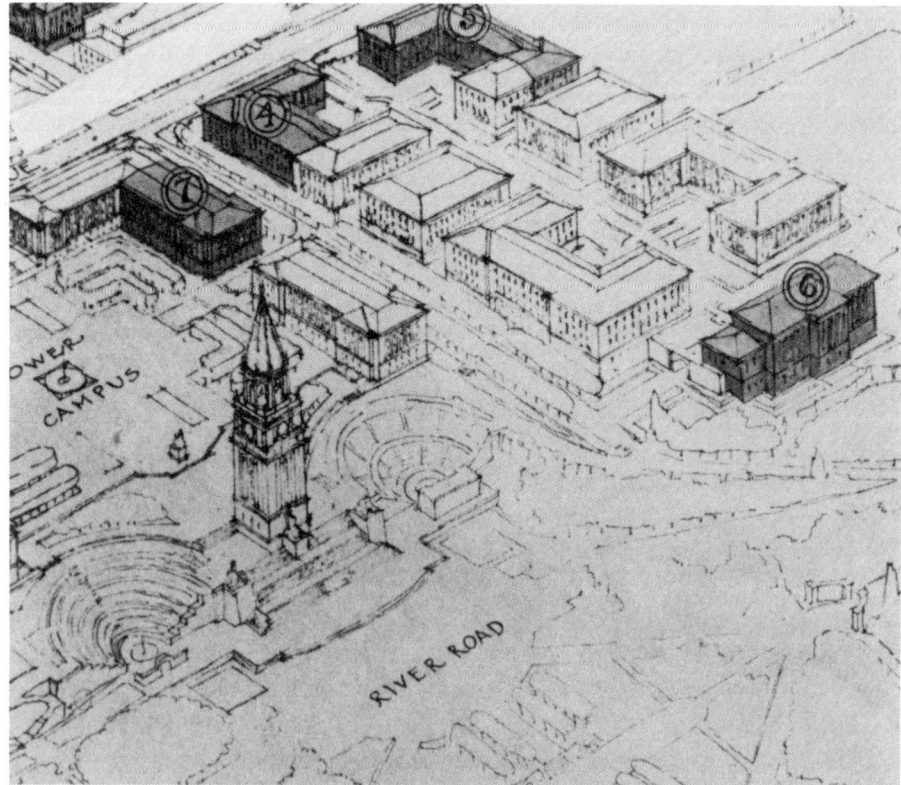

FIGURE 6:3 Sketches of buildings proposed for the first stage of Cass Gilbert's revised plan: (4) Institute of Anatomy; (5) Millard Hall; (6) Elliot Hospital; (7) Biology Building. Courtesy Mn U Archives.

Despite the fact that funds for the Elliot Memorial Hospital had been available for several years, construction had still not begun. In 1909, in accordance with Cass Gilbert's overall plan for the campus, the Board of Regents decided finally that the Elliot Hospital should be located overlooking the Mississippi River on the north side of Essex Street, between Church and Union Streets. They at first intended to place the anatomy building and new medical science building on the same block, but in November 1909 the executive faculty recommended that the whole of the block on which the Elliot Hospital was to be placed be left clear for the future expansion of the university hospital, and that the new anatomy and medical science buildings should be located on the block across Delaware Street to the north, between Delaware Street and Washington Avenue. With some reluctance the Board of Regents agreed to the change in site.[23]

During 1908 the university acquired land, which was primarily residential property, by purchase and condemnation, property extending south from the old campus to the river bluff and west as far as Union Street. Although the Elliot

Memorial Hospital would not be ready until the autumn of 1911, the university officially opened its hospital to patients on 22 March 1909. The regents made available three houses located on the newly acquired property, and they were equipped with beds; in the course of the next year an additional three houses were added. While dividing clinics, patient rooms, nurses' residence, and laundry and kitchen facilities among six houses was less than ideal, the faculty was glad to be getting on with the establishment of their own clinics. The original three houses were located at 200 and 304 State Street, and at 303 Washington Avenue. The largest house, that at 303 Washington Avenue, had formerly been the Phi Kappa Psi fraternity house. The three houses were equipped with twenty-four hospital beds. In the large house at 303 Washington Avenue the bedrooms were converted into wards. The operating room was on the first floor where there was also a delivery room and a kitchen in which meals for patients could be heated, the preparation and cooking of the food being done in another house. Because the staircase at 303 Washington Avenue was too narrow to permit patients to be carried up or down on stretchers, physicians or medical students carried patients in their arms to and from the operating room. Later the university also assigned to the hospital a house at 119 State Street; it was equipped with eighteen beds. The nursing staff consisted of five graduate nurses under the superintendent of nurses, Bertha Erdmann, who served also as chief surgical nurse. A sister of the professor of anatomy, Dr. Charles Erdmann, Miss Erdmann had gone to New York City for additional study in nursing education at Columbia Teacher's College.

The clinical staff of the university hospital was organized into three divisions, medicine, surgery, and obstetrics, with the chief of each division being the professor in charge of the corresponding department in the College of Medicine and Surgery. Thus Charles Lyman Greene was chief of the medical division, James E. Moore of the surgical division, and Parks Ritchie of the obstetrics division. Each chief of clinic could appoint two assistant chiefs of clinic who were in daily attendance at the hospital and were assigned patients in rotation. In addition twelve physicians were appointed to the staff for three month terms as *clinical associates,* so that they might study the patients under their charge with the aid of modern diagnostic methods and supported by trained laboratory personnel.

Finally senior medical students were brought into the hospital to participate in the examination, care, and treatment of patients under the supervision of the staff. The students each recorded their observations of the patient, and were asked to make recommendations for treatment.[24] Thus in 1909 Minnesota medical students began to enjoy a form of clinical clerkship similar to that which William Osler had developed for medical students at Johns Hopkins in 1895.

On opening day, 22 March 1909, the professor of surgery, James E. Moore, conducted the first clinic at the university hospital, assisted by Arthur T. Mann. In the presence of four other physicians and twenty-three senior medical students, Dr. Moore operated in the former Phi Kappa Psi fraternity house on two patients, one from Marietta, Minnesota for appendicitis, the other from Sandstone, Minnesota

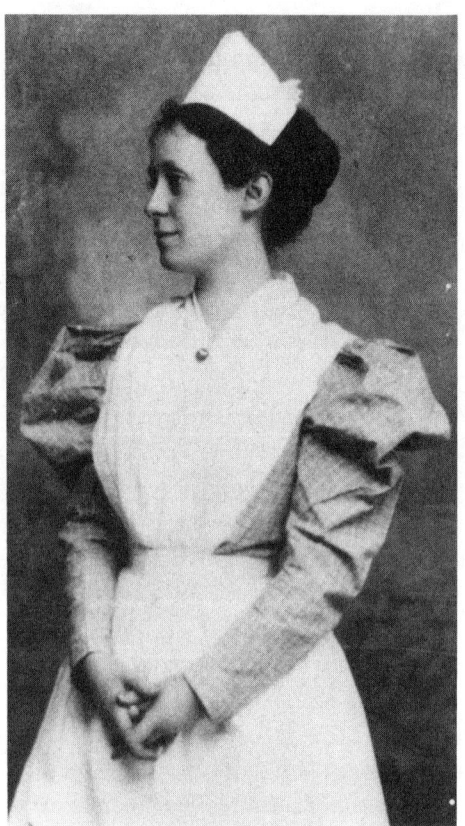

FIGURE 6:4 Louise Powell, circa 1910. Courtesy Mn U Archives.

for tuberculosis of the shoulder joint with extensive cold abscesses in the surrounding tissues.[25] By the first of May the university hospital had admitted forty-seven patients, thirteen of them medical cases and thirty-four surgical cases, while thirty-two surgical operations had been performed. The following December the *Northwestern Lancet* reported that, in its temporary quarters, with a limited number of beds, the university hospital was nonetheless being run "in the true hospital spirit. Everything about the buildings is scrupulously clean. Everything, of course, is new in the line of equipment, nurses are plentiful, and attending surgeons and physicians are to be found each day."[26] In the spring of 1910 Bertha Erdmann, suffering from consumption, resigned as superintendent of nurses and soon after died. In June 1910 Louise M. Powell was appointed superintendent of nurses.[27]

Early in the summer of 1910 the Board of Regents assigned an additional house, the Matson House at 324 Union Street, to the hospital, where twenty-two beds were installed for the use of medical patients. The house at 200 State Street, which contained sixteen beds and was formerly used for medical patients, was now used for patients with special ophthalmological or otolaryngological problems. The Board of Regents also assigned a building at 417-419 Delaware Street for use as a nurses' home. In June 1910 the hospital was caring for about thirty-six patients daily, divided about evenly between medical and surgical cases with a few obstetric cases.[28] In August Dr. Louis B. Baldwin became superintendent of the university hospital and took up his residence in the house at 304 State Street.

The temporary hospital service developed in the six houses proved its value from the beginning. When the faculty became able to offer clinics to the medical students, and to bring the medical students into the hospital to participate in the care of patients, they realized how much they had been missing previously in not having their own hospital for clinical teaching. Furthermore, the opening of the university hospital revealed the great number of poor patients in need of medical care throughout the state. From the time the hospital opened there was a waiting list for admission and the capacity of the several houses was strained to the utmost.

In April 1910 the contractor broke ground for the construction of the Elliot Memorial building. The architect, William M. Kenyon of Minneapolis, working more for love than profit, sought to provide the best possible hospital building that could be created with the funds available, adapting its exterior dimensions and design to the overall plan for the campus developed by Cass Gilbert. By June 1910 the foundations were laid, and by January 1911 the building was nearly completed, but no funds had been provided for its equipment. The Board of Regents was obliged to make an emergency request to the legislature at its 1911 session for $54,000 to equip the Elliot Hospital and the outpatient department and for $33,700 to maintain both it and the temporary university hospital through July 1911. For the succeeding biennium of 1911-13 the Board of Regents requested $159,200 to maintain the university hospital.[29]

On 5 September 1911 the dedication ceremonies for the Elliot Memorial Hospital were held in the University Chapel, with Dean Wesbrook presiding. The occasion was a particularly happy one marked by many expressions of high regard for the medical faculty and warm feeling for the university. After Dean Wesbrook's welcoming remarks, James E. Moore described the history of the Elliot bequest and of the movement that it sparked to create a greater campus for the university. Next, in his dedication address, President George Edgar Vincent referred to the origin of hospitals as charitable institutions in the Middle Ages. Frank M. Elliot spoke on behalf of the Elliot family, and Elbert L. Carpenter for the donors of the site, while Charles Lyman Greene described the role that the Elliot Memorial Hospital would play in the clinical education of medical students. Among other speeches William J. Mayo described the economic contribution that the university hospital might make to the state as a whole by restoring to health many poor persons who would otherwise become public charges. "Now that the economic value of every individual is definitely established," said Dr. Mayo, "the poor and the crippled will not only have the care needed for their comfort, but they will also receive the skilled assistance necessary to restore them to a condition of usefulness which will bring revenue to the state." And on that sunlit September day in 1911 he concluded with emphasis, *"Enlightened socialism is the keynote of modern civilization."*[30]

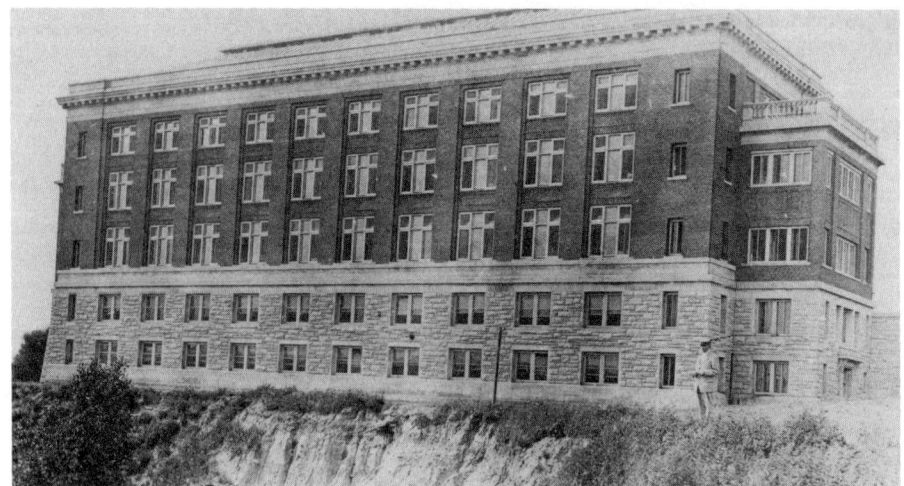

FIGURE 6:5   Elliot Hospital, 1912, south view. Courtesy Dr. Jesse Barron.

When the ceremonies in the University Chapel were over, the speakers and audience walked in a body from the chapel to the new Elliot Memorial Hospital, pausing on the way to lay the cornerstone for the new Institute of Anatomy then under construction on the southeast corner of Washington Avenue and Church Street. The cornerstone of the new Millard Hall, which was also then under construction, had been laid by Dean Wesbrook on 16 August in a very quiet ceremony.[31] At the hospital there was a brief ceremony of unveiling two memorial plaques, one to commemorate the Elliot gift, the other bearing the names of the donors of the site, and then the keys of the building were given to the superintendent, Dr. Louis Baldwin. When the assembled group toured the hospital, they found a bright and cheerful modern fireproof brick building of four stories, commanding a broad view over the Mississippi River. The surgical rooms were spacious, with seating space for a large group of students. "No hospital in either of the Twin Cities," observed the editor of the *Journal-Lancet,* "is so attractive, either in location or construction . . . ."[32]

On 19 September, two weeks after the dedication, the Elliot Memorial Hospital opened to receive patients. Of the 120 beds, the department of medicine was assigned 60 beds, surgery 40 beds, and obstetrics 20 beds. The hospital did not admit more specialized kinds of cases, such as eye, ear, nose, or throat patients, nor dermatological patients, because if it had been subdivided into a larger number of services, the resultant clinics would have been too small to be useful for teaching purposes. The first patients admitted were transferred from the temporary university hospitals. During the two and a half years of its existence the temporary hospital had admitted 951 patients. Even after the opening of the Elliot Memorial building the university hospital continued to use the house at 303

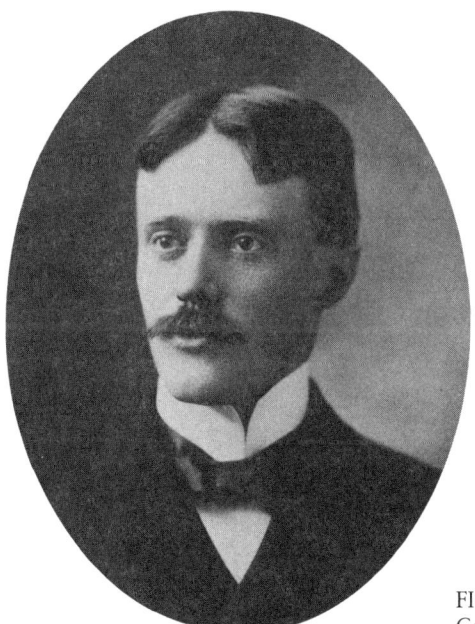

FIGURE 6:6 Louis Baldwin, 1897. Courtesy Mn U Archives.

Washington Avenue as a detention hospital for emergency and contagious cases. The need for an isolation hospital for contagious cases became urgent even before the Elliot Hospital opened. At the beginning of September there was an outbreak of diphtheria in the university hospital, confirmed first on 2 September when a positive diphtheria culture was obtained from the throat of a patient, Serena Offerdahl. Immediately all of Frank Wesbrook's knowledge and experience of diphtheria epidemics was needed to deal with an epidemic on his own home ground. The staff took cultures from the throats of all patients and nurses and from the wound surfaces in two burn cases. The throat cultures revealed ten patients, five nurses, and one interne infected with diphtheria. Among them, nine patients and three nurses developed clinical diphtheria and were treated promptly with diphtheria antitoxin. Both those sick with diphtheria and those who remained well but who had positive throat cultures, were isolated at 303 Washington Avenue until two successive negative cultures were obtained from their throats. They were then transferred to 324 Union Street where their quarantine was continued until two more negative throat cultures were obtained, when they were moved to the Elliot Hospital. On 25 September quarantine was lifted on the last diphtheria patient, a nurse, and the epidemic was over.[33]

When he came as superintendent of the university hospital in August 1910 Dr. Louis Baldwin realized that the Elliot building, when completed, would not be large enough to house such services as kitchen and laundry, essential to a hospital, so he asked the Board of Regents to assign the Madsen Flats, a two-storied brick-veneer frame building at 417–419 Delaware Street, for the use of the hospital. In the basement of the Madsen Flats Dr. Baldwin installed a large steam boiler and machinery for a hospital laundry, while the remainder of the building became a nurses' home. From the beginning Dr. Baldwin recognized that the Madsen Flats were unsuitable for their combined uses. The large boiler in the basement created a high risk of fire, and the operation of the laundry six days a week was accompanied by noise and pervasive smells. Nurses lived also in an old frame house at 324 Union Street which was similarly a fire trap. In his first report Dr. Baldwin emphasized that both buildings were dangerous and that a proper nurses' home should be built as soon as possible, with separate provision for the hospital laundry.[34] As superintendent of nurses, Louise Powell felt even more keenly the dangers and discomforts of the nurses' residences. In 1914, when more than thirty nursing students were enrolled in the school for nurses, Miss Powell reported that the need for a nurses' home was urgent both to "relieve our crowded, unsanitary housing conditions," and to provide proper teaching equipment.[35] Nevertheless, a proper residence for nurses would be a long time in coming. In 1916 Miss Powell noted that although the nursing school provided a nursing service indispensable to the university hospital, it still was not properly housed. "At the end of six years," she wrote, "our housing is still unsanitary, uncomfortable, and inadequate, our teaching equipment as meager as it was six years ago."[36]

NOTES

1. On 31 May 1905 the Board of Regents authorized its executive committee to confer with Mr. Trask about the purpose to which Mrs. Elliot's legacy should be devoted. Board of Regents, Minutes, 1888–1905, p. 579.

2. College of Medicine and Surgery, Executive Committee, Minutes, 13 November 1905 [Book 9, p. 13].

3. College of Medicine and Surgery, Executive Commitee, Minutes, 26 November 1906 [Book 9, pp. 80–81].

4. Frank M. Elliot, "The Elliot endowment," in University of Minnesota, *The university hospitals of the University of Minnesota, history and dedication* (Minneapolis, 1912), pp. 18–25, p. 20.

5. George Douglas Head et al., "A vital matter," *Minn. Alumni Wkly,* 1907, 6, no. 15, 1,3–5, p. 1.

6. Ibid., p. 4.

7. Ibid.

8. [Editorial], "It is a fact," *Minn. Alumni Wkly,* 1907, 6, no. 15, 3.

9. Elliot (n.4), pp. 20–21.

10. The hospital committee consisted of Arthur E. Benjamin, Abraham B. Cates, Warren Dennis, Charles L. Greene, George D. Head, Thomas G. Lee, James E. Moore, Parks Ritchie, Thomas S. Roberts, Frank C. Todd, and Frank F. Wesbrook. The hospital site committee included Drs. Benjamin, Head, Lee, Moore, Roberts, Todd and Wesbrook.

11. Elbert L. Carpenter, "The donors of the hospital site," in University of Minnesota, *University hospitals* (n. 4), pp. 25–26.

12. [Editorial], "Medical alumni active," *Minn. Alumni Wkly,* 1907, 6, no. 22, p. 3.

13. F. F. Wesbrook [for the hospital committee] to the Hon. James T. Wyman, Presi-

dent of the Board of Regents, 26 April 1907, in College of Medicine and Surgery, Executive Committee, Minutes, 15 May 1907 [Book 9], pp. 85-89.

14. Ibid., p. 89.

15. Board of Regents, Minutes, 10 June 1908, pp. 5-6.

16. In September Dean Wesbrook reported that the dental college wanted to take over the faculty room and chart room in Millard Hall, to use the large amphitheater two morning hours per week, and to transform the lower lecture room into a dental operating room. College of Medicine and Surgery, Executive Committee, Minutes, 14 September 1907 [Book 9, p. 103].

17. Ibid., 14 December 1907 [Book 9, p. 127].

18. "Anatomy building at the 'U' burns," *Minneapolis Journal,* 6 October 1908.

19. College of Medicine and Surgery, Executive Committee, Minutes, 11 November 1908 [Book 12, p. 2-23, p. 9].

20. College of Medicine and Surgery, Executive Faculty, Minutes, 16 December 1908 [Book 12, p. 37].

21. The committee's foresight was later ignored. Although the medical buildings today extend one block east of Union Street, their further expansion eastward has been prevented by the location of a group of large student dormitories south of Washington Avenue, between Harvard Street and Oak Street. As a result the medical campus is extremely congested, and its main parking ramp is located three blocks away on the east side of Oak Street.

22. College of Medicine and Surgery, Executive Committee, Minutes, 10 February 1909 [Book 12, pp. 55-59].

23. College of Medicine and Surgery, Executive Faculty, Minutes, 24 November 1909 and 14 December 1909.

24. "New hospital will be model . . . . Senior medical students to have opportunity to observe cases," *Minneapolis Journal,* 12 May 1909, p. 13, col. 3.

25. "The first clinic at the state university hospital," *J. Minn. St. med. Ass. & Northwest. Lancet,* 1909, *29,* 180-181.

26. "The university hospital," *J. Minn. St. med. Ass. & Northwest. Lancet,* 1909, *29,* 538-539.

27. A native of Staunton, Virginia, Miss Powell graduated in nursing from St. Luke's Hospital in Richmond, Virginia. Later she worked in various hospitals and nursing schools, including the Columbia school where she studied under the great pioneer of nursing education in America, Adelaide Nutting.

28. College of Medicine and Surgery, Executive Faculty, Minutes, 3 June 1910.

29. [Editorial], "The needs of the College of Medicine and Surgery," *Minn. Alumni Wkly,* 1911, *10* (no. 18), 18-23, pp. 21-22.

30. William J. Mayo, "The economic value to the state of the university hospital," in University of Minnesota, *University hospitals* (n.4), pp. 41-45.

31. "Laying the cornerstone," *Minn. Alumni Wkly,* 1911, *11,* no. 1, 12.

32. "Dedication of the new university hospital," *J. Minn. St. med. Ass. & Northwest. Lancet,* 1911, *31,* 444-445.

33. L. B. Baldwin to R. O. Beard, Secretary, the Hospital Committee in College of Medicine and Surgery, Executive Faculty, Minutes, 25 October 1911 [Book #18, pt. 1].

34. L. B. Baldwin to Dean F. F. Wesbrook, report to 31 July 1912, in University of Minnesota, *The president's report 1911-1912* (Minneapolis, 1913), pp. 121-123.

35. Louise M. Powell, "The school for nurses," in University of Minnesota, *The president's report 1913-1914* (Minneapolis, 1915) pp. 102-103.

36. Louise M. Powell, "The School for Nurses," in University of Minnesota, *The president's report for the year 1915-1916* (Minneapolis, 1917) pp. 81-83, p. 83.

CHAPTER 7

The College of Medicine and Surgery under Dean Wesbrook

One of Frank Wesbrook's first concerns on assuming the deanship in 1906 was the reorganization of the College of Medicine and Surgery into a form that would be more efficient and more easily administered. The faculty consisted of a large number of independent professors, who much of the time went their own way, while the affairs of the college were managed by a small executive committee that was not broadly representative of the faculty. At a meeting of the executive committee on 22 November 1906 Dean Wesbrook called attention to the need for the teaching staff of large departments to meet together to coordinate their didactic, laboratory, and clinical teaching. He also appointed a committee to develop a plan for reorganization of the faculty.[1] The following week Dean Wesbrook asked the heads of the large departments such as medicine, surgery, obstetrics, gynecology, and nervous and mental diseases to call meetings of their respective staffs to make recommendations for the coordination of work in their departments as a step toward the coordination of the work in all departments.[2] The plan developed by the reorganization committee called for the creation of various departments within the college, so the following year, on 20 November 1907, Dean Wesbrook appointed a second committee with Dr. W. A. Jones as chairman, to plan the reorganization of the faculty into formal departments that would serve as administrative units of the college.[3] One year later Dr. Jones presented the reorganization plan to a special meeting of the executive committee. The plan called for the creation of two faculties: an executive faculty and a general faculty. The executive faculty was to consist of the heads of some thirteen departments of instruction, namely, departments of: anatomy; surgery; histology and embryology; medicine; physiology; obstetrics; chemistry; gynecology; materia medica, pharmacology, and therapeutics; ophthalmology, otology, rhinology, and laryngology; pathology, bacteriology, and hygiene; dermatology; nervous and mental diseases. Each department would be responsible for courses in its field, or elective courses allied to it, so that no course would be taught without falling under the jurisdiction of a particular department. Each department would be represented at meetings of the executive faculty by its chief or alternate, and the executive faculty was to meet regularly on the first Wednesday of each month from August to May. The president of the university or the dean of the college might call special meetings of the executive faculty at any time. The executive faculty would conduct all the executive business of the college.

The general faculty would include the whole teaching staff of the college from professors to clinical instructors and laboratory instructors. It would meet regularly twice a year in September and February, but the president or the dean might call special meetings at any time. The general faculty was to be responsible for the educational work and policy of the college.

The chief of each department was to hold three meetings annually of the members of his department, within the two weeks before the meetings of the executive faculty in September, January, and May, and he might call special meetings at any time. The members of each department were to keep records of the standing and attendance of students and the combined records of the staff would determine the standing of the students in the department. The decision to pass or condition a student was to be a decision of the department as a whole to be reported for final action to the executive faculty.

The dean was to preside over both the executive and general faculties, and might at his pleasure attend a meeting of any department. A secretary was to be elected by the executive faculty for a term of two years and would act as the recording officer for both the executive and general faculties.[4]

The plan for reorganization was approved by the executive committee at the meeting on 11 November and presented to the faculty of the college on 23 November 1908. At the meeting several of the older members of the faculty, including Frederick Dunsmoor, expressed reservations about the proposed reorganization because it would deprive those members of the faculty who were not heads of departments of a faculty vote. For men who had participated in the founding of the school in 1888 and who had been voting members of the faculty through the whole of the twenty years since, it was not easy to be deprived of an effective vote in the affairs of the college. What made the feeling more acute was that three St. Paul members of the original faculty, Parks Ritchie, Alexander Stone, and Eugene Riggs, each said that the St. Paul representative on the reorganization committee, Archibald Maclaren, had not consulted with them in the preparation of the committee's report. Other members of the faculty expressed fear that where several subjects were grouped together under one department, not all might receive adequate attention. In answer to such objections, Thomas Lee said that a similar condensation of departments had occurred in many leading medical schools, although the particular grouping of subjects might vary in different schools according to local conditions. In the end the senior professors gave up their objections gracefully. The faculty voted to adopt the reorganization plan with various amendments made in the course of the meeting, the most important of which was the elimination of dermatology as a separate department and its inclusion under the Department of Surgery.

The incorporation of dermatology into surgery reduced the number of departments to twelve, and created an exact balance between the six basic science departments and the six clinical departments. Previously the professors of the basic medical sciences had been a minority among the larger group of professors of clinical subjects. The balance between basic science and clinical departments established in 1908 was reminiscent of the balance struck between the number of St. Paul and Minneapolis members on the original faculty in 1888, and in 1908 it may have represented an equally significant balance of forces in the life of the college.

The passage of the reorganization plan without a serious division of the faculty was probably a tribute to the tact and patience of Dean Wesbrook, who was sensitive to the outlook of the senior faculty members. As if in response to the feeling that in the rapid development of the college the efforts and sacrifices of its founders were in danger of being forgotten, Dean Wesbrook arranged an "Historical Evening" for 8 December 1908 to recall the origins and early history of medical teaching in Minnesota. The particular occasion for the Historical Evening was the merger into the College of Medicine and Surgery of the last-remaining private medical college in Minnesota, namely, the Hamline University Medical School.

On 30 January 1908 C. A. McCollum, dean of the Hamline University Medical School, wrote to Dean Wesbrook to propose a merger of the Hamline medical department into that of the University of Minnesota. The Hamline medical department proposed that the University of Minnesota should accept students matriculated in the current freshman, sophomore, and junior medical classes at Hamline, with their individual standings certified by their Hamline teachers. As each class graduated the University of Minnesota was to certify the Hamline medical students to Hamline University, which would award their medical degrees. On 7 February the executive faculty accepted the general proposition for the admission of Hamline medical students, but stipulated that the Hamline students must satisfy all requirements of the University of Minnesota subsequent to their matriculation, and must proceed to graduation within four years after the merger.[5] The Minneapolis College of Physicians and Surgeons, the corporate body that conducted the medical department of Hamline University, agreed not to continue as a medical school, nor to permit its building and grounds in Minneapolis to be used as a medical school, unless by the University of Minnesota. It agreed to sell its microscopes and other equipment to the University of Minnesota at prices to be set by a joint committee of the two institutions. The College of Physicians and Surgeons agreed further that immediately following the merger and the sale of their property, they would surrender their charter of incorporation to the University of Minnesota.

The Hamline medical department also proposed that various members of their faculty should be appointed to the faculty of the College of Medicine and Surgery, but the executive faculty demurred until each proposed appointment could be reviewed by appropriate members of the college. Dean Wesbrook called a meeting of the college faculty for the evening of 20 February, for the purpose of going over the terms of the proposal item by item, and the faculty approved the proposal with only minor changes.[6] The proposal was then presented to the Board of Regents at its meeting on 4 March and approved by them. Eight members of the Hamline medical faculty were appointed to the medical faculty of the university, and in the fall of 1908 the Hamline medical students were admitted to the University of Minnesota.

On Tuesday, 8 December 1908 the Historical Evening took place in the University Chapel. President Northrop presided and the members of the Board of Regents attended together with many faculty, alumni, and students. In his opening remarks President Northrop said that the College of Medicine and Surgery was " . . . not only a credit to the University and a credit to the state, but . . . is an institution that compares favorably with any medical college within the limits of the United States."[7] The principal speaker, Richard Olding Beard, described at length the history of medical education in Minnesota.[8] Alexander Stone spoke briefly on the history of the St. Paul Medical College and Frederick A. Dunsmoor on that of the Minnesota Hospital College.[9] James T. Moore described the history of the Minneapolis College of Physicians and Surgeons which in 1897 had become the department of medicine of Hamline University, and C. A. McCollum outlined the events of the merger with the university.[10] Former Dean Parks Ritchie described the background to the founding of the Department of Medicine at the university in 1888.[11] The Hon. John Lind, president of the Board of Regents, discussed the relation of the Board of Regents to the college.[12] Mr. Lind said that if the legislature would grant a modest request that the Board of Regents was about to make on behalf of the medical college, it would become possible to begin research, and he appealed for the private endowment of scholarships for medical research. William J. Mayo, chairman of the medical committee of the regents, discussed the clinical needs of the college and promised "within a few years we shall have a clinical hospital equal to any that any medical institution in the country can show."[13] Dean Wesbrook looked to the future when a university hospital would combine the charitable care of the sick poor with the advancement of medical science.[14] "The state's College of medicine and surgery [Dean Wesbrook said] should stand in the position of consultant to the various medical practitioners throughout the state. It is possible to create a people's institution in Minnesota which will do more for her citizens than can be done in older communities where many institutions are already in the field . . . ."[15]

In May 1909 the Board of Regents acted to amalgamate the College of Homeopathic Medicine and Surgery with the College of Medicine and Surgery. The number of students in the homeopathic college had dropped to such a low level that the university was not justified in continuing it as a separate college. To compensate for the elimination of the homeopathic college, two new chairs were established in the College of Medicine and Surgery to teach homeopathic materia medica and homeopathic therapeutics. Any medical student who wished might take the homeopathic courses in place of the regular courses (he was not permitted to take both), and at graduation would receive a diploma indicating that he was a homeopathic physician and surgeon. Nevertheless, no students chose to take

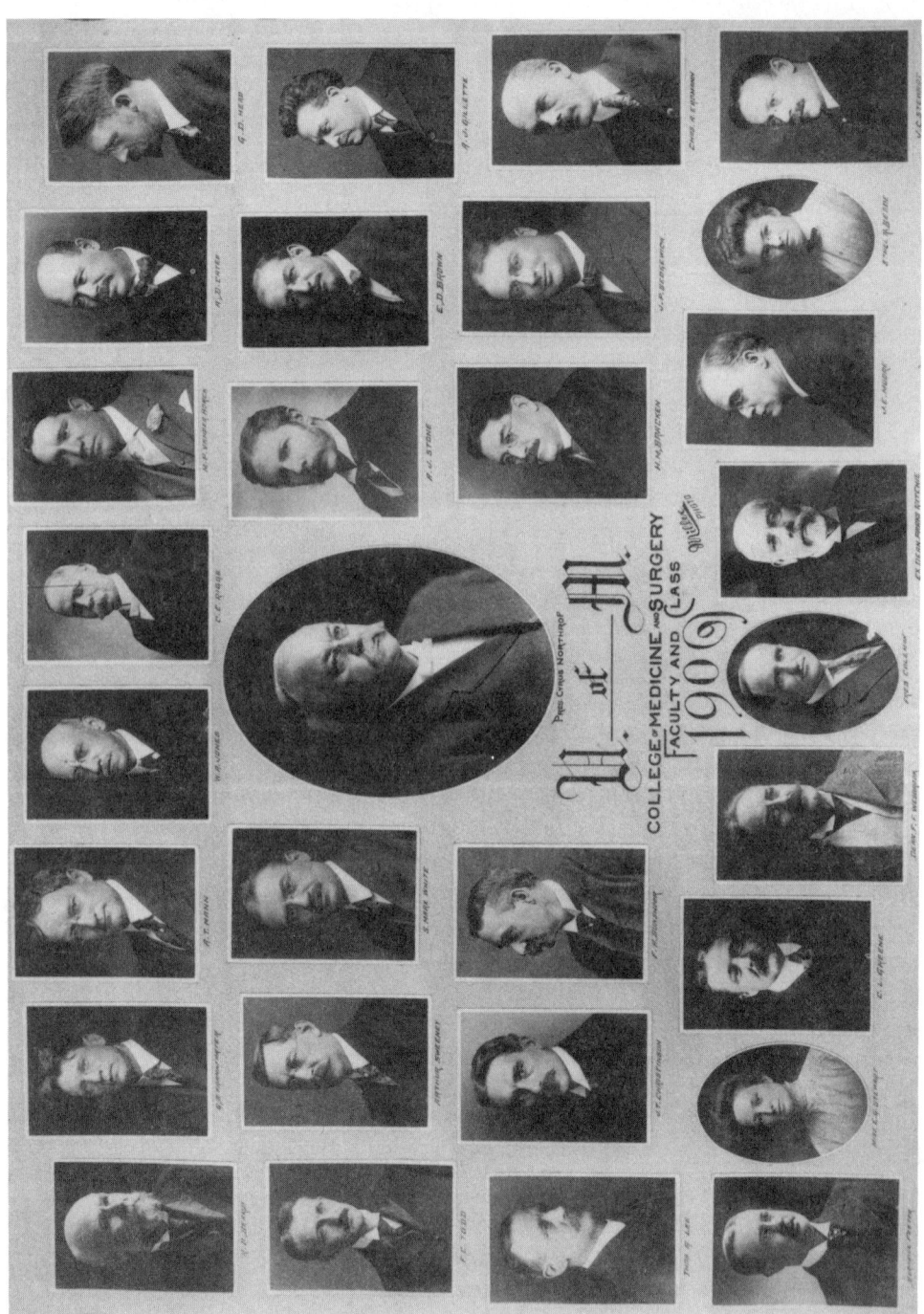

FIGURE 7:1 Medical faculty, 1909. Courtesy Mn U Archives.

homeopathic courses. The homeopathic professors, confronted with empty classrooms, did not lecture, and presently the two chairs were abolished.

In May 1909 Abraham Flexner visited the College of Medicine and Surgery in the course of his survey of medical schools of the United States and Canada for the Carnegie Foundation for the Advancement of Teaching. In his published report Flexner described the laboratories at Minnesota for the scientific branches of medicine as "excellent, exceedingly attractive, and well organized." He noted that for clinical education Minnesota had previously relied on municipal hospitals and unpaid clinical teachers with, he said, "the usual results," but that the university was about to build a teaching hospital and had already opened a temporary hospital. Also to its credit, the chiefs of medicine and surgery were provided salaries. Although the university still had to fulfill its plans for an adequate teaching hospital, Flexner thought that Minnesota was the "first state in the Union that may fairly be considered to have solved the most perplexing problems connected with medical education and practice . . . ."[16]

On Christmas Eve 1909 fire broke out in Millard Hall and, before it was brought under control, burned out the entire third floor and the amphitheater on the second floor. The fire destroyed the laboratory and lecture charts of the Department of Pharmacology, while the head of the department, Edgar D. Brown, lost his personal library, notes, and other papers. The dental college also lost its laboratories and teaching clinics. On Christmas morning a group of nearly forty students went to work under the direction of Dr. Brown, Dean Alfred Owre of the dental college, and other members of the faculty to salvage whatever equipment could be saved and to make the intact portion of the building usable by enclosing it with a temporary wooden roof covered with tarpaper.[17] At the beginning of the New Year, classes went on without interruption in improvised lecture rooms and laboratories. The losses from the fire were heavy, especially in the medical library. Several hundred books were damaged by water and nearly six hundred volumes of periodicals burned.[18] The medical library was moved temporarily to the Institute of Public Health and Pathology until Millard Hall could be repaired.

Two months after the fire, on the morning of 25 February, Dr. James Moore was lecturing to the junior medical class, beneath the temporary wooden roof on the third floor of Millard Hall. A high wind had been blowing all morning, and in the midst of the lecture the students were startled by a sudden impact on the roof. Dr. Moore remarked that it sounded like a brick, but continued his lecture. Ten minutes later a portion of a brick and mortar gable crashed through the wooden roof, burying Dr. Moore beneath a pile of rubble. When the medical students pulled Dr. Moore from the rubble, he was unconscious and blood was pouring from his ears. As soon as Dean Wesbrook learned of the disaster he hurried from his office in the Institute of Public Health and Pathology to Millard Hall where he and other members of the faculty gave emergency treatment to Dr. Moore and two students, Edward Ziegler and David Berkman, who were seriously injured. Within ten minutes they were on their way in carriages to the university hospital. Fortunately, despite the severe blows on the head that he received, Dr. Moore did

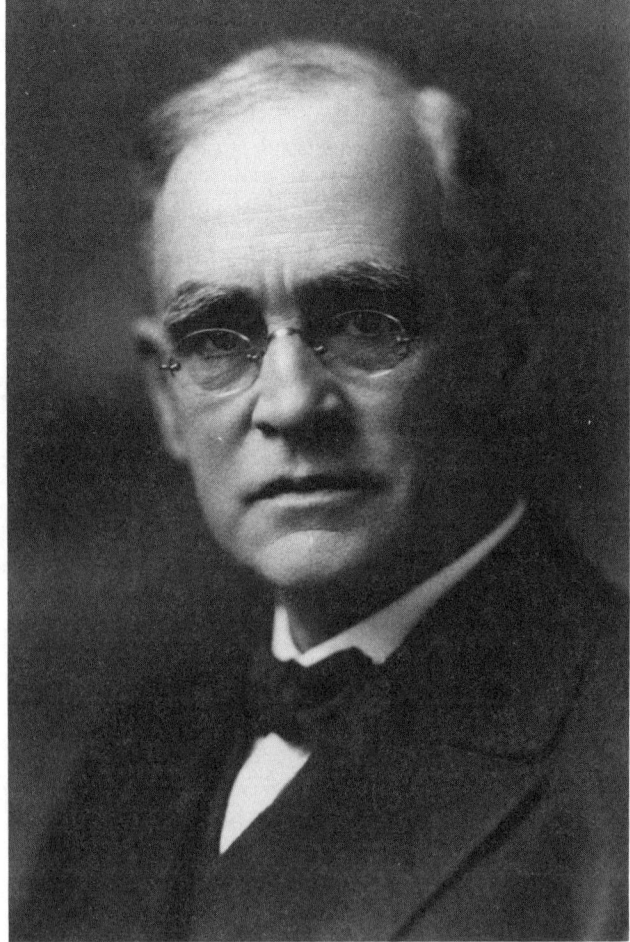

FIGURE 7:2 James E. Moore, circa 1910. Courtesy Mn U Archives.

not suffer a fracture of the skull, and about two hours after the accident recovered consciousness. The incident revealed the ties that bound together students and faculty at that time. The *Minneapolis Journal* reported: "Although the students had no way of knowing whether the remaining part of the wall would fall, not one left the room until Dr. Moore was carried out. The two men most seriously injured, Edward Ziegler and David Berkman, assisted in carrying Dr. Moore from the room."[19]

In December 1910 the Board of Regents elected George Edgar Vincent president of the University of Minnesota. Then forty-six years of age, Vincent was born in Rockford, Illinois, the only child of the Rev. John Heyl Vincent, a minister in the Methodist Episcopal Church. The Rev. Vincent founded the Chautauqua Institution in 1874. As a child, growing up in an atmosphere of enlightened evan-

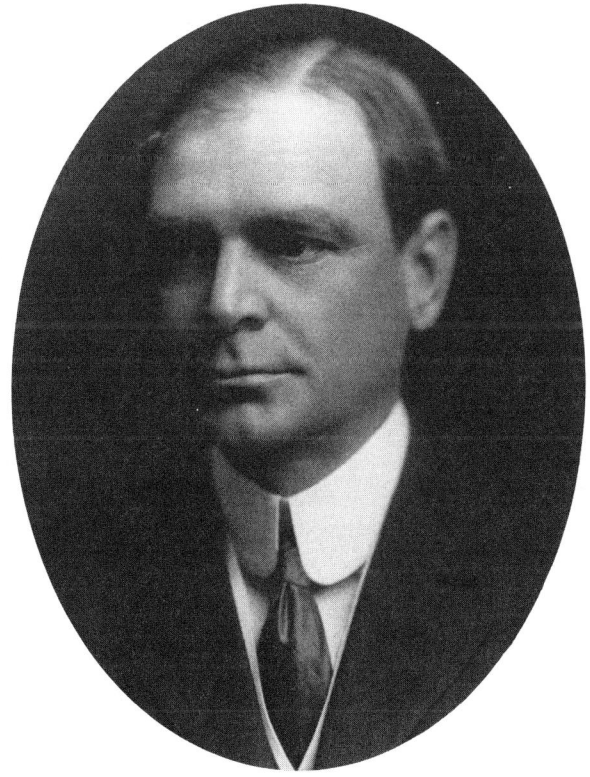

FIGURE 7:3 George Edgar Vincent, circa 1911. Courtesy Mn U Archives.

gelism, George Edgar Vincent was influenced deeply by his father and by the many famous persons he met in connection with the Chautauqua Institution, an educational endeavor for adults seeking to improve their minds. He was educated at Yale College where he was graduated B.A. in 1885. After graduation he assisted his father with the institution, becoming in 1886 literary editor of the Chautauqua Press and in 1888 vice principal of instruction. Through his Chautauqua work Vincent met William Rainey Harper, president of the University of Chicago, who persuaded him to begin graduate study in sociology at Chicago, where in 1896 Vincent received the Ph.D. and was appointed to the faculty.[20]

The appointment of George Edgar Vincent as president of the University of Minnesota caused considerable stir in the Twin Cities. When the appointment was announced Mrs. Vincent and the children were returning from Europe on board the *Mauretania,* and that circumstance alone suggested the atmosphere of cosmopolitan life that the Vincents were to bring with them to Minneapolis. Mrs. Vincent was accustomed to travel widely, and frequently to remote and romantic-sounding places in the Rocky Mountains or Central America. The children, two girls and a boy, were attractive and intelligent, and participated in sports

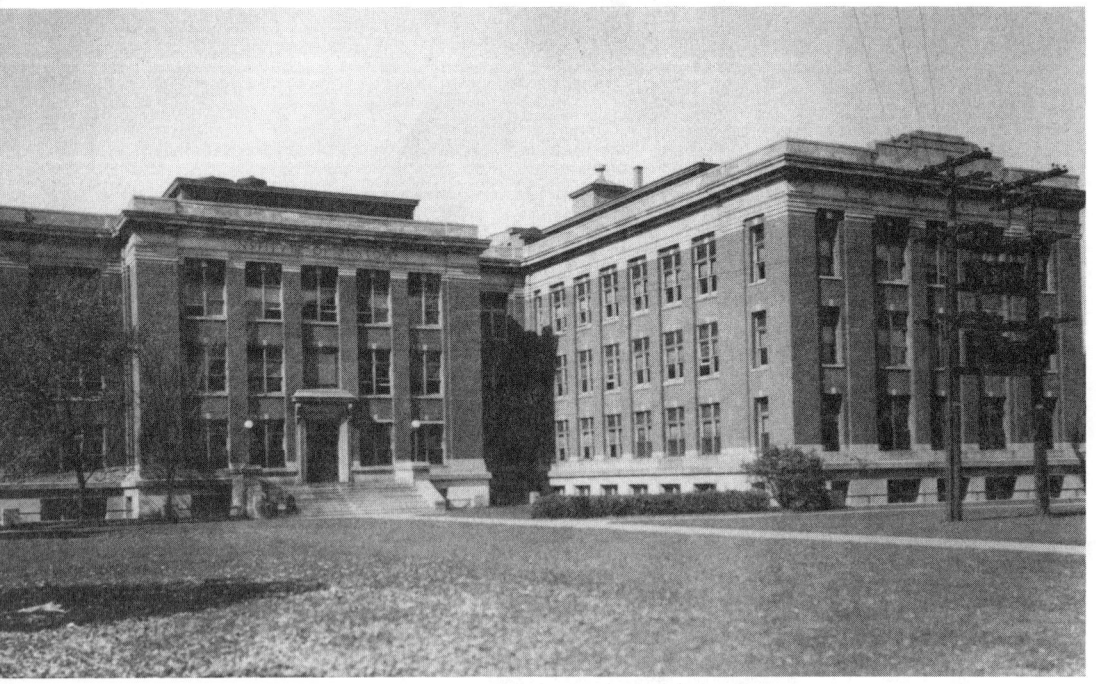

FIGURE 7:4 Institute of Anatomy: "the greatest and most complete" anatomical laboratory in the world. Courtesy Mn U Archives.

and social activities. Soon after the Vincents arrived in Minneapolis in April 1911 and took up residence in the former home of Governor Pillsbury, Mrs. Vincent began to dazzle Twin Cities society with her brilliant parties. On the third floor of the old Pillsbury mansion she created a ballroom, equipped with a player piano, in which she encouraged awkward undergraduates to dance. Frequently there were amateur theatrical entertainments organized by the hostess.

The inauguration of President Vincent in October 1911 continued over four days, beginning with a torchlight procession of alumni and students on Tuesday evening, 17 October, which proved to be an extraordinary demonstration of loyalty and affection for the university. "The illumination of torches, lanterns, searchlights and fireworks, the marching and countermarching of thousands of alumni and students, led by the university band and singing their college songs and with it all the general manifestation of enthusiasm and delight" would more than anything else, thought the *Pioneer Press,* ensure the future of the university.[21] At the conclusion of the parade there was a magnificent display of fireworks. The inaugural exercises the next afternoon were followed by a banquet attended by 1,100 persons, and addresses at the University Chapel in the evening. The succession of brilliant events ended Friday evening with a concert by the Minneapolis Sym-

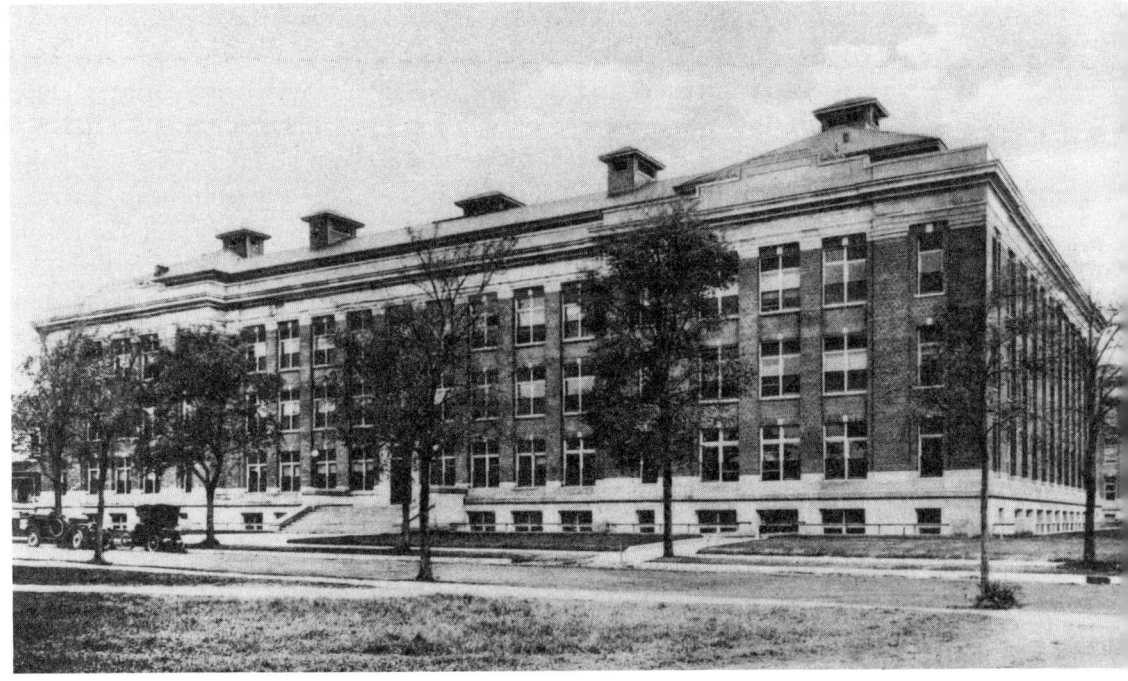

FIGURE 7:5 Millard Hall, 1912. Courtesy Mn U Archives.

phony Orchestra. Seldom has a university president been inaugurated with as much ceremony or more enthusiastic expressions of confidence in his leadership.

In his inauguration address President Vincent stated, among other things, his belief "that buildings are but the shell of the University; its real life lies in its men." He added, "Only great men and women can make a University great. Better inspired investigators and teachers in barracks than a staff of industrious mediocrity in marble palaces."[22] Thus, in a few sentences buried in the midst of a speech of splendid generalities about the value and purpose of university education, President Vincent hinted at what would be his attitude toward the building program embodied in the extension of the university campus, and in particular toward the development of the new medical campus.

President Vincent's critical attitude toward expenditure on buildings was to affect the College of Medicine and Surgery because the planned move to new buildings on a new campus was unavoidably costly. In January 1911, after Vincent had accepted the presidency but several months before he arrived in Minneapolis, the executive faculty learned that the lowest bids for the construction of the Institute of Anatomy and the new Millard Hall were almost $100,000 more than the legislature had appropriated for the two buildings.[23] The executive faculty thereupon voted to ask the Board of Regents to increase the legislative request for the new Institute of Public Health from $200,000 to $300,000.[24] Later that month the Board of Regents asked the legislature for an emergency appropriation to cover the additional cost of building the Institute of Anatomy and the new Millard Hall and for the maintenance and equipment of those two buildings and the Elliot Hospital.[25] Construction of the Institute of Anatomy began in May 1911 and that of the new Millard Hall the following autumn. Both buildings were practically completed by August 1912 and ready to be used when the term began that fall.

In March 1912 the executive faculty decided to invite President Vincent to meet with them to discuss the needs of the college. At that time the faculty considered that they needed urgently an outpatient building, a nurses' home, and a service building, all in relation to the Elliot Hospital at an estimated cost of $250,000, a new building on the medical campus for the Institute of Public Health and Pathology to cost $300,000, and a psychiatric hospital to cost $60,000. They also wished to plan for separate hospital buildings for infectious diseases, children's diseases, and for eye, ear, nose, and throat diseases, but made no estimate of their possible cost.[26]

On 11 September 1912 when the executive faculty held their regular monthly dinner meeting at the Minneapolis Club, President Vincent attended. Although he took little part in the discussion, Vincent asked the faculty to provide nominations to the university senate that the Board of Regents was about to establish.[27] President Vincent was not present at the next meeting in October when the executive faculty considered in detail its needs for an enlarged budget and additional buildings. At that meeting the faculty prepared a memorial on development to submit to the president and the Board of Regents. They noted:

> The University has the opportunity to serve as the center for medical education in the Northwest and it should rise to this opportunity. The position of the University as the sole and sufficing medium of medical education in the state of Minnesota—a position practically unique in America—places upon the University and upon its faculty of medicine, in particular, the responsibility of maintaining the high rank which the College has attained among teaching institutions—a rank which cannot be maintained unless the mechanism of efficient teaching be secured.[28]

At present, the memorial continued, the salaries paid to the teaching staff were inadequate, and many of the clinical teachers were not paid at all. The faculty recommended a scale of minimum salaries for each level of appointment and the extension of the payroll to include those teachers who presently were not paid. They also recommended the establishment of a summer quarter term to permit medical teaching and research to continue throughout the year.

The faculty's most expensive recommendations were for new buildings. With the creation of the new medical campus, the Institute of Public Health and Pathology became a half mile distant from the other medical buildings. At the same time the building had become inadequate for both the Department of Pathology and Bacteriology and the laboratories of the State Board of Health, which it contained. They therefore recommended a new building for pathology, bacteriology, and public health on the new medical campus at an estimated cost of $325,000. They recommended also the building of a residence for nurses to cost $75,000, and a new building for the dispensary or outpatient department to cost $100,000. Furthermore, at the end of its first year the Elliot Memorial building was already inadequate to the needs of the university hospital. It could provide no facilities for the care of eye, ear, nose, and throat diseases, for children's diseases, or for nervous diseases. Taken together such deficiencies left an enormous gap in the clinical education that the college could provide. The faculty, therefore, recommended that the university request $150,000 for an additional hospital pavilion for children's diseases and nervous diseases, and the use of one of the houses of the former temporary hospital for diseases of the eye, ear, nose, and throat. Finally, they recommended that $50,000 be requested to build a fifty-bed isolation hospital for contagious diseases.

The list of buildings thus itemized came to a total cost of $775,000 but they represented only the most immediate needs of the college. In future the university hospital would need additional buildings for obstetrical patients, for nervous diseases, for a tuberculosis clinic, and for an addition to the projected nurses' home at a projected total cost of $165,000. In future the faculty also planned for a separate building for public health at a cost of $400,000 and the completion of the Institute of Anatomy and Millard Hall to their original planned size at a cost of $175,000. Altogether the immediate and future needs for medical buildings added up to a total of $1,615,000.[29]

The buildings contemplated by the College of Medicine and Surgery were reasonable if the university hospital were to serve as a general hospital for indigent patients from throughout the state of Minnesota and if the transfer of the college to the new medical campus were to be carried through in a logical and consistent manner. Although the proposed building program may have been large when compared to the earlier scale of building at Minnesota, it was modest when compared to the outlays for new medical buildings at other universities at that time. Washington University at St. Louis had spent one and a half million dollars on its hospital alone.[30] Nevertheless, urgently needed though they might be, when the medical faculty's proposals for new buildings came before President Vincent, they struck him as outrageous. George Edgar Vincent believed in men, not buildings. Although the University of Minnesota possessed a remarkable group of men among the medical faculty, President Vincent did not recognize their value. At a special meeting of the executive faculty on 5 December 1912, Dean Wesbrook reported that President Vincent proposed to complete the Institute of Anatomy for the use of the Department of Pathology and Bacteriology and the State Board of Health, and that requests for appropriations for a hospital service building remained in doubt. Vincent was in effect cancelling the planned development of the new medical campus, when the new campus was just well begun. The executive faculty then requested that President Vincent and William Mayo meet with them before the meeting of the Board of Regents on 11 December.[31]

In response to the executive faculty's request, President Vincent met with them in the new Millard Hall on the afternoon of Monday, 9 December. During the hour before the meeting, President Vincent inspected the university dispensary at Seven Corners together with Dean Wesbrook and Drs. Louis Baldwin and Jennings Litzenberg. At the executive faculty meeting Dr. Baldwin said that attendance at the dispensary had risen recently to 150 or 160 per day from 126 the previous month. President Vincent noted that the outpatient service was limited to two hours per day. James Moore explained that because the clinicians were unpaid, they could come to the dispensary only for those few hours that they could spare from their practice. President Vincent said that he appreciated the need for a hospital service building to free the first floor of the Elliot Hospital for beds and he mentioned the need to cut down "the unwieldy faculty," although he did not say why he thought the medical faculty was unwieldy. He emphasized the need for agreement in drawing up the legislative request. The president then stated his own view of the needs of the university as a whole. They were:

1. To relieve from routine duties those men on the faculty who are able to do research, and pay them salaries that will make them feel that they are appreciated.

2. To bring in other able men to join them.

President Vincent said that he regarded the plan for the new campus prepared by Cass Gilbert "as one of the great dangers of the University." If the university were to cover the campus with buildings, said Vincent, they did not want a president but rather a construction engineer. He wanted to secure big men and pay our own men well, but that could not be done unless the buildings were cut down "to the inside limit."

When James Moore inquired whether the $50,000 for a hospital service building could not be requested in addition to a wing to the Anatomy Building to house pathology and bacteriology, President Vincent replied that if it were, others would clamor for increases in their appropriations. "Every building we get houses only very limited departments." Said Vincent, "These two buildings are not being economically used. It is a pity that there cannot be a concentration of departments in these buildings so that we can have the building matters out of the way and get down to work." Vincent did not allow for the fact that the Institute of Anatomy and the new Millard Hall had been completed only the previous summer and the departments were still in process of settling themselves into them.

When Dean Wesbrook pointed out that the wing to be added to the Institute of Anatomy would only take the place of the Institute of Public Health and Pathology building, which was to be given up, and that only truly additional buildings should be charged to the college, President Vincent replied angrily:

> If I were doing it, I would put two departments in the Anatomy building, Anatomy and Pathology; I would put the Board of Health in the second and third floors of the

new wing, and the Dispensary in the first floor and basement. You could do that perfectly well if you can treat Dr. Lee with alum or something to make him shrink.[32]

Thomas George Lee, then fifty-two years of age, was five years older than George Edgar Vincent. As a young man he had pursued graduate study in anatomy at the University of Wurzburg, Harvard University, and the University of Munich. In the twenty years since he had come to Minnesota in 1892, Dr. Lee had worked steadily and successfully to develop well-equipped laboratories for histology, embryology, and anatomy. During that time he had earned three sabbatical years, but had been granted none. In the spring of 1910 he spent two and a half months visiting anatomical institutes in Great Britain, France, Germany, and Italy to learn features of design and equipment that might be incorporated in the Institute of Anatomy, then being planned so that when completed it would be one of the most modern anatomical laboratories. Almost as President Vincent was proposing to shrink Dr. Lee "with alum or something," Dr. Charles S. Minot, in delivering his inaugural lecture at the University of Berlin in the presence of the Kaiser Wilhelm and other dignitaries, was describing the new Institute of Anatomy at the University of Minnesota as "the greatest and most complete" anatomical laboratory in the world.[33] Although Dr. Lee had reduced his teaching load somewhat while he was overseeing the planning and equipment of the Institute of Anatomy, he had continued through 1911 and 1912 to deliver four to five lectures per week and to spend five to ten hours each week in laboratory teaching. Dr. Lee carried out significant research himself on comparative embryology, and encouraged students to pursue research. It was Dr. Lee who launched Louis B. Wilson on a research career and, according to Wilson, Dr. Lee also was responsible for starting the famous botanist Bror Eric Dahlgren on his career.[34] Dr. Lee likewise encouraged Hal Downey, the future father of American hematology, in his early studies on blood cells. Thomas George Lee was one of the big men whom President Vincent said he wished to encourage, but Vincent seemed oblivious to Lee's worth.

In response to President Vincent's verbal assault, Dr. Lee said that while he was perfectly willing to do whatever was for the good of the college, they should not retard the normal growth of anatomy. President Vincent replied that there was plenty of room for anatomy for six or eight years and plenty of room then for research.[35]

When Jennings Litzenberg asked President Vincent how they might relieve the overcrowded state of the university dispensary, Vincent said that it could be placed in the proposed new wing of the Anatomy Building as he had suggested. When Dean Wesbrook asked whether the college might hope for any increase in the support fund for the university hospital, President Vincent said the present fund was sufficient, and he advised keeping within the existing appropriation to avoid criticism from enemies of scientific medicine.

When President Vincent left the meeting of the executive faculty that December afternoon, the prospect before Dean Wesbrook and the six department heads

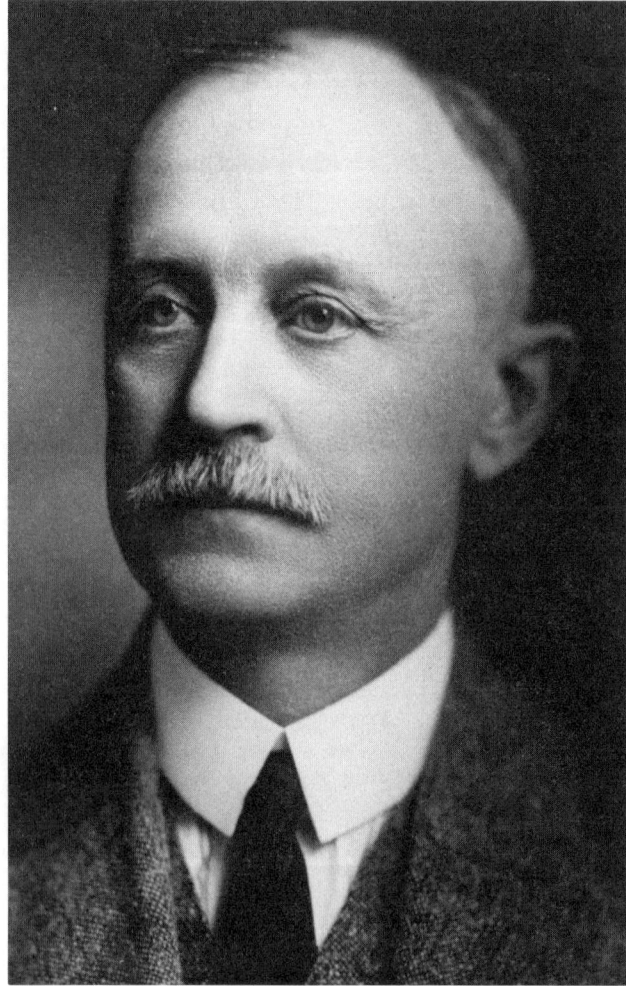

FIGURE 7:6   Thomas G. Lee, 1915. Courtesy Mn U Archives.

present must have seemed bleak indeed. Their outline of urgent needs, drawn up in October with much thought and labor, had been swept aside. President Vincent had treated not only their plans and hopes, but even their immediate and obvious needs, with contempt. But, whatever may have been their feelings, they were too strong in their faith to allow themselves the luxury of discouragement. After the president had gone, the faculty members went to examine the basement of the south wing of Millard Hall and Dr. Frank Todd suggested that the present dispensary building at Seven Corners be sold and the money thus obtained be used to build as much as possible of the south wing of Millard Hall in order to locate the outpatient department in it. The executive faculty then decided to accept a new wing on the Anatomy Building in exchange for the Institute of Public

Health and Pathology Building, to ask the Board of Regents to request $50,000 for a hospital service building, and to recommend the sale of the old dispensary to help pay for part of the south wing of Millard Hall.[36]

The years of rapid growth of the college had come to an abrupt end. Its past achievements and its current high national reputation were alike ignored by a reckless and ambitious president, whose superficial brilliance obscured for the moment his profoundly bad judgment.[37]

NOTES

1. College of Medicine and Surgery, Executive Committee, Minutes, 22 November 1906 [Book 9, pp. 69–73].
2. Ibid., 26 November 1906 [Book 9, p. 79].
3. Ibid., 20 November 1907 [Book 9, pp. 117–119]. The committee consisted of Richard O. Beard, W. A. Jones, Archibald MacLaren, and Frank C. Todd.
4. Ibid., 11 November 1908 [Book 12, pp. 11–15].
5. College of Medicine and Surgery, Executive Faculty, Minutes, 7 February 1908.
6. College of Medicine and Surgery General Faculty, Minutes, 20 February 1908.
7. "The unification of medical teaching in the state of Minnesota: an historical evening," *J. Minn. St. med. Ass. & Northwest. Lancet*, 1909, *29*, 24–54, p. 24.
8. Ibid., pp. 24–42.
9. Ibid., pp. 42–43.
10. Ibid., pp. 46–47.
11. Ibid., pp. 47–48.
12. Ibid., pp. 48–50.
13. Ibid., pp. 50–51.
14. Ibid., pp. 51–54.
15. Ibid., p. 52.
16. Abraham Flexner, *Medical education in the United States and Canada*, p. 248.
17. "Repairing the burned Millard Hall," *Minneapolis Journal*, 1 January 1910, p. 6, col. 3; "The burning of Millard Hall," *J. Minn. St. med. Ass. & Northwest. Lancet*, 1910, *30*, 17–18.
18. The loss to the dental and medical colleges was estimated at $9,755, and to the library alone, $3,379. College of Medicine and Surgery, Executive Faculty, Minutes, 9 February 1910 [Book 13, pp. 43–54, pp. 50–52].
19. "Wall crashes on University class," *Minneapolis Journal*, 26 February 1910, p. 6., col. 5.
20. George Edgar Vincent, *The social mind and education*.
21. *St. Paul Pioneer Press*, 18 October 1911.
22. George Edgar Vincent, "Inaugural address," *Minn. Alumni Wkly*, 1911, *11* (no. 6) 41–50, p. 44.
23. College of Medicine and Surgery, Executive Faculty, Minutes, 5 January 1911 [Book 18, pt. 1, p. 3].
24. Ibid., p. 4.
25. Ibid., 13 March 1911 [Book 18, pt. 1].
26. Ibid., 13 March 1912 [Book 18, pt. 1].
27. Ibid., 11 September 1912 [Book 18, pt. 1].
28. Ibid., 3 October 1912 [Book 18, pt. 1].
29. Ibid.

30. Richard Olding Beard, "The teaching hospital," *Minn. Alumni Wkly,* 1911, *10* (no. 20), 4–5.

31. College of Medicine and Surgery, Executive Faculty, Minutes, 5 December 1912 [Book 18, pt. II].

32. Vincent's words are given within quotation marks in the Executive Faculty minutes. College of Medicine and Surgery, Executive Faculty, Minutes, 9 December 1912 [Book 18, pt. II].

33. "Greatest institute of anatomy in the world is that at University of Minnesota, Harvard professor tells German Kaiser," *Minneapolis Journal,* 11 December 1912, p. 6, col. 2. Cf. Charles Sedgwick Minot, "Antritts vorlesung," *Science,* 1912, n.s. *36,* 771–776, pp. 775–776.

34. Louis B. Wilson, "Pioneers in research," *Minn. Alumni Wkly,* 1940, *39* (no. 29), 481–482.

35. In 1910, when Richard Olding Beard sought to locate one of the clinical departments in the new anatomy building then being planned, Thomas Lee " . . . called attention to the fact that the Anatomical Building was conceived of, carried to the Regents, and by the Regents to the Legislature, and by the Legislature granted for the puposes of Anatomy only, and that it always had been known as the Anatomical building, and that there would be no space in said building beyond the needs of the Department of Anatomy." Executive Faculty, Minutes, 9 February 1910 [Book 13, pp. 43–54, p. 46].

36. Ibid., 9 December 1912 [Book 18, pt. II].

37. My estimate of George Edgar Vincent is quite different from that of James Gray, the historian of the university, who described Vincent in terms of extravagant eulogy. See James Gray, *The University of Minnesota 1851–1951,* pp. 147–155. One can only judge the man by the effects of his actions. Gray had great admiration and affection for Vincent. In September 1916, when Gray was packing to go to Harvard, his father died suddenly, placing the family in financial straits, and Gray thought he must go to work in a bank. At that juncture President Vincent obtained a scholarship for Gray to enter the University of Minnesota, and was kind to him in many ways. James Gray, "The temper of fellowship: Some highly personal footnotes to the story of the university," ms. in the Gray papers.

CHAPTER 8

The Convulsion of 1913 and the Appointment of Dean Lyon

Shortly after George Edgar Vincent arrived in Minneapolis in April 1911 to assume the presidency of the University of Minnesota, he sought to bring about a reorganization of the College of Medicine and Surgery, although it is not clear in what respects Vincent thought the college needed reorganization. The publication of the Flexner report in 1910 had suggested reorganization or closure for many medical schools, but not for Minnesota of which Flexner gave a favorable account.[1] Flexner observed at the time of his visit in 1909 that at Minnesota the clinical teaching had already been reorganized with the chiefs in medicine and surgery placed on salaries.[2] Through 1911 and 1912 President Vincent conferred repeatedly with Dean Wesbrook about the possibility of reorganization, but Wesbrook steadfastly opposed it, pointing out that such changes in the faculty as might be desirable could be achieved on an individual basis, without announcing or attempting an overall reorganization.[3] There is no record of their conversations, but Wesbrook may have argued that the college had already undergone one reorganization in 1908, that its faculty was generally of high quality, and that it was recognized throughout the country as one of the leading medical schools in the United States. Wesbrook knew that the time had come when, with the availability of the Elliot Memorial Hospital, full-time salaried appointments in the clinical departments might be desirable, but the university did not have funds to pay the level of salaries required for full-time clinical appointments. Nor was the Elliot Hospital by itself nearly large enough to receive the number of patients needed to occupy the whole time of a clinical chief. In 1912 no medical school in the United States had as yet made full-time clinical appointments, and when the Johns Hopkins University undertook to make such appointments in October 1913 they were only enabled to do so with the aid of $1,500,000 given by the Rockefeller General Education Board to endow clinical chairs. The chiefs of medicine and surgery at Johns Hopkins were each to receive salaries of $10,000 per year, almost three times the salaries paid for the same positions at Minnesota. In 1912 the feasibility of full-time clinical appointments at Minnesota had become even more re-

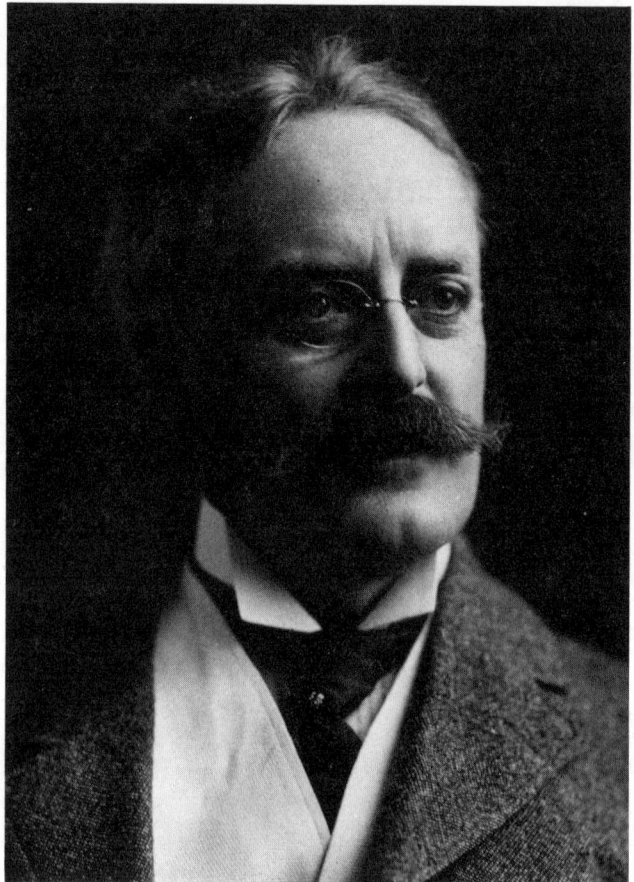

FIGURE 8:1   Frank F. Wesbrook, 1912. Courtesy Mn U Archives.

mote because of a sharp cut in the legislative appropriation for the university in 1911.

When, on 18 May 1911, Dean Wesbrook prepared the budget for the College of Medicine and Surgery for 1911–1912, he assumed on the basis of the budget of the previous year that the college would receive $110,780 for the year. Instead the Board of Regents was able to provide only $91,235, or $19,545 less than Wesbrook had expected. Such a large budget cut required a reduction in the supply budgets for the three laboratory departments, and the clinical salaries and the costs of the outpatient department had to be paid from the hospital maintenance budget instead of from the college budget. The inroads thus made on the hospital maintenance fund by clinical salaries and the outpatient dispensary naturally left less money to pay the costs of patients, or for necessary hospital equipment. The reduction in the college budget meant that there could be no increases in faculty salaries. Laboratory teachers would tend to leave the university and clinical teachers would be discouraged, especially because in 1910 the Regents Salary Committee had promised to give salary needs priority in their requests to the legislature.[4]

President Vincent was, therefore, contemplating changes in a medical faculty that was partly paid and partly unpaid, but the paid portion was poorly paid. Except for the chiefs of departments, the clinical faculty were for the most part not paid at all. In the scientific departments the faculty were paid badly, and had not received even the modest increases they had been led to expect. Nevertheless, President Vincent remained determined to reorganize the medical faculty to reduce, he said, its unwieldy size, although, since the faculty members that he proposed to get rid of were not paid, their removal would achieve no economy. Furthermore, as experience was soon to show, President Vincent had not based his judgment that the clinical faculty was too large on any careful analysis of how many clinical teachers were needed to do the teaching that had to be done. Within a year after the reorganization, the university was obliged to appoint additional clinical teachers. The medical faculty was soon as large as it had been before, and presently it became larger. Dr. S. Marx White, who was on the faculty at the time and who was Dean Wesbrook's personal physician and close friend, recalled the situation:

> Dr. Wesbrook had many sessions with the president and, at one time, had come to a definite agreement that reorganization would be fostered as rapidly as could be done but no specific announcement would be made. Within a few days after this definite agreement had been made, the president spoke at a meeting in St. Paul. Evidently his enthusiasm mounted with his well-known rapid-fire diction. His memory slipped momentarily, for he announced that he was about to reorganize the medical school. This, of course, came as a severe shock in many quarters.[5]

Some writers on the history of the school have said that the reorganization was intended to promote research. If it were, it did not succeed in doing so. Research had been carried on at Minnesota before 1913, especially in the fields of bacteriology, histology, and embryology. The pace of research did not quicken after 1913; it may even have slowed down. Such research as was done continued to be done in the same departments and frequently by the same men as were doing research before 1913. Furthermore, the changes that occurred in the reorganization did not particularly encourage research. Dr. Thomas G. Lee, who had himself done research and had encouraged such men as Louis B. Wilson and Hal Downey to become investigators, was demoted from the headship of the Department of Anatomy. By contrast with Dr. Lee, a scientific investigator, who was demoted and officially ignored after 1913, Dr. Richard Olding Beard, who had never done any research and never would do any, flourished in the affairs of the school following the reorganization. Even in President Vincent's own list of criteria for appointment to the new faculty, research was mentioned only incidentally.

On 7 January 1913 President Vincent met with the executive faculty to explain "the plan for reducing the number of the clinical staff and increasing the teaching efficiency of the college."[6] His aim, he said, was to concentrate the teaching in the smallest number of faculty needed for the work. President Vincent also stated emphatically "that both this and the proposal to house the department of Pathology and Bacteriology and the State Board of Health in the wing of the Anatomy building originated with the Board of Regents and are administrative measures."[7] The latter statement meant that Dean Wesbrook was not to be considered responsible for either proposal. The consequence of President Vincent's initiative in two measures that affected the College of Medicine and Surgery so profoundly was to take control of the affairs of the college out of the hands of its dean. In the circumstances Dean Wesbrook was left with no option but to resign, although he did not make the reorganization the public reason for his resignation.

A few weeks earlier, at the beginning of December 1912, the government of British Columbia had approached Dean Wesbrook to learn whether he might be interested in becoming president of the new University of British Columbia. Five days after President Vincent's meeting with the executive faculty on 7 January, Dr. Wesbrook wrote to Dr. Henry Esson Young, Minister of Education for the Province of British Columbia, to say that he had obtained President Vincent's consent to be away from Minneapolis for two to three weeks in order to come to Vancouver to look over the plans for the proposed university. Within a few days Dr. and Mrs. Wesbrook boarded the train for Vancouver where Dr. Wesbrook met with the provincial cabinet on 27 January. After his return to Minneapolis Wesbrook telegraphed his acceptance of the presidency of the University of British Columbia on 14 February.[8] Probably at the same time Wesbrook offered his resignation at Minnesota to take effect 30 June 1913.

Meanwhile, on 11 January the executive faculty met again to consider the recommendation of the heads of the clinical departments for a reduction in the number of faculty in accordance with the request of President Vincent and the Board of Regents. The executive faculty voted its understanding that the skeleton faculty list that they were submitting to President Vincent was submitted on the understanding that salaries were to be paid to all clinical men.[9] The heads of each of the departments (medicine; surgery; obstetrics and gynecology; eye, ear, nose, and throat; mental and nervous diseases; and anatomy) then presented a list of faculty positions for their respective departments. The faculty also approved the reestablishment of a department of pharmacology and the division of the department of pathology and bacteriology into two departments, one of pathology, the other of public health and bacteriology. At the conclusion of the meeting the members of the executive faculty signed the following joint letter of resignation:

CRISIS AND REORGANIZATION

January 11, 1913

The President
The University of Minnesota

Sir:
In order to promote and accelerate the reorganization of the work and the concentration of the Faculty, the undersigned respectfully submit their resignations to take effect at the pleasure of the President.

(Signed)
F. F. Wesbrook
J. E. Moore
Chas. L. Greene
Richard Olding Beard
Thomas G. Lee

Frank C. Todd
Louis B. Baldwin
A. B. Cates
J. B. Johnston
C. Eugene Riggs[10]

Two days later on 15 January President Vincent and Regent William J. Mayo met with the general faculty of the College of Medicine and Surgery, and President Vincent outlined to the faculty the plans for reorganization. A committee on reorganization, consisting of three members of the present faculty and three graduates of the college practicing in the state outside the Twin Cities, was to be appointed. The committee on reorganization would nominate heads of departments. These nominated heads of departments would then be associated with the reorganization committee in appointing the faculty in the various departments.

There are two features of President Vincent's plan for reorganization that went well beyond his previously stated aim to reduce the size of a medical faculty that he declared to be unwieldy. The sweeping nature of the proposed reorganization implied President Vincent's complete contempt for the College of Medicine and Surgery in its existing form. He dismissed alike its high national standing and its scientific achievements. His actions almost convey the impression that President Vincent was deeply jealous of the college and of its dean, Frank Wesbrook. Because the college was already outstanding before he came, Vincent could not improve it. If he supported the plans that the college had already laid out for its future development, Vincent would have been supporting and strengthening the hands of Dean Wesbrook. From Vincent's standpoint Wesbrook was already too strong and independent a figure in the university. Wesbrook had proven exceedingly effective in gaining the support of the legislature for new medical buildings and for the expansion of the campus, whereas in his initial dealings with the legislature, Vincent had been ineffective. The contrast was striking and to Vincent may have been galling.

The departure of Dean Wesbrook may have been convenient for President Vincent by removing an obstacle to his plans for reorganization, but for the University of Minnesota it was a disaster. There followed long dreary years of stagnation in the development of the school, of endless quarrels among the faculty and between the medical faculty and the medical profession in the Twin Cities and throughout the state. Elsewhere in the United States medical schools developed rapidly, gaining new laboratories, new hospitals, and money to support research and full-time clinical appointments. At Minnesota no comparable developments occurred for almost fifteen years. The stagnation and turmoil after Wesbrook's departure stand in striking contrast to the rapid and on the whole peaceful development of the school that had occurred during the years of his deanship.

The second striking feature of the reorganization was that the alumni representatives on the reorganization committee were to be from *outside the Twin Cities*. The reorganization was intended to break the strong link that had existed previously between the college and the medical profession in the Twin Cities. Such an aim may have been particularly attractive to Regent William J. Mayo because the Mayo Clinic at Rochester was in competition with the medical profession of the Twin Cities for referred patients from throughout Minnesota. As the university hospital developed, Dean Wesbrook envisioned that the hospital would receive indigent patients from throughout the state and that its staff would act as consultants to the medical profession throughout the state. At Rochester the Mayos had provided free treatment to poor patients at St. Mary's Hospital from wherever they might come, and through such practice they had developed the surgical skills that brought to them a steady flow of paying patients. Dr. William Mayo foresaw clearly that the future would bring an ever larger role for the corporate practice of medicine in which various specialists worked together in a large clinic, using the facilities of a large hospital. Although the Elliot Hospital at the University of Minnesota was still small and received only charity patients, Dr. Mayo could foresee that as the university hospital grew and drew ever larger numbers of poor patients, the members of its staff would develop such medical and surgical skill that they would be sought out by private patients who paid for their care, just as had occurred at the Johns Hopkins Hospital in Baltimore and at St. Mary's Hospital in Rochester. Such a development would occur all the more easily at Minneapolis because of the strong links between the College of Medicine and Surgery and the Twin Cities medical profession, so many of whom had served, or were serving, on the medical faculty, or who were graduates of the college. Dr. Mayo may, therefore, have been happy to join President Vincent in slowing down the growth of the university hospital and in doing whatever might be done to sever the links between the college and the medical profession of the Twin Cities. In 1912 the concept of conflict of interest was not well developed, and it may have seemed perfectly natural to Dr. Mayo to use his position as a member of the Board of Regents to promote a policy that would prove beneficial to the Mayo Clinic, even if it were detrimental to the university for which as a regent he was responsible. The role of Dr. Mayo in the reorganization is difficult to assess, but President Vincent could not have carried out such a sweeping reorganization of the medical college without Mayo's consent and support.

At the meeting of the general faculty on 15 January President Vincent stated the principles to be used in selecting members of the faculty. They were:

1. Personality and character, including ability for team play, social service, etc.

2. Teaching power. The members of the faculty should be specialists in practice as well as in teaching.

3. Capacity, training, prestige, indicated in part by contributions to science.

4. Past service to the college.[11]

The noteworthy feature of President Vincent's criteria for faculty appointment is the relatively minor importance assigned by him to research or scholarship. By contrast "personality" and "ability for team play" came first on his list. Such position and emphasis strengthens the impression that President Vincent wanted primarily a medical faculty that would be compliant to his wishes. The reorganization was intended to destroy the capacity for initiative, and the intellectual and moral independence that had previously characterized the medical faculty.

The next day, 16 January, the Board of Regents appointed to the committee on reorganization President Vincent and Dean Wesbrook, James E. Moore and Charles L. Greene from the medical faculty, Louis B. Wilson of Rochester, Edward L. Tuohy of Duluth, and Theodore B. Bratrud of Warren.[12]

On 2 February, Parks Ritchie died suddenly from a stroke at the age of sixty-seven and the next day Richard Olding Beard, acting in Dean Wesbrook's absence, called a special meeting of the executive faculty to pass in Dr. Ritchie's memory a resolution that said in part:

> He entered into the work of medical education in 1885 and has continued the teaching of obstetrics for twenty-eight years. Until his election to the Deanship of this College, he carried his share of the burden of medical teaching without remuneration.
>
> He filled the office of Dean with constant devotion to its interests during a difficult constructive period in the history of the College, for nine years.[13]

At the next meeting of the executive faculty on 12 February Dean Wesbrook read a letter written by Dr. Ritchie before his death, offering his resignation as professor of obstetrics and gynecology to take effect at the close of the current academic year.[14]

When the executive faculty met on 1 March a committee that had been appointed to prepare plans for hospital facilities under the new reorganization of the medical school submitted a report. The committee, chaired by Jennings Litzenberg recommended that the university offer to reduce its representation in the city hospitals of Minneapolis and St. Paul with the understanding that one half of all patients admitted to those hospitals be assigned to the medical school, which would assume responsibility for their professional care. Because it was not clear how patients were to be assigned to the medical school, the committee recommended that the superintendents of the two city hospitals and the university hospital should confer to decide on a plan for assigning cases to respective services in the city hospitals. The committee recommended, thirdly, that the university should nominate the staff for the university services in each of the city hospitals, but they did not say whether the governing boards of their hospitals had agreed to appoint to their staffs physicians nominated by the university.[15]

President Vincent was present at the meeting on 1 March 1913 and gave a lengthy explanation of why the funds for the new wing of the anatomy building intended to house the Departments of Pathology and Public Health and Bacteriology had been omitted from the university's legislative request in 1913. Vincent said that the burning of the school of mines building created a need for a new building for the school of mines, which the university had decided to request instead of a new wing for the anatomy building. The university was also committed to build a new biology building. The Institute of Public Health and Pathology would, therefore, remain in its present building a half mile distant from the university hospital and other medical buildings. President Vincent evidently felt some compunction about breaking the promise he had given previously that the university would request a new wing for the anatomy building because he offered to call a special meeting of the the Board of Regents "to discuss the claims of the Medical School on account of the previous arrangement regarding Pathology."[16] Vincent stated also that the abandonment of the new wing for the anatomy building that had been intended to house pathology would not give pathology any future priority over the need for additional clinical facilities.[17] To Charles L. Greene, James E. Moore, and other members of the clinical faculty, the need for additional clinical facilities was already clearly apparent, and indeed urgent, as the memorandum of the medical faculty of October 1912 had stated. Their words had evidently fallen on deaf ears. Now President Vincent was saying that the faculty might in future have to choose between a new wing on the anatomy building and additional clinical facilities. In presenting the possibility of such a choice, was he seeking to create a division between the basic science members and the clinical members of the medical faculty? Or was George Edgar Vincent too innocent to realize the divisive implications in the choice he was presenting? President Vincent stated also that it was impossible to get a special appropriation for a new building for the school of mines, because the appropriations committee of the legislature had stated that day that no addition could be made to the university budget.

The executive faculty then adjourned for a meeting of the general faculty of the College of Medicine and Surgery held in Millard Hall at eight o'clock in the evening. The meeting was called at the request of President Vincent to discuss the general problems facing the reorganized faculty. President Vincent addressed the meeting, stating first "that the initiative in development and appointments remains always with the faculty," a curious statement after Vincent had ignored and frustrated the initiatives of the medical faculty for development put forward the previous October. Vincent continued:

> The relation of this college to the University presents some problems. The reorganization is in no sense disciplinary or a reflection on this college. It is most difficult to preserve the unity of the whole University. In the legislative budget an addition to the

support funds of $250,000 a year has been asked for, in consequence of which the building program had to be cut to the quick. The University is going to get all they ask for, and this will prove the best policy in the long run.

The departments of Anatomy and Physiology ought to be primarily University departments, carrying on research and adapting themselves to the medical teaching. These departments should be charged in part to the general University budget, thus relieving the budget of this college. This is thrown out merely as a suggestion.

We must lay increasing stress upon research work in clinical medicine, making this college a center for this work in the northwest, and to push forward in biological research in connection with the University graduate work.

The plan for cooperation with the Mayo Clinic and the publication of [a] scientific journal offers new opportunities for scientific work in the college.

We should develop a great central medical library for the northwest with branches in other cities.

The problem of clinical salaries is a most difficult one. A memorial has been received from the clinical men. A meeting should be held and the whole evening spent in discussing this question.[18]

The president expressed his regret at the loss of Dean Wesbrook, but said that he had made a wise choice in accepting the larger opportunities offered him. Perhaps the sincerity of President Vincent's speech may be gauged from his concluding statement because he had placed Dean Wesbrook in such a position that Wesbrook was forced to leave. In other respects President Vincent's statements were equally at variance with the effect of his actions.

After President Vincent's speech, Jennings Litzenberg described the severely overcrowded state of the university dispensary and added that in its first year and a half the obstetrical clinic had completely outgrown the facilities available for it in the university hospital. Dr. Hynes described the particularly overcrowded state of the medical clinic at the dispensary where he said it was impossible to teach students to listen to heart sounds because there were too many surrounding noises. Arthur Hamilton said that the division of nervous and mental diseases had one room at the dispensary in which to attempt to care for as many as twenty-four patients, and in which both men and women patients had to be examined. Not one of the 6,000 beds for mental patients in the state hospitals was available for university teaching. The university hospital ought be be provided with a psychiatric clinic with at least one hundred beds. "Harvard, Johns Hopkins, Michigan and Pennsylvania," said Dr. Hamilton, "have large hospitals at their disposal. Very few colleges have such poor facilities as Minnesota for the study of mental cases."[19]

Julius Parker Sedgwick, chief of the division of pediatrics, said that although every member of the staff in pediatrics had had work published in the best foreign and American journals, "There is not a teaching bed in the University Hospital open for children."[20] Beds for children were available in the city hospitals, but research could not be carried out effectively in those hospitals. S. Marx White of the department of medicine noted that only some of the departments were equipped for teaching and research, that the university needed a hospital of 400 to 500 beds to provide adequate clinics in all departments, and that the university

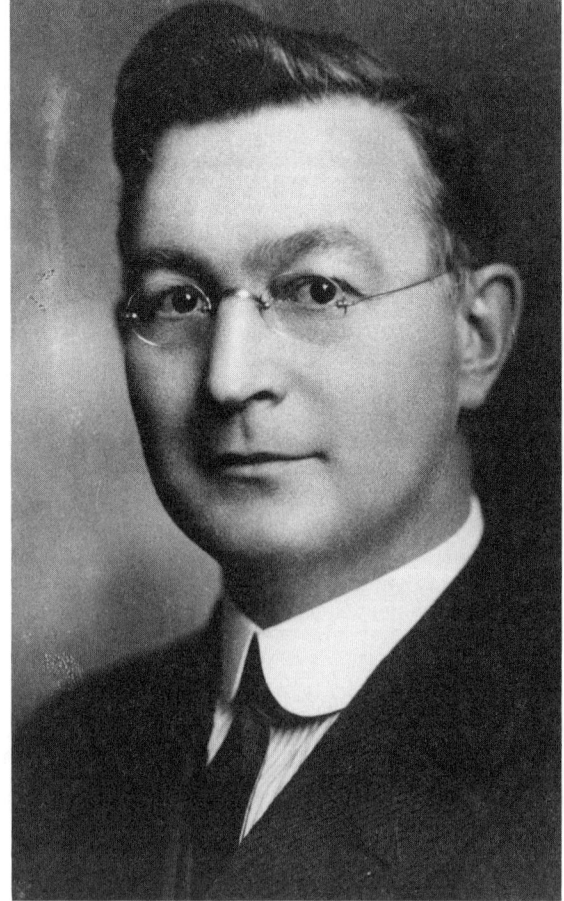

FIGURE 8:2   Clarence M. Jackson, 1916. Courtesy Mn U Archives.

dispensary should be on the campus. George D. Head suggested, "Public health and preventive medical movements must emanate from the medical school. Large sums of money can properly be asked for to enable the school to do this work. It is impossible for the faculty to live up to its opportunities without provision for proper clinical salaries." He urged the need to establish a tuberculosis pavilion on campus in connection with the university hospital.

Finally, in closing, President Vincent "pointed out that one of the first things for the administrative board to do is to prepare a definite program of symmetrical progressive development for a term of years."[21] Three months before, President Vincent had rejected such a program when it was presented to him by the exccutive faculty.

On 22 March 1913 the executive faculty recommended the appointment of Dr. Clarence M. Jackson, dean of the University of Missouri Medical School, as professor of anatomy and director of the Department of Anatomy.[22] In the reorganization Thomas G. Lee had been appointed professor of comparative anatomy in the Department of Anatomy, but the headship of the department had been left vacant. Then at the age of thirty-eight, Dr. Jackson had been graduated M.D. from the University of Missouri in 1900 and immediately appointed assistant professor of anatomy and histology. During the summers of 1900 and 1901 he pursued graduate study in anatomy at the University of Chicago under Henry H. Donaldson and in 1903–04 spent eighteen months at the universities of Leipzig and Berlin where he studied the effects of undernutrition and refeeding on the bone marrow of rabbits and pigeons. At the time of his appointment at Minnesota, Dr. Jackson had published on average about one paper per year since 1900.[23] His appointment may have been influenced by his association with Henry H. Donaldson at the University of Chicago because President Vincent probably consulted his former colleagues at Chicago about new appointments at Minnesota, but Elexious T. Bell, who had come to Minnesota from Missouri in 1910, is said to have helped persuade his former teacher, Dr. Jackson, to accept the headship of anatomy at Minnesota.[24]

The reorganization of the medical faculty had also left vacant the directorships of the Departments of Pharmacology and Physiology. For director of pharmacology President Vincent sought to appoint Reid Hunt, who was then chief of the division of pharmacology of the Hygienic Laboratory of the United States Public Health and Marine Hospital Service at Washington, D.C. In 1913 at the age of forty-three, Hunt was a well-established investigator in the field of pharmacology, and for that reason he was sought not only by Minnesota but also by Harvard where that same year he was appointed professor of pharmacology and head of the department.

For the directorship of the Department of Physiology, President Vincent hoped to appoint Walter B. Cannon, professor of physiology at Harvard University. Both President Vincent and Dr. William J. Mayo wrote to Dr. Cannon to offer to appoint him both director of the Department of Physiology and dean of the medical school, but Cannon decided to remain at Harvard.[25]

In the reorganization of the medical school a new office of secretary of the medical school was established, the secretary to be appointed by the Board of Regents instead of being elected by the faculty. The secretary was to act as an assistant to the dean and to exercise general oversight of the medical buildings, except for the university hospital, and to be responsible for the accounts and business administration of the medical school. The first and only secretary to be appointed was Richard Olding Beard, and with his passionate preoccupation with detail and not inconsiderable sense of self-importance, the position may have suited him. At any rate, Dr. Beard was induced at first to take a benign view of the reorganization and the events that followed from it.

On 6 May 1913, the reorganization having been completed, the administrative board, which replaced the executive faculty in the new organization of the school of medicine, met formally for the first time. Both President Vincent and

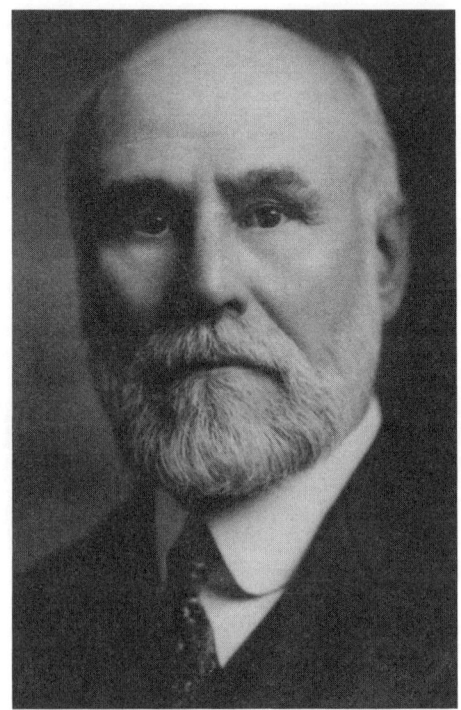

FIGURE 8:3 Richard Olding Beard, 1908. Courtesy Mn U Archives.

Dean Wesbrook were present. One of their first acts was to postpone the establishment of the separate Departments of Pathology and of Public Health and Bacteriology called for in the new plan of organization, and to retain for the time being the existing Department of Pathology, Bacteriology and Public Health. Among other business dealt with at this meeting, the salary committee reported their recommendation that all faculty members in the clinical departments, who were devoting a certain minimum proportion of time to teaching, should be paid a salary according to their rank. The report presented a schedule of salaries paid in other medical schools, but discussion of the report revealed that the university had no money to pay such salaries to clinical faculty.

On 6 May the administrative board also discussed the desirability of appointing a new dean to succeed Dean Wesbrook. After mentioning various possible candidates from outside the university, members of the board suggested that a dean might be obtained from among the present members of the faculty. According to the minutes President Vincent "concurred in the selection, if possible, of any desirable member of the faculty, but stated his view that Dr. Mayo should be consulted before a candidate was finally proposed to the Board . . . ."[26] Among candidates from within the faculty the names of Charles Lyman Greene and S. Marx White were discussed, but Dr. Greene declined to be considered. A committee consisting of President Vincent, Dean Wesbrook, and Dr. Greene was suggested to discuss with Dr. White his possible candidacy for the deanship.

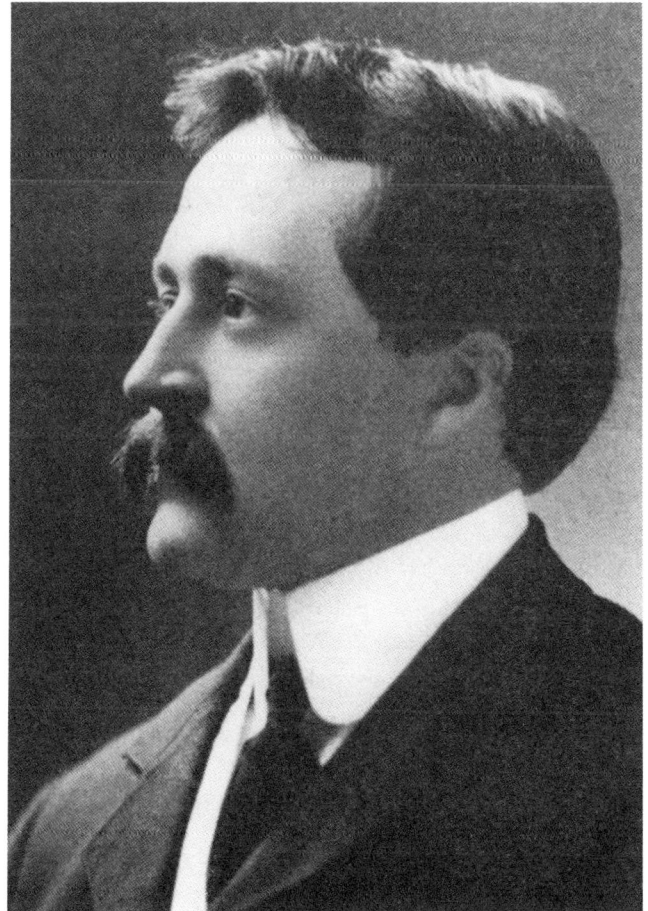

FIGURE 8:4   Charles Lyman Greene, 1908. Courtesy Mn U Archives.

By the time of the next meeting of the administrative board on 28 May, Dean Wesbrook had left for British Columbia and Dr. Beard presided as acting dean. The board once again discussed the possibility of nominating a candidate for the deanship and proceeded to cast ballots for nominees. After three ballots, six of eight votes were cast for Charles Lyman Greene. Dr. Greene said that his acceptance of the nomination, if it were confirmed by President Vincent and the Board of Regents, "would depend upon assurances to be had from the Administration of the University with reference to the present and future needs of the School," but that if he were to accept the nomination, he would make the deanship "the principal interest in his life work."[27] In a letter to President Vincent and in conversation with him, Dr. Greene made his acceptance of the deanship conditional on Vincent's support for an expansion of the university hospital to 300 beds, the building of a nurses' home, and the payment of salaries to clinical members

CRISIS AND REORGANIZATION

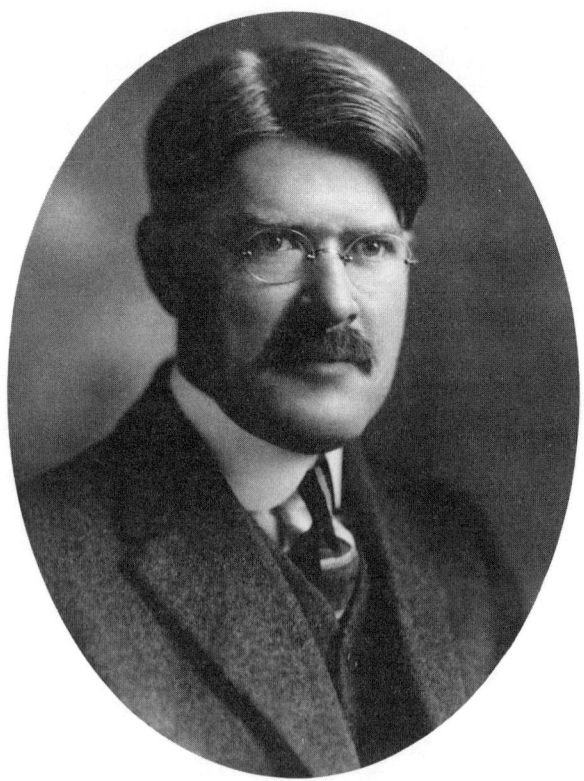

FIGURE 8:5   Elias P. Lyon, 1914. Courtesy Mn U Archives.

of the faculty who devoted half their time to clinical teaching.[28] On the evening of 10 June 1913, Dr. Greene met with President Vincent and William J. Mayo to discuss his conditions, but Vincent and Mayo refused to give the assurances that Dr. Greene requested so he was unable to consider the appointment. When the administrative board met the next evening, President Vincent described the results of his and Dr. Mayo's conversation with Dr. Greene and proposed Elias P. Lyon of St. Louis for the deanship. The administrative board then voted to nominate Dr. Lyon to be dean of the medical school and director of the Department of Physiology.[29] In order to provide for a salary for Dr. Lyon, William J. Mayo, who was present, suggested the omission of part of the salary increases proposed for the heads of the Departments of Medicine and Surgery and for Richard Beard and Harold E. Robertson, and the omission of any new or increased salaries for members of the faculty in the clinical departments.[30] Part of the price paid for the appointment of Elias P. Lyon as dean was thus the abandonment of any attempt to provide salaries for members of the clinical departments, even though the promise of salaries for the clinical members of the faculty had been part of the original understanding on which the faculty had agreed to cooperate in the reorganization of the medical school. It is curious that in planning the reorganization of the medical school President Vincent evidently had not set aside funds for the new appointments contemplated as part of the reorganization.

When he came to Minnesota as dean of the medical school in August 1913, Elias Potter Lyon was forty-five years old.[31] In 1907 Dr. Lyon had been appointed dean of the St. Louis University Medical School and served in that position for six years before he came to Minnesota. He was interested in medical education and had published a number of articles on questions facing medical schools.

One of Lyon's first acts as dean was to recommend by telegram to the administrative board at its meeting on 3 July 1913 the appointment of Arthur Hirschfelder of Johns Hopkins University as professor of pharmacology.[32] Dean Lyon was responding to the recommendation of a medical school search committee, chaired by Charles Lyman Greene, who at the meeting of the American Medical Association held at Minneapolis in June 1913 had been impressed by a paper delivered by Dr. Hirshfelder on the use of diuretics in heart disease.[33] After the meeting Dr. Greene, who was himself keenly interested in diseases of the heart, read Dr. Hirschfelder's recently published book, *Diseases of the heart and aorta,* which likewise impressed him by its evidence of the great potential value of pharmacology to clinical medicine.[34]

During the summer of 1913 President Vincent regularly attended and presided over meetings of the administrative board, even after Dean Lyon arrived in August to assume his responsibilities. When the board met on 15 September President Vincent attended, but Dean Lyon was in the chair. On 20 October the board met at Dean Lyon's house where the dean and Mrs. Lyon entertained the members at dinner. On this occasion President Vincent again occupied the chair, and among other matters the board decided to hold its regular meeting on the first Thursday of each month. Richard Olding Beard, as secretary of the faculty, proposed the creation of two central storerooms for the medical school, one in Millard Hall for glassware and chemicals, the other in the Institute of Anatomy for stains, special glassware, and special chemicals. The storerooms were to take the place of the storerooms kept previously by individual departments. Only the Institute of Public Health and Pathology was to retain its storeroom temporarily "on account of its present remoteness."[35] The workshops, art rooms, photographic rooms, and animal rooms of the medical school were also to be unified, again except for such rooms in the Institute of Public Health and Pathology. All budgets for supplies, previously allocated to departments, were to be merged into a common supply budget to be administered by the secretary. Dr. Beard's recommendations, which clearly gave him a larger role in the administration of the medical school, were approved unanimously by the administrative board. Since the central storerooms diminished significantly the independence of the department heads, the unanimity of the board in favor of the change is curious. Perhaps the presence of President Vincent was helpful in discouraging opposition. The measure reflected Dr. Beard's considerably greater influence in the medical school following the reorganization. Others, who had served the medical school faithfully for many years, now exerted little influence. Dr. Thomas Lee was omitted from all committees, including even the library committee, when Dean Lyon made his committee appointments in December 1913.

At the same meeting Dr. Beard reported a deficit of $900 in the medical school supplies budget, the deficit having been created by the transfer of that amount to help provide salaries for new appointees to the faculty. According to the minutes, "President Vincent offered an explanation of the existing financial conditions, of the action by which the deficit was taxed upon the Medical School budget, and of the necessity of the acceptance of the obligation by the School." But the administrative board voted " . . . to enter its protest with the President against the continued submission of the Medical School to sacrifices of its salary and supplies budgets."[36]

Such were the immediate results of the reorganization of 1913 — reduced budgets and dissension among the members of the administrative board. The damage done to the medical school was immense; the bitterness of the reorganization would haunt its halls and corrode its life for decades. The new research activity promised to result from the reorganization was slow in coming, and, when it did come, occurred more in spite of the reorganization than because of it. The research that was done in the years immediately after 1913 was carried out largely by men who had been trained, encouraged, or appointed by Frank Wesbrook or Thomas Lee. The saddest fact about the medical school during the years after 1913 was that during years when great sums of money were being poured into medical schools, such as those of Washington University at St. Louis, Johns Hopkins, Yale, Harvard, and many other universities, for new or expanded hospitals and laboratories, and for salaries for clinical faculty, the medical school at Minnesota stagnated. The only building added to the Elliot Hospital was a service building. The nurses continued to live in their cramped and dismal quarters. The Institute of Anatomy and Millard Hall remained unfinished. Except for the heads of departments, the clinical teachers remained largely unpaid.

NOTES

1. Abraham Flexner, *Medical education in the United States and Canada*, pp. 247–249.

2. Ibid., p. 248. The salaries in 1909 were $3,000 per year for part-time service, and in 1910 were increased to $3,500.

3. S. Marx White, "Frank F. Wesbrook, M.D. Action in medical education and public health in Minnesota," *J.-Lancet*, 1960, *80,* 259–264, p. 263.

4. College of Medicine and Surgery, Executive Faculty, Minutes, 30 March 1912 [Book 18, pt. II].

5. Ibid.

6. Ibid., 7 January 1913 [vol. 19].

7. Ibid.

8. William C. Gibson, *Wesbrook and his university*, pp. 53–55.

9. College of Medicine and Surgery, Executive Faculty, Minutes, 11 January 1913 [vol. 19].
10. Ibid.
11. College of Medicine and Surgery, General Faculty, Minutes, 15 January 1913 [vol. 19].
12. Board of Regents, Minutes, 16 January 1913.
13. College of Medicine and Surgery, Executive Faculty, Minutes, 3 February 1913 [vol. 19].
14. Ibid., 12 February 1913 [vol. 19].
15. Ibid., 1 March 1913 [vol. 19].
16. Ibid.
17. Ibid.
18. College of Medicine and Surgery, General Faculty, Minutes, 1 March 1913 [vol. 19].
19. Ibid.
20. Ibid.
21. Ibid.
22. College of Medicine and Surgery, Executive Faculty, Minutes, 22 March 1913 [vol. 19].
23. E. A. Boyden, "Clarence Martin Jackson," *Anat. Rec.*, 1947, *98,* 317–324, pp. 320–321.
24. J. Arthur Myers, "Tommy Bell," *J.-Lancet,* 1964, *84,* 237–238.
25. George E. Vincent to Walter B. Cannon, 6 March 1913, and 17 March 1913, Cannon papers. Cf. Saul Benison, A. Clifford Barger, Elin L. Wolfe, *Walter B. Cannon: the life and times of a young scientist,* pp. 337–338.
26. School of Medicine, Administrative Board, Minutes, 6 May 1913 [Bk. I].
27. Ibid., 28 May 1913 [Bk. I].
28. In 1917 Dr. Greene described publicly the conditions that he had attached to his acceptance of the deanship. See Charles Lyman Greene, "The present unfortunate situation of the Medical School of the University of Minnesota," *J.-Lancet,* 1917, *37,* 149–156.
29. School of Medicine, Administrative Board, Minutes, 11 June 1913 [Bk. I].
30. The administrative board then voted to revise the proposed budget as follows:

Dr. J. E. Moore, omission of increase in amount of	$500.
Dr. R. O. Beard, omission of increase in amount of	500.
Dr. H. E. Robertson, omission of part of increase in amount of	250.
Omission of proposed new instructor in bacteriology	1,200.
Omission of proposed salary for Dr. F. C. Todd	1,000.
Omission of proposed salary for Dr. A. S. Hamilton	1,000.
Omission of proposed salary for Dr. J. P. Sedgwick	1,000.
Omission of proposed salary for Dr. A. T. Mann	400.
Reserved for Dean's salary	2,500.
Total retrenchments	$ 8,350.
Salary for Dr. E. P. Lyon, Dean and Director of the Department of Physiology	$6,000.
Increase of salary for Dr. F. H. Scott, promised "on his surrender of offer from College in Canada"	250.
Reserve	2,100.
	$ 8,350.

Ibid.

31. Lyon was born 20 October 1867 on a farm near Hillsdale, Michigan and was educated at the Hillsdale High School and Hillsdale College where he was graduated B.S. in 1891 and B.A. in 1892. After a period of teaching in preparatory schools at Chicago, Lyon began graduate study in physiology under Jacques Loeb at the University of Chicago, where he received his Ph.D. degree in 1897. He then became head of the department of biology at the Bradley Polytechnic Institute at Peoria, Illinois. In 1900 Professor Loeb invited Lyon to return to the department of physiology at the University of Chicago, where he remained until 1904 when he was appointed professor and chairman of the department of physiology at the St. Louis University Medical School.

32. School of Medicine, Administrative Board, Minutes, 3 July 1913 [Bk. I].

33. Arthur D. Hirshfelder, "Diuretics in cardiac disease: A general review," *J. Am. med. Ass.*, 1913, *61*, 340–344.

34. In 1913 Arthur Hirschfelder was only thirty-three years of age. A native of San Francisco, where his father was professor of medicine at the Cooper Lane Medical College, Hirschfelder was educated at the University of California where he received a B.S. degree in 1897 at the age of eighteen. He then went to Germany to begin the study of medicine at Heidelberg, but after two years returned to the United States to complete his medical education at Johns Hopkins where he was graduated M.D. in 1903. In October 1905 Dr. Hirschfelder became director of the physiological laboratory of the medical clinic at the Johns Hopkins Hospital, where during the next several years he carried out the investigations on cardiac physiology, blood pressure, and electrocardiography that so impressed Dr. Greene. A. McGehee Harvey, "Arthur D. Hirschfelder—Johns Hopkins's first full-time cardiologist," *Johns Hopk. med. J.*, 1978, *143*, 129–139, p. 136. Cf. Arthur Douglas Hirschfelder, *Diseases of the heart and aorta*.

35. School of Medicine, Administrative Board, Minutes, 20 October 1913 [Bk. I, pp. 67–79].

36. School of Medicine, Administrative Board, Minutes, 4 December 1913 [Bk. I, pp. 80–89].

CHAPTER 9

Affiliation of the University with the Mayo Foundation, 1915–1917

At a meeting of the executive faculty on 1 March 1913, when the College of Medicine and Surgery was in the throes of reorganization, President Vincent referred to a "plan for cooperation with the Mayo Clinic."[1] Vincent's passing reference to such a plan must have been based on conversations or correspondence with William J. Mayo, but he did not then mention what the plan consisted of, nor how it had been developed.

A year later almost to the day, James Moore, reporting as chairman of a committee to consider graduate degrees in surgery, recommended the establishment of a master's degree in surgery to be awarded to surgeons who had been in practice for five years and who had spent one year in resident work in surgery at the university. Candidates for the degree would also be required to submit and defend a thesis. The administrative board did not act immediately on the recommendation, but referred the plan for the master's degree in surgery back to the committee.[2] Dr. Moore's proposal for a graduate degree in surgery reflected the great development of surgery during the preceding quarter century following upon the introduction of antiseptic and aseptic surgery. A graduate degree in surgery was also one of the ideas discussed in the founding of the American College of Surgeons and at its first convocation at Chicago in November 1913.[3] Moore was one of the surgeons invited to Washington, D.C. in May 1913 to participate in the organization of the college, and supported wholeheartedly its aim to establish standards of training for the practice of surgery.[4] The idea for a college of surgeons had originated with Franklin Martin who in 1910 had organized the first Clinical Congress of Surgeons of North America at Chicago, a meeting that, in place of the reading and discussion of papers, consisted of demonstrations of surgical operations at various Chicago hospitals. Earlier in 1896 Dr. Martin had founded at Chicago the Post-graduate Medical School and Hospital to help medical practitioners learn surgery by giving them the opportunity to watch surgical operations and to hear lectures from experienced surgeons. After the publication of the Flexner report in 1910, Martin realized that it would be better for the young doctor to continue in surgical training immediately following the internship instead of attempting to learn surgery by trial and error upon his unfortunate patients. In an organized program the student, already a graduate physician, could assume responsibility for patients and learn to give surgical care under supervision.[5] Nevertheless, when the American College of Surgeons was organized in 1913, there were few opportunities for graduate training in surgery in the United States. At the Johns Hopkins Hospital a distinguished group of residents had learned surgery under William Stewart Halsted. Many American surgeons were self-taught, their education extended by visits to the clinics of other surgeons in the United States or in Europe. A growing number became assistants to experienced surgeons and were taught by them, but frequently such young men were more exploited by their preceptors than educated.[6]

At the same meeting of the executive faculty in March 1914, Frank Todd similarly proposed a two-year graduate course for physicians in diseases of the eye, ear, nose, and throat, leading to a degree which would probably also be a master's degree. The purpose of the degree would be to train specialists in eye, ear, nose, and throat diseases and secondly "to provide our department with assistants who will devote their full time in the work of the division."[7] Dr. Todd said that the only such course in America was offered at the University of Michigan, and Michigan did not grant a degree. In England Oxford University granted the degree of doctor of ophthalmology for similar training. In the United States most physicians who called themselves specialists in eye, ear, nose, and throat diseases had taken only a six weeks' course. Dr. Todd said that such men were very incompetent, and there was consequently need to establish an organized university course to provide proper training for specialists in eye, ear, nose, and throat disease. Such a course would help to distinguish a real ophthalmologist from the six weeks ophthalmologist. Meanwhile the eye, ear, nose, and throat clinic at the dispensary was receiving more than forty patients a day, or 1,100 per month, many of whom required a considerable amount of the attending physicians' time, and Dr. Todd was having difficulty in getting enough physicians to carry on the clinic. If a master's degree course in ophthalmology and otology were established, Dr. Todd expected that those taking the course would devote their full time to it and would spend a large part of every afternoon at work on patients at the dispensary. Dr. Todd's proposal was likewise referred to the committee on the degree in surgery, to which committee Todd was added. A month later, on 6 April 1914, Dr. Todd sent a copy of his proposal to William J. Mayo, with whom he, Dean Lyon, and James E. Moore had discussed such graduate medical training during the summer and fall of 1913.[8]

On 30 July 1914 the administrative board recommended the establishment of nine teaching fellowships to be distributed among the various clinical departments and divisions, with two assigned to the division of eye, ear, nose, and throat.[9] At the same meeting the committee on teaching fellowships, chaired by Dr. Moore, recommended that a graduate school in medicine be established.[10] Candidates for graduate study in medicine would have to possess the M.D. degree and have completed a year of internship at an approved hospital. The graduate course should cover a period of three years, leading to the degree of doctor of science in a clinical subject, as for example, doctor of science in surgery. In some specialties a two-year course might be offered, for which a certificate of proficiency would be given in place of a degree.

Meanwhile plans for the further development of the Elliot Hospital had been at a standstill for more than a year, and the medical school was suffering for lack of facilities for clinical teaching. In December 1913, on a motion by James E. Moore, chief of surgery, seconded by Charles Lyman Greene, chief of medicine, the administrative board established a committee on hospital and clinical development with Dr. Moore as chairman.[11] About June 1914 this committee sent to Regent Mayo a long communication in which they described their urgent need for enlargement of the university hospital and for new facilities for the outpatient department. The committee said: "The time is come when we must either develop a completely controlled clinic or frankly admit an enforced mediocrity and lose our standing as a Class A + school."[12] Although the school was equipped to teach the basic medical sciences, it was unable to meet its obligations to provide clinical instruction for the students, and the committee emphasized that the school could not depend for clinical teaching on the city hospitals of St. Paul and Minneapolis. Speaking directly to Dr. Mayo, the committee said of the need for enlargement of the university hospital: "No one indeed, can better appreciate its truth than you, who have personally experienced the value and necessity of complete clinical control as indispensable to the upbuilding of a great clinic . . . ." The committee emphasized the need to enlarge the number of clinical clerkships in the hospital, and to use small group teaching as much as possible.[13] Clinical research, the committee said, could be carried on only in a clinic of sufficient size by men who possessed some freedom from routine work. Nevertheless, in pediatrics there was no clinical service in the university hospital, and the beds for children in other Twin City hospitals were too scattered to permit an effective pediatric service. The school needed at least fifty beds for children's diseases in the university hospital. The study of diseases of the eye, ear, nose, and throat, and of nervous and mental diseases was similarly hampered by a lack of beds in the university hospital. The clinical facilities for surgery, genitourinary diseases, and obstetrics should be two or three times greater than they were. The university also badly needed a separate hospital building for contagious diseases, both to protect patients in the university hospital and for students at the university.

The committee described the university dispensary at Seven Corners as "a poorly constructed, ramshackle building" with such inadequate space and insufficient equipment that some of the best physicians were unwilling to continue to work there. Even more acute was the need for a nurses' residence. "At the present time," the committee said, "these women are housed in ordinary dwellings which are neither decently comfortable nor even safe. Indeed the chief dormitory carries the University Hospital laundry in its basement and has already once been on fire."[14] The committee asked that the Board of Regents request an appropriation

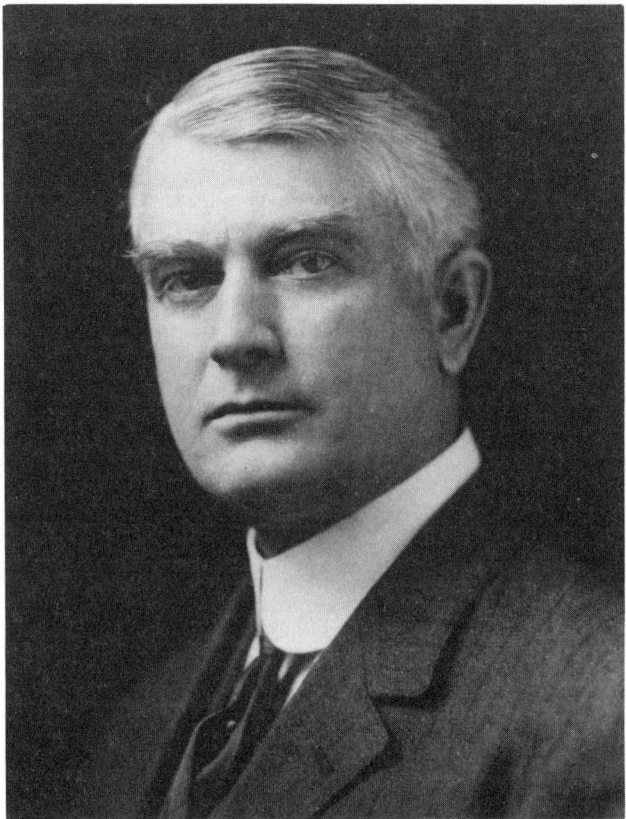

FIGURE 9:1   William J. Mayo, circa 1914. Courtesy Mn U Archives.

for a hospital building to house the outpatient department on the ground floor and approximately 200 beds for contagious diseases, neurological diseases, sick children, and internal medicine on two upper floors. The building should also contain a lecture room on each of the three hospital floors for the presentation of patients before small groups of medical students, and two clinical laboratories. The superintendent of the Elliot Hospital, Dr. Baldwin, estimated that the proposed nurses' residence and hospital addition would cost $375,000. The committee summed up their appeal to Dr. Mayo:

> . . . it is futile to attempt any extended postgraduate instruction, secure anything approaching our possibilities in the way of productive research or even to satisfy the requirement of modern undergraduate instruction, until these facilities are available and we firmly believe that they represent the greatest need of our University.
>
> We, therefore, ask your support not only with President Vincent and the Board of Regents but also in the halls of the legislature.[15]

The committee's appeal to Dr. Mayo apparently led in July 1914 to a conference between Dr. Mayo and members of the committee. On 30 July the chairman

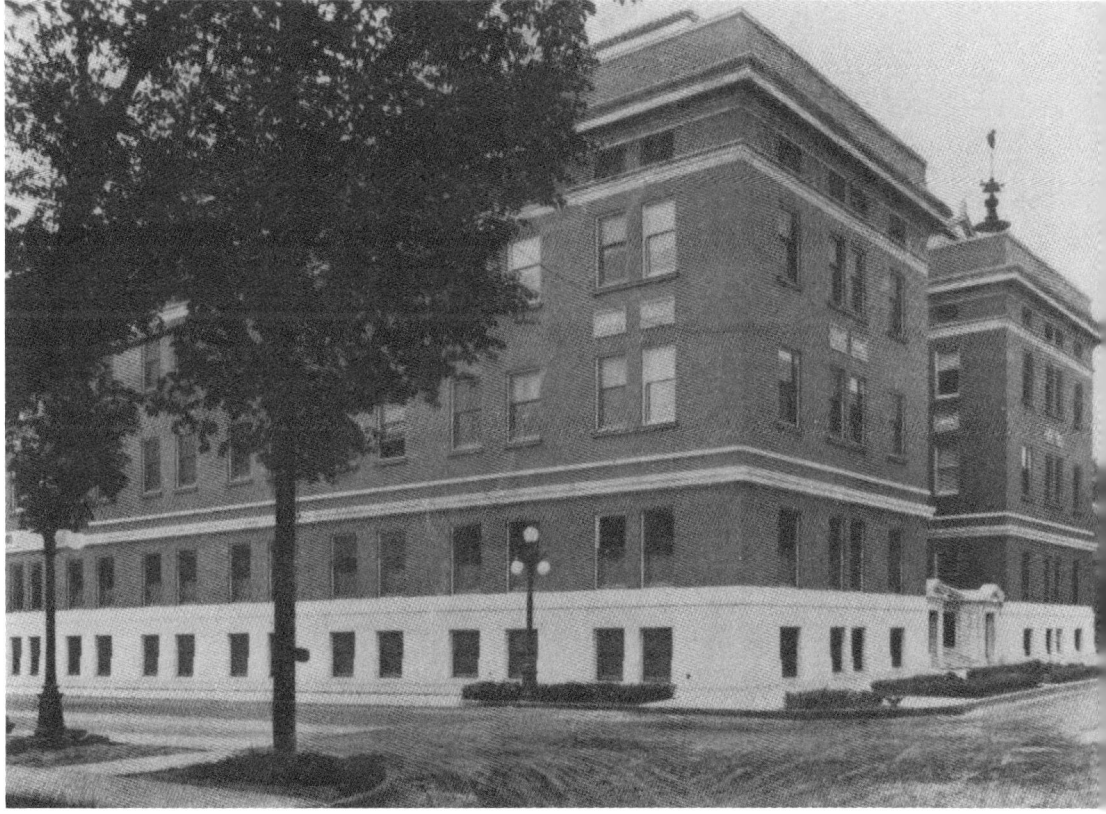

FIGURE 9:2 Mayo Clinic, the new building, 1914. *Journal-Lancet*, 1914.

of the committee, Dr. Moore, reported to the administrative board that at their conference Dr. Mayo had agreed to support a request for a legislative appropriation for a contagious disease infirmary to cost $100,000, a building for the school of nurses to cost $100,000, and an extension of the university hospital to cost $200,000 to house the outpatient department and to create clinical services for children's diseases and nervous and mental diseases.[16]

Dean Lyon felt sufficiently strongly about the urgency of the need to expand that he referred to it in a speech before the Minnesota State Medical Association at the beginning of October. He emphasized the inadequacy of the Elliot Hospital and said that its capacity should be doubled or tripled.[17] Dean Lyon asked the members of the State Medical Association to back the medical school "in the modest request it is about to make for the extension of its clinical facilities."[18]

During the autumn of 1914 discussion of a possible relationship of the medical school with the Mayo Clinic went forward. On 6 March 1914 the Mayo Clinic moved out of the scattered collection of offices and laboratories, improvised from converted stores and other buildings and connected by temporary passageways,

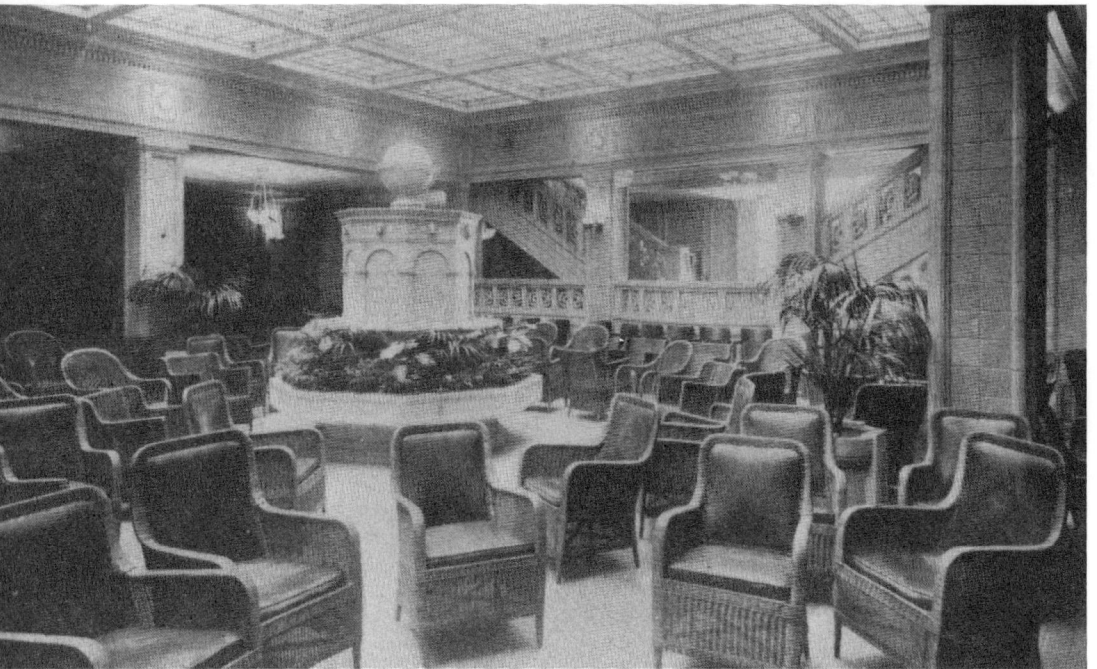

FIGURE 9:3 Mayo Clinic, Waiting Room, 1914. *Journal-Lancet,* 1914.

in which the Mayo brothers and their partners had been carrying on their burgeoning practice, into a magnificent new four-story brick building. From the marble staircase that greeted the visitor on entrance, and the large, marble-paneled waiting room furnished with a marble fountain in the center banked with palms on the first floor, to the third-floor reading room furnished with oriental rugs and an assembly room for the staff dominated by large portraits of William and Charles Mayo flanking the fireplace, the building struck a note of opulent grandeur. But the new clinic building was as impressive for its highly organized and integrated facilities as for its public display. Designed by the St. Paul architects Ellerbe and Round to meet the specifications of Mayo partner Henry Plummer, the building was intended to bring all the diverse capabilities of modern scientific medicine to bear upon the care of the patient. On the ground floor were outpatient clinics and an orthopedic surgery clinic together with laboratories, dressing rooms, and a diet-kitchen for gastroenterologic work, a pharmacy, sterilizing rooms, and an office for medical records and statistics. Dr. Plummer had developed a system both for keeping complete and accurate patient records and for gaining immediate access to them. On the first floor, examination and consulting rooms surrounded on three sides the great marble waiting room with its fountain and palms. On the second floor were specialty clinics, clinical laboratories, x-ray equipment, and a library of x-ray photographs. The third floor was divided among laboratories for pathology, histology and physiological chemistry, editorial offices, and a library with stacks, reading room, and assembly room. On the fourth floor was a pathological museum, photographic service and various technical workshops, while in a roofhouse were animal houses and runways together with laboratory facilities for experimental surgery and physiology.[19] When the new building was dedicated Dr. William Mayo said that it was for the scientific investigation of disease as well as for the cure of the sick and suffering.

The whole complex organization of the Mayo Clinic had grown out of the medical practice of Dr. William Worrall Mayo and his two sons in the twenty-five years since St. Mary's Hospital had opened at Rochester in the fall of 1889, with William Worrall Mayo as consulting physician and his two sons as the attending staff. From the beginning St. Mary's Hospital had charged all patients who could pay, and at rates that were sufficient to keep the hospital self-supporting. The Mayos equipped the operating room at St. Mary's and the Sisters of St. Francis admitted no patient until he had been examined by one of the Mayos so that the Mayos controlled St. Mary's Hospital. For their part, the Mayos decided to attend patients at no other hospital than St. Mary's. In 1894 the elder son, William J. Mayo, visited the Johns Hopkins Hospital where in William Osler's clinic he saw how the clinical laboratory could be used effectively for the diagnosis of disease. Dr. Mayo saw also how the permanent organization of the various services in the Johns Hopkins Hospital, each under a single head with long-term paid residents as their assistants, permitted the creation of an organized and highly efficient clinic. Furthermore, at Johns Hopkins all members of the medical and surgical staff pursued research as an integral part of their hospital work. The following year the senior Dr. Mayo and and his younger son, Charles, also went to Baltimore and thereafter the Mayo brothers visited the Johns Hopkins clinics in succession, spending most of their time in William Stewart Halsted's surgical clinic, where Halsted and his associates were refining the new techniques of aseptic surgery.

At St. Mary's Hospital in Rochester the Mayo brothers applied all that they learned from visits to Johns Hopkins and to clinics at Chicago, New York, and Boston. In the early 1890s most of their surgical operations were gynecological, but they operated also for appendicitis. In 1900 the Mayos performed 186 operations for appendicitis and by the year 1905 they were performing more than a thousand such operations annually. As their reputation for surgical skill grew, patients began to come to them from a distance and their practice became predominantly surgical. In 1890 William Mayo performed his first gallbladder operation. During the year 1895 the Mayos performed 10 operations for gallbladder; in 1900, 75; and in 1905, 324 operations. By 1903 the Mayos had also done thirty-five radical operations for hernia without a death. In 1895 William Mayo performed his first operation on the stomach to relieve obstruction of the pylorus. The result was successful and encouraged the Mayos to operate for stomach cancer, and then for ulcers of the stomach and duodenum. In 1905 William J. Mayo performed 217 operations on the stomach and duodenum; all told that year the Mayos performed more than two thousand abdominal operations at St. Mary's

Hospital. The Mayos also operated for tuberculous glands and joints, and for varicose veins. In 1895 they began to do Halsted's radical operation for breast cancer, and during 1905 performed fifty-four such operations. In 1890 the Mayos performed their first operation on an emergency basis to remove a greatly enlarged goitre and by 1904 Charles Mayo had performed sixty-eight operations for goitre with only two deaths.

During the 1890s the growing reputation of the Mayo brothers as surgeons drew patients from throughout southern Minnesota and the Dakotas. By 1905 they were becoming known throughout the United States for their remarkably low rates of mortality in operations, as well as for their success in performing new surgical procedures. As early as 1892, to meet the demands of their growing practice, the Mayos took into partnership Augustus W. Stinchfield, and in 1893 they added Charles Mayo's brother-in-law, Christopher Graham. In 1898 Melvin C. Millet became a resident at St. Mary's Hospital under the Mayos, in 1901 he was promoted to attending physician. Also in 1901 the Mayos hired Henry Plummer to take charge of their clinical laboratory, including the x-ray equipment which was at that time in a rudimentary state. In 1903 E. Starr Judd became an assistant surgeon to Charles Mayo, and presently began to perform operations independently. In 1904 the growing volume of surgical work required a third addition to St. Mary's Hospital.

In 1899 William J. Mayo was elected to the American Surgical Association and in 1905 he was elected president of the American Medical Association, honors indicative of his national reputation. By 1901 surgeons were beginning to come from Chicago, New York, and other distant American cities to watch the Mayos operate. In 1903 the Polish surgeon Johann von Mikulicz-Radecki visited Rochester, the first of many surgeons to come from abroad to observe the Mayos' surgical techniques. In 1906 a group of visiting surgeons was present so regularly in Rochester that they formed a club called "The Surgeons Club."

In 1905 when Louis B. Wilson moved from the university and the State Board of Health Laboratory to join the Mayos at Rochester, he began systematically to collect, examine, and preserve all pathological specimens removed during surgical operations or at autopsy. By 1914 the large volume of surgery performed at St. Mary's Hospital had generated a great pathological collection, invaluable for research. Also by 1914, Charles Mayo had moved to the forefront of the exacting field of thyroid surgery, and Henry Plummer had become an authority on all aspects of thyroid disease then so common throughout the goiter belt that extended through Minnesota, Iowa and other midwestern states. In February 1914 the Mayos appointed a chemist, Edward C. Kendall, to pursue research on the isolation of the thyroid hormone and by 1915 Kendall had obtained the pure hormone which he named *thyroxine*.

In 1914, in addition to the Mayo brothers and Dr. Judd as operating surgeons, the Mayo Clinic possessed a diagnostic staff of seventeen physicians and eleven clinical assistants. Most of the staff came from the medical schools of the University of Minnesota, the Johns Hopkins University, and the University of Toronto. Al-

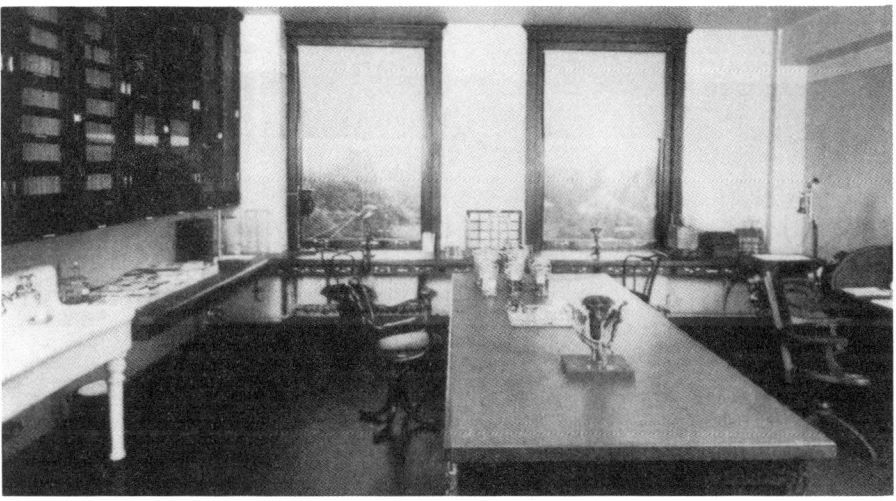

FIGURE 9:4   Mayo Clinic, pathology laboratory, 1914. *Journal-Lancet*, 1914.

though originally the Mayos had hired young doctors simply to help them with the examination and care of patients, they realized presently that they had a responsibility to educate them, and in 1912 decided that they would designate them as fellows of the Mayo Clinic instead of calling them interns or assistants. Each fellow was to pursue a three-year program in which he spent a year each in pathology, diagnosis, and surgery. The Mayos began then to appoint a sufficient number of fellows that each would have a third of his time to devote to laboratory work.

In 1912 when the Mayo Clinic was still in scattered, improvised, and often cramped offices and laboratories, Louis B. Wilson said that they could provide for only a limited number of men to study the pathological material of the clinic on a volunteer basis.[20] In 1914 with the greatly expanded laboratories and pathological museum available in the new building, the Mayo Clinic was able to provide many more opportunities for physicians to study their pathological collections for diagnosis and research, or as part of their training in surgery.

On 8 October 1914 Dean Lyon raised the question of relations with the Mayo Clinic at a meeting of the administrative board and, on motion, the board requested Dean Lyon to appoint a committee to consist of three members of the board and of President Vincent and Dean Lyon, ex officio, to confer with a committee of the medical school alumni and subsequently with the Doctors Mayo. Dean Lyon then appointed a committee consisting of Richard Olding Beard, chairman, James E. Moore, and Jennings C. Litzenberg, together with himself and President Vincent, and on 14 November 1914 the committee met with the advisory committee of the Medical Alumni Association to discuss a possible affiliation of the medical school with the Mayo Clinic.[21] At the request of President Vincent, Dr. Beard told the meeting that in the informal discussions carried on so far, a possible affiliation with the Mayo Clinic might include an exchange of fellowships, a combination of graduate courses and opportunities for research, elective courses at Rochester for advanced undergraduates, an exchange of laboratory workers and lecturers, the use of St. Mary's Hospital at Rochester for internships, and the establishment of a joint medical journal. The representatives of the alumni agreed that the committee of the medical school should seek a conference with the Doctors Mayo to explore the possibilities of affiliation with the Mayo Clinic, and then hold a further conference with the advisory committee of the Medical Alumni Association. Although in the minutes of the conference recorded by Dr. Beard, it is stated that the conference generally favored affiliation in graduate work, the accuracy of the minutes on this point was questioned at the second conference with the medical alumni on 19 January 1915.[22] The conference did not favor affiliation for undergraduate students. It favored an exchange of workers between the two institutions, and possible internships at Rochester. Almost everyone present opposed the proposal for a joint medical journal.[23]

Dr. Beard sent the minutes of the conference with the medical alumni to Dr. Mayo who, on 19 November, held a meeting of the administrative board of the Mayo Clinic to consider them. The Mayo Clinic board agreed with almost all the conclusions of the 14 November conference. They approved an exchange of fellowships, a combination of opportunities for graduate study, and an exchange both of laboratory investigators and special lecturers. They agreed to leave the question of elective courses at Rochester for advanced undergraduates to be discussed later in the light of experience with graduate students. They offered to set aside half of the internships at St. Mary's Hospital for medical graduates of the university. The question of a joint medical journal, they decided, could wait. In general the Mayo Clinic men seemed willing, perhaps even anxious, to modify the details of the proposed affiliation to meet the wishes of the medical school and the medical alumni.[24]

On the morning of Sunday, 22 November, Dr. Beard met with the staff of the Mayo Clinic at Rochester where he presented a verbal summary of the results of the 14 November conference to supplement the minutes sent previously to Dr. Mayo. Dr. Beard said that, although the fact was not noted in the minutes, some members of the alumni did object to affiliation between the university and the Mayo Clinic, but a majority were in favor of such an affiliation.[25] He did not explain the reasons for the objections, nor why they were not recorded in the minutes. Although Dr. Beard may have misjudged the breadth and intensity of opposition to affiliation among the alumni, the depth of feeling that would appear later may not yet have existed in November 1914. That afternoon at William Mayo's house, Dr. Beard met with alumni and former students then on the staff of the Mayo Clinic, and he discussed the proposed affiliation "quite freely in all its bearings." He asked each of the younger alumni how he thought the medical students would regard affiliation with the Mayo Clinic, and each thought that the students would welcome eagerly such an addition to their opportunities for clinical education. Several of the alumni also suggested that it would be good for members of the Mayo Clinic staff to have an opportunity to do occasional undergraduate teaching.[26]

During the following week the staff of the Mayo Clinic discussed the proposed affiliation informally among themselves and all were evidently in favor of it. Many thought it would be wise to start with a small number of graduate students "so as not to block the efficiency either of the instruction or of the Clinic."[27]

The next Sunday, 29 November 1914, the full medical school committee, including President Vincent and Dean Lyon, were at Rochester for a conference with a corresponding committee of the Mayo Clinic.[28] At the conference William Mayo said that an endowment had already been created to support the educational and scientific work carried on at the Mayo Clinic. The fund was to be added to from year to year, and he proposed that if an affiliation between the clinic and the university were established, this fund should come ultimately under the control of the Board of Regents. The endowment fund would not be used to maintain the business of the clinic, and if the clinic were to decline or fail, the endowment fund would nonetheless continue to be used for educational and scientific purposes under the control of the Board of Regents. For the present the endowment fund would be allowed to grow, while the educational and scientific work of the clinic would be supported by an annual budget from the clinic's income. Dr. Mayo proposed that the Mayo Clinic staff should name a board of trustees or directors to administer its educational and scientific work, the nominees to such a board to be submitted to the administrative board of the medical school for their approval and afterwards to be confirmed by the Board of Regents of the university.

After discussion of the various features of the proposed affiliation, including a proposal for joint publication of "a quarterly bulletin or report of scientific or clinical articles," which had aroused strong objections at the 14 November conference with alumni representatives, Dr. Beard suggested that a principal objection to affiliation derived from the fact that the Mayo Clinic was a private business. To meet this objection Dr. Beard suggested that the scientific and educational work of the Mayo Clinic should be separated from its business side by the creation of a Mayo Foundation for the promotion of medical education and research. The board of directors or trustees, that Dr. Mayo had mentioned, might then be appointed to carry on the work of the foundation. The creation of such a foundation would remove any possibility that in future the university might incur a responsibility for the maintenance of the Mayo Clinic. The university would be affiliated with the Mayo Foundation, not with the Mayo Clinic.

Although the concept of the Mayo Foundation was presented to the conference by Dr. Beard, the idea had originated with President Vincent who then spoke upon the great advantages inherent in the plan. "Dr. Mayo met the suggestion very hospitably and promised to confer with his associates with reference to it . . . ."[29] The next day Dr. Mayo wrote to President Vincent that he and his colleagues had discussed the idea of a Mayo foundation to support medical education and research and thought it "an exceedingly good one," because it would separate the educational and research work from the practical work of the clinic. Mayo added that he would incorporate such a foundation at once, and then appoint a scientific committee to direct its activities.[30]

On 3 December Dr. Beard's committee reported to the administrative board on the results of their conference on 14 November with the committee of the Medical Alumni Association. After extensive discussion the board instructed the committee to send their report to Dr. Mayo for his approval, and then to distribute copies of the approved report to members of the administrative board.[31] On 16 December the administrative board held a special meeting, with President Vincent in the chair, to consider the report. The professor of medicine, Charles Lyman Greene, was absent. The board first voted unanimously to approve the principle of affiliation between the medical school and such an institution as the Mayo Clinic, and then discussed the report in detail, making various amendments to it. George Head suggested that it would be better to have the endowment fund, which at the conference on 29 November Dr. Mayo had offered to provide, placed under the control of the Mayo Foundation in case the Mayo Clinic should at any time be discontinued. Some members of the administrative board asked who the board of trustees of the Mayo Foundation would be. Dean Lyon asked whether the board should consist wholly of physicians, and whether the university should not be represented on it. The next day Dr. Beard wrote to Dr. Mayo to tell him that the administrative board had approved the principle of affiliation.[32] When the administrative board met next on 14 January 1915, Dr. Beard's committee reported that the changes proposed in their report at the December meeting had been accepted by Dr. Mayo. The revised report was appended to the minutes.[33]

In its report the committee stated that the Mayo Foundation for the Promotion of Medical Education and Research had been created, and would in future be supported by an endowment fund provided for it. In order to permit the income of the endowment to be added to the principal, the Mayo Clinic would for the present provide an annual budget for the support of the Mayo Foundation. If the proposed affiliation between the University of Minnesota and the Mayo Foundation should prove on trial to be satisfactory, the endowment fund of the Mayo Foundation would ultimately be placed "as to the investment and general supervision of expenditures" under the control of the Board of Regents of the university. The endowment fund of the Mayo Foundation was to be independent of the Mayo Clinic. The Mayo Foundation was to be carried on in affiliation with the medical school of the University of Minnesota, its work being directed by a board of trustees to consist of the founders, that is, William and Charles Mayo, and six physicians or medical scientists, five to be nominated by the Mayo Clinic and one to be nominated by the medical school and approved by the Mayo Clinic.

The proposed affiliation between the Mayo Foundation and the University of Minnesota would be for the conduct of graduate medical education with exchanges of students and fellows between the university and the Mayo Foundation, the students being registered in the graduate school of the university and paying fees to the university.

In an atmosphere of good will the proposed agreement might have been accepted by the faculty of the medical school, the medical alumni, and the medical profession of Minnesota, but the reserves of good will had become severely depleted by events of the preceding two years. Many members of the faculty were embittered by the arbitrary and unjust treatment they had received in the reorganization of 1913. They distrusted President Vincent, and suspected that Dr. Mayo was using his position as a regent to prevent the development of the clinical departments of the medical school and of the university hospital. Since 1912 the president and Board of Regents had failed to request appropriations for additions to the Elliot Hospital or for a nurses' residence, all of which were badly needed. In the summer of 1914 Regent Mayo had promised Dr. James E. Moore's committee on hospital and clinical development that he would support legislative requests in the amount of $400,000 for a contagious disease infirmary, a nurses' residence, and an extension of the Elliot Hospital to provide 200 additional beds to create clinical services for children's diseases and for nervous and mental diseases.

In January 1915 the administrative board learned that at their annual meeting on 8 December 1914, with Dr. Mayo present, the Board of Regents had decided to request only $100,000 for a contagious disease infirmary, which the students on the agricultural campus in St. Paul had requested independently the year before.[34] Although the contagious disease infirmary was to be built in connection with the university hospital, the sum requested was only a quarter of what Dr. Mayo had promised to support the previous July. It provided nothing for the outpatient department, for enlarged clinical services in the university hospital, or for a nurses' residence. The news struck clinical members of the medical faculty like a slap in the face. They could not believe that the Board of Regents, of which Dr. Mayo was a leading member, would fail to include a building request that he supported unequivocally. To the clinical members of the faculty such news confirmed what they had feared since 1912, namely, that Dr. Mayo would use his power as a regent ruthlessly, to prevent the development of the clinical departments in the medical school.

Undeterred by any sense of disappointment among clinical members of the faculty, Dr. Beard and Dean Lyon proceeded with the discussion of the proposed affiliation between the medical school and the Mayo Foundation. At the meeting of the administrative board on 14 January 1915, Dr. Beard presented the revised report of his committee, which he said had been accepted by Dr. Mayo, and it was appended to the minutes. Dr. Beard said also that during the coming week he planned to hold conferences with the advisory committee of the Medical Alumni Association and with the general faculty.[35]

When the medical school committee met with the advisory committee of the Medical Alumni Association on the evening of Tuesday, 19 January 1915, the alumni representatives pointed out that the minutes of the previous conference on 14 November, recorded by Dr. Beard, were incorrect in conveying the impression that the conference had approved the proposed affiliation. The conference voted that the secretaries of both the medical school and the alumni committee should join in the preparation of the minutes. In an atmosphere of such mistrust the conference produced little agreement. It was finally proposed that the question of a temporary affiliation with the Mayo Foundation should be submitted to the advisory committee of the Medical Alumni Association for advice.[36] After the conference the alumni committee met privately and passed unanimously a resolution in which they stated their doubts of the wisdom of affiliation between the university and any private institution, but approved a temporary arrangement between the university and the Mayo Foundation restricted to interchange of opportunities for graduate study and members of the teaching staffs. The secretary was directed to send the resolution to President Vincent and to Dean Lyon.[37]

Two days later on Thursday, 21 January, the general faculty of the medical school met to discuss the proposed relationship between the medical school and the Mayo Foundation. President Vincent presided. Dr. Beard read the proposals for the relationship and various faculty members asked questions. President Vincent was asked about the effect of the proposed relationship upon the clinical development of the medical school. He replied that the idea that an affiliation with the Mayo Clinic might retard the development of the university hospital had not occurred to him until it was suggested by certain medical men, but he did not see why it should have such an influence. Vincent suggested that in future the enlargement of the university hospital must depend upon private gifts as well as state support, or upon charges to patients.[38] Vincent was curiously oblivious to the significance of the repeated failure of the Board of Regents to submit requests for expansion of the university hospital, nor did he explain why the legislature should not be asked to support the development of a hospital which would be of benefit to the people of the whole state.

Charles Lyman Greene urged that the question should be studied very carefully, and should have more time devoted to it. The faculty decided to adjourn for two weeks and then meet to vote upon the question. When they met again on the evening of Friday, 5 February, with President Vincent in the chair, Dean Lyon presented a resolution calling for an affiliation with the Mayo Foundation for a trial period, during which the affiliation might be terminated on one year's notice by either party. After discussion the resolution was voted on by ballot, and passed, with thirty-nine votes for and twenty-six votes against. Many of the negative votes may have been by clinical members of the faculty, most of whom were opposed to affiliation, but who were a minority in the general faculty. In the basic science departments every teacher down to the level of instructor belonged to the general faculty, but in the clinical departments only teachers at the rank of assistant professor and above were included. The clinical assistants possessed no vote in the general faculty. The faculty vote did not have the effect of settling the question of affiliation, because it did not express the views of the clinicians who would be affected most directly by affiliation. Indeed, the clinical teachers had not been represented adequately on the committee responsible for the negotiations leading up to affiliation. Dr. Beard had never engaged in clinical teaching, while Dean Lyon and President Vincent were not physicians. The professor of surgery, James

E. Moore, was on the committee to negotiate with the Mayo Clinic, but the professor of medicine, Charles Lyman Greene, was not.

On 8 February 1915 the Mayo Foundation for Medical Education and Research was incorporated at Rochester, the incorporators being William J. Mayo, Charles H. Mayo, Henry S. Plummer, Edward Starr Judd, and Donald C. Balfour, all partners in the Mayo Clinic. The same day at Minneapolis the administrative board of the medical school by a vote of eight to one authorized Dr. Beard's committee to prepare formal resolutions to be presented to the Board of Regents for the purpose of recommending an affiliation of the University of Minnesota with the Mayo Foundation. The dissenting vote was that of Charles Lyman Greene.[39]

Appalled at the relentless progress toward the proposed affiliation with the Mayo Foundation, with its ominous implications for the future of the clinical departments of the medical school, Dr. Greene now prepared to make public his opposition to the affiliation. In 1911 Dean Wesbrook recorded his impression of Dr. Greene as an enthusiastic and stimulating teacher, who possessed charm, but who was also " . . . forceful and not inclined to compromise with wrong or doubtful issues."[40] To Dr. Greene the proposed Mayo affiliation was extremely doubtful and Dr. Mayo's role in promoting it clearly wrong. Moreover, Greene was expressing a general feeling of deep resentment against Mayo among the faculty of the clinical departments who thought that he was using his power as a regent improperly to prevent the clinical development of the medical school. They believed also that he was acting to prevent the further development of the nursing school, which was considered superior to the nurses' training program operated by St. Mary's Hospital at Rochester. Whether the university clinicians were correct in their interpretation of Dr. Mayo's motives or not, they were in a good position to judge the effect of his actions or inactions as a regent. For more than three years the Board of Regents had failed consistently to request appropriations urgently needed by the medical school and the nursing school. And in medical matters the Board of Regents was accustomed to act on the advice of Regent Mayo.

On 27 January 1915 Dr. Greene wrote a long, confidential letter to his former teacher at the University of Michigan, Dr. Victor C. Vaughan, who was planning to come to the Twin Cities on 30 January.[41] To Dr. Vaughan, Dr. Greene described Dr. Mayo's persistent refusal as regent to develop the clinical departments of the medical school by expansion of the university hospital and outpatient department, culminating in the breaking of his promise of the previous summer to support a legislative request for $400,000 for clinical buildings. Dr. Greene said that 90 percent of the faculty in the clinical departments were opposed on principle to an affiliation with a pay clinic, but many of the faculty in the scientific departments favored the idea because they thought that students at the Mayo Clinic would have to come to them for graduate instruction. Calmly, Dr. Greene listed the arguments both for and against the proposed Mayo affiliation. He thought that the plans for graduate medical education put forward by Dean Lyon and adopted by the medical school in 1914 were premature, so long as the clinical facilities at the university remained so limited.[42]

On 15 February the *Minnesota Alumni Weekly* published the affiliation proposal as it had been approved by the general faculty on 21 January, and commented: "the fact that two fifths of the faculty opposed its adoption shows that there is room for an honest difference of opinion on the question . . . ." The editor thought that the university would be wise to go slow "until all reasonable doubt as to the wisdom of the plan has been removed."[43] The debate over affiliation moved next into the pages of the *Journal-Lancet,* which was also the journal of the Minnesota State Medical Association. On 15 March 1915 Dr. Beard's committee published in the *Journal-Lancet* a statement describing and defending the affiliation, and in the same issue Charles Lyman Greene published a detailed criticism of the proposed affiliation agreement. In their statement Dr. Beard's committee referred to the need for expansion of clinical facilities at the university and for a building for the nursing school, but suggested that the state could not afford to provide the necessary appropriations.[44] The committee did not know what the state could or could not provide, because the Board of Regents had not requested the funds from the legislature. For the 1916–17 biennium the Board of Regents made no requests for buildings apart from the request for $100,000 for a contagious disease infirmary.[45] The committee said that the medical school would "have to accept the fulfillment of these needs by piecemeal and with as much grace of patience as it can muster."[46] Thus four years after the completion of the Elliot Hospital, the committee saw little hope for the future. From their pessimism, an outside observer might have supposed that the state of Minnesota was in a serious economic decline.

The committee described enthusiastically the need for graduate medical education in the United States, especially because the outbreak of war in Europe now prevented American doctors from going to European medical schools. Graduate medical education was especially necessary for the training of specialists. A six-week course in a polyclinic was no longer sufficient, whether taken in Europe or the United States. For such reasons the medical school had established its Graduate School in Medicine, which would offer physicians opportunities to pursue problems in medical research or to pursue a course of graduate study leading either to a master of science or a doctor of science degree. Yet graduate study in medicine required a wealth of clinical and laboratory material which the university did not itself possess, but which was available at Rochester in the Mayo Clinic. For some years the Mayo Clinic had given a few doctors opportunities to study informally and in 1910 the clinic had begun to offer graduate fellowships each for a period of three years. Up to 1915 some ninety-five physicians had pursued graduate medical study at the clinic with the aid of such fellowships. The committee referred to the trial affiliation with the newly created Mayo Foundation. The affiliation was for the joint conduct of graduate medical education, including the interchange of graduate students and graduate teachers. The courses offered at Rochester would be approved by the graduate committee of the medical school and by the dean of the graduate school, and degrees awarded for graduate study would be conferred by the University of Minnesota. If at the end of a trial period the Mayo Foundation and the university were to agree on a permanent affiliation, the trustees of the Mayo Foundation endowment would surrender it to the control of the Board of Regents of the university with the stipulation that it be used to support the educational and research work of the foundation at Rochester. Among other things, the committee stated: "The Foundation; its work, its workers and its finances, will be definitely separate from the clinic."[47] In appraising the proposed affiliation the committee said: "Such a gift to medical education and research is so unusual and looms so large in its possibilities that one marvels that its benefits should need statement."[48] Among its benefits the committee emphasized the creation of a graduate school in medicine that would be unique in the United States.[49]

When the committee came to possible objections to the proposed affiliation they hinted darkly that there were objections "which it is better not to define."[50] Nevertheless, "medical men and medical educators, of lofty purpose" might object to the affiliation because the Mayo Foundation derived its financial support and its scientific material from the Mayo Clinic, which was a private enterprise operated for profit. The committee contended that the same objection would apply to every clinical teacher who engaged in the private practice of medicine. The committee took particular pains to answer the objection that the Mayo Foundation was inseparable from the Mayo Clinic. They argued that the scientific and research work at Rochester was separate from the care of paying patients. The Mayo Foundation would support medical research and teaching, but would have nothing to do with the care and treatment of paying patients, which would be the responsibility of the Mayo Clinic. Again they compared the role of the Mayo Clinic to that of part-time clinical teachers in the medical school.

To the fear that affiliation would stop the development of clinical facilities at the university, the committee said that while they believed the fear to be without foundation, " . . . no assurance to the contrary can, with propriety, be given. The administration cannot commit future Boards of Regents or future legislatures to any program of clinical development."[51] The words were undoubtedly President George Edgar Vincent's. The committee did not explain why the present Board of Regents could not commit itself to particular steps in clinical development that were needed immediately and urgently, nor why they had failed to do so during four years of Vincent's administration. The committee thought "the natural stimulus to the growth of the Medical School which the affiliation must be, will insure the speedier completion of the absolutely essential laboratory of the clinical teacher."[52]

Among his reasons for opposition to the Mayo affiliation, Charles Lyman Greene emphasized that affiliation would convey to the Mayo Clinic, a private firm, "an amount of prestige, power, authority, rights and privileges such as are without modern precedent."[53] He rejected the analogy, drawn by the committee, between the Mayo Clinic and part-time clinical teachers at the medical school.

The medical school had years before withdrawn its clinics from private and even from semi-public hospitals in the Twin Cities. No faculty member was permitted to teach in his private clinic or office. At the university dispensary no physician was permitted to refer a patient to his own office, and the university hospital admitted no paying patients.

Dr. Greene suggested that William J. Mayo, who was chiefly responsible for the organization and management of the Mayo Clinic, was concerned to perpetuate the clinics by means of an endowment combined with a university affiliation. "Indeed, it would be necessary," said Dr. Greene, "that the mantle of some great University be thrown over their clinic in order that it might be made attractive to men of recognized preeminence who would serve as heads of the different departments, and who otherwise are in great measure unobtainable."[54] The effect of affiliation with the University of Minnesota would be, thought Dr. Greene, to increase greatly the profits of the Mayo Clinic which were estimated already to exceed a million and a half dollars annually. Nevertheless, he added, "One of the irritating features attending the promotion of the affiliation project has been the apparent disregard of the immense value of the gift contemplated by the University."[55]

Under the proposed affiliation the university would delegate to the Mayo Foundation the same powers to give academic credit for work done in the Mayo Clinic, or at St. Mary's Hospital, and the same right to recommend graduate students for degrees as the medical school possessed. The university's power to confirm or reject nominations to the Board of Scientific Directors of the Mayo Foundation was purely formal. Dr. Greene emphasized that the distinction drawn between the Mayo Foundation and the Mayo Clinic was not real because the board of trustees which controlled the Mayo Foundation were the Mayo brothers and their partners, who also owned the Mayo Clinic. Although Dr. Greene was correct, the separate corporate identity of the Mayo Foundation did permit its finances to be kept separate from the business operations of the Mayo Clinic, and, if it were operated in good faith, the Mayo Foundation could serve the educational and research purposes for which it was created.

Dr. Greene pointed out accurately that the endowment provided by William and Charles Mayo for the Mayo Foundation involved no gift to the university for its own use. The income from the endowment would be spent at Rochester. Dr. Greene might have added that at Rochester the clinical fellows supported by the Mayo Foundation would help to care for patients in the Mayo Clinic and at St. Mary's Hospital so that they could hardly fail to contribute to the work of the Mayo Clinic. Fellows who published the results of their research, whether in clinic or laboratory, would contribute to the prestige of the Mayo Clinic, and thereby to its ability to attract patients and earn income. The affiliation might also bring surgical prestige to the university, but Dr. Greene feared that the affiliation might be used as a substitute for the development of the university hospital into a complete clinic on the campus. On 8 February 1915 the *Minneapolis Tribune* had announced that the affiliation would mean that legislative appropriations for the university, otherwise urgently needed, might be avoided or deferred.[56] Affiliation must, therefore, mean a weakening of the medical school, and if the medical school were to "remain in irons . . . deprived of necessary funds for clinical development," Dr. Greene thought that it ought to become a half school with all clinical teaching taken over by the Mayo Clinic.[57]

In a separate article, opposing the affiliation, George Douglas Head emphasized the extraordinary position in which William J. Mayo would be placed by the proposed affiliation, because as a regent he would frequently be called upon to decide matters that would vitally affect both the university and the Mayo Foundation. Dr. Head asked: "Is it wise to place such large powers in the hands of one of its regents?"[58] Like Dr. Greene, Dr. Head believed that under the affiliation agreement the university could not exercise effective control over the education its students might receive as fellows of the Mayo Foundation.

Meanwhile, medical societies in the Twin Cities and elsewhere in the state were beginning to express opposition to the Mayo affiliation. On 22 February the Ramsey County Medical Society adopted unanimously a resolution to be sent to the Board of Regents to protest the Mayo affiliation, their grounds of objection being essentially similar to those expressed by Dr. Greene, namely, that the affiliation would convey "an incalculable gift of power, prestige and ultimate financial benefit" to a private medical firm, and would check the normal growth of the medical school and damage its morale.[59] In March 1915 the *St. Paul Medical Journal* commented editorially that the affairs of the Mayo Clinic were its own business, but when its chief was also a member of the Board of Regents of the university, an affiliation between the Mayo Clinic and the university became " . . . entirely suitable for public discussion."

> Why the President of the University and the Dean of the Medical Faculty and Dr. Mayo himself cannot any of them see the impropriety of carrying on these negotiations under the existing circumstances we are at a loss to understand. We are quite sure that the Board of Regents would not for a moment consider it proper to let a large and profitable business contract to one of its own members—and yet are they not asked to do a very similar thing?

The *St. Paul Medical Journal* emphasized that the endowment fund was not a gift to the university but to the Mayo Foundation at Rochester, where the expenditures of the foundation would also support the work of the Mayo Clinic and tend to increase its income. The editorial noted that in a newspaper interview Dean Lyon had said that " . . . one advantage of the proposed affiliation would be that it would no longer be necessary to ask the legislature for large appropriations for the development of the clinical facilities of the medical school, as those would be furnished at Rochester." The latter consequence of the affiliation explained, said the editor, why almost all the clinical teachers of the medical school opposed the Mayo affiliation.[60]

On 16 February the board of directors of the General Alumni Association, concerned at the implications of the proposed Mayo affiliation, held a meeting, at which Guy Stanton Ford, dean of the graduate school, Jennings C. Litzenberg of the medical school, and Louis B. Wilson of the Mayo Foundation made statements concerning the proposed affiliation, and answered questions. After discussion the board recommended to the Board of Regents that action upon the proposed affiliation with the Mayo Foundation be postponed for at least two months.[61]

On 1 March 1915 the *Minneapolis Journal* stated editorially that it was receiving reports "that indicate new suppression at the University as regards the Mayo proposal . . . ." Among other questions, the *Minneapolis Journal* asked: "Should Dr. Mayo resign as regent while he submits a proposal that involves his private interest?"[62] Two days later Dean Lyon was quoted in the *St. Paul Pioneer Press* as saying that "leading educators" favored the idea of the Mayo affiliation, a report which evoked a letter to the editor from Charles Lyman Greene. Dr. Greene questioned whether the various educators in other parts of the country knew that the Mayo Foundation was controlled completely by the Mayo firm, that none of the foundation fund would be spent outside the Mayo Clinic, or that the proposed Mayo affiliation was to be a substitute for the university's own clinical development.[63] On 8 March Dean Lyon replied to Dr. Greene in vigorous terms in the pages of the *St. Paul Dispatch*. Said Dean Lyon:

> Dr. Greene says not a dollar of the fund would belong to the university. I say every dollar of it would belong to the university.
>
> Dr. Greene ways the foundation would not be separate from the Mayo clinic. I say it would.
>
> Dr. Greene says the foundation would be controlled by the Mayo firm. I say the foundation would be controlled by the Board of Regents.
>
> Dr. Greene says "this proposition is avowedly a substitute for the natural and indispensable growth of the medical school on the campus." I say that it is not such a substitute.

On the last point Dean Lyon was contradicting what he himself was quoted as saying in the *Minneapolis Tribune* on 8 February.[64] After contrasting Dr. Greene's views with his own on several more points, Dean Lyon said, "Now it is evident that either Dr. Greene is wrong or I am wrong. If he were right, I am frank in saying I should be opposed to affiliation. It is up to him to prove his statements. I shall do my best to prove mine."[65] Brave words,—but in attempting to sustain them Dean Lyon was obliged to ignore or gloss over awkward facts. Since the governing board of the Mayo Foundation consisted of the partners of the Mayo Clinic it was difficult to establish the independence of the foundation from the clinic, but Dean Lyon did his best. He may have been misled. Several times Dean Lyon used the words "I am authorized to say . . . ." He emphasized that the scientific work of the Mayo Clinic was carried on separately from the care of patients. Some of the laboratory workers had nothing to do with patients, and devoted their full time to research. That was strictly true. For instance, Dr. Edward Kendall, the chemist who in 1915 isolated thyroxine at the Mayo Clinic, was not a physician, and could have nothing to do with the care of patients. Nevertheless, it was not the whole truth. Most of the research done at the Mayo Clinic was clinical investigation carried out by clinicians engaged in the care of patients. Almost all of the fellows supported by the Mayo Clinic served as assistants in the care of patients at the clinic and at St. Mary's Hospital. The same was to be true of fellows to be supported by the Mayo Foundation. Nonetheless, Dean Lyon said: "This scientific work can easily be separated from the medical work involved in the treatment and care of patients." Further on, he added: "I am authorized to say that the division of functions will be along the lines indicated, and that the private business of the Mayo clinic will stand in no closer relation to the foundation than does the private business of part time university professors to the medical school." Dean Lyon then asked why the Mayo Foundation should be separated from the Mayo Clinic if the foundation were owned and controlled by the clinic. He said that at the conclusion of the trial period " . . . the endowment fund of the foundation will become the absolute property of the university, subject to two restrictions as to the use of the income: (1) it is to be used only for medical research and education. (2) It is to be used in Rochester, Minn." In certain unstated eventualities, Dean Lyon hinted, the second restriction might be waived.[66]

Throughout his long and vigorous reply to Dr. Greene, Dean Lyon did not pursue Greene's point that the Mayo affiliation was to be a substitute for clinical development on the campus. The most effective answer to Dr. Greene would have been to outline plans for the expansion of the university hospital and outpatient department, but Dean Lyon had no such plans. His contradiction of Dr. Greene on the effect of the affiliation on clinical development at the university, therefore, was mere bluster. Dr. Greene was right. In the minds of Dean Lyon and President Vincent the Mayo affiliation *was* a substitute for clinical development on the campus.

Dean Lyon attached sufficient importance to his reply to Dr. Greene in the *St. Paul Dispatch* that he sent a copy of it to the Alumni Association with a letter in which he restated his main points: (1) the Mayo endowment fund was to belong to the university, (2) the Mayo Foundation was to be separate from the Mayo Clinic, and (3) the Mayo Foundation was to be controlled by the Board of Regents.[67] In the end none of Dean Lyon's stout assertions were fulfilled. The Mayo endowment never came to the university for its own use; the Mayo Foundation remained inseparable from the Mayo Clinic; and any control exerted by the Board of Regents over the Mayo Foundation was purely nominal. So long as William Mayo remained a regent, the reverse was more nearly true; the Mayo Foundation controlled the Board of Regents in medical matters.

The spectacle of the dean of the medical school arguing with the head of the Department of Medicine in the pages of the *St. Paul Dispatch* was a public indication of the deep division within the medical school over the Mayo affiliation. The determination of the university administration, represented by President Vincent and Dean Lyon, to achieve affiliation over the objections of a large part of the medical faculty, and an overwhelming majority of the medical profession, is striking. Did they ever pause to balance the possible benefits of affiliation against the growing toll of costs? Was the Mayo affiliation worth the damage to the medical school that it entailed? Did they ask themselves such questions? In the heat of battle evidently they did not. Throughout President Vincent acted as a faithful servant of Dr. Mayo. Nothing interrupted the university administration's drive toward affiliation, nor the growth of opposition to it.

On 22 March a petition signed by more than two hundred Minneapolis and St. Paul physicians, including many of the most eminent among the medical profession of the Twin Cities, was sent to the Board of Regents, asking them to drop the proposed Mayo affiliation.[68] The next day the board of directors of the General Alumni Association voted to advise the Board of Regents that the university should not accept any gift with a condition that deprived the regents of absolute control of the gift, or that would "even tend to remove the major part of the graduate work (or undergraduate work) of any department or college from the University campus."[69] The alumni thought, too, that the principles of any permanent affiliation should be settled before entering upon a temporary affiliation.

A week later on 29 March, evidently influenced by the alumni directors resolution, Representative Paul W. Guilford of Minneapolis introduced into the Minnesota legislature a bill which forbade the university to "affiliate or unite with, or delegate any of its teaching functions to any person, firm or corporation not under the exclusive supervision and control of the board of regents."[70] The bill was immediately endorsed by the medical societies of Ramsey County, Hennepin County, St. Louis County, and Blue Earth County, and by many individual physicians throughout the state. Early in April committees of the Hennepin County and Ramsey County medical societies sent circular letters to every member of the legislature urging passage of the Guilford bill.[71]

On 4 April 1915 Dean Lyon published ten replies he had received from leading medical educators throughout the United States to his request for their candid opinion concerning the value of the proposed Mayo affiliation to the University of Minnesota.[72] Typical of Dean Lyon's letters of inquiry may have been that to Dr. Victor C. Vaughan, dean of the College of Medicine and Surgery at the University of Michigan at Ann Arbor, in which he asked whether an affiliation for graduate medical teaching between "the Mayo institutions at Rochester" and the university would be of advantage or disadvantage to medical education, and whether it would be of advantage or disadvantage to the university itself.[73] Dean Lyon did not trouble Dean Vaughan with details of the proposed affiliation, the dissension it was creating among the faculty at Minnesota, nor its possible implications for the development of clinical facilities on the university campus. In his reply Dean Vaughan showed an equally blithe disregard of such factors, even though Charles Lyman Greene had described them to Dean Vaughan in some detail in his long and anguished letter of 27 January. Dean Vaughan wrote: " . . . the University of Minnesota should accept the very liberal offer made by the Mayo Clinic. It would certainly give the University a unique position among the medical schools of the country. It would enable you to carry on a great work in clinical medicine. I cannot understand how there can be any difference of opinion on this matter."[74] Other replies to Dean Lyon's inquiries were similarly sanguine. Dr. John B. Murphy, professor of surgery at Northwestern University wrote: "In the Mayo institutions you have, first, the highest class of surgery in enormous quantity under observations every day, under one roof, with the least possible percentage of waste of time to the postgraduate student and practitioner."[75] Dr. A. W. Myers, professor of anatomy at Leland Stanford University referred to the proposed Mayo affiliation as "that magnificent gift," which he considered absolutely unique.[76] Others too wrote under the impression that the Mayo endowment was to be a gift to the University of Minnesota for the purpose of developing graduate medical education. On 5 April 1915 the *Minneapolis Tribune* commented editorially: "An offer has been made by certain scientific men interested in the relief of human suffering, to devote the annual income from $1,500,000 to medical research in connection with the University of Minnesota."[77] To the editorial writer of the *Tribune* the $90,000 annual income that might be anticipated from such an endowment "would secure the entire time and trained energies of thirty scientists at $3,000 yearly or of fifteen at $6,000 yearly." His impressions of the kind of work that the Mayo Foundation would support may have been remote from the actual work of the Mayo Clinic, but he did share the assumption that the endowment would constitute a gift to the university. There was, in fact, widespread public confusion about the nature of the proposed Mayo affiliation. On 6 April 1915 the *Minneapolis Journal* asked editorially: "Exactly what is the Mayo proposition as to the State University? The public has never been presented with the formal proposition." The writer thought that the apparent desire to act with secrecy gave "a bad color to the whole affair."[78]

Meanwhile members of the Board of Regents began to campaign against the Guilford bill introduced to the legislature on 4 April. On 6 April C. G. Schulz, state superintendent of education and ex officio member of the Board of Regents, said that the Guilford bill would probably prevent clinical teaching at the St. Paul and Minneaplis city hospitals, joint work with the State Board of Health, and similar medical activities. Mr. Schulz thought that the bill would likewise prevent the university from sending agriculture students to farms to gain practical experience, or engineering students to industrial plants, where they would be in charge of persons not under the direct control of the Board of Regents. For years students in the School of Mines had spent part of each year at mines on the Iron Range in northern Minnesota, or in other states, and the proposed law, according to Mr. Schulz, would prohibit such work.[79] That same day the *St. Paul Dispatch* in an editorial described the Guilford bill as "a vicious and reactionary measure." The editorial writer thought that the bill would deprive the Board of Regents of the exercise of their judgment and intelligence. He suggested that the passage of such a measure might bring about the resignation of the Board of Regents in a body.[80]

The next day the supporters and opponents of the Guilford bill spoke at a joint hearing of the Senate Committee on Education and the House University Committee. Many physicians from the Twin Cities were present as was also Louis B.

Wilson from the Mayo Clinic and E. L. Tuohy from Duluth. The debate centered on the merits of the proposed Mayo affiliation, but as the discussion went on there was increasing doubt as to what the Mayo proposal was.[81] In answer to questions Dr. Wilson acknowledged that the proposed Mayo affiliation did not involve a gift of money to the university. By contrast Dean Lyon compared the Mayo Foundation endowment to the Shevlin and Gilfillan endowment funds given to the university for specific purposes, a comparison which was immediately challenged by E. L. Tuohy and by Soren P. Rees of Minneapolis. President Vincent described the manifold harm that the Guilford bill would do to the university by preventing it from giving students credit for courses taken or experience gained outside the university. Louis B. Wilson described the need for graduate medical education to provide adequate training for medical specialists. He referred disparagingly to physicians who went to Europe to attend the "medical quick lunch counter" at Vienna for two or three months and returned with a certificate and a "beer breath." At the Mayo Clinic they required three years of graduate work for specialist training, and for the coming year they had fifty-three applications for thirty-six fellowship positions.

In answer to questions concerning the availability of clinical material in the Twin Cities as compared with Rochester, Dr. Rees said that in Twin Cities hospitals there were 1,689 free beds whereas at Rochester there were 250 to 300 hospital beds, but they were not free beds. "We are not operating on beds or diagnosing beds," replied Louis B. Wilson. "We are dealing with patients and 30,000 were treated last year. None of them were charity patients to be looked over by undergraduate students." "This seems contradictory," commented Dr. Tuohy. "We are told of the great opportunity for clinical work at Rochester, and then in the next breath we are told there are no beds and no opportunity for students to observe patients."[82]

Behind the sharp exchange of words between Drs. Wilson and Tuohy lay a real and important issue. The Mayo Clinic was in 1915 almost exclusively a surgical clinic, offering general surgery and the various surgical specialties. In fact, the growth of the clinic at that time depended significantly on the development of new surgical specialties. After 1910 the number of operations in general surgery, primarily abdominal surgery, performed at the Mayo Clinic had tended to level off, but the total number of operations performed at the clinic had continued to grow because of a continued rapid increase in the number of operations on the thyroid gland and in orthopedic surgery. In 1912 the Mayo Clinic began to do thoracic surgery and ear surgery, in 1915 they introduced neurosurgery, and in 1919 they began operations on the nose and antrum.[83] By contrast, while the Mayo Clinic from 1900 to 1915 brought general diagnosis and surgical treatment at Rochester to a very high level, they were obliged to reduce the medical treatment that they could offer in hospitals to a very low level. Almost all hospital beds at Rochester were reserved for surgical patients, and the Mayo physicians were accustomed to refer patients needing medical treatment to their home physicians or to other institutions. In 1915 the Mayo Clinic did not provide services in obstetrics, children's diseases, infectious diseases, dermatology, or nervous and mental diseases. During 1914 the clinic cared for only about 200 medical patients as compared with more than 30,000 surgical patients.[84]

In 1915 the Mayo Clinic was nearly overwhelmed by an avalanche of patients that had begun in 1912 when the rate of growth of the business of the clinic accelerated. The number of patients registered at the clinic increased from 14,000 in 1912 to 31,000 in 1915, and the number of surgical operations performed from 9,000 to 15,000. By 1915 the staff of the Mayo Clinic must have been working under great pressure. They badly needed additional physicians to assist with the care of the increased numbers of patients. The various laboratory and diagnostic services were also working under great pressure, and needed additional staff. If the Mayo Clinic could offer a university affiliation in addition to appointment at the clinic, Dr. Mayo and his colleagues may have thought that the clinic could more easily attract first-rate people.

To clarify the terms of the proposed Mayo affiliation, Dean Lyon prepared an official statement based on the resolution adopted by the administrative board on 6 March and authorized by Dr. William Mayo, but it was not sufficient to remove public confusion.[85] As a result of the conflicting arguments offered at the hearing before the combined house-senate committee on 7 April, the Minnesota State Senate appointed a special committee to study both the proposed affiliation and the effect that the Guilford bill, if passed, would exert on the university. On Friday, 9 April the senate committee met with President Vincent, Fred P. Snyder, president of the Board of Regents, and other university officials in President Vincent's office. The committee asked for a definitive statement by the Mayos on the terms of their proposal to the university, and especially on the question of the control and use of the endowment fund.[86] Immediately after the meeting Dean Lyon and Dr. Beard left for Rochester to confer with the Doctors Mayo.[87] The same day the Mayo brothers and other trustees of the Mayo Foundation issued their own statement at Rochester on the terms of their proposal to the university. On the question of the endowment fund for the Mayo Foundation, the trustees said that if a permanent affiliation of the foundation with the University of Minnesota were achieved, the endowment would be placed in the hands of the Board of Regents subject to certain conditions. Its income must be used for the promotion of medical education and research, and the Mayo Foundation must be maintained at Rochester, Minnesota. While the educational and scientific work of the foundation was to be conducted and directed from Rochester, the Mayo trustees said that appropriations from the endowment income might be used to support medical research elsewhere in the state, or anywhere that should be desirable in a medical investigation.[88]

On Sunday, 11 April, the *Minneapolis Journal* announced that the Mayo Foundation was already in operation with an endowment of $1,500,000. A reporter for the *Journal* had traveled to Rochester where he had interviewed the Doctors Mayo, their attorney and financial manager, Burt W. Eaton, and others. He then wrote a colorful account of the Mayo Clinic, and of the gradual development of the Mayo brothers' ideas for the endowment of medical education and research.[89] The next day the university committees of the Minnesota legislature held a second public hearing on a bill intended to prevent the Mayo affiliation, now amended to read: " . . . this act shall not be so construed as to disable the [Board of Regents] from employing or authorizing the employment of instructors, lecturers or teachers who shall devote a part only of their time or service to the educational work of any department of the University."[90] At the hearing most of the speakers discussed the proposed Mayo affiliation instead of the bill. Three speakers representing the medical societies of eight rural counties protested against the Mayo affiliation, while the gentle Dr. Arthur Sweeney of St. Paul made "a strong and conciliatory plea" in favor of it. Dr. Sweeney thought that the motives of the Mayos were entirely altruistic, and the objection that the university should not delegate its teaching functions to a private corporation was not supported by modern practice. Recently Yale and St. Louis universities had formed affiliations with private hospitals.[91] The Reverend J. N. Kildal spoke against the affiliation on several grounds, one of which was that it would require the university to affiliate with St. Mary's Hospital in Rochester, a Catholic institution. Dr. Wilson of the Mayo Clinic declared that the clinic was " . . . in a position to carry out the work of studying cases in a way not afforded by any other institution in the country," but Dr. George Head of Minneapolis questioned whether the Mayo Clinic could carry on research in internal medicine effectively. The report of the Mayo Clinic, said Dr. Head, showed that they had had only 178 medical cases during the year, whereas in the Twin Cities there were approximately 1,500 medical cases available at all times. When Louis Wilson was asked whether he thought the opposition to the affiliation was honest, he replied that he would diagnose it as "hysteria."[92]

When Charles Lyman Greene spoke he noted that whereas 30,000 patients were treated at Rochester during the year, the university free dispensary received between 40,000 and 50,000 visits annually. The Mayo Clinic was doing remarkably good work, but the university was also doing work that in quality and quantity would compare favorably with that done at Rochester. At the conclusion of his remarks, Dr. Greene was subjected to a vigorous cross-examination by Regents Pierce Butler, George M. Gillette, and others, but evidently Dr. Greene managed to reply calmly and effectively. Among other statements, Dr. Greene said that a majority of the teaching staff of the medical school opposed the affiliation, but that fact was not reflected in the faculty vote of thirty-nine to twenty-six in favor of affiliation, because a large portion of the clinical teaching staff had no vote. The cross-examination of Dr. Greene revealed the large number of physicians who were devoting time to teaching in the medical school without pay.[93] The impressions created by the debate at the hearing on 12 April may have varied. Two days later Dean Lyon wrote to William J. Mayo: "You have doubtless heard all about the last hearing and know that we need fear no trouble from the Guilford law. There are already signs that the opponents acknowledge their defeat."[94] He went on to discuss how the scientific directors of the Mayo Foundation should be chosen.

But Charles Lyman Greene was not finished yet. On 15 April Dr. Greene issued a statement, expressing the views of the medical societies of eighteen Minnesota counties in opposition to the proposed Mayo affiliation. Dr. Greene noted that the temporary affiliation proposed for three or four years might be extended indefinitely, and that, therefore, the features of the temporary affiliation were more important than the proposals for a possible future permanent arrangement. Dr. Greene noted that at the legislative hearings Louis B. Wilson, speaking on behalf of the Mayo Clinic, had said that " . . . all graduate students must and do act as assistants in the private clinic during the greater part of their stay, and being picked men they represent and actually are most valuable to the clinic in which they act as assistants."[95] The Mayo Clinic, Dr. Greene said, was on Dr. Wilson's own evidence almost entirely a surgical clinic, and Dr. Greene suggested that for the most part the patients suffered from chronic conditions and the operations performed were elective. The clinic "was deficient with respect to diversity of material, cases of acute disease—infectious or otherwise, and the all important emergency services."[96]

Dr. Greene's letter, published in the two leading Minneapolis newspapers, spurred Dean Lyon to immediate action. He sent a special delivery letter to Louis B. Wilson at Rochester, enclosing a copy of Dr. Greene's statement as it appeared in the *Minneapolis Tribune,* and Dr. Wilson spent all his available time the next day in writing a reply to Dr. Greene. That evening he wrote to Dean Lyon that he had not had an opportunity to show the statement to Dr. Mayo, nor even to decide in his own mind how to use it or whether it should be used at all.[97] In the end Dr. Wilson did not publish it, but his unpublished reply does reveal his thinking on the issues in affiliation. Whereas Dr. Greene charged that under the affiliation Minnesota medical graduates would not have any greater claim upon a Mayo Foundation fellowship than graduates of other medical schools, Dr. Wilson replied that under affiliation every Mayo Foundation fellow would become a student of the University of Minnesota which would thus become the alma mater of a group of men who had received their highest special medical training at Minnesota. On the question of a money gift Dr. Wilson said " . . . upon affiliation, the graduate education and research of the Mayo Foundation will become a part of the University and will require a 'money gift' from the Mayo Clinic of approximately $100,000 per annum."[98] He did not reply to Dr. Greene's charge that the Mayo Foundation fellows contributed to the work of the Mayo Clinic, and that, therefore, the money provided for their stipends might be considered a payment for services rendered rather than a gift. Dr. Wilson said that the reason for the existence of the Mayo Foundation at Rochester was the presence of the patients there. "These cannot be transferred elsewhere. Since they are an asset for scientific study exceeding in value many times the endowment fund, it is obvious that the fund must be expended where the patients congregate."[99] Similarly, since the clinical work of the Mayo Foundation was based upon the clinical material of the Mayo Clinic, the scientific directors of the foundation must be acceptable to the Mayo Clinic.

In answer to Dr. Greene's point that the fellows acted as assistants in the Mayo Clinic and were very valuable to it, Dr. Wilson said that the reason for the existence of the Mayo Foundation was to give men who were preparing themselves for medical specialties access "to the unequalled clinical facilities of the Mayo Clinic." He said that about one fifth of the fellows devoted their full time, and one half more than half their time "to research which has no relation to the patients in the clinic but concerns only specimens or data accumulated from previous patients."[100] Dr. Wilson said that it would be possible to fill every temporary position in the Mayo Clinic with volunteers or with physicians who would pay for the privilege of working at the clinic. The purpose of the fellowships was to enable young physicians, who could not do without an income, to take advantage of the opportunities for special medical training at Rochester. On the question of the value of the fellows to the Mayo Clinic, Dr. Wilson may have been slightly disingenuous. While the clinic might have been able to fill its temporary positions with volunteers, such volunteers would be older physicians who, being unpaid, could not be asked to work as long or as hard in the care of patients as young doctors on fellowships.

Dr. Wilson described in some detail the rich clinical material at Rochester. He emphasized the high proportion of autopsies performed on patients who died at the clinic. He said that the accumulated diagnostic material dealt with every disease known in North America, and that while in 1914 operations were performed on 14,000 patients, 18,000 were not operated upon. A large majority of the 18,000, he said, were medical cases. After listing the various surgical and diagnostic services of the Mayo Clinic, Dr. Wilson wrote:

> With the above clinical material at its command and with extensive and well-equipped laboratories of clinical medicine, pathology, bacteriology, experimental chemistry and experimental surgery and physiology, all of which are supplemented by a well selected and thoroughly organized library of over 4,000 volumes to which additions costing approximately $10,000 per year are being made, the Mayo Foundation feels justified in offering to graduate physicians courses fitting them for the practice of the specialties of pathology and bacteriology, clinical and experimental medicine, orthopedic surgery, urology, ophthalmology and otology, rhinology and laryngology, and roentgenology.[101]

The controversy over the Mayo affiliation at the legislative hearings and in published statements also attracted editorial comment in Minnesota newspapers. On 19 April the *Minneapolis Tribune* devoted an editorial to the opposition to what they called "the Mayo gift," which, they asserted, arose from physicians who were "commercial competitors of the Mayos," and were, therefore, not disinterested. The editorial stated that in contrast to the physicians opposing the Mayo affiliation the Mayos had not sought to present their side of the case to the public. They had " . . . remained consistently aloof and have given out no information except such statements as were explicitly requested of them by the legislative committee."[102] The editorial overlooked the fact that Louis B. Wilson had testified at legislative hearings on behalf of the Mayo Foundation, and it showed bias by referring to the proposed affiliation as a gift, and by suggesting that the opponents of affiliation had misrepresented it, but it was true that the Mayos had appeared to remain aloof from the controversy. That seeming aloofness was not indifference. There is much evidence that Dr. William J. Mayo was deeply determined to achieve affiliation. If he did not come to the Twin Cities to participate in the controversy, he did not need to. The president of the university, the dean of the medical school, and the secretary of the medical faculty were acting essentially as his agents, advocating and defending the affiliation, and keeping him informed by letter and by telephone. Mayo's colleagues on the Board of Regents included shrewd and experienced lawyers who attacked the opponents of affiliation by ferocious cross-examination at legislative hearings. Dr. Mayo may also have possessed allies in the publishers and editors of the *Minneapolis Tribune,* the *St. Paul Pioneer Press,* and the *St. Paul Dispatch.* All three newspapers attacked the opponents of affiliation editorially, and with evident sympathy for the Mayos.[103] The *Minneapolis Journal* was more neutral, asking that the exact nature of the proposed affiliation be made public, but opposing legislation to prevent the Board of Regents from entering into such an arrangement.[104]

On 19 April a Minneapolis attorney, Einar Hoidale, expressed his opposition to the Mayo affiliation. Although Mr. Hoidale said that his first impression was that the apparently generous offer of the Mayos should be accepted, on more careful examination he thought that acceptance of the proposition would be a serious mistake. As a state institution the university's only proper function was to advance the public interest. The affiliation was not proper for the university because it would constitute a partnership between a state institution and a business corporation operated for profit. By entering into affiliation, the university " . . . would give to one unit of a competitive profession an undue advantage over all others in the same profession by placing its stamp of approval upon the Rochester firm, and by throwing to that firm the prestige of its indorsement." Mr. Hoidale questioned the double role of William Mayo as a regent of the university and leader of the Mayo Foundation.[105] He went on to draw a parallel with the position in which a hypothetical Minneapolis lawyer, whom he called Henry Brown, might be if a half dozen of the brightest and most successful lawyers formed a partnership for carrying on a law business on a large scale, and if after achieving great success, they were to establish a foundation which then sought affiliation with the university law school: "Why not affiliate?" asked Mr. Hoidale, "All this great law firm asks is that the state put the seal of indorsement upon its work. A blind man can see that this would result in giving to this concern a dignity, standing and prestige that would spell blasted hopes for Mr. Brown." In such a situation Hoidale said that the state, by affiliation, would have aided in the development of a monopoly of the legal business. "It is the most ingenious device imaginable," said Mr. Hoidale, "for creating a special privilege and perpetuating a monopoly."[106]

On 20 April 1915 the Minnesota Senate passed the anti-affiliation bill by a vote of thirty-six to thirty-one, but because the legislative session ended the following day, the House could not consider the bill, and it did not become law.[107] On 4 May six members of the Board of Regents, including Governor W. S. Hammond, traveled to Rochester to inspect the laboratories of the Mayo Clinic and St. Mary's Hospital.[108] Two days later, on 6 May, the Board of Regents decided to open their meetings to the public, and to refer the proposed affiliation with the Mayo Foundation to a committee consisting of all the regents with the exception of Regent Mayo. At the same time they referred an affiliation proposal from the Swedish Hospital of Minneapolis to the administrative board of the medical school.[109]

At the university on 12 May 1915 the Board of Regents held a public hearing on the question of affiliation, attended by thirty-five persons in addition to the regents. At the hearing a Minneapolis attorney, C. J. Traxler, suggested that the affiliation might be illegal. Regent Pierce Butler asked questions concerning the nature of the opposition to the Mayo proposal and the amounts of money that had been contributed by Twin Cities physicians to oppose it. Mr. Butler had been told that a group of Minneapolis and St. Paul physicians had each pledged $100 to fight the proposal, but it turned out that no such pledges had been given, and the most that any physician had contributed was $10.[110] At the hearing various physicians spoke against the affiliation. Dr. H. B. Sweetser of Minneapolis said that the Mayo affiliation would interfere seriously with the clinical development of the medical school because it would remove the incentive of the clinical instructors to contribute their time. A public statement of reasons for objection to the affiliation was submitted by a committee of sixteen Twin Cities physicians.[111] In an analysis of documents in the case, the *Minnesota Alumni Weekly* noted: "The fact that the proposed union is . . . a substitute for the early completion of our controlled campus clinic and must so operate is a body blow to the clinical faculty of the School of Medicine."[112]

Despite such adverse testimony, on Thursday, 27 May, the executive committee of the Board of Regents approved the proposal for affiliation of the University of Minnesota with the Mayo Foundation and published the complete proposal.[113] On Saturday, 5 June, just nine days after the publication of the final terms of the Mayo affiliation proposal, the executive committee of the Board of Regents held a public hearing on the proposal, at which Charles Lyman Greene again testified in opposition to affiliation, but said he had not had sufficient time to study the terms of the revised proposal published on 27 May. The regents asked Dr. Greene about his course in leading opposition to the affiliation proposal before the regents had acted. Dr. Greene and Regent Pierce Butler engaged in a sharp exchange of words and Butler asked Greene, "Will you continue in the harness if this plan is carried out?"[114] Dr. Greene replied that he would not make any promise. The same day the executive committee approved a report prepared by a subcommittee recommending affiliation with the Mayo Foundation for an initial period of six years.[115] The report was to be considered by the full Board of Regents at its meeting on Wednesday, 9 June. On Monday, 7 June, the Hennepin County Medical Society at a special meeting voted 200 to 10 that the proposed affiliation, even in its revised form, was not a gift to the university, but a contract between the university and the Mayo Foundation, or between the Board of Regents and one of its own members. The society petitioned the Board of Regents not to enter into such a affiliation so long as Dr. Mayo was a regent of the university because " . . . his conflicting interests as a member of the Mayo Clinic, one of the founders of the Mayo Foundation, and at the same time a member of the Board of Regents may, and most probably would, lead to dangerous impediments to the future growth and welfare of the medical department of the university."[116] In its petition the society added that the university was already operating a graduate school in medicine, and credit for its pioneering work in graduate medical education should not be obscured by affiliation with " . . . a distinctly surgical clinic."[117] The society noted that one reason given for considering the Mayo affiliation was that the Board of Regents was unwilling to ask the state legislature to provide for the expansion of the university hospital into a complete clinic. They estimated the cost of a clinical hospital, nurses' home, and additional service building at $350,000, which would give facilities "infinitely superior to those at Rochester and . . . in proper relation to the fundamental laboratories." They said: "The university hospital is primarily devoted to the relief of the sick poor of the state of Minnesota and to teaching and research. It stands absolutely separate and apart from any business undertaking and makes return in overflowing measure and with peculiar directness in the form of public service."[118] Despite the petitions against and objections to the Mayo affiliation, the Board of Regents at its meeting on June 9 decided unanimously to implement the Mayo affiliation.[119]

Once their decision to enter into the Mayo affiliation was taken, the Board of Regents turned upon those who opposed affiliation. They demanded the resignation of the head of the Department of Medicine, Charles Lyman Greene, who led the opposition to affiliation, and passed a resolution: " . . . that the new plans for developing the graduate medical work of the University should not hereafter be opposed by any member of the faculty of the Medical School, but, on the other hand, should have the loyal support of all members thereof."[120] This resolution was clearly intended to silence opposition to the Mayo affiliation among members of the medical faculty, and thereby to infringe upon freedom of speech and their academic freedom as members of the faculty. The next evening, the members of the Department of Medicine, now without Dr. Greene, met and twelve members signed a call for a meeting of the general faculty of the medical school to be held in mid-July. Shortly thereafter six members of the medical faculty submitted their resignations.[121] In an effort to hold the faculty together, Dean Lyon held the six resignations, and about the end of June wrote to President Vincent as follows:

> Some doubt has arisen as to the exact intent of the Board of Regents as expressed in their resolution adopted at the June meeting. I have told those interested in the matter that it is my understanding that no abridgment of proper academic freedom was intended by the resolution, and that all members of the medical faculty who are willing to give the plan of graduate work adopted by the regents a fair trial, may continue as members of the faculty with complete self respect.[122]

Dean Lyon was attempting at once to deny the restrictive effect of the regents' resolution on the freedom of speech of the medical faculty and to suggest tactfully to the regents that they had gone too far. On 3 July 1915 President Vincent replied tersely:

My dear Dean Lyon,
 I presented to the Board your letter in which you reported the interpretation you have placed upon the recent resolution of the Board. The Regents authorized me to say that your interpretation is officially sanctioned.

Sincerely yours,
G. E. Vincent[123]

On 12 July the administrative board asked Dean Lyon to confer personally with each member of the faculty who had resigned to ask the reason for their resignation, and to report back to them.[124] The next day Fred B. Snyder, president of the Board of Regents, was quoted in the newspapers as saying that the board would not interpret the resolution. He added: "The resolution does not refer to anything that may have taken place in the past, but it does mean that if any member of the faculty . . . feels that he cannot cooperate in trying out the plan, he is not wanted."[125]

When the administrative board met again on 23 July, Dean Lyon reported that five faculty members, Drs. Freeman, Gilfillan, Head, Hoff, and Hynes were unwilling to withdraw their resignations, and the board accepted them with regret.[126] All of those who resigned were alumni of the medical school, who may have felt most keenly a restriction on their right to speak about medical school affairs. When the general faculty of the medical school met two days later, Dean Lyon read to the meeting his letter to President Vincent and Vincent's reply. S. Marx White then moved that since Dean Lyon's interpretation of the Board of Regents resolution of 9 June "disposed of the question so far as faculty action could carry," the faculty should accept the interpretation as satisfactory.[127] The faculty thus made the best of a bad situation, but it is not clear that they had succeeded in cancelling the intimidating effect of the regents' resolution. Members of the faculty thereafter did not venture to speak out against the Mayo affiliation. On 6 August the administrative board accepted with regret a sixth resignation, that of Alexander R. Hall of St. Paul, instructor in medicine.

A year later, Dr. George Douglas Head, one of those who resigned, commented that the regents' resolution "was a direct blow at the freedom of speech and action of the clinical teachers in the School. It was an attempt in advance of the trial period to coerce those men into submission, and to close their mouths to a discussion of its merits and objections." Many of the faculty affected, Dr. Head noted, were alumni of the school who had ". . . grown up in its service, had sacrificed much in its interest, and loved its ideals and traditions." In October 1915, even after more than a year, the Board of Regents had not rescinded its motion. Dr. Head reflected sadly:

> I can see how in the heat of the controversy such a resolution might have been passed. It is difficult to understand how a board of fair-minded men having the best interests of a great institution of learning at heart, knowing the value of free interchange of opinion and discussion, and the blighting effect of coercion upon the spirit of its teaching force, can continue to hold this club over its faculty members. It is a direct violation of one of the most highly prized laws governing rights of teachers in higher institutions of learning.[128]

Unfortunately the regents in 1916 were not all fair-minded men, and placed little value on freedom of thought or discussion.

On 28 July 1915 the Board of Regents appointed fifteen members of the Mayo Foundation staff to the graduate faculty. In August the medical school reported an unprecedented increase in the number of applications for admission to the freshman year, but the school was obliged to limit the size of the entering class to eighty because of the limited facilities for clinical teaching in the third and fourth years.[129] The ability of the school to provide clinical instruction in medicine, previously limited, had been reduced significantly by the loss of seven members of the Department of Medicine. In October Dean Ford of the graduate school announced that the first exchange of students between the university and the Mayo Foundation would begin in January 1916.

At the beginning of July, in the immediate wake of the resignations of Dr. Greene and five other members of the Department of Medicine, President Vincent and Dean Lyon were faced with an urgent need to find a new head for the department. Characteristically, President Vincent decided that he must import the new professor from one of the older medical centers on the East coast. On 4 July, even before acting on the resignations, Vincent left by train for the East to interview possible candidates for vacant positions in the medical faculty. On 13 September the committee appointed to recommend a successor to Dr. Greene submitted the names of Leonard G. Rowntree of Johns Hopkins University and G. Canby Robinson of Washington University at St. Louis as their first and second choices respectively.[130] The committee recommended also that the new professor of medicine should serve practically full time, but be permitted to maintain a restricted consultation practice. "Consultation," they said, "is interpreted to include referred cases in hospital in which the consultant remains in active co-operation with the physician originally in charge of the case."[131] During October Dr. Rowntree visited Minneapolis to look over the situation. He also visited Rochester where Dr. Mayo assured him as a regent of the university of his full support.[132] On his return to Baltimore Dr. Rowntree wrote to Dean Lyon to express his willingness to accept the appointment on condition that he and other university clinicians be permitted to do consultation work, that a laboratory be provided for the Department of Medicine in the university hospital, and that a position for a resident physician be created on the medical staff. The medical school accepted his conditions. Early in January 1916 Dr. Rowntree arrived in Minneapolis with his family.

In March 1916 the medical school's committee on hospital and clinical development recommended the adoption of a per diem payment plan for patients

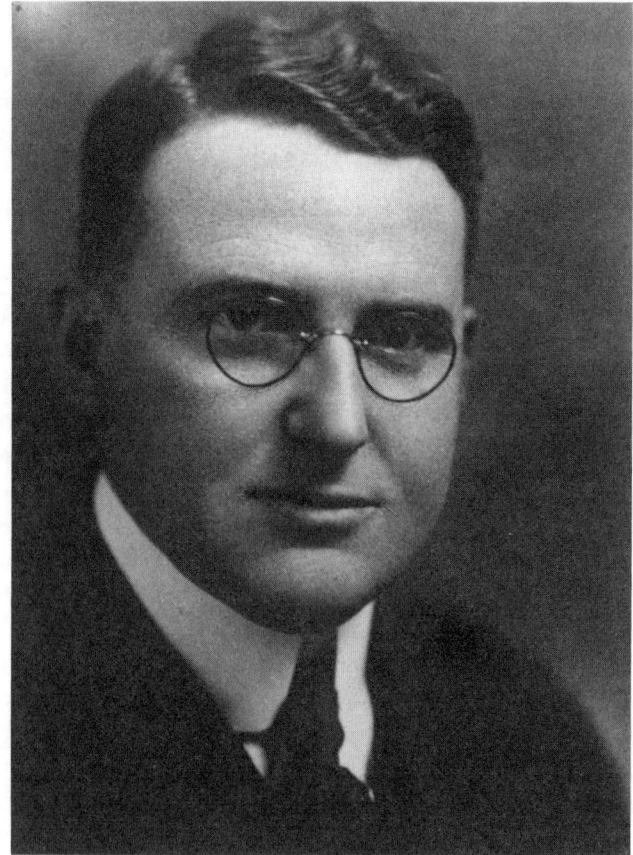

FIGURE 9:5   Leonard G. Rowntree, 1916. Courtesy Mn U Archives.

in the buildings of the university hospital outside the Elliot Memorial building. Under the per diem plan, patients would pay for their room and board in the hospital, but would receive free medical or surgical care. The committee recommended also that, within a restricted number of hospital rooms, patients should pay the full costs for their care. Finally the committee recommended that in cooperation with the Board of Regents and the Minneapolis Civic and Commerce Association the medical school should make plans to raise funds for hospital buildings from private donors. The committee did *not* suggest that the Board of Regents should ask the Minnesota legislature for the necessary funds.[133]

On 28 April 1916 the Minneapolis Civic and Commerce Association sent a letter to 200 prominent Minnesota physicians inviting them to attend a meeting to discuss the need to increase the clinical facilities of the University of Minnesota Medical School. The letter noted that the Board of Regents had been forced to limit the number of students admitted to the school and said that the university hospital needed 355 more beds to provide adequate clinical facilities for the medical school. Such expansion of the university hospital would cost from $575,000 to $700,000 and an additional $190,000 annually to maintain the enlarged hospital as a free institution. Because the administrative board of the medical school thought that appropriations on such a scale could not be obtained from the legislature, some other means, namely, private gifts, must be found to provide the additional buildings required. After the gift for hospital buildings was obtained, the question of funds for maintenance would remain. To meet this problem, the association said that the administrative board of the medical school had suggested "the taking of patients in the new buildings who would pay the full per diem cost of maintenance." Such patients would be referred by physicians to the university hospital for investigation, diagnosis, or treatment. The administrative board had suggested also that in order to obtain full-time clinical teachers, the clinical teachers should " . . . be allowed to take upon the University Campus only, a limited number of pay patients for consultation purposes."[134]

The *Journal-Lancet,* which reflected opinion among the medical profession, immediately published a long editorial on the proposal to admit paying patients to the university hospital, predicting strenuous opposition from both public and private hospitals in the Twin Cities. The *Journal-Lancet* was strongly in favor of enlargement of the clinical facilities at the university and the completion of the university hospital. They likewise supported an effort to obtain private gifts for new hospital buildings, but they were adamantly opposed to the admission of paying patients. The *Journal-Lancet* thought that the state had a moral obligation to support the university in all its departments. They objected similarly to the idea that full-time clinical teachers might supplement their meager salaries by fees from a limited number of patients referred to them. They thought it unlikely that such a scheme would win the approval of the legislature.[135]

At a special meeting on 4 October 1916 the Hennepin County Medical Society discussed the proposal to admit paying patients to the university hospital. There were 130 persons present, including representatives of the Minneapolis Civic and Commerce Association. The first speaker was Leonard Rowntree, who said that among physicians in the East the University of Minnesota was recognized as a great medical teaching center, but the medical school was not thought to be as productive scientifically as it might be. When he had come to Minnesota Dr. Rowntree had found that the reason for the school's relative lack of productivity in research was that the faculty were too few for the work they had to do, and the clinical facilities were insufficient. The university hospital was too small, and the medical school could not attract faculty unless it was enlarged. Dr. Rowntree thought also that a medical professor could not be a leader in his work if he did not engage to some degree in the practice of medicine. He urged the need for development at the university, and invited the Minneapolis physicians to participate in that development. Dr. Rowntree concluded, "We do not want the repetition of conditions that exist in St. Louis. Five years ago St. Louis promised to become a great medical center. The University and the profession split, and they have never gotten anywhere. We do not want that condition here."[136] Dr. Rowntree's words must have sounded strangely in the ears of the assembled physicians of Hennepin County. The reorganization of the medical school in 1913 was designed to shrink a medical faculty that Dr. Rowntree now said was too small, and to divide it from the medical profession of the Twin Cities. Moreover, in 1915 the Mayo affiliation had been introduced over the medical profession's united opposition. Previously despised, dismissed, and ignored, their cooperation was now invited, and said to be essential.

S. Marx White, speaking for a committee of the medical faculty, similarly urged the need for development of the university hospital. The Elliot Hospital was too small to permit clinical investigation or an adequate number of clinical clerkships. Dr. White said that legislative support had been and would continue to be inadequate because of opposition from other university departments and from the state at large. To make up for lack of legislative support, Dr. White recommended the admission to the university hospital of per diem patients, who paid a daily rate for hospital charges but not for medical or surgical care. Dr. White said that the best clinical teachers could not be obtained for the highest salary then paid by the university. The medical school needed both to obtain full-time clinical teachers and to prevent abuse of their position by such teachers "to secure large and very lucrative practices."[137] To avoid the latter difficulty the medical school had developed a plan to limit the number of private patients in an enlarged university hospital to 15 percent of its capacity. If the enlarged university hospital were to contain 550 beds, the number of beds available for private patients would be eighty-three which, Dr. White thought, would not cause much excitement among hospital superintendents in the Twin Cities. Dr. White proposed further that all fees for full-time members of the medical faculty should be collected in a central office, with regular accounting to university authorities. He concluded by suggesting that the development of the university hospital would "put the Medical School in such a position that nothing can overshadow it," and would make the Twin Cities the medical center of the Northwest.[138]

Despite Dr. White's plea, Dr. W. A. Jones, editor of the *Journal-Lancet*, who spoke next, was opposed completely to the admission of paying patients to a state-supported hospital, which the university hospital must always be. He was also emphatically against allowing full-time members of the medical faculty to supplement their salaries by seeing private patients. Dr. Jones thought that the state should provide full-time medical teachers with sufficient salaries, as they did in every other hospital and institution that belonged to the state. He thought that the university and the medical profession should be working together to persuade the legislature to provide funds for adequate faculty salaries. Dr. Jones said that there existed a division of feeling between the university medical faculty and the medical profession outside the university, which he regretted "because we all ought to stand together and all ought to do the same work . . . ."[139] Dr. Jones thought that the university's requests should be directed to the legislature.

With some diffidence because of his position as a former teacher in the medical school, George Head rose to speak. He recalled the history of the school and after referring to the impropriety of the Mayo affiliation, urged a resolution to condemn "this attempt to place upon state property in state buildings accommodations for the care of the private practice of any physician."[140] Dr. Frederick A. Dunsmoor recalled that when he had first become interested in medical teaching thirty-eight years before, he had tried to combine hospital training with the didactic lectures because he realized that clinical education was essential for the training of effective physicians. Up until the reorganization of the medical college, said Dr. Dunsmoor, "we had nearly 3,000 beds with patients in them under the care of reasonably well-educated and thoroughly devoted men, who did not give a thought to their salary."[141]

Dean Lyon spoke for the medical school. He sought to begin with points on which they might agree. Although the primary function of the medical school was to train medical practitioners, the medical practitioner of the future must be trained scientifically by men who were themselves engaged in scientific research. Although he himself was a physiologist, and although physiology needed much development at the university, he thought that the most urgent need of the medical school was the extension of the university hospital. The hospital needed more beds. As to teaching, anatomy and physiology had formerly been taught by physicians in active practice who devoted a few hours a week to lectures on these subjects. Now they were taught by full-time men. The clinical departments, too, must now be led by full-time teachers who were active in research, but clinical teachers were supposed to teach the facts of active practice. Was it wise, therefore, to isolate them completely from practice? Said Dean Lyon: "What is the middle ground, then, between these two alternatives? On the one hand, to withdraw him [the clinical teacher] entirely? Shall we say that these men chosen from all the world shall treat only the sick poor of the state, or shall we say that they shall have some touch with the medical profession and active practice."[142] Dean Lyon said that he himself had changed his opinion. Formerly he had thought that the clinical teacher should work entirely with nonpaying patients in a laboratory setting completely apart from ordinary medical practice; but as he came to recognize that clinical teachers should be in active touch with their profession, he realized that such isolation would not work. Dean Lyon said that they were seeking " . . . a proper limitation, one that shall be fair to the doctors and which shall add to the efficiency of full time men, and yet leave them with you as active practitioners . . . If you can help us to reach a conclusion which is fair to all, along these lines, you will do a great thing."[143]

Dean Lyon's simple and sincere appeal did not go unheeded, but it could not remove the great, awkward fact of the Mayo affiliation, which he, probably little knowing what he was doing, had worked so hard to achieve. Soren P. Rees, a member of the medical faculty, said that he had opposed the affiliation. He feared that, like the affiliation, the plan to admit paying patients to the university hospital would "breed discord and feeling and unfairness, so that the School may lose the unanimous support of the profession."[144]

George Head asked Dean Lyon: "What makes the Administrative Board feel that the State will not grant a reasonable request of the University for enlarged hospital facilities? that is, have any attempts been made to secure appropriations and failed?"[145] Dean Lyon replied that he had tried for a contagious hospital but failed, and that the last legislature had given nothing to the university. Dean Lyon admitted that the medical school had made no appeal to the alumni for support, saying that the Board of Regents considered it unwise for every separate interest in the university to go to the legislature to lobby on its own behalf. The administrative policy of the Board of Regents thus prevented the university's requests on behalf of the medical school from receiving the political support needed for their favorable consideration. When Dr. Head asked Dean Lyon whether it was wise to attempt to introduce a plan for private medical practice on the campus over the opposition of the medical profession instead of asking them to join in an appeal to the legislature for the funds needed for additional hospital facilties at the university, Dean Lyon, somewhat nettled, replied that, while he regretted the difference of opinion between the medical school and some members of the profession, he did not think that the profession ought to run the school. Dr. Head then suggested that Dean Lyon might " . . . have misinterpreted the interest that medical men have shown . . . in connection with the affiliation of a year ago and the plan now before us?"[146] Dr. Head said that the medical men did not want to run the medical school, but to avoid harm to the university. He recalled that the year before the charge was very freely made that opposition to the Mayo affiliation arose simply from jealousy of the Mayo Clinic, a charge that Dr. Head called "untruthful." Dr. Head urged: " . . . let us all get on common ground and discuss this thing as one honest man discusses it with another, and not on the ground of saying to the man who opposes our argument that it is a purely personal and selfish motive that he has in doing this or in that."[147] Other physicians spoke in support of Dr. Head.[148]

When the Minnesota State Medical Association met in mid-October 1915 they unanimously rejected the plan to receive paying patients at the university hospital as "unsound in principle, bad public policy, and contrary to the established ideals upon which the Medical School was founded."[149] The Medical Alumni Association also rejected the plan in similar terms.[150] Probably as a result of the discussion at the meeting of the Hennepin County Medical Society on 4 October, the Minneapolis Civic and Commerce Association made no report on the medical school's plan to receive paying patients at the university.

On 2 November 1916 the administrative board, evidently despairing of help from the Minneapolis Civic and Commerce Association, recommended to the Board of Regents that the board request $200,000 from the legislature for a hospital for contagious diseases. They referred the question of maintenance to the Board of Regents on the understanding that the proposed addition to the university hospital would *not* admit patients from whom the physicians in charge would receive fees.[151] The administrative board also asked the regents to request an appropriation to build the wings of the Institute of Anatomy and of Millard Hall to house the Department of Pathology, Bacteriology, and Public Health and the laboratories of the State Board of Health.[152] Nothing came of their requests.

On 23 November 1916 S. Marx White, chairman of the medical school's subcommittee on hospital extension, submitted a lengthy report, emphasizing the urgent need to enlarge the university hospital and stating that the size of classes must be limited mainly by the lack of hospital beds.[153] The 140 to 160 students in the third and fourth years could not be adequately supplied with patients for study from 192 beds. Even the major clinics in medicine, surgery, and obstetrics were "not large enough to permit the grouping of cases for effective teaching." The special clinics offered "a mere pittance of opportunity." The outpatient department failed as a feeder to the hospital because the hospital was "not big enough to be fed."[154] The Minneapolis City Hospital was a valuable addition for clinical teaching, but its function was limited to the earlier type of demonstrative clinic. It was not satisfactory for clinical investigation, or for the study of patients by medical students. It was chiefly valuable for the opportunity it gave students to see acute cases, emergencies, accidents, and contagious diseases.[155]

The smallness of the university hospital also placed a serious limitation on clinical teachers. Although the policy of appointing a number of full-time clinical teachers was either accepted or under consideration at leading American medical schools, full-time clinical teachers needed not only an adequate salary but also sufficient opportunity to care for patients to maintain their clinical skills and to permit them to carry on clinical investigation. Without an adequate hospital clinical teachers could not do their work, nor could they carry on the graduate medical education to which the medical school was committed. The report estimated that the university hospital should be enlarged to 555 beds, which would be sufficient for the clinical needs of the school. The larger hospital would also require larger administrative and service quarters and a proper residence for nurses. The buildings required were estimated to cost about $750,000, and an annual budget of $295,000 for maintenance. The committee proposed the raising of a fund of one and a half million dollars, half of which would become a building fund for the university hospital while the other half would become an endowment fund, the income of which would be used for clinical salaries and fellowships.

The committee said that they had conferred with members of the legislature friendly to the university who said firmly that the legislature would not provide additional hospital buildings with an annual budget for their maintenance. The legislature might, however, provide funds for a hospital building if they did not have to provide annually for its maintenance. The committee, therefore, recommended that the Board of Regents request from the legislature $200,000 for a hospital building to be used primarily for contagious diseases, and that the cost of maintaining the building be met by per diem charges to patients. The committee dismissed the arguments against the per diem method of hospital support as "largely theoretical and somewhat obscure" because the per diem beds of other hospitals were in demand, but the per diem charges were so close to costs that per diem patients were a liability to the hospitals. "The argument of competition with these hospitals for patients of this class," said the committee, " does not seem substantial."[156]

The committee thought that some beds in the university hospital should be set aside for private patients who paid fees for their medical or surgical care. The income derived from such fees could be used to help pay the salaries of full-time clinical teachers. As an alternative to an enlarged university hospital the committee considered the possibility of a private hospital near the university campus with a staff composed of part-time members of the clinical faculty, but after weighing the pros and cons of such a plan, decided against it.

The committee's recommendations in sum were to seek additional state funds for hospital construction but to supplement them with funds to be raised by private subscription, to place 80 percent of additional hospital beds on a per diem basis, and to devote the other 20 percent to paying patients. The income from per diem charges would add to the support funds of the hospital, while the professional fees from paying patients would be placed in a fund for clinical research. The salaries of full-time clinical teachers and research workers should be paid from the support funds of the university, reinforced by endowment funds.[157]

The plan for clinical expansion submitted by Dr. White's subcommittee was approved by the administrative board, and became known through the Minnesota medical community. Some members of the administrative board seem to have considered the plan substantially identical with the plan for clinical expansion put forward by Charles Lyman Greene when he was offered the deanship of the medical school in June 1913. When Dr. Greene learned of the alleged identity between the two plans, he was horrified. On 10 February 1917 he wrote a letter of protest to the editor of the *Journal-Lancet* because not only was the plan of Dr. White's subcommittee very different from the 1913 plan of Dr. Greene, but Dr. Greene disapproved strongly of the new plan.[158]

Dr. Greene said that in order to succeed, a state-supported medical school needed the support both of the medical profession in the state and of its alumni. The policy of such a school should not be dominated by entangling alliances, and the teaching of members of the faculty should be kept entirely separate from their private medical practice so that no one might claim that the state university gave special privileges to any group of men. A state university medical school needed to emphasize undergraduate medical teaching because its primary function was the training of medical practitioners for the state. It should promote research as much as it could, but until the needs of undergraduate medical education were met fully, such a school should not undertake any elaborate scheme of graduate medical education. Undergraduate medical students should be taught at the bedside by physicians on half-time appointments, who should be paid something for their teaching. The growth of the medical school should be achieved by legislative appropriations, "making the character of the work done and the great and direct service given to the State the justification for legislative requests and for the active support of our alumni and of the physicians of the State . . . ."[159] The policies outlined by Dr. Greene had been followed successfully, he noted, by Dean Wesbrook and President Northrop. "With Dr. Northrop's withdrawal," said Dr. Greene, "came the almost complete arrest of clinical development and lean years for the University as a whole, chargeable, not to legislative parsimony, as has been stated so persistently, but to a complete change of policy . . . ."[160]

The most striking example of change of policy, thought Dr. Greene, was the affiliation with the Mayo Foundation.[161] If the affiliation became permanent, the endowment for the Mayo Foundation would be transferred to the Board of Regents, but that would only mean, said Dr. Greene, that the regents would act gratuitously as trustees without controlling the activities of the Mayo Foundation. The Mayo partners, acting as the governing board of the Mayo Foundation, nominated teachers, decided the expenditures of funds, and determined the nature of the work to be undertaken. Dr. Greene emphasized that the research work and graduate teaching of the Mayo Foundation were "inextricably fused" with the business of the Mayo Clinic, so that the affiliation with the Mayo Foundation was really with the Mayo Clinic. Although the endowment of the Mayo Foundation had been acclaimed as a gift to the university, the experience of a year and a half of affiliation had demonstrated practically that no part of the Mayo Foundation income could be used for the medical school, as the authorities of the school had come to recognize, said Dr. Greene, in putting forward their new plan for clinical expansion.

Dr. Greene considered that the new plan to add 355 beds to the university hospital was a breach of faith with the medical profession of the state and the alumni of the medical school, because from the time that the plans for the university hospital were first laid both groups had been assured that the hospital would be free to the sick poor of the state and open to them alone. Dr. Greene said that the alleged necessity for the plan would not exist if it were not "that proper and timely requests for administrative action concerning appropriations had been denied and that the forces normally available for support had been alienated, deliberately and cynically."[162] Dr. Greene was hinting that in the reorganization of the medical school in 1913, President Vincent had sought deliberately to alienate the medical profession and the medical alumni. If it were not the intent, that had certainly been the effect of Vincent's actions. Dr. Greene said that the chief obstacle to the enlargement of the university hospital was the failure of the Board of Regents to ask the legislature for the money. He thought that such a request would have received the support of the alumni and the medical profession.[163]

Dr. Greene's fundamental objection to paying patients at the university hospital was that it would place the university in direct competition with the medical profession and with the private hospitals, that is, in competition with many citizens who paid taxes to support the university. He thought that the university hospital should provide a complete, but free, clinic and the heads of major clinical departments should be "*generously* salaried full-time men," so that they might conduct research, and devote time to teaching. Finally Dr. Greene said that the six years since 1911 had been for the medical school "a period of continuing and progressive demoralization . . . ."[164]

In the next issue of the *Journal-Lancet* on 15 March 1917 appeared a letter entitled "Why the Mayo affiliation with the University should be terminated" signed by seventy-eight Minnesota physicians, including thirty-five medical alumni and twenty-two former members of the faculty.[165] Twenty-eight signers had never been connected with the university. The signers were also sponsors of a bill introduced into the legislature that would require the Board of Regents to terminate the affiliation with the Mayo Foundation, and the statement contained their reasons for seeking such a law. The statement asserted that the medical school was no longer self-governing or well organized, and was torn by discord. Because of the gag rule imposed by the regents in 1915, it was impossible for them to obtain the opinion of the medical faculty on how the Mayo affiliation was working, and therefore alumni and friends of the school outside the faculty were compelled to speak. The Mayo affiliation was an entering wedge that separated the university from the medical profession of Minnesota and from the alumni, who had come to distrust President Vincent, the Board of Regents, and Dean Lyon. The affiliation emphasized research and graduate medical education at the expense of undergraduate medical teaching. Worst of all, the affiliation agreement, unless revoked, committed the university to maintain the work of the Mayo Foundation permanently at Rochester, and although the initial affiliation was for six years only, it would become permanent automatically unless revoked by the Board of Regents or by the Mayos before 1 September 1921. The fact that the work of the Mayo Foundation must be carried out forever at Rochester denied the Board of Regents effective control of it, and the service rendered by the Mayo Foundation was not to the university but to the Mayo Clinic.

The revival of controversy over the Mayo affiliation prompted the Mayo Foundation on 19 March to prepare a private reply to the charges published in the *Journal-Lancet* four days earlier.[166] After a brief review of the events leading up to the affiliation and of the work being conducted by the Mayo Foundation, the document said that the Doctors Mayo were willing to give up their right to terminate the contract at the end of the six-year trial period, while leaving the university free to terminate the contract if it wished. The Mayos were also willing immediately to turn the Mayo Foundation endowment over to the Board of Regents as trustees. The document denied that all the income of the Mayo Foundation must be spent in Rochester. The foundation's work in graduate medical education and research was to be carried on at Rochester, but funds might be spent elsewhere in support of medical investigation. Although true, the claim was misleading by what the document did not say, namely, that in no circumstances would the Mayo Foundation support graduate medical education anywhere but at Rochester. It would provide no fellowships for work in the medical school at Minneapolis.

Against the objection that the state should not ally itself with a private corporation, the document said that if the Board of Regents took over the Mayo Foundation, the foundation would then have the same relation to the university as the hospitals in the Twin Cities that provided opportunities for clinical training for the undergraduate medical students.

The document blamed the opposition on the history of bitter strife among various factions at the medical school, the resentment of men deposed in the reorganization of 1913, and the further resentment of those who had been defeated in their opposition to affiliation in 1915. It did not admit that there might be reasonable grounds for objection to the Mayo affiliation. The statement concluded:

> The Doctors Mayo have been the victims of a merciless campaign of vilification. The men who have engendered the attack profess to believe the worst of them, that it is merely a scheme to make money, yet it must be apparent to everyone that they have the money, and if money were the object they would keep it rather than give it to the University. They have not plead for sympathy, but they do ask for justice and fair treatment, and hope that no one will think so poorly of them as to believe that they have no motive except to add to those forces which will benefit suffering humanity.[167]

Despite the confusion and contradiction in the last sentence, the final message of the statement is clear: the Mayos were the victims of false and malicious attacks. Now the remarkable feature of the speeches, resolutions, editorials, and public statements issued in opposition to the Mayo affiliation was that they almost invariably referred to the Doctors Mayo with respect for their great achievements in surgery, their honesty, and even their generosity. The opposition to affiliation had been based upon questions of public policy, and whatever passions may have figured in the controversy it could not be described accurately as "a merciless campaign of vilification." The opponents of affiliation had not charged that it was merely a scheme to make money, but a plan to endow the Mayo Clinic so as to perpetuate it. They had pointed out accurately that the additional prestige conferred by connection with the university would prove immensely profitable to the Mayo Clinic, a factor that the Mayo Foundation statement did not consider at all. The troublesome feature of the Mayo Foundation statement is that in it the foundation itself was vilifying its opponents without attempting to answer their central arguments, and was doing so in a private statement which would not be subjected to public analysis and refutation. The Mayos seem to have suffered from their own illusions, perhaps their own passions. Although they lived in the manner of the millionaires that they were, with mansions, yachts, servants, and automobiles, they cherished the belief that they lived modestly and humbly. They described the endowment of the Mayo Foundation as their life savings, but it was only a part, and possibly a small part, of their total wealth. The Mayo Foundation was created, they said, to "benefit suffering humanity." Perhaps in the long run it did, but it also produced large, immediate, and tangible benefits to the Mayo Clinic, and the Mayos could not bring themselves to admit the existence of such benefits.

On 1 April 1917 the affairs of the medical school and the Mayo affiliation again filled the pages of the *Journal-Lancet*. In addition to a long and carefully balanced editorial on the medical school controversy, Dean Lyon and Dr. Beard published a letter presenting the plan for extension of the university hospital, the plan criticized by Charles Lyman Greene a month earlier.[168] The circular letter entitled "Why the Mayo affiliation with the University should be terminated," which had been distributed widely among the Minnesota medical profession and had appeared in the *Journal-Lancet* on 15 March, had provoked an immediate reaction from the medical school. On 13 March the administrative board had held a special meeting at which they appointed a committee to prepare a reply which was presented to a special meeting of the general faculty on the evening of Monday, 19 March.[169] The faculty voted to sign the statement and to invite faculty members not present to add their signatures. Dr. Soren Rees moved that a committee be appointed to confer with a committee of the signers of the pamphlet "Why the Mayo affiliation should be terminated," but the motion lost. There was to be no peace. When the medical school's reply appeared in the *Journal-Lancet* it bore the names of seventy-seven members of the faculty, although not that of Dr. Rees.[170] The faculty asserted that the medical school was "a well-organized effective working unit," unembarrassed by any outside influence. Within the school there were healthy differences of opinion on questions of policy, but the faculty trusted each other and expressed their opinions freely. The medical school had not deteriorated. The student body had increased from 180 in 1912 to 263 in 1916; the dispensary had moved to larger quarters in Millard Hall where in 1916 it had received 50,320 patient visits; a social service department and a psychologic and psychiatric clinic had been established; the scientific departments had been strengthened and the curriculum broadened.

On the clinical side the faculty noted that the headship of the Department of Medicine had been placed on practically a full-time basis; a metabolism laboratory had been equipped; the dispensary staff had grown from eleven to twenty-six, and special clinics for tuberculosis and syphilis had been established; clinical clerkships had been expanded to give each senior student four months hospital service; and the medical school had formed an affiliation with the State Hospital for the Crippled and Deformed at Phalen Park to provide students with clinical training in orthopedic surgery. Graduate study was proceeding in the scientific departments and had begun in the clinical departments, where there were ten teaching fellowships and several scholarships. Graduate work in the clinical departments was not at the expense of undergraduate teaching but tended to reinforce it. The teaching fellows were very effective teaching assistants. Departments of ophthalmology and otolaryngology and of pediatrics had been established. Although it was true that the summer school for practicing physicians had been discontinued, lectures and clinics at the medical school remained open to practitioners throughout the year.

The catalogue of achievements and improvements at the medical school is, nevertheless, less impressive than the striking manner in which the faculty closed ranks in the face of outside criticism. Keenly aware though they might be of the deficiencies of the medical school, the faculty remained fiercely loyal. The *Journal-Lancet* also published official statements on behalf of the Board of Regents and the Mayo Foundation, dated 19 March. In their statement on behalf of the Mayo Foundation, the Doctors Mayo agreed to turn the Mayo Foundation endowment, then about $1,600,000, over to the Board of Regents.[171] On 22 March, two days after the Doctors Mayo had announced their willingness to turn over the Mayo Foundation endowment to the Board of Regents immediately, joint committees of the Minnesota House and Senate held an open hearing in the Senate Chamber on the bill to require the regents to dissolve the Mayo affiliation. Nine physicians and three laymen spoke in favor of the bill, presenting essentially the arguments published in the *Journal-Lancet* the week before. The speakers presented evidence that Minnesota physicians were overwhelmingly in favor of the bill.[172] President Vincent and Regents Fred B. Snyder and William J. Mayo spoke against the bill. When Dr. Mayo rose to speak the Senate Chamber fell silent. He began by saying that he had hesitated to appear before the committee, but there was so much misunderstanding and so many misstatements concerning the purposes of the Mayo Foundation that he wished to offer an explanation. He recalled his boyhood and the influence of his father, Dr. William Worrall Mayo, whom William and Charles Mayo had helped " . . . just as a farmer boy would help his father who was a farmer . . . ." The elder Mayo had believed that the surplus money taken for the care of the sick should go back to the people. Dr. Mayo referred to the success of their clinic, the beginning of their graduate school in medicine, and the growth through investment of their savings which by 1915 had accumulated $1,500,000. He denied that there was any self interest in their offer of the fund to the university. He said that the money came from the people, not from the medical profession, and would go back to the people. Dr. Mayo said that as the plan for the Mayo affiliation proceeded various objections had been met and restrictions had been withdrawn until now he and his brother required only that the graduate work be done at Rochester, although part of the fund could be used to support medical research elsewhere.

To me [said Dr. Mayo] Lincoln's inaugural address has always been a very wonderful thing. In that address Lincoln said "that these dead have not died in vain" [*sic*] I am thinking now of the people who have died needlessly, of the people whose deaths could have been prevented. And I want to ask in what better way can money be spent than in using it in an effort to train men to prevent unnecessary deaths "that these dead have not died in vain."

Dr. Mayo concluded by asking the committee to visit Rochester to judge the graduate work being done there under the Mayo Foundation.

Dr. Mayo's speech has been described as a "lost oration," but a substantial portion of it was recorded by the reporter for the *Minneapolis Journal*.[173] As a speech it was tremendously effective. Dr. Mayo presented himself and his brother as simple men who in their calling followed naturally in their father's footsteps. His reference to a farmer's following his father in the business of farming struck a responsive chord among the legislators, many of whom were rural or had grown up on farms. By emphasizing that the Mayo Clinic provided much free medical care to poor patients and did not force the collection of their bills, Dr. Mayo asserted that he and his brother were not grasping and avaricious. The Mayos may have been generous, but their policy of not forcing collections was also sound business policy and good public relations. They knew that the resentment created by efforts to enforce payment cost more than it was worth. Since most of their patients paid, they could overlook the few who did not and help those who could not. Nevertheless, in his speech Dr. Mayo implied further that because he and his brother were generous and did not force collections, there could be no element of self-interest in their endowment of the Mayo Foundation. He did not attempt to deal with the reasoned arguments of his critics, and asserted that he had no obligation to do so. His quotation, or misquotation, from Lincoln's Gettysburg address was a strongly emotional appeal to his audience, but of uncertain relevance to the question at hand. But mere reason was of little account in the hush of the Minnesota Senate Chamber that evening as Dr. Mayo concluded his speech.

Nevertheless, the defeat of the anti-Mayo affiliation bill probably depended as much on the strong representations made by Dean Ford of the graduate school and Dean Lyon of the medical school. On 26 March, four days after Dr. Mayo's speech, they sent a joint statement to the members of the legislature in which they reviewed the work in graduate medical education carried out during the first two years of the Mayo affiliation and urged that the university should be permitted to continue the educational experiment undertaken for the six years that had been planned.[174] The next day Fred B. Snyder, president of the Board of Regents, again testified before the legislature against the bill and a group of sixty-four prominent citizens of Minneapolis sent a statement to legislators in protest against the bill.[175] By the end of March 1917 it was clear that the bill could not pass the legislature, but its backers planned to introduce an amended bill to prevent the regents from entering into a permanent affiliation without the consent of the legislature.[176] On 5 April the Minnesota House by a large vote refused to consider the anti-Mayo affiliation bill.[177] On 1 May the *Journal-Lancet*, noting that public opinion supported the Mayo affiliation, announced that it had no desire to discuss the affiliation further, and would refuse to publish any more letters or affirmations concerning it.[178]

The entrance of the United States into the First World War on 6 April 1917 also tended to submerge the differences over the Mayo affiliation, and the Doctors Mayo themselves wished to do something to remove the causes of controversy. On 21 June the *St. Paul Daily News* announced that the Mayos were about to propose a new plan of affiliation to the Board of Regents. The Doctors Mayo would transfer the Mayo Foundation endowment immediately from the trustees who then held it to the Board of Regents. They would also propose that the agreement between the university and the Mayo Foundation be for twenty-five years rather than in perpetuity, and that the university be given more latitude to spend the income from the endowment. On 1 July the *Journal-Lancet* commented editorially: "The new plan will be unobjectionable to very many who strenuously opposed the old one. It shows a liberal and generous attitude of the Mayos toward the

State . . . ."[179] The warm editorial response of the *Journal-Lancet* to news of the new plan evidently caused Dr. William Mayo to send an outline of the proposed changes to the editor, Dr. W. A. Jones, who replied on 9 July in a long letter that is historically interesting for its analysis of the reasons for opposition to the Mayo affiliation. Dr. Jones said that the opponents fell into three groups: first, those who had been injured by the reorganization of the medical faculty, for which they held Dr. Mayo responsible, and who considered the reorganization as a step preliminary to the Mayo affiliation; second, a group of physicians, perhaps largely surgeons "whose prejudices against the Mayo Clinic knew no bounds;" and finally those who had conscientious scruples against the affiliation. Dr. Jones thought that most members of the first two groups were willing to forget their grievances " . . . but many in the third class will not change their views, although they may accept a reasonable compromise along the lines now under consideration." He suggested that if the controversy were renewed the third group would dominate the opposition, and that their objection was to an affiliation between the university, as a state institution, and the Mayo Clinic as a private firm, while Dr. Mayo was a regent of the university. Dr. Jones thought that the third group of men would be numerous, and that their contention was right. The law in Minnesota prohibited public boards from having financial dealings with one of their own members, and in any renewed controversy the law might be invoked to annul the affiliation between the university and the Mayo Clinic. Nevertheless, even if the Mayo affiliation were contrary to the law, Dr. Jones thought that its opponents might be persuaded to forego their objections because the Mayo Clinic was capable of giving such aid to medical education as the medical school might never be able to develop by itself. "Therefore," said Jones, "the affiliation finds justification in its own power for good, and ample financial return for any financial benefits to private individuals which may inhere in the proposed relation of such individuals to the State . . . . " Dr. Jones suggested that the legislature might be asked to confirm any revised affiliation agreement entered into by the Board of Regents in order "to remove all conscientious objections to the affiliation . . . ." He concluded:

> . . . I think the fullest faith should be placed in the conscientiousness of most men who have opposed the affiliation, and that their strength should not be minimized. With such an attitude toward them they can be won over to an honest trial of the plan for a period long enough to determine its value; and I do not think serious objection will be raised to the twenty-five year period.[180]

Under the terms of the new plan which the Mayos offered to the Board of Regents in July 1917, the Board of Regents could at the end of twenty-five years decide to spend the income of the Mayo Foundation for graduate medical education or medical research at places other than Rochester, although in order to protect students who might be enrolled in programs at Rochester, the regents would have to give three years' notice of its intention to move graduate medical education from Rochester. The total period that graduate medical education under the foundation must remain at Rochester was, therefore, twenty-eight years, and a decision to move the work from Rochester would require approval by three-quarters of the full membership of the Board of Regents. As before, the endowment income was to be added to the principal until the principal should exceed $2,000,000, when the income could begin to be used for the work of the Mayo Foundation. Meanwhile the Mayos would support the work of the foundation with an annual budget. Twenty percent of the endowment income was to be kept in reserve each year as a contingency fund to support emergency research needs, half for such needs outside the state and half for needs either within or outside the state. The Board of Regents accepted the Mayo proposals, and the new agreements were signed on 17 September 1917.[181]

Even before the outbreak of war on 6 April, both of the Mayo brothers had joined the Army Reserve Corps and during the summer of 1917 they began to go alternately to Washington as advisors to the Surgeon-General. On 1 October, following the new affiliation agreement, the *Journal-Lancet* commented editorially that in view of the war and the service in the war of both William and Charles Mayo ". . . it is well to close the affiliation controversy."[182]

NOTES

1. College of Medicine and Surgery, Executive Faculty, Minutes, 1 March 1913.
2. School of Medicine, Administrative Board, Minutes, 5 March 1914.
3. Among his proposals for a college of surgeons Franklin Martin of Chicago included "a supplementary degree for operating surgeons." Loyal Davis, *Fellowship of surgeons: a history of the American College of Surgeons.* Cf. Rosemary Stevens, *American medicine and the public interest,* pp. 77–92.
4. Davis, *Fellowship of surgeons* (n. 3), pp. 477–479. Amos W. Abbott of Minneapolis and Archibald Maclaren of St. Paul, both of whom were members of the Department of Surgery at Minnesota, were also invited to attend the Washington meeting on 5 May 1913 at which plans for the formation of the college were presented.
5. Ibid., pp. 39–68.
6. Ibid., p. 143.
7. Ibid.
8. Mayo Clinic, Rochester, Minn., *Sketch of the history of the Mayo Clinic and the Mayo Foundation,* p. 144. Cf. Dr. Todd's letter to James E. Moore in School of Medicine, Administrative Board, Minutes, 5 March 1914.
9. School of Medicine, Administrative Board, Minutes, 23 May and 30 July 1914.
10. Ibid. The committee on teaching fellowships recommended that the administrative board create a committee on the graduate school to confer with the graduate school of the university on graduate medical education.
11. The committee was composed of nine members of the administrative board, including Dr. Greene. Ibid., 4 December 1913.
12. "Communication addressed to Dr. Wm. J. Mayo, Regent, by the hospital committee of the Medical School of the University of Minnesota," [1914] Medical School [papers], Miscellaneous Correspondence 1883–1948, pp. 1–2.
13. Ibid., p. 3–4.
14. Ibid., p. 12.

15. Ibid., pp. 18–19.

16. School of Medicine, Administrative Board, Minutes, 30 July 1914.

17. E. P. Lyon, "Medical education and the medical profession," *J.-Lancet,* 1915, *35,* 81–87, p. 84.

18. Ibid.

19. Richard Olding Beard, "The Mayo Clinic building at Rochester," *J.-Lancet,* 1914, *34,* 425–434; Helen Clapesattle, *The Doctors Mayo,* pp. 528–533.

20. Louis B. Wilson, "Graduate instruction in medicine," *St. Paul med. J.* , 1912, *14,* 287–295.

21. "Minutes of a conference between the advisory committee of the Medical Alumni Association and a committee of the administrative board of the Medical School on Saturday, November 14th [1914], at 8 p.m. in the office of President Vincent," Medical School [papers], Affiliation with the Mayo Foundation, 1914. The advisory committee of the Medical Alumni Association consisted of Drs. E. L. Tuohy, Paul D. Cook, Herbert W. James, Harry G. Irvine, J. C. Boehm, and E. R. Hare.

22. Ibid. The conclusions of the conference were also published in Mayo Clinic, *Sketch of the history* (n. 8), p. 145. Cf. Minutes of the second conference between the committee of the Medical School on relations with the Mayo Foundation and the advisory committee of the Medical Alumni Association, Tuesday, 19 January 1915, Medical School [papers], Affiliation with the Mayo Foundation, January - 9 April 1915.

23. "Memoranda of a conference held at Dr. W. J. Mayo's residence, Nov. 19, 1914, of the administrative board of the Mayo Clinic concerning the affiliation of the clinic with the medical department of the state university," Medical School [papers], Affliation with the Mayo Foundation, 1914. Doctors William J. Mayo, Henry S. Plummer, E. Starr Judd, and Louis B. Wilson, and Mr. Harry J. Harwick were present.

24. Ibid.

25. "Memoranda of a conference of the staff of the Mayo Clinic with Dr. R. O. Beard of the faculty of the Medical School of the University of Minnesota held in the Mayo Clinic Building, November 22nd, 1914," ibid.

26. Ibid.

27. Ibid.

28. "Minutes of a conference between the committee of the Medical School and the committee of the Mayo Clinic at Rochester, on November 29th, 1914," ibid. The committee of the Mayo Clinic included Drs. William J. Mayo, Charles H. Mayo, Louis B. Wilson, Henry S. Plummer, E. Starr Judd, and Emil H. Beckman.

29. Ibid.

30. Mayo Clinic, *Sketch of the history* (n. 8), pp. 146–147.

31. School of Medicine, Administrative Board, Minutes, 3 December 1914.

32. Mayo Clinic, *Sketch of the history* (n.8), p. 147.

33. School of Medicine, Administrative Board, Minutes, 14 January 1915.

34. Board of Regents, Supplement to the Minutes for 8 December 1914, p. 62. University of Minnesota, Administrative Services, Central Files.

35. School of Medicine, Administrative Board, Minutes, 14 January 1915.

36. [Minutes of the second conference between the committee of the Medical School on relations with the Mayo Foundation and the advisory committee of the Medical Alumni Association, Tuesday, 19 January 1915. Secretaries: Dr. Richard O. Beard for the Medical School, and Dr. Herbert W. Jones for the Medical Alumni], Medical School [papers], Affiliation with the Mayo Foundation, January - 9 April 1915.

37. [Minutes of the advisory committee of the Medical Alumni Association, 19 January 1915], ibid.

38. School of Medicine, General Faculty, Minutes, 21 January 1915 [Minutes of the general faculty are interfiled with administrative board minutes].
39. School of Medicine, Administrative Board, Minutes, 8 December 1915.
40. "Charles Lyman Greene, general remarks," initialed F.F.W. [esbrook], personnel records, University of Minnesota.
41. Greene to Vaughan, 27 January 1915, Vaughan papers. Dr. Vaughan was to lecture at the university on Saturday morning, 30 January 1915, and speak at a meeting of Michigan medical alumni at the University Club in St. Paul in the evening.
42. Ibid.
43. "The Mayo Foundation proposition," *Minn. Alumni Wkly*, 1915, *14* (no. 20), 1–4, p. 4.
44. Richard Olding Beard et al. [Committee of the Medical School upon the proposed relations of the school with the Mayo Foundation], "The Medical School of the University of Minnesota and the Mayo Foundation for the promotion of medical education and research," *J.-Lancet*, 1915, *35*, 123–141. Charles Lyman Greene, "University-Mayo affiliation," ibid., 142–147. Both statements were published also on 22 March in the *Minnesota Alumni Weekly*, 1915, *14* (no. 25), 8–14.
45. Board of Regents, Supplement to the Minutes for 8 December 1914, p. 62. University of Minnesota, Administrative Services, Central Files.
46. Beard et al. (n. 44) p. 136.
47. Ibid., p. 139.
48. Ibid.
49. Ibid., p. 140.
50. The committee was hinting that opposition to affiliation arose in large part from professional jealousy on the part of physicians. In this respect the committee was less generous than its opponents who, whatever they may have thought privately, did not question the motives of Dr. Mayo or other members of the Mayo Clinic.
51. Ibid., p. 141.
52. Ibid.
53. Greene (n. 44), pp. 142–147.
54. Ibid.
55. Ibid.
56. *Minneapolis Tribune*, 8 February 1915.
57. Greene (n. 44), p. 146.
58. George Douglas Head, "The principles of affiliation," *J.-Lancet*, 1915, *35*, 149–151, p. 150.
59. "Ramsey County Medical Society," *St. Paul med. J.*, 1915, *17*, 209–210. Cf. *St. Paul Pioneer Press*, 23 February 1915.
60. "Editorial. The proposed affiliation between the Mayo Foundation and the Medical Department of the University of Minnesota," *St. Paul med. J.*, 1915, *17*, 212–214.
61. "In regard to the Mayo Foundation affiliation," *Minn. Alumni Wkly*, 1915, *14* (21), 12.
62. "The Mayo Foundation," *Minneapolis Journal*, 1 March 1915.
63. Greene to the Editor of the Dispatch, *St. Paul Dispatch*, 5 March 1915.
64. Dean Lyon said that the statement in the *Minneapolis Tribune* on 8 February "was written by a reporter and never seen by any member of the committee until it appeared in print," but he had apparently not attempted to correct it in the *Minneapolis Tribune* and did not say it was untrue. Elias P. Lyon, "Reply to Dr. Greene," Medical School [papers], Affiliation with the Mayo Foundation, January - 9 April 1915.
65. "Opposition to the Mayo Foundation laid to misinformation by Medical Dean," *St. Paul Dispatch*, 8 March 1915.

66. Ibid.
67. Lyon to the Alumni Executive Committee, 9 March 1915, Medical School [papers], Affiliation with the Mayo Foundation, January—9 April 1915.
68. "Physicians ask regents to reject foundation offer . . . ," *Minneapolis Journal*, 23 March 1915, p. 11.
69. "Alumni action on Mayo Foundation proposal," *Minn. Alumni Wkly*, 1915, *14* (no. 26), 10–11, p. 11.
70. "Alumni directors oppose 'U' gifts with any 'strings'," *Minneapolis Journal*, 29 March 1915.
71. "Physicians urge bill to defeat Mayo proposal," ibid., 4 April 1915.
72. "America's leading medical educators endorse Mayo gift," ibid., The respondents included Lewellys F. Barker, Arthur Dean Bevan, Walter B. Cannon, William T. Councilman, Samuel W. Lambert, John B. Murphy, A. W. Myers, Henry S. Pritchett, and William H. Welch.
73. Lyon to Vaughan, 15 February 1915, Vaughan papers.
74. Vaughan to Lyon, 1 March 1915 [copy], Vaughan Papers.
75. "Medical educators . . . ." *Minneapolis Tribune*, 4 April 1915.
76. Ibid.
77. "The Right of Humanity," ibid., 5 April 1915.
78. "What is the proposition?" ibid., 6 April 1915.
79. "Anti-Mayo bill would cripple Minnesota 'U'," *St. Paul Dispatch*, 6 April 1915.
80. "Do not shackle the board," ibid.
81. "Mayo Foundation debated without definite details of what proposal means," *Minneapolis Journal*, 7 April 1915.
82. Ibid.
83. Mayo Clinic, *Sketch of the history* (n. 8), pp. 17–50.
84. Ibid., p. 66.
85. "An official statement by Dean Lyon on the proposed Mayo gift to the University," *Minneapolis Tribune*, 8 April 1915.
86. "New statement on permanent Mayo merger promised," *Minneapolis Journal*, 9 April 1915.
87. "Beard and Lyon sent to confer with Drs. Mayo," *St. Paul Dispatch*, 9 April 1915.
88. William J. Mayo et al., "To whom it may concern, Rochester, Minn., April 9, 1915," Medical School [papers], Affiliation with the Mayo Foundation, January - April 9, 1915. The document was published in the *Minneapolis Tribune* on 13 April 1915.
89. "Mayo Foundation is already in operation with $1,500,000 fund," *Minneapolis Journal*, 11 April 1915, pp. 1, 3.
90. "Senate Committee approves," *Minn. Alumni Wkly*, 1915, *14* (no. 29), pp. 4–5.
91. "Second public hearing on University bill," ibid., pp. 5–8, p. 5.
92. Ibid., p. 7.
93. Ibid.
94. Lyon to Mayo, 14 April 1915, Medical School [papers], Affiliation with the Mayo Foundation, 11 April 1915 - 13 June 1917.
95. "Statement opposes special privilege to Mayos' school," *Minneapolis Journal*, 15 April 1915; "Medical societies oppose Mayo plan," *Minneapolis Tribune*, 15 April 1915.
96. Ibid.
97. Wilson to Lyon, 16 April 1915, Medical School [papers], Affiliation with the Mayo Foundation, 11 April 1915 - 13 June 1917.
98. Ibid. "Reply to Chas. Lyman Greene."
99. Ibid.
100. Ibid.

101. Ibid.
102. "A message to the legislature," *Minneapolis Tribune,* 19 April 1915.
103. Ibid. See also the editorials: "The right of humanity," *Minneapolis Tribune,* 5 April 1915; "Do not shackle the Board [of Regents]," *St. Paul Dispatch,* 6 April 1915; "Affiliation with the Mayo Foundation a necessity," *St. Paul Pioneer Press,* 6 April 1915; "In a magnificent isolation," ibid., 11 April 1915; "An inexcusable imputation," *Minneapolis Tribune,* 14 April 1915.
104. "Let's have the proposition," *Minneapolis Journal,* 7 April 1915; "Dr. Mayo clears the air," ibid., 9 April 1915; "No call for legislation," ibid., 19 April 1915.
105. "Attorney attacks foundation plan," ibid., 19 April 1915.
106. Ibid.
107. "Senate passes anti-Mayo bill by 5 majority," *St. Paul Pioneer Press,* 21 April 1915.
108. "Regents inspect clinic," *Minneapolis Journal,* 4 May 1915.
109. "Regents' meetings public; Mayo plan is referred," ibid., 6 May 1915, p. 1.
110. "Fight on legality of Mayo compact hinted at hearing," ibid., 15 May 1915, p. 4.
111. "Present status of the proposed University of Minnesota-Mayo Foundation affiliation," *Minn. Alumni Wkly,* 1915, *14* (no. 33), 9–12.
112. Ibid., p. 12.
113. "Mayo proposal as modified is made public," *Minneapolis Journal,* 27 May 1915, pp. 1, 21.
114. "Foundation foe sharply quizzed at Mayo hearing," ibid., 5 June 1915, p. 1.
115. "Mayo plan is unanimously recommended," ibid., 6 June 1915, p. 1.
116. "Mayo Foundation union with the University is opposed while physician remains a Regent," ibid., 8 June 1915, p. 9.
117. Ibid.
118. Ibid.
119. "Regents accept Mayo plan by a unanimous vote," ibid., 9 June 1915, p. 1.
120. Board of Regents, Minutes, 9 June 1915.
121. Those who resigned were Drs. Charles D. Freeman, James S. Gilfallan, Robert A. Hall, George D. Head, Peder A. Hoff, and John E. Hynes. Four, Drs. Gilfallan, Head, Hoff, and Hynes, were in the Department of Medicine. Dr. Freeman was instructor in dermatology and genitourinary diseases, and Dr. Hall was assistant professor of pharmacology.
122. Dean Lyon's letter is quoted in School of Medicine, General Faculty, Minutes, 30 July 1915.
123. Ibid.
124. School of Medicine, Administrative Board, Minutes, 12 July 1915.
125. "Clear resignation action delay at 'U'," *Minneapolis Journal,* 13 July 1915, p. 10.
126. School of Medicine, Administrative Board, Minutes, 28 July 1915.
127. School of Medicine, General Faculty, Minutes, 30 July 1915.
128. George Douglas Head, "The state and medical education," *J.-Lancet,* 1916, *36,* 557–561.
129. School of Medicine, Administrative Board, Minutes, 6 August 1915.
130. Ibid., 13 September 1915.
131. Ibid.
132. Leonard G. Rowntree, *Amid masters of twentieth century medicine*, pp. 185–191.
133. School of Medicine, Administrative Board, Minutes, 3 March 1916.
134. "A new proposition regarding the University Hospital," *Minn. Alumni Wkly,* 1916, *15* (no. 35), pp. 5–6.

135. [Editorial] "Pay patients in public hospitals," *J.-Lancet*, 1916, *36*, 328–329.

136. "A joint discussion on another step in the reorganization of the Medical School of the University of Minnesota," *J.-Lancet*, 1916, *36*, 615–634, p. 617.

137. Ibid., p. 618.

138. Ibid.

139. Ibid., p. 619.

140. Ibid., p. 621.

141. Ibid., p. 623.

142. Ibid., p. 624.

143. Ibid., p. 626.

144. Ibid.

145. Ibid., p. 628.

146. Ibid., p. 629.

147. Ibid. Cf. "Physicians oppose plan," *Minn. Alumni Wkly*, 1915, *16* (no. 2), p. 2.

148. "A joint discussion," (n. 137), pp. 630, 634. Cf. "State Medical Association dissents," *Minn. Alumni Wkly*, 1916, *16* (no. 3), pp. 11–12.

149. Minnesota State Medical Association, "Minutes of the forty-eighth annual meeting, held at Minneapolis, October 11, 12, and 13, 1915," *J.-Lancet*, 1916, *36*, 648–671, pp. 666–671.

150. Herbert W. Jones, "Medical alumni official action," *Minn. Alumni Wkly*, 1916, *16* (no. 6), p. 2.

151. School of Medicine, Administrative Board, Minutes, 2 November 1916.

152. Ibid.

153. Sub-Committee on Hospital Extension, Committee on Hospital and Clinical Development, "The needs and obligations of the Medical School," 13 pp. in ibid., 23 November 1916.

154. Ibid., p. 1.

155. Ibid.

156. Ibid., p. 8.

157. Ibid., pp. 12–13.

158. Charles Lyman Greene, "The present unfortunate situation of the Medical School of the University of Minnesota," *J.-Lancet*, 1917, *37*, 149–157.

159. Ibid., p. 149.

160. Ibid., p. 151.

161. Ibid., pp. 151–152.

162. Ibid.

163. Ibid.

164. Ibid.

165. "Why the Mayo affiliation with the university should be terminated," *J.-Lancet*, 1917, *37*, 198–200. The document was also published in the *Minnesota Alumni Weekly*, 1916–17, *16* (no. 24), 5–7.

166. [Mayo Foundation], "Statement concerning the Mayo Foundation and its affiliation with the Graduate Medical School of the University of Minnesota. March 19, 1917. Personal communication. Not for publication," 10 pp., President's Office, Papers, 1911–1945. The document, although unsigned, is on the letterhead of the Mayo Foundation, and may, therefore, have been written by its director, Louis B. Wilson, or possibly by William Mayo himself.

167. Ibid.

168. [Editorial]. "The Medical School Controversy," *J.-Lancet*, 1917, *37*, 234–236; Elias P. Lyon and R. O. Beard, "A reply from the Medical School of the University of Minnesota," ibid., p. 237.

169. School of Medicine, Administrative Board, Minutes, 13 March, 16 March, 19 March 1917, General Faculty, Minutes, 19 March 1917.

170. [Administrative Board and General Faculty], "A reply to charges against the Medical School of the University of Minnesota," *J.-Lancet,* 1917, *37,* 237–239.

171. William J. Mayo and Charles H. Mayo to Honorable F. B. Snyder, President of the Board of Regents in "Official statements University of Minnesota," *J.-Lancet,* 1917, *37,* 239–240. Cf. "The Mayo Foundation," *Minn. Alumni Wkly,* 1916–17, *26* (no. 25), 7–8.

172. "Hearing on the Mayo bill," *Minn. Alumni Wkly,* 1916–17, *16* (no. 25), 1–2.

173. "Mayos offer to give the University $1,500,000 fund. Senate committee considers proposal of sole control by regents. Representatives of profession oppose linking education with private concern," *Minneapolis Journal,* 23 March 1917, p. 1.

174. "Mayo affiliation brings wide fame to University say two school's deans," ibid., 26 March 1917, p. 6.

175. "Anti-Mayo bill's defeat predicted by legislators," ibid., 27 March 1917, p. 3.

176. "Mayo bill friends forecast its doom," ibid., 30 March 1917, p. 1.

177. "Anti-Mayo bill is believed killed," ibid., 5 April 1917, p. 15.

178. [Editorial] "The anti-affiliation bill," *J.-Lancet,* 1917, *37,* 313.

179. [Editorial], "A new Mayo plan," ibid., p. 449.

180. Jones to Mayo, 9 July 1917, copy to Burton in President's Office, Papers, 1911–1945.

181. "The Mayo proposition accepted," *Minn. Alumni Wkly,* 1917–18, *17* (no. 2), 5–8.

182. [Editorial], "The Mayo affiliation," *J.-Lancet,* 1917, *37,* 647–648, p. 647.

CHAPTER 10

The Medical School in the First World War 1917–1919

In October 1915, eighteen months before the entrance of the United States into the First World War, but when its eventual involvement was foreseen as probable, Surgeon-General William C. Gorgas asked Dr. William J. Mayo to organize a base hospital. In the late summer of 1914, during the early weeks of the war, a group of Americans living at Paris had organized a "Section for the Wounded" in the Lycée Pasteur. This hospital became attached to the French *Service de Santé* and later to the United States Army as Red Cross Military Hospital No. 1. It cared for wounded soldiers from the first battle of the Marne until the end of the war.

During the first battle of the Marne, various Americans living at Paris carried wounded soldiers in their automobiles from the battlefield to the American hospital at the Lycée Pasteur. From such individual efforts two volunteer corps of American ambulance drivers developed: the *Ambulance Américaine* at Neuilly-sur-Seine and the *Formation Harjes,* also known as *Section Sanitaire No. 5.* Several hundred young Americans volunteered to serve in these two organizations, driving small Ford ambulances contributed by their countrymen at home.

On 27 November 1914, on behalf of the Medical Board of the Ambulance, Dr. Joseph A. Blake suggested to certain American medical schools that each of them should send over a corps of surgeons and nurses to work in the American Hospital at Paris for a three-month period. The first such unit, organized by Dr. George Crile from the Lakeside Hospital of Western Reserve University at Cleveland, Ohio, served from January to April 1915, and was succeeded by similar units from Harvard University and then from the University of Pennsylvania.

In the summer of 1915, James E. Moore considered the possibility of organizing a University of Minnesota unit to become responsible for the university section of the American Ambulance for a three-month period in 1916, and he wrote to George Crile to learn the arrangements needed for such a unit and the costs involved.[1] From Boston Harvey Cushing wrote that the three university units that had gone to France had each paid their own expenses with funds raised from local donors.[2] Dr. Moore was evidently unable in 1915 to raise sufficient funds to send a privately sponsored unit from Minnesota.

Such volunteer hospital units proved particularly effective because the doctors and nurses came from the staff of a single hospital in the United States, knew each other, and were accustomed to work together. In October 1915 Dr. Crile pointed out that a similar plan of organization might be used for base hospitals organized by the United States Army Medical Reserve Corps to be ready for use in case of war.[3] Surgeon General Gorgas authorized three members of the Army Medical Reserve Corps, Dr. George W. Crile of Cleveland, Dr. Harvey Cushing of Boston, and Dr. J. M. Swan of Rochester, New York, to organize base hospitals. The surgeon general's action brought an immediate protest from the American Red Cross, which by its charter was responsible for the organization of volunteer medical assistance to the armed forces in time of war.

In December 1915 the American Red Cross separated its work into two departments, civil and military relief, and placed a United States Army medical officer, Colonel Jefferson R. Kean, in charge of the Department of Military Relief. The surgeon general and the Red Cross then decided that the Red Cross should organize the base hospitals, but that they should be organized on a military basis. The personnel of a base hospital were to be officers and enlisted men in the United States Army Reserve Corps, so that when called into active service the base hospital staff would become completely part of the army. In February 1916 Colonel Kean began to visit leading physicians at hospitals or medical schools in various cities to ask them each to organize a base hospital.[4] In October 1916 Colonel Kean asked William J. Mayo to organize such a base hospital for Minnesota.

Dr. Mayo thought that a base hospital was properly a project for the University of Minnesota Medical School and should be organized under its auspices. He offered to collaborate with the university and to provide from the Mayo Clinic half of the medical and surgical staff and as many enlisted men and nurses as might be required. The university accepted Dr. Mayo's offer and Arthur A. Law, associate professor of surgery, who had served as a medical officer with the United States Army in the Philippines during the Spanish-American War and the Philippine insurrection, was appointed director of the proposed hospital, which was designated Base Hospital No. 26.

In 1916, in anticipation of war, the United States War Department was feverishly buying supplies and equipment for an expanded army and navy. Because of the urgency to equip the fighting forces, it possessed neither funds, nor time, nor attention to devote to the purchase of equipment and supplies for base hospitals to meet possible future needs. Nevertheless, in 1914 Americans had witnessed the pitiful consequences of medical unpreparedness during the first Battle of the Marne. The American Red Cross, therefore, resolved to raise from private gifts the funds needed to buy the beds and bedding, the medical and surgical supplies, and all other items of equipment needed for each of the proposed 500-bed base hospitals.

During the winter of 1916–17 the university made little progress with its plans for a base hospital. In December 1916, Dean Lyon and Dr. Law attended a conference of American medical schools in the office of the secretary of war at Washington and in March 1917 the school decided to offer lectures on military medicine.[5] During March the medical school was preoccupied with the renewed controversy over the Mayo affiliation and with the charges that the school was demoralized and deteriorating, but on 31 March, with war imminent, the university announced that it would organize a 500-bed base hospital, the equipment for which would cost $30,000. The Doctors Mayo had given $15,000 and a group of Minneapolis citizens had undertaken to raise the other $15,000.[6] On 1 April Surgeon General Gorgas asked the university to begin to organize Base Hospital No. 26, and with the declaration of war by the United States on 6 April the organization of the hospital became urgent.

The next day, 7 April, Dr. Law reported to the administrative board that funds for the base hospital had been secured. Eleven of the staff would be from the Mayo Clinic while the remainder would be from the medical school. Base Hospital No. 26 would be one of forty base hospitals that had been pledged. Together they would be capable of caring for the medical and surgical needs of 600,000 men. The administrative board decided that junior and senior medical students who volunteered to serve in the university base hospital should be given time credit for their period of service. In view of the probable urgent need for trained medical men in the army and navy the administrative board decided to stand ready to keep the school operating continuously through the summers of 1917 and 1918. They decided to ask the surgeon general whether medical students in the junior and senior classes should be encouraged to enlist or to continue in medical study, and what special courses might be offered to graduate students to fit them for army or navy medical service.[7] The surgeon general advised against the enlistment of medical students who had not completed their undergraduate work, but the administrative board decided that junior and senior students should still be permitted to go with the base hospital. Students would receive medical instruction in the base hospital and time credits for their period of service. If they passed the final examinations, students would also receive subject credits for their work in the base hospital. Dean Lyon appointed a committee of three to be responsible for the clinical and military training of junior students who enlisted. In May twenty students who were completing their junior year decided to enlist in Base Hospital No. 26. On the last day of the term the class gave a banquet for its enlisted members at the West Hotel in Minneapolis. At the end of the evening, after toasts and songs, the enlisted students passed in line before their classmates and solemnly shook their hands.[8]

When the fund of $30,000 for the base hospital was raised in mid-April, the Red Cross donated an additional $10,000 worth of surgical supplies. Dr. Louis Baldwin, superintendent of the university hospital, volunteered to serve as purchasing agent, and acted with such efficiency that, despite the confusion of wartime, the equipment of the hospital was completely assembled on 10 July. The

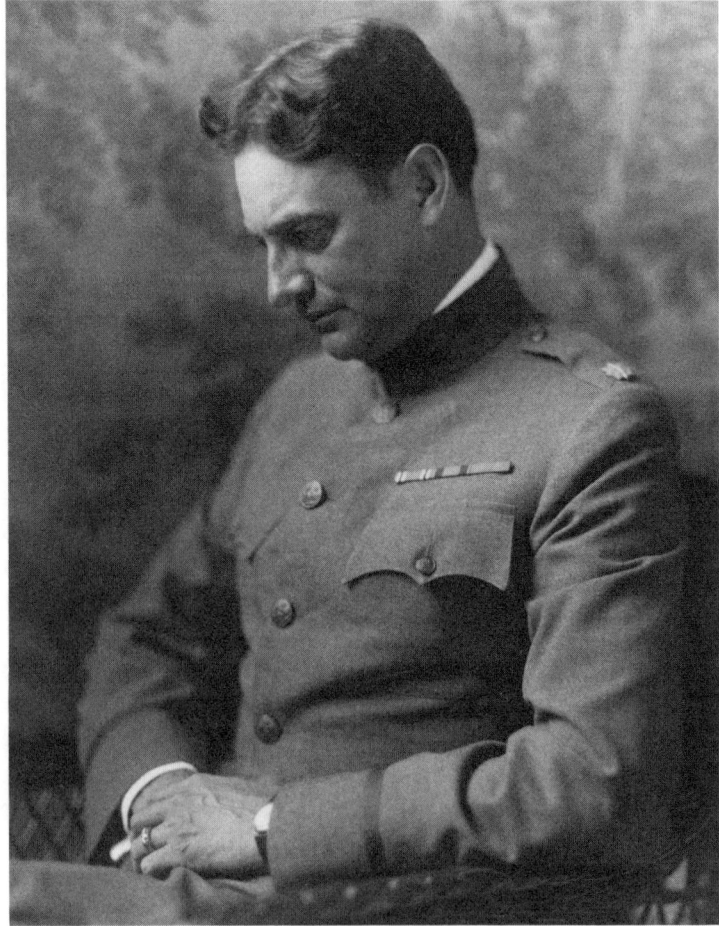

FIGURE 10:1   Major Arthur A. Law. Courtesy Mn U Archives.

hospital continued to receive additional gifts. Mrs. Edmund Pennington of Minneapolis, together with the Office Men's Club, organized a patriotic baseball game which raised $3,600 for a contingency fund. Major Law used the fund to purchase specialized instruments and scientific apparatus which, although not required by the government, were desired by the medical and surgical staff to increase their effectiveness. Mrs. Charles Pillsbury of Minneapolis gave the hospital her Packard touring car, the Minikahda Club gave a Ford touring car, and Mr. C. C. Bovey a motorcycle with side car. Other Minneapolis citizens donated two complete army motor ambulances.[9]

The recruitment of the hospital staff was completed by 1 July. Major Law was to be chief surgeon as well as director of the hospital. S. Marx White, professor of medicine, was commissioned, also with the rank of major, as chief of medicine

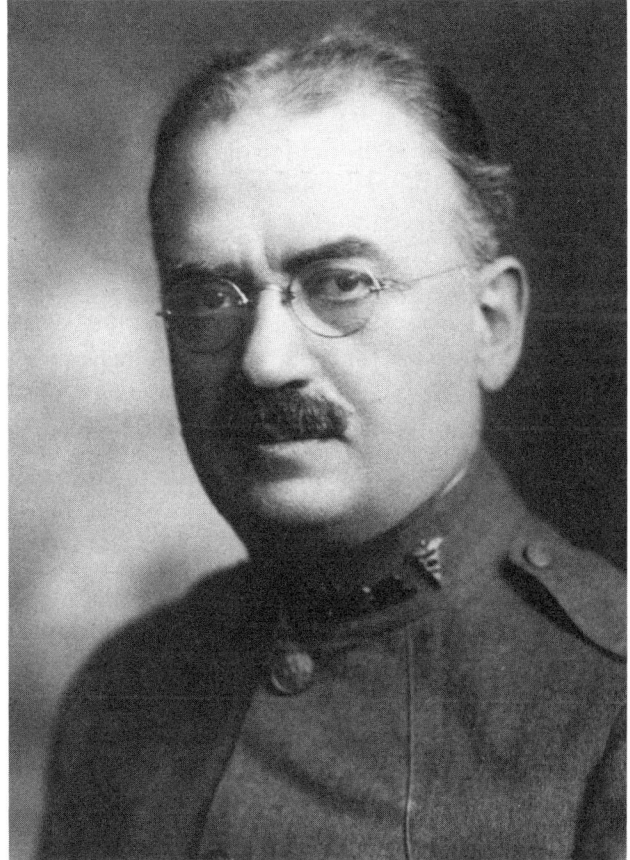

FIGURE 10:2   Major S. Marx White. Courtesy Mn U Archives.

for the hospital. Fourteen officers of the staff were from the University of Minnesota and eight were from the Mayo Clinic. The 153 enlisted personnel, chosen from 1,500 applicants, included trained wireless operators, telegraphers, engineers of various kinds, carpenters, machinists, constructors of x-ray apparatus, telephone constructors, plumbers, undertakers, plasterers, ambulance drivers, pharmacists, male nurses, tailors, barbers, stenographers, and clerks. With such an array of skills, Base Hospital No. 26 was prepared to create the facilities of a modern hospital in almost any circumstances in which they might be placed. By 10 July 1917 the hospital was fully equipped, recruited, and ready for duty, but the War Department was not yet ready to use it. Months of tedious waiting followed.

The chaplain to the base hospital was the Right Reverend W. P. Remington, who had recently been appointed bishop of South Dakota in the Episcopal church. On Sunday, 9 December, Major Law asked all members of the hospital staff to attend a drumhead service conducted by Bishop Remington in St. Paul's

Episcopal Church, Minneapolis. As the choir sang "Soldiers of Christ, Arise" the staff and enlisted men marched to the pews reserved for them in front of the church. In his sermon Bishop Remington compared the position of the United States in the war to that of David going forth to meet the heavily armed Goliath, but he spoke not of warfare, but of the need to deal with the devastation of war — to do everything that could be done to mitigate its horrors. To the men of Base Hospital No. 26 he said: " . . . It is not a playday jaunt we are going on, for, though we are not going to the firing line, we are enlisting for a service which requires high courage, untiring energy and unbounded cheerfulness. Ministering to wounded men is no easy task."[10] The next day, the War Department telegraphed Major Law to mobilize the hospital, and mobilization was completed by 15 December.

During the fall of 1917, the senior medical students who had enlisted in the base hospital continued to pursue the normal work of the senior year in the medical school. Shortly before the mobilization order came, the senior class had requested that any student who at the end of the year applied for a commission in the army, navy, or Medical Reserve Corps should be awarded the M.D. degree as soon as the government accepted him for service, without waiting for the year of internship then required at Minnesota for the M.D. degree. In reply the administrative board urged the students, so long as there was no immediate call to service, either to perform their year of internship or to serve in the base hospital.[11] The board thought that service in the base hospital would be valuable as practical medical experience. After the mobilization order was received, they appointed a committee of three of the hospital staff who were also members of the medical faculty, Major Arthur Law, Major S. Marx White, and Captain Moses Barron, to conduct the educational work of the base hospital on behalf of the medical school. Major Law was to teach surgery and the surgical specialties, Major White medicine, and Captain Barron laboratory work.[12]

When Base Hospital No. 26 was mobilized in December 1917 its complement of 185 men was quartered at the university. The large laboratories in Millard Hall and the auditorium in the Main Engineering building were cleared out to serve as barracks for the men. They were fed at the Men's Union. The men were issued uniforms, blankets, and cots, and came under military discipline.[13] All the equipment for the hospital was assembled and ready to go. The period of waiting at the university was fortunately brief. On 26 December the hospital staff boarded the train for Fort McPherson near Atlanta, Georgia.[14]

At Fort McPherson the hospital came under the military command of Colonel Joseph H. Ford, while Major Law served as director of the hospital. On 30 March 1918 Unit "V" from Baylor University at Dallas, Texas, under the command of Major Mark E. Lott was attached to Base Hospital No. 26, thereby approximately doubling the size of the hospital unit to make it sufficient for a 1,000-bed hospital. Thenceforward Base Hospital No. 26 was a composite Minnesota-Texas unit with the colorful contrasts and strengths inherent in that diversity. At Fort McPherson both officers and men began basic military training. The senior medi-

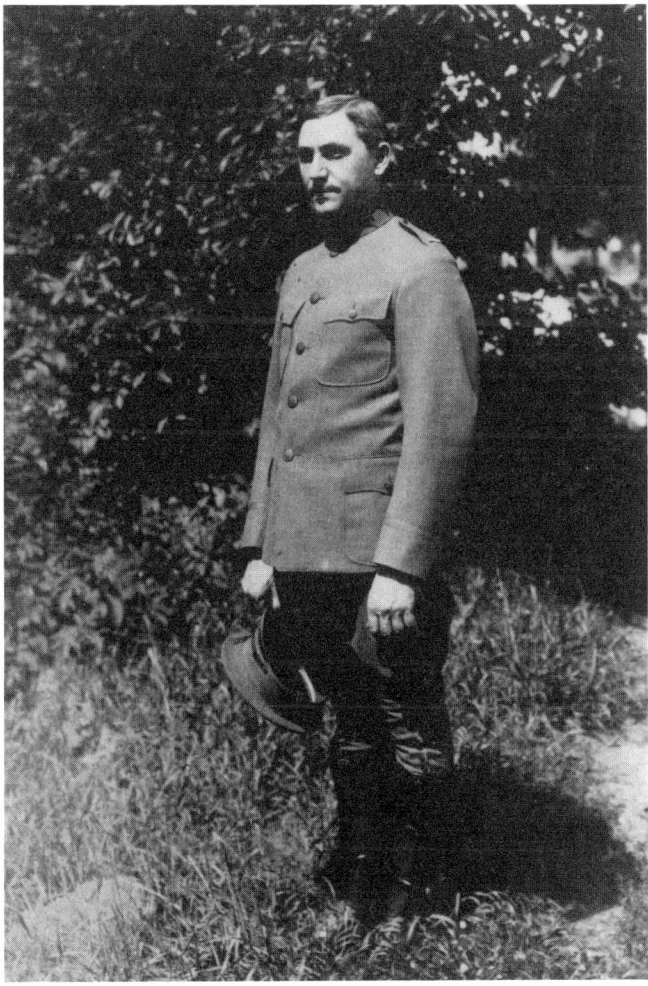

FIGURE 10:3   Captain Moses Barron. Courtesy Dr. Jesse Barron.

cal students, now reduced to thirteen in number, were given charge of the infirmary. They also went daily to the officers' quarters for medical lectures from their former professors. Captain Zimmerman taught surgery. Major White and Captains Beard, Mussey, and Barron lectured on obstetrics and gynecology. Major Law entertained them with reminiscences of the Philippines. In March 1918 the father of one of the hospital enlisted men reported that Base Hospital No. 26 was a crack unit. He spoke highly of the officers and men. He had watched them go through the manual of arms, put up their shelter tents, and go through first aid procedures. He had also observed them "in the study and lecture room where they work many hours daily."[15] In late March Major Law wrote that he and his fellow teachers " . . . have worked much harder down here on the lectures than we ever did at

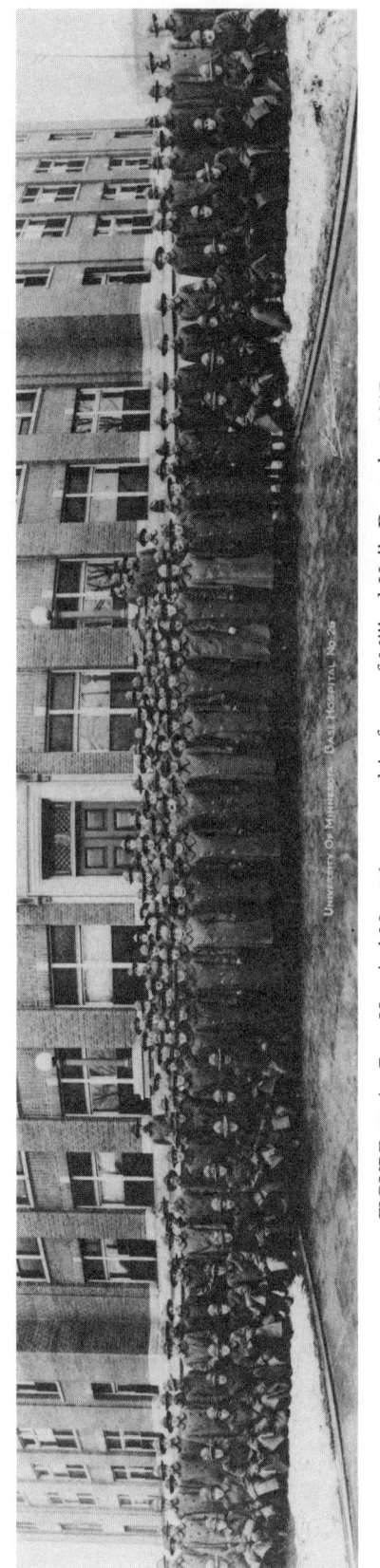

FIGURE 10:4 Base Hospital No. 26 mustered in front of Millard Hall, December 1917. Courtesy Dr. Jesse Barron.

home . . . ."[16] In May 1918, Dr. Beard, assistant dean of the medical school, wrote to Major Law and other members of the medical faculty to remind them that in a week's time they would need to submit grades for the senior medical students, a necessity that they seem to have forgotten. Suddenly that meant examinations. The faculty gave the students three days to prepare, and during those three days the students studied their notes all day under the pines back of the camp and through most of the nights in the mess hall. Finally they took the examinations and passed them satisfactorily. On 17 May Major Law and his colleagues put the grades in the mail to go to Minneapolis.[17] The only requirement remaining for their medical degree was an adequate internship.[18]

Two days later, the personnel of Base Hospital No. 26, now consisting of 36 officers and 207 enlisted men, boarded a train at Fort McPherson to travel north to Camp Merritt, New Jersey. On 5 June the officers and men sailed from Hoboken aboard the *Adriatic*. The same day a corps of one hundred nurses sailed from New York on the *Baltic*, which joined the same convoy as the *Adriatic*. With them were six militarized civilian women, including a dietitian, a laboratory technician, and four secretaries.

On 16 June the officers and men of Base Hospital No. 26 disembarked at Liverpool on a beautiful summer day to travel southward across England by train, arriving at Southampton in the evening. After twenty-four hours in a rest camp they boarded a small steamboat to cross the channel, landing at Le Havre on 18 June. Late that night they boarded a train which took them to Allerey, a village of some 800 people, about eleven miles north of the town of Chalons-sur-Saone on the line of the Paris, Lyon, and Mediterranean Railroad.

At Allerey, located behind the central section of the front, the American Expeditionary Force planned to create a great hospital center that would ultimately contain ten base hospitals. Base Hospital No. 26 was the first to arrive at Allerey, preceded only by the engineers who had come about two weeks before to lay out roads and drains and to begin to erect the long, low, prefabricated wooden buildings that were to house the hospitals. When the train backed into the railway spur running down the middle of the Allerey Hospital Center that June evening, the Minnesotans and Texans found themselves looking at rows of wooden huts spread across broad, low muddy fields.

The men of Base Hospital No. 26 came to Allerey just before supper time, and because they had been living almost entirely on travel rations supplemented by hot coffee at railway stations during the five days since they had landed at Liverpool, supper was very much on their minds. The mess departments found the mess hall partly finished, a kitchen with one stove half set up, a few cooking utensils, and no food. The cooks quickly finished setting up the stove, got a fire going, and brought up the remainder of their travel rations from the train. The engineers lent them flour, bacon, and potatoes. Supper that evening at Allerey was not a feast, but it was the first hot meal that Base Hospital No. 26 had had for several days. Next morning for their first breakfast in camp they had coffee, fried bacon, griddlecakes and syrup, which tasted very good to them.

At Allerey the engineers had laid out ten sections, each section to contain a base hospital arranged in two rows of five sections each on either side of a broad central roadway with the railway spur passing down its middle. Other branch roads led around and between the wooden huts of each section. Each base hospital was built to accommodate a thousand patients but had to be prepared to house an additional thousand in tents, if needed in a crisis. The prefabricated wooden buildings were set on weak foundations that tended to settle, and as the buildings settled cracks appeared in their walls.

A base hospital was a unit complete in itself, intended to be housed in fifty-five buildings. When Base Hospital No. 26 arrived at Allerey only forty of the fifty-five buildings needed had been put up, and the buildings erected were completely unfurnished. The carpenters, electricians and other artificers went immediately to work. First, for the kitchens they set up stoves and constructed serving tables, mess tables, benches, and so forth. They made a serviceable sink from an old packing case lined with tin obtained by pounding out bacon cans and soldering them together. In the nurses' and officers' quarters they moved partitions to accommodate two persons to a room. For the administration building they constructed desks, files, chairs, and tables. During the first month they had only hammers and saws and a few antiquated French tools of little use, but then they received a whole kit of tools donated by the Morrison Company of Minneapolis and began to produce much finer furniture. For Captain Moses Barron they made a post-mortem table, built according to his own plans, which Captain Barron declared to be the best post-mortem table in the world. For Colonel Ford, who became commander of the whole Allerey Center, they made office furniture that the colonel said was the best piece of camp-constructed furniture he had ever seen.[19]

Initially water was obtained from wells in the village of Allerey, but as time permitted the center created a system of piped running water supplied from wells dug on the site. For a long time the men had to remove liquid wastes in barrels or in a tank wagon, but eventually they build a sewage system to dispose of it. Feces and urine were at first carried off in pails and buried in pits. Later the solids were burned and the liquids poured into the sewers. Electricity was generated by small 25 kilowatt generating plants, which proved inadequate. At night there was often not enough power to illuminate the receiving stations, wards, and operating rooms, and to supply the x-ray equipment. Despite the risk of fire, they were forced frequently to use kerosene lanterns.

At the beginning of July, Captain Moses Barron set up the hospital laboratory. For equipment he requisitioned a portable field laboratory, and the artificers made for him a microscope warming stage from a metal cigarette box, the post-mortem table aforementioned, and a water still from biscuit tins. When the laboratory was set up, the staff began to make media and to sterilize bandages. The still supplied distilled water to the operating room and the dispensary. The laboratory was immediately important because when the surgeons arrived at Allerey on 20 June they found no equipment for the operating room and no medical supply depot from which to obtain it. After hurried trips to surrounding towns, they assembled a few of the more essential items of equipment, including two small autoclaves, and began to make sterilized dressings in order to have a supply on hand when the wounded would begin to arrive. The autoclaves had been working night and day for forty-eight hours and the surgeons were proud of the growing supply of dressings when Captain Barron said he thought it would be a good idea to examine the dressings for sterility. A day or two later he reported that the dressings were not sterile. They had to be resterilized, but in different autoclaves. Until their own sterilizing equipment arrived, the surgeons sent dressings by truck to Dijon where they were sterilized at Base Hospital No. 17.

On 20 July, Major White, then in command of Base Hospital No. 26 in the absence of Major Law, who was at the front with a surgical team, received a telegram to announce the impending arrival of a large convoy of sick and wounded men from the front. At this point the contingency fund raised by the Minneapolis ladies assumed critical importance. Major White was faced with an immediate crisis because all of the equipment for Base Hospital No. 26, so generously donated and carefully assembled at Minneapolis the year before, had still not arrived from the United States. "All we had," recalled Dr. White, "were the barracks which would house two thousand beds. We had the beds, mattresses, pillows, blankets, and that was all . . . . Some surgical instruments had been secured but there was very little with which to work . . . ."[20] He sent Captain Moses Barron to Is-sur-Tille with two trucks borrowed from the engineers to bring back medical supplies and surgical dressings, and 2,000 francs from the contingency fund. Captain Barron persuaded the commanding officer of the depot at Is-sur-Tille to provide three truck loads of supplies. He borrowed the third truck needed to transport them from the motor transport officer at Is-sur-Tille and returned to camp that night, reaching Allerey at 1:30 a.m. The equipment thus obtained included three army operating room tables, two army sterilizers, one single burner kerosene stove, and an assortment of operating room equipment. Major White also sent Captain Gilbert J. Thomas and Lieutenant Thaddeus L. Szlapka to Lyon, Dijon, and other cities for drugs, surgical dressings, and other equipment to supplement the supplies obtained by Captain Barron at Is-sur-Tille. They obtained several bolts of gauze, a few pounds of compressed cotton, six dozen surgical skin needles, and about three dozen tubes of silkworm-gut and catgut at a cost of about $5,000, paid out of the contingent fund of the hospital. In response to urgent telegrams, the Red Cross at Paris sent boxes of gauze supplies to Allerey, and Captain Thomas took the gauze to Dijon to be sterilized at Base Hospital No. 17. As a result said Major White, " . . . no man who came to the unit lost his life because of any essential thing."[21]

At three o'clock in the afternoon of 23 July 1918, the first train bearing wounded men from the Chateau Thierry region pulled into the Allerey Hospital Center. Among the 398 patients on board, 327 were surgical patients. Most of them had already been operated on at evacuation hospitals near the front, so that only twelve needed primary operations. In the operating room the instruments

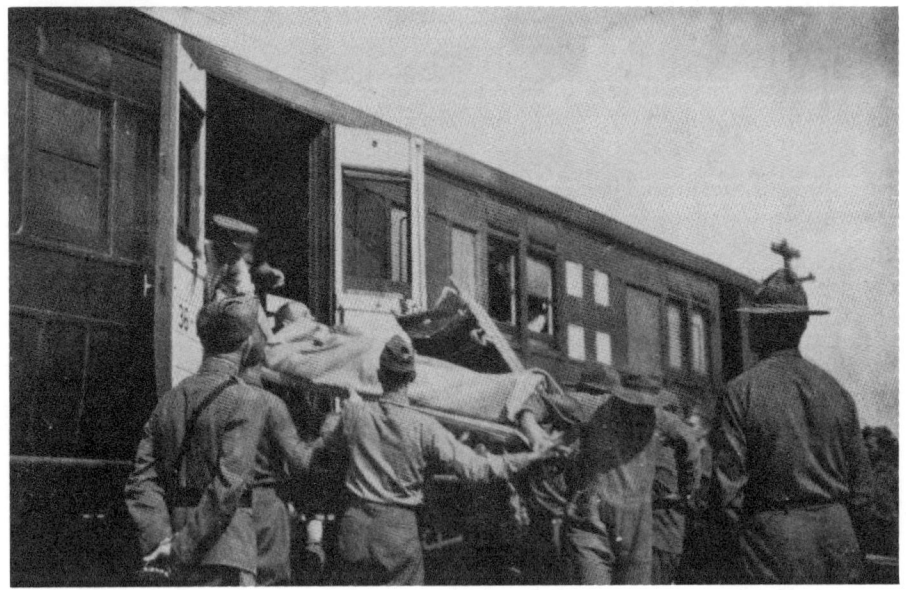

FIGURE 10:5   Unloading the wounded at Allerey. *History of Base Hospital No. 26.*

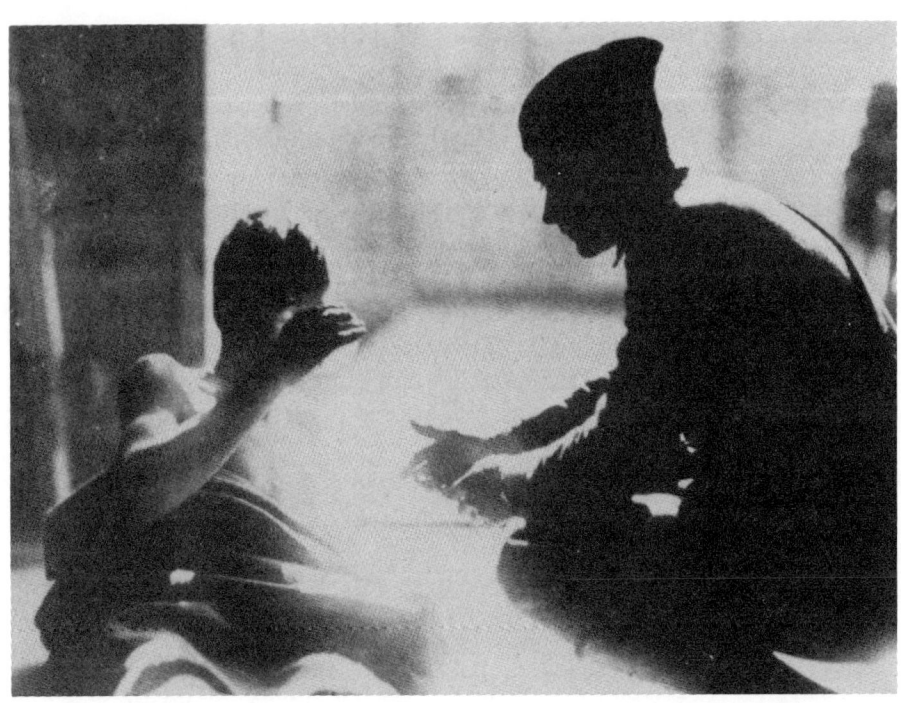

FIGURE 10:6   The Bishop at work. *History of Base Hospital No. 26.*

and gloves were suspended in socks and boiled in a five-gallon, enameled covered kettle on the one-burner kerosene stove.

On 30 July the second convoy of patients arrived from evacuation hospitals where relatively few had been operated on. During the next twenty-four hours at Base Hospital No. 26, two surgical teams, using four operating room tables, debrided the wounds of seventy-five patients. In the operating room as patients went under anesthesia they frequently reenacted the charge over the top that had led to their being wounded.

After 30 July hospital trains arrived steadily, usually arriving at night, and often three in one night. The Red Cross women were always on hand to serve hot coffee and chocolate to the wounded. Most patients who came to Allerey had already been debrided in the forward hospital so that few debridements were needed. Both then and later, Base Hospital No. 26 received very few patients with gas gangrene and only one with tetanus, who was treated successfully with tetanus antitoxin. When wounds were subjected to proper debridement, the surgeons encountered little trouble with pyogenic infection. Again the laboratory proved useful to the surgeons because they became accustomed to make bacterial cultures from open wounds before attempting to close them. If the bacterial count were not more than one in ten fields, the wound was closed, but if a hemolytic streptococcus proved to be present, the wound was kept open until the organism had disappeared. Although the results of bacteriological tests usually corresponded closely to the clinical appearance of a wound, in patients in whom the wounds showed clinical evidence of streptococcal infection, the surgeons learned to leave the wound open even though the results of bacteriological examination were negative. They irrigated severely infected wounds with Carrel-Dakin solution, a buffered solution of sodium hypochlorite recommended by Alexis Carrel and Henry Dakin for the antiseptic treatment of wounds.

Early in August 1918, Base Hospital No. 26 received large convoys of wounded until the hospital contained more than 1,350 patients. At one point Major Law uttered words that remained forever imprinted on the memories of everyone at Base Hospital No. 26. "We'll take a thousand today, a thousand tomorrow, and a thousand the next day; we can't do it, but by God we will." And they did. In such crisis conditions they accommodated the lightly wounded men and convalescents in large tents erected behind the ward buildings. By mid-September the number of patients had dropped to about 300, but then convoys of wounded began to pour in as a result of the large-scale American offensive and by mid-October Base Hospital No. 26 contained almost 1,900 patients. On 7 October Major Law wrote to his chief at Minneapolis, Dr. Moore, describing the conditions under which they worked:

> . . . As I was operating this afternoon and Miss Larson put on my accustomed mask and gown, my mind harked back to the amphitheatre of the University, and we spoke of you and wondered what you would think of this big operating room, with its numerous tables, its crudities, yet its efficiency; its compo-board partitions, yet its radiators and steam heat; its beautiful instruments in crude cases . . . . This operating room

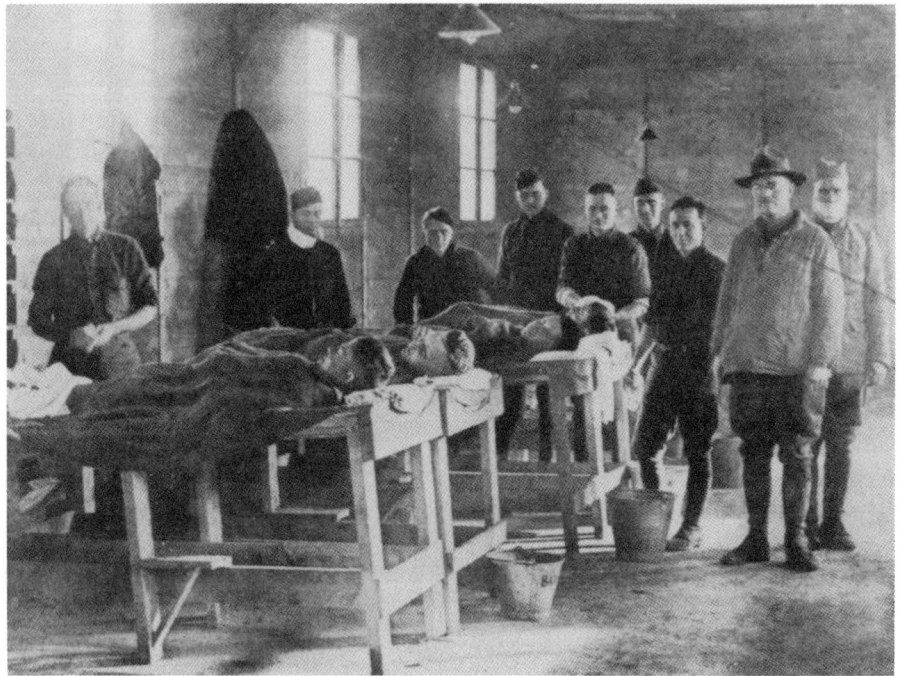

FIGURE 10:7 Bathing the wounded. *History of Base Hospital No. 26.*

has been brought to the "nth" degree of efficiency, yet with all non-essentials eliminated. It is the same throughout this colossal hospital. We have the essentials, but have sloughed the non-essentials. When you think . . . that the complete hospital has ten times as many patients as yours on the campus, you may marvel that thirty professional men and one hundred nurses can administer so huge a hospital. That they do it, and that our results are as fine as any I have ever seen, is an expression of what men and women can do when they must.[22]

On 21 October they were caring for 1,191 surgical patients. From the arrival of the first convoy of patients on 23 July until Base Hospital No. 26 closed in January 1919, the surgical service performed 1,021 operations including 660 secondary closures, 178 debridements, and 84 removals of foreign bodies, as well as various special operations. Apart from the treatment of war wounds they performed twenty-two appendectomies, removed one gallbladder, and repaired forty-four hernias. Throughout the great stress of surgical work the thirteen senior medical students from Minnesota worked as assistants to the ward surgeons, giving invaluable help — surely an adequate internship!

On 15 July 1918 Base Hospital No. 25 from the Cincinnati Medical College arrived at Allerey to become the second base hospital at the center. It was followed by five base hospitals in succession:

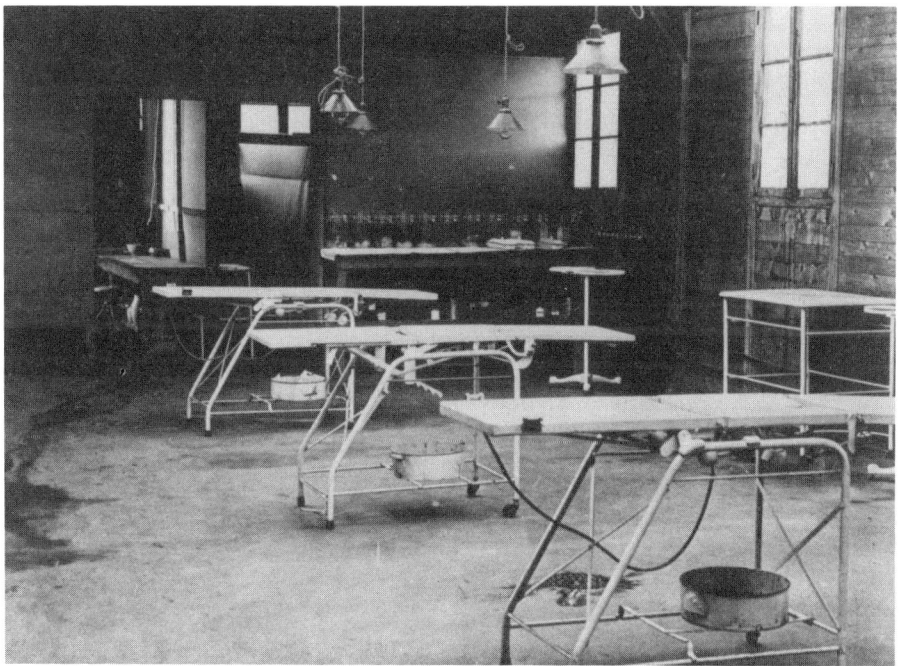

FIGURE 10:8   Operating room, Base Hospital No. 26. Courtesy Dr. Jesse Barron.

5 August—Base Hospital No. 49, University of Nebraska;

19 September—Evacuation Hospital No. 19, Fort Riley, Kansas;

28 September—Base Hospital No. 70, Fort Riley, Kansas;

30 September—Base Hospital No. 56, Fort Oglethorpe, Georgia;

30 November— Base Hospital No. 97, El Paso, Texas.

Three days after Base Hospital No. 26 arrived at Allerey on 20 June 1918, its commanding officer, Colonel Joseph Ford, was appointed commanding officer of the whole Allerey Hospital Center, and Major Arthur Law became the hospital commander. As commander of the Allerey Center, Colonel Ford needed quickly to develop a headquarters staff so he took with him several officers from Base Hospital 26. During the first few weeks, when Base Hospital No. 26 was the only hospital at the Allerey complex, such officers did double duty in the hospital and the headquarters. On 28 July Captain Moses Barron was detached as laboratory officer of Base Hospital No. 26 to become laboratory officer for the center, but until Captain Barron could establish a central laboratory the laboratory at Base Hospital No. 26 served the whole camp. On 28 August, when Base Hospital No. 26 finally received its equipment from Minneapolis, it possessed an abundance of both equipment and chemical supplies and was able to contribute a considerable amount of apparatus and stains to Captain Barron's central laboratory.

In the autumn of 1918 the weather in France became rainy and almost constantly cloudy. During the latter half of September, when fighting on the American front became intensified, in addition to the flood of wounded soldiers that poured into Allerey, numbers of men began to be sent back from the evacuation hospitals as suffering from influenza. Sometimes three to five hospital trains came into the Allerey Center daily. Frequently on arrival in one of the base hospitals at Allerey, they were found to have pneumonia. During this period Base Hospital No. 26 received many very ill soldiers and a very large proportion of those most severely wounded.[23] Because practically all of the sick or wounded German prisoners sent to Allerey were admitted to Base Hospital No. 26, the hospital received 222 German prisoners of whom 90 percent were surgical patients. One of the senior medics, Harold Diehl, recalled his impressions of the first wounded Austrian soldiers he saw. "Our propagandists had painted such realistic pictures of the monsters in enemy uniforms," said Dr. Diehl, "that it was quite a surprise to find that these wounded prisoners were just immature and homesick boys who didn't know what it was all about and were glad to be out of it."[24] Six of the prisoners died, including an Austrian colonel. On 24 September 1918, the first case of diphtheria at Allerey occurred in Base Hospital No. 26. On 1 October two more cases appeared, followed by one on 5 October, one on 8 October, and three on 9 October. Cases of diphtheria appeared most frequently in the pneumonia ward where there were many patients who had been gassed. With the appearance of diphtheria, the wards containing diphtheria patients were quarantined and throat cultures began to be taken routinely from both patients and attendants in order to detect carriers. Diphtheria continued to appear within the ward and, despite the quarantine, carriers of diphtheria were discovered in two tents connected with the ward. Nevertheless, the quarantine was effective on the whole because other tents, kept isolated from the diphtheria ward, remained uninfected.[25] The crowded state of the wards, containing seventy beds although designed for only fifty, favored the spread of diphtheria.

To control the epidemic Moses Barron adopted a modification of the measures taken by Frank Wesbrook in 1911 to control the diphtheria epidemic in the Elliot Hospital at the University of Minnesota. As the sole intern at the Elliot Hospital in 1911, Moses Barron had himself contracted diphtheria so that he had personal experience of the kind of measures required. When it became clear that there was a diphtheria epidemic at Allerey, Base Hospital No. 56 became an isolation hospital and all clinical and carrier cases of diphtheria were moved there and subjected to strict isolation. In order to diagnose cases of diphtheria early, throat cultures were taken frequently, especially from patients who had been gassed. The effects of gassing were very similar to those of diphtheria because a severely gassed patient often developed a fibrino-purulent membrane over the lining of the larynx and trachea from the epiglottis down into the bronchi and bronchioles. Similarly, serious cases of diphtheria had the infection in the lining of the larynx often without any apparent infection in the throat. Sometimes the diphtheria was superimposed on the effects of gassing. Although about a third of the diphtheria carriers, iden-

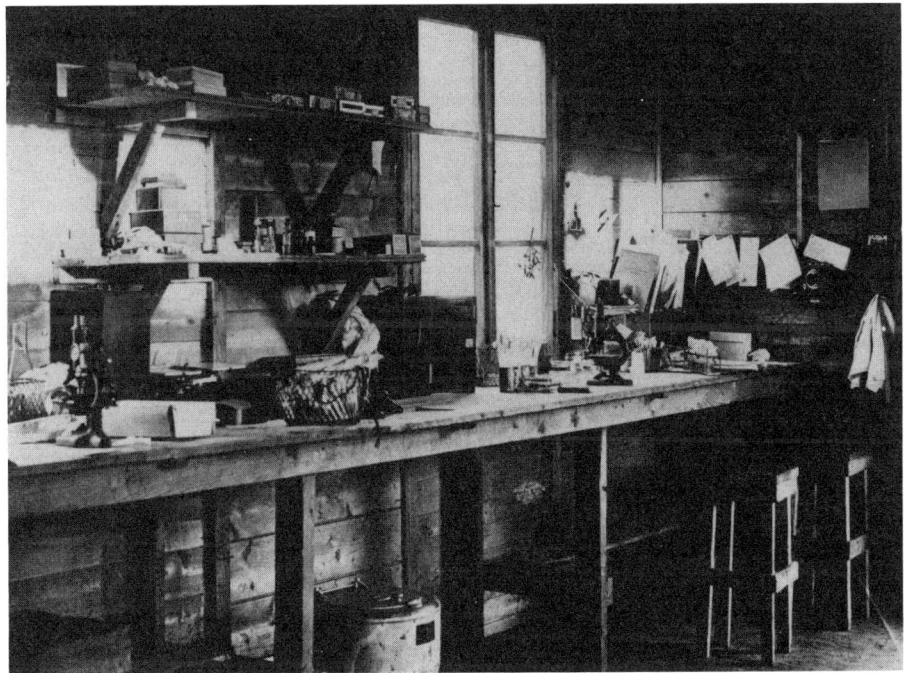

FIGURE 10:9   Laboratory, Base Hospital No. 26. Courtesy Dr. Jesse Barron.

tified by means of throat cultures, were patients who had been gassed, only about 5 percent of the clinical cases of diphtheria had been gassed.

The throat cultures were all examined at the central laboratory rather than in the laboratories of the individual base hospitals. In late November one to seven new cases of diphtheria were appearing each day, and Captain Barron decided to include as clinical cases of diphtheria all patients with positive throat cultures who showed even the slightest symptoms of sore throat. When a clinical case of diphtheria appeared in a ward, the ward was isolated and throat cultures were taken from all patients and attendants. Within twenty-four hours usually one or more carriers were identified, who were then moved to the isolation hospital, but as growing numbers of carriers were identified from day to day, Moses Barron realized that in the interval of time before carriers could be identified by throat culture they were infecting other persons in the ward. Therefore, in a ward where diphtheria had appeared, he began to have patients wear face masks during the day and isolated them as much as possible from each other, until the ward was shown to be free of diphtheria. From 29 November to 9 December the central laboratory examined 600 to 1,300 throat cultures daily. About 1 percent proved to be diphtheria carriers, a proportion no higher than that in a normal unexposed population. Since the most important factor in controlling the epidemic was early diagnosis, an order was issued that throats of all patients and personnel should

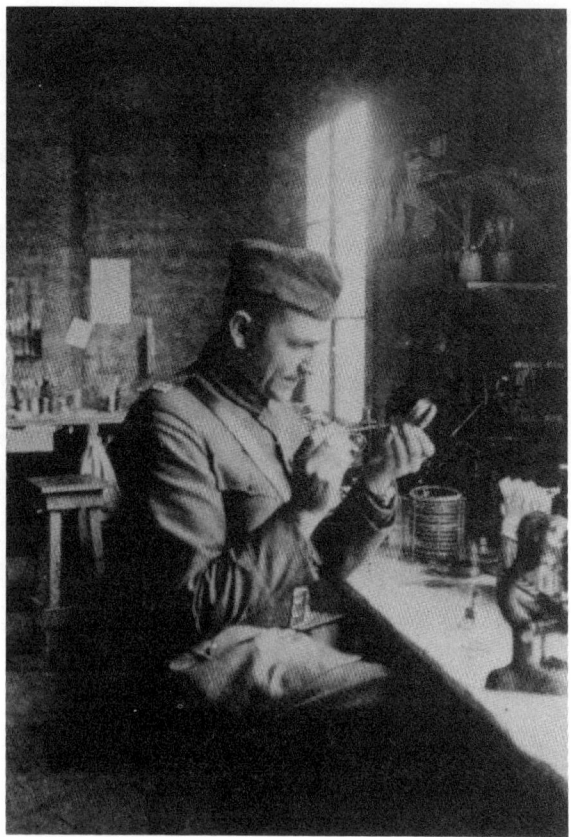

FIGURE 10:10   Captain Barron at work. Courtesy Dr. Jesse Barron.

be inspected daily, and throat cultures taken from any showing signs of soreness or inflammation. By a combination of early diagnosis through daily throat examinations of the whole camp, individual quarantine by mask and cubicle in wards where diphtheria had appeared, and the isolation of clinical cases of diphtheria and diphtheria carriers in Base Hospital No. 56, the epidemic was brought under control and came practically to an end by late December 1918.[26]

Thus in circumstances very different from, and far more difficult than, those that had existed at the Elliot Hospital in 1911, Moses Barron stamped out the diphtheria epidemic at Allerey in 1918. Perhaps as important as the particular measures taken was the scientific, investigative attitude adopted towards the problems posed by the epidemic. That was the attitude which Frank Wesbrook had attempted to inculcate in his bacteriology and pathology classes at Minnesota. On 20 October 1918 the *Minneapolis Journal* reported that Frank Wesbrook, at the age of fifty, was dying at Vancouver. He had wanted very much to take part in the war but could not because of his age and his health. Since 1914 he had given

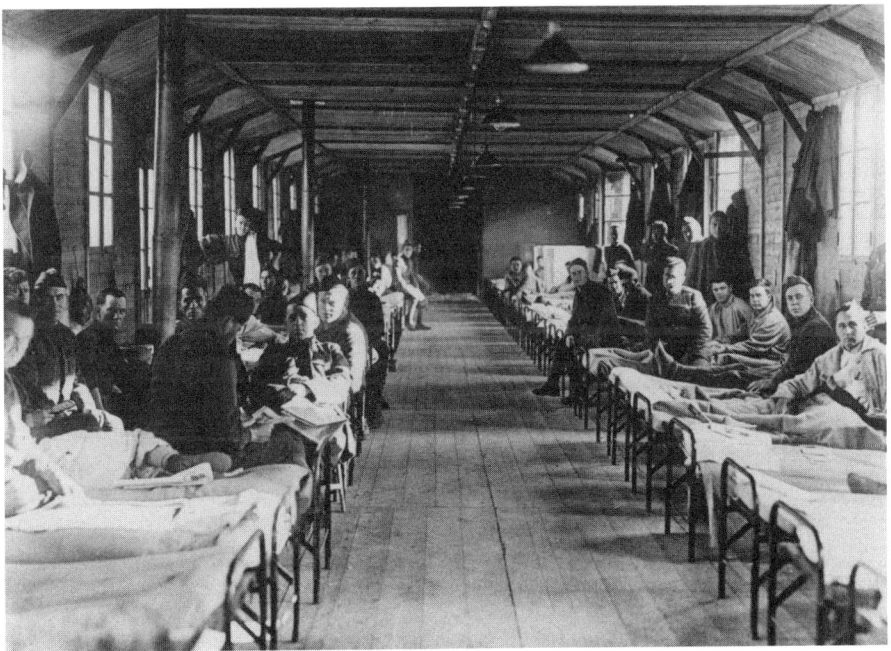

FIGURE 10:11   Ward, Base Hospital No. 26. Courtesy Dr. Jesse Barron.

all of his income that he did not need for immediate living expenses to the government of Canada to help pay for the war.[27] Through his former students and colleagues, Moses Barron, S. Marx White, and others, Frank Wesbrook may have contributed more than he knew to the care of the wounded in the war.

In December 1918 and early January 1919 wounded and convalescent soldiers were gradually evacuated from Base Hospital No. 26 and sent home. Several of the officers, including Colonel Law, Major White, and the chaplain, Captain Remington, were detached to go home. Lieutenant Colonel John S. Staley remained in command of the hospital until demobilization. On 10 January 1919, Base Hospital No. 26 ceased to function as a hospital. In its brief life as an active hospital it had cared for more than 5,700 sick and wounded soldiers, including 3,050 surgical cases. The surgeons performed 1,021 surgical operations. At the Allerey Hospital Center, Base Hospital No. 26 was responsible for most of the surgery and all of the ophthalmology. There were thirty-three deaths from surgical conditions, a mortality of slightly more than 1 percent.

One of the senior medical students who had served with Base Hospital No. 26, Harold Diehl, did not return directly to the United States. Discharged from the army in France by special request, Diehl volunteered to join the American Red Cross Commission to Poland, where he worked under a fellow Minnesotan and former student of Dean Wesbrook, Albert J. Chesley. In April 1919 he was assigned to Bialystock, which the Red Cross had selected for their headquarters in

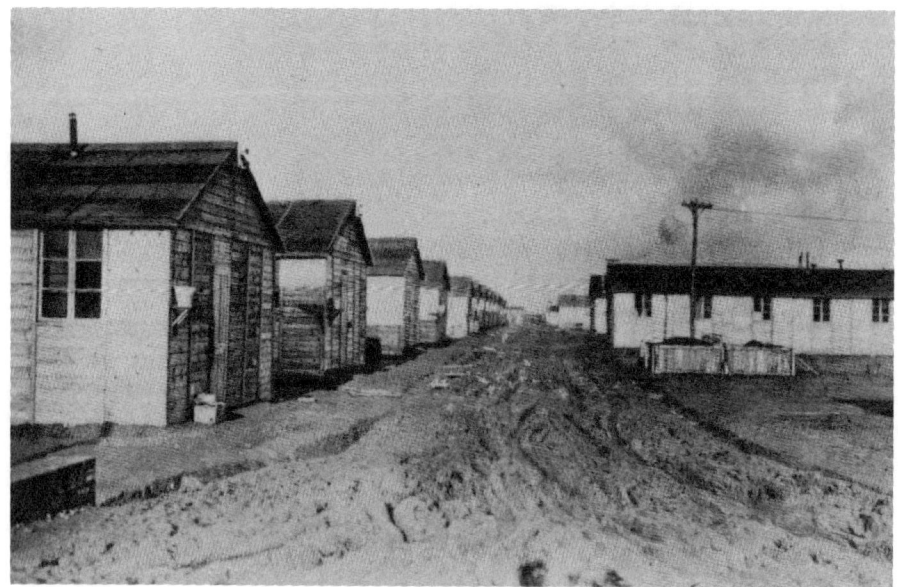
FIGURE 10:12   Mud at Allerey, Autumn 1918. *History of Base Hospital No. 26.*

eastern Poland. At Bialystock a group of wrecked buildings in filthy condition were turned over to the Red Cross. The Red Cross had to set to work to establish themselves in Poland and to turn their meager accommodations into an effective headquarters. Young Dr. Diehl revealed both an extraordinary ability to organize and to obtain the cooperation of men and women. Diehl showed such striking capacity for leadership that Chesley placed him in charge of the Bialystock headquarters, where his judgment, tact, and firmness soon established his authority in the midst of chaotic conditions. "He had medical officers under him," wrote Dr. Chesley later, "who had from ten to thirty years experience but they recognized his marked ability as an organizer and administrator and were loyal to him, never objecting to his discipline."[28] As the Bolshevik armies advanced across Poland during the summer of 1920, Dr. Diehl oversaw the evacuation of some 600 wounded from the Military Surgical Hospital, additional sick from the Wilno Typhus Hospital, and 800 children from the Bialystock Orphanage. Through these terrible days, according to Dr. Chesley, Dr. Diehl " . . . visited all the points of greatest danger and distress and set a fine example for the other workers who were not lacking in courage or resourcefulness, yet needed his presence."[29] Within a mere two years after he had completed his medical course, and a year after his service with Base Hospital No. 26, Harold Diehl achieved great distinction in his work with the Red Cross in war-torn Poland.

Although Base Hospital No. 26 was a special contribution of the medical school in the First World War, it was only part of what the school contributed to the war effort. By February 1918 some fifty-one members of the medical faculty, about one-third of the whole faculty, were in active service with the army or the navy. Twenty-nine were commissioned in the Army Medical Reserve Corps, of whom thirteen were with Base Hospital No. 26. Lieutenant Colonel Frank C. Todd was in charge of the division of head surgery of the base hospital at Camp Dodge, Iowa. On 6 July 1919 Colonel Todd died suddenly and unexpectedly at Chicago as he was preparing to go to France to command a base hospital. Lieutenant Colonel Louis B. Baldwin served at the surgeon general's office in Washington, while Major Harold E. Robertson was stationed in France, first at Army Laboratory No. 1 for six months and then for another six months at the Central Medical Department Laboratory at Dijon. Major Arthur T. Mann served as chief of surgery at Camp Dodge, Iowa. Major Julius P. Sedgwick led a commission of the American Red Cross to France to rescue and care for children in the war zone.

At home the remaining two-thirds of the faculty carried on the work of teaching classes as best they could. Under the strain of carrying on the teaching of surgery almost alone, James E. Moore fell ill in the spring of 1918 and died on 2 November of pernicious anemia, perhaps as much a casualty of the war as if he had gone to France. The size of the medical classes was not reduced significantly by the war because medical students were placed in the reserve and were to be drafted only after graduation in order to maintain a supply of medical officers if the war should be prolonged. The medical students in the reserve were, however, merged into the Students' Army Training corps where they did their share of K. P. and guard duty. At the Elliot Hospital the assistant superintendent of nurses, Miss Marion L. Vannier, conducted a training course for naval hospital corpsmen in groups of 100 at a time, and was responsible for training some 400 hospital corpsmen for the navy.

NOTES

1. Crile to Moore, 2 August 1915, Moore papers. In addition to providing details of the organization and staff required, Dr. Crile said that the expenses of the Cleveland unit were under $8,000, and that $10,000 should be sufficient to cover any expenses.

2. Cushing to Moore, 2 August 1915, Moore papers.

3. G. W. Crile, "The unit plan of organization of the Medical Reserve Corps of the U.S.A. for service in base hospitals," *Surg. Gynec. Obstet.*, 1916, 22, 68–69.

4. Jefferson R. Kean, "Development of Red Cross Medical Department units," in U. S. Surgeon-General's Office, *The Medical Department of the United States Army in the World War*, I, 92–105.

5. School of Medicine, Administrative Board, Minutes, 22 December 1915 and 1 March 1917.

6. "$5,000 raised for Base Hospital; aid of citizens asked," *Minneapolis Journal*, 31 March 1917.

7. School of Medicine, Administrative Board, Minutes, 7 April 1917.

8. "The senior medics' story," in U. S. Army, Base Hospital no. 26, Allerey, *History of Base Hospital 26*, pp. 96–101, p. 96.

9. Motor transport was pooled by the American Expeditionary Force and the vehicles never reached Base Hospital No. 26 in France.

10. School of Medicine, Administrative Board, Minutes, 6 December 1917.

11. Ibid.

12. Ibid., 26 December 1917.

13. Arthur A. Law, "History of the University of Minnesota Base Hospital No. 26," *J.-Lancet,* 1918, *38,* 16–18. Cf. "Base Hospital takes University quarters," *Minneapolis Journal,* 15 December 1917, p. 7, col. 3.

14. "Medical unit goes to training camp," *Minneapolis Journal,* 27 December 1917, p. 1, col. 2.

15. "Base Hospital 26 crack unit, says visitor at camp," *Minneapolis Journal,* 14 March 1918, p. 13, col. 2.

16. Law to Moore, 27 March 1918, Moore papers.

17. Law to Moore, 17 May 1918, Moore Papers.

18. "The senior medics' story" (n. 8).

19. "The artificers," in *History of Base Hospital No. 26* (n. 8), pp. 77–79.

20. S. Marx White, "Highlights of old Base Hospital No. 26," *Bull. Minn. med. Fndn,* 1942, *3* (no. 2), 7.

21. Ibid.

22. Law to Moore, 7 October 1918, Moore papers.

23. "Medical service," in *History of Base Hospital No. 26* (n. 8), pp. 26–28.

24. Harold S. Diehl, "How U.S. General Hospital No. 26 came to be organized at Minnesota," *Bull. Minn. med. Fndn,* 1942, *3* (no. 2), 4–6, p. 4.

25. Moses Barron and George H. Bigelow, "Diphtheria at a hospital center," *J. infect. Dis.,* 1919, *25,* 58–73, p. 59.

26. Ibid., pp. 70–73.

27. "Former Dean in Minnesota dying," *Minneapolis Journal,* 20 October 1918, p. 1, col. 2.

28. Chesley to Coffman, 13 August 1921, Harold S. Diehl personnel record, University of Minnesota.

29. Ibid.

CHAPTER 11

Renewed Controversy and Continued Stagnation 1919–1923

When Arthur Law and S. Marx White returned to the medical school in January 1919, they found the school struggling with the same problems as before the war. The Elliot Hospital still possessed the same 200-bed capacity that it had possessed since the completion of the service building in 1914, and no means had been found to expand it. Under President Vincent the Board of Regents had been generally unwilling to ask the legislature for funds for buildings, and except for the service building, nothing had been built on the medical campus since 1912. The Institute of Anatomy and Millard Hall remained unfinished, blank walls showing where the south wings of each were to be added. The nurses and nursing students were still crowded into several old houses near the hospital.

When President Burton assumed office in 1917, he was confronted with the consequences of the foolish neglect of building needs throughout the university during the six years of President Vincent's administration. Between 1911 and 1917 enrollment at the university had increased from 6,100 to 14,800 students, but legislative appropriations for buildings had dropped from $1,762,000 obtained by President Northrop for the 1911–13 biennium to $125,000 for the 1917–19 biennium. The outbreak of the First World War in Europe in August 1914 had brought legislative appropriations for university buildings to an almost complete halt in 1915, but that made the sharply reduced appropriations for buildings in the preceding two years even more unfortunate. To meet a situation that was becoming increasingly serious in 1918, President Burton proposed a comprehensive building plan to extend over a ten-year period from 1919 to 1929 and to cost almost $7,000,000. Among the proposed medical buildings included in the plan were the south wings of the Institute of Anatomy and Millard Hall, two hospital pavilions, and an addition to the hospital service building which together were estimated to cost $675,000. President Burton proposed that the comprehensive building plan be financed by a special state property tax of 35/100 mills during the ten-year period 1919 through 1928.[1] In November 1918 the Board of Regents approved the comprehensive building plan, which was then presented to the legislature during the 1919 session. The legislature appropriated $503,000 for buildings for the 1919–20 biennium and approved in principle the comprehensive building plan under which the sum of $560,000 was made available each year for ten years beginning 1 July 1920, or $5,600,000 for the decade.[2]

In 1919 the university was also impoverished in other respects by years of insufficient legislative appropriations. The Board of Regents' failure to request building funds had not been compensated for by any conspicuous success in obtaining funds for operating expenses, and the monetary inflation that occurred during the war years had almost doubled the cost of living. Faculty salaries, already low before the war, had become seriously inadequate. In 1919 President Burton requested and obtained from the legislature an increase of $500,000 in the annual maintenance budget of the university, and devoted almost the whole amount to increases in faculty salaries. Despite the increase, the maintenance budget proved insufficient almost immediately. In the fall of 1919 the university received a flood of new students. Enrollment was 46 percent above that of the year before, and every part of the university was placed under great strain. Between the increased costs for supplies and the need to appoint additional instructors, who could not be obtained at the salary rates then prevailing at the University of Minnesota, President Burton found it impossible to prepare a budget for 1920–21. In March 1920 the university administration advised the Board of Regents to ask the governor to call a special session of the legislature to deal with the situation. The Board of Regents refused, and the university was then obliged to prepare a budget which included no increase in faculty salaries except when needed to retain faculty members who had received offers from elsewhere. The Board of Regents planned to request an emergency appropriation from the legislature as soon as it convened in 1921.

In 1921 the legislature passed an emergency appropriation of $546,000, which provided for no salary increase, but increased the annual appropriation for maintenance of the university from $1,865,000 to $3,000,000.[3] The onset of the economic depression of 1921, which was especially severe in agriculture, made the legislature unwilling to provide the full university request.

The financial difficulties of the university were reflected in a number of significant departures of faculty. In 1920 President Burton himself left to become president of the University of Michigan, confessing frankly that the larger salary and more secure financial basis of the University of Michigan were important to him. In the medical school the Department of Medicine in 1918 lost Dr. Francis Blake to Yale. In November 1919 Dean Lyon arranged that the chief of the Department of Medicine,[4] Dr. Leonard Rowntree, should spend the spring and summer quarters of each year at Rochester, working in the Mayo Clinic, and that half of his salary of $8,000 should be paid by the Mayo Foundation. Several months prior to this arrangement, Dr. Rowntree learned that Dr. Mayo was willing to pay him an annual salary of $20,000, more than double what he was receiving at the university, if he would move to the Mayo Clinic.[5] Such an offer to Dr.

Rowntree raised in sharp relief the difficulties inherent in full-time clinical appointments, especially at the University of Minnesota. The university could not afford to pay salaries to clinical faculty members that would come even close to what they might earn in private practice. A further difficulty at Minnesota, apart from the question of income, was that the Elliot Hospital was too small to keep the clinical faculty sufficiently occupied in the care of patients, or to provide patients in the numbers needed for clinical research. Leonard Rowntree said that from his viewpoint Minneapolis suffered from the disadvantage that there was no provision on the university campus for private practice so that he lost much time in visiting hospitals away from the campus. Such practice at hospitals away from the campus was hardly consistent with even the loosest interpretation of a fulltime clinical appointment. Another disadvantage of the university mentioned by Dr. Rowntree was that the medical school failed to support research adequately.[6] Nevertheless, the immediately fascinating attraction to Rochester for Dr. Rowntree may have been the prospect of a much larger income and the opportunity to work in a larger hospital.

When in August 1919 President Burton learned of the Mayo offer to Dr. Rowntree, he consulted with Dr. William Mayo, and on 4 September proposed to the Board of Regents that the university seek from private sources a half million dollars to build a hospital on the campus for private patients and per diem patients. The Board of Regents approved the proposal and President Burton attempted to raise the money.

In November 1919 President Burton met with Abraham Flexner at New York City to explore the possibility of a grant from the Rockefeller General Education Board to the medical school. On his return to Minnesota, Burton wrote to Flexner to make official application for a grant, leaving the amount to be determined after Flexner had an opportunity to visit Minneapolis to study the situation of the medical school.[7] Flexner himself did not come to Minneapolis, but in March 1920 George Edgar Vincent, formerly president of the University of Minnesota and now president of the Rockefeller Foundation, and Dr. Richard M. Pearce, director of the foundation's Division of Medical Education, came. On the train from Chicago to Minneapolis President Vincent and Dean Lyon talked together, and Vincent told Lyon then that because of the forthcoming departure of President Burton, the controversies of the medical school with the medical profession, and uncertainties about the attitude of the next Minnesota legislature, there was no probability at that time of a grant for the medical school from the General Education Board.[8] At Minneapolis Vincent repeated his discouraging message to President Burton. He and Dr. Pearce also met at Dean Lyon's house with President Burton, Dean Lyon, and members of the medical school's hospital committee. At that conference the faculty representatives said that they could obtain no increase in state maintenance for the university hospital, but that they were going to seek construction funds for two additional pavilions to add 350 hospital beds. They also described to Vincent and Pearce their conception of a full-time clinical appointment, namely, that in addition to their university salaries, the chiefs of clinical departments should be permitted to take consultation patients for additional fees, a full-time plan different from that advocated by Abraham Flexner and the General Education Board. Vincent and Pearce did not commit themselves to accept the Minnesota interpretation of full-time.[9] Later Dean Lyon wrote to Dr. Pearce to urge that Minnesota should be developed as a genuine university medical school with emphasis on research. Its already favorable development, its geographical location as the single medical school in a vast area of the Northwest, and its development of graduate medical education both at Minneapolis and Rochester together laid a foundation for further development. He outlined the faculty's plans for development, all contingent upon hoped-for legislative appropriations and private gifts, and defended the Minnesota plan for geographic full-time.[10] At Dr. Pearce's request the chief of medicine, Dr. Leonard Rowntree, also wrote to him outlining the needs and hopes for hospital expansion in much the same terms as Dean Lyon, but noting specifically the need for an amphitheater in which to hold large clinics, and a clinical laboratory for the medical students.[11] Despite pleas from Minnesota, the Rockefeller men took no further steps. They evidently judged that there existed at Minnesota deep-seated obstacles to the further development of the medical school.

The proposal that Dr. Rowntree should spend half the year at Rochester was a compromise intended to retain him at least half of the year at Minneapolis, but it failed. Dr. Rowntree went to Rochester for the spring and summer of 1920, but by July he resigned as chief of the Department of Medicine so that he could work full time at the Mayo Clinic and be chief of medicine in the Mayo Foundation; this change allowed him to remain a professor of medicine in the graduate school of the University of Minnesota because of the affiliation between the university and the foundation.[12]

In the spring of 1920 the head of the Department of Pathology at the medical school, Dr. Harold E. Robertson, was similarly invited to spend the three summer months of June, July and August at the Mayo Clinic doing post-mortem work.[13] At Rochester during the summer of 1920 Dr. Robertson breathed such new life into the weekly clinico-pathological conferences of the Mayo Clinic by his merciless exposure of the clinician's errors, that at the end of the summer Dr. William Mayo invited him to come permanently to the clinic.[14] In the spring of 1921 Dr. Robertson resigned to move to Rochester. Meanwhile, Dr. S. Marx White was appointed chief of medicine in 1920 to replace Dr. Rowntree, and in 1921 Dr. Elexious T. Bell was promoted to succeed Dr. Robertson as head of pathology.

In the fall of 1920 the sense of concern and frustration created by the loss of faculty members coupled with the repeated failures of efforts to expand the university hospital boiled over at a luncheon meeting held by the Medical Alumni Association in conjunction with the annual meeting of the Minnesota State Medical Association in St. Paul. At the luncheon a committee of medical alumni, chaired by Dr. George D. Head of Minneapolis, reported on the results of their study of conditions at the medical school. The committee had been appointed two years before at the 1918 meeting of the Medical Alumni Association in Duluth, but, because of the war, had not begun its work until the fall of 1919. During a period of some six to eight months the committee had conferred with President Burton, Dean Lyon, Assistant Dean Beard, the superintendent of the university hospital, Dr. Louis Baldwin, other members of the medical faculty, senior students, house officers, and alumni.[15]

Dr. Head's committee argued that although the primary purpose of the medical school was to train general practitioners for the state, the development of graduate medical education both at the university and at the Mayo Foundation was causing the needs of undergraduate medical education to be neglected. The committee argued further that the effect of the Board of Regents' resolution of June 1915, which required all members of the medical faculty to support the Mayo affiliation, had acted " . . . to disorganize administration, nullify leadership, demoralize discipline, and crush initiative."[16] The committee thought that the basic medical sciences were being taught in the medical school too much as pure sciences with insufficient regard to their application in medical practice, and too much of the teaching was done by young and inexperienced members of the faculty. The rapid development of graduate medical education under the Mayo Foundation at Rochester completely overshadowed the efforts to develop graduate medical education in the medical school. Nevertheless, even the relatively small number of graduate medical fellows at the university were too many for the limited amount of clinical material available in the Elliot Hospital. By contrast, the large numbers of patients in the city hospitals of Minneapolis and St. Paul remained almost entirely unused for graduate medical education. The committee thought that the two city hospitals should be used more fully for graduate medical training and that the university hospital should be enlarged, but should continue to be a charity hospital as the Elliot Memorial Hospital was when planned. They objected to the university hospital's being used for either per diem or private patients because by so doing the medical school lost the support of the medical profession of the state and the medical alumni. The committee supported the medical school's plan to have the State Board of Control build a psychiatric hospital on the campus—a hospital in which medical care would be provided by members of the medical faculty. The committee also wished to see built on the campus a hospital pavilion for patients suspected of being in the early stages of tuberculosis.

At least some of the defects in the medical school, the committee thought, derived from the fact that Dean Lyon was not a physician, and therefore lacked both intimate knowledge of, and sympathy with, the needs of practicing physicians. The medical school was isolated from its alumni who, in sharp contrast to the past, had not for four years been consulted at all concerning the educational policies of the school or its interests.

When Dr. Head presented the findings of his committee to the luncheon of the Medical Alumni Association on 1 October 1920, the allegations of the committee were challenged sharply by certain other alumni. There were particularly vigorous exchanges between George Head and Louis B. Wilson. According to the *Journal-Lancet:*

> There was a general discussion that was a joy and treat to the listener, especially if he loved a fight, for evidently there was a fight . . . . The lie was passed back and forth with a good deal of freedom. The defense and the prosecution were very much in evidence, and the impression left on the majority of the members of the Alumni Association was a very unfortunate one . . . . At all events, it was an outspoken plainly worded effort to improve the medical situation at the university as it exists today. Perhaps it will clarify the atmosphere, or at least blot out the flame that has been smoldering for two or three years . . . the denial or suppression of the truth will not accomplish the end.[17]

The day after this exchange, Louis Wilson wrote to George Head to state his objections to the committee's report. He offered to provide accurate details on the work of the Mayo Foundation in order to correct the report before it was published, and went on to object to the implication of the report that the medical school was doing poor work. As director of the Mayo Foundation, Dr. Wilson knew that the records of Minnesota medical graduates compared favorably with those of graduates of the best medical schools in the United States. Minnesota students were particularly well trained in anatomy, pathology, and bacteriology, and their training in obstetrics and pediatrics was equal to that of other good schools. He insisted that good graduate medical education would tend to improve the quality of undergraduate work, not harm it. Nevertheless, Louis Wilson agreed that the medical school faced serious problems. The basic science departments were "undermanned and pitifully underpaid," and were kept going only by the personal sacrifice of the faculty. If they did not receive help soon, their morale would break and they would degenerate.[18]

Despite the debate at the luncheon meeting on 1 October, the Medical Alumni Association adopted the report of Dr. Head's committee, without a dissenting vote, on the understanding that the figures for the number of postgraduate fellows and students at the Mayo Foundation would be corrected with up-to-date figures when the report was published. On 19 October Dr. Head sent a copy of the report to the new university president, Lotus D. Coffman.[19] In December the *Minnesota Alumni Weekly* reprinted the *Journal-Lancet* account accompanied by editorial comment that began, "The poor medical school!" and said: "The malignity of the controversy has become so acute that the University's medical standing is in jeopardy."[20] The full report of Dr. Head's committee appeared in the December 1920 issue of *Minnesota Medicine.*[21] The report was reprinted in January 1921 in the *Minnesota Alumni Weekly* together with a letter from Dean Lyon to Regent Sommers in which Dean Lyon replied to the criticisms in the report.[22]

To the criticism that the emphasis on graduate medical education was at the expense of undergraduate instruction, Dean Lyon said that the teaching fellows provided instruction for undergraduates. He thought that the medical school possessed as much initiative as ever in educational matters although it was apparently not free "to work the Legislature." Dean Lyon defended his own record as reflected in " . . . the liberal curriculum, the improved dispensary, the greater use of the library, the student internship, the better integration of the school with the University, the comprehensive program of graduate work." The criticism that the basic medical sciences were taught too much as science, with insufficient attention to their applications in medical practice, Dean Lyon said was a common criticism everywhere, but that Minnesota tried to combine pure science with its practical applications. He denied that the heads of departments were doing too little teaching. He thought that the city hospitals of Minneapolis and St. Paul might be used more fully, but it was too strong to say that they were almost unutilized. The city hospitals should be brought fully under control of the medical school and should be used for both undergraduate and graduate medical instruction. After replies to other criticisms, Dean Lyon referred to what he considered the hostile attitude of the Medical Alumni Association.

> . . . I am frank to express the belief that as a result of the reorganization (which took place before my time) and as a further result of the Mayo controversy, the controlling element of the alumni association has taken such a hostile attitude that it has been impossible to work with them. It is not true that no efforts were made to do so.[23]

Dean Lyon's comments reveal the yawning gulf of bitterness that separated him from leading members of the medical alumni. The situation revealed by the controversy was sufficiently serious that the university administration could not ignore it. On 11 November the administrative board of the medical school asked President Coffman to appoint an external committee to study the report of the alumni committee and make recommendations concerning it.[24] In January the Board of Regents authorized such a special survey and President Coffman then wrote to three eminent medical men: Dr. Frank Billings of Chicago, Dr. Victor Vaughan, dean of the University of Michigan Medical School, and Dr. William H. Welch of Johns Hopkins University to ask them to serve as a committee of three to survey the medical school and make recommendations.[25] Dr. Welch declined to serve so Dr. John M. T. Finney, clinical professor of surgery at Johns Hopkins, was invited in his place.

The survey team came to Minneapolis where they spent several days, interviewing Dean Lyon, Dean Ford of the graduate school, members of the medical faculty, and students. They met with a committee of the medical alumni, and with any medical men in Minneapolis and St. Paul who cared to talk with them. Among such physicians, they interviewed several of the men who had not been reappointed in the reorganization of 1913. They also visited the laboratories and clinics of the medical school, including the Elliot Memorial Hospital and the city hospitals of Minneapolis and St. Paul. From the Twin Cities the committee went to Rochester where they had a long meeting with Dr. William J. Mayo and the heads of departments in both the Mayo Foundation and the Mayo Clinic, and learned of the various lines of research being pursued at the Mayo Foundation.

Although the purpose of an external survey committee was obviously to obtain a detached viewpoint on the affairs of the medical school and its relationships with the Mayo Foundation and the Mayo Clinic, the composition of the committee casts some doubt upon its complete detachment. Had William H. Welch served on the committee, he might have been a detached and impartial observer, but the members of the actual committee that served possessed the common characteristic that they were close personal friends of the Doctors Mayo. Victor Vaughan had been for many years dean of the medical school of which William Mayo was an alumnus and in 1915 had demonstrated his unswerving loyalty to the Mayos. As a fellow surgeon, Dr. John Finney knew Dr. Mayo well and had been associated with him closely in the affairs of the American College of Surgeons and in the Army Medical Department during the war. Frank Billings had known both of the Mayos for many years, and was a particularly close friend of Charles Mayo with whom he had been a fellow student at the Northwestern University Medical School in Chicago. Whatever effort they might make to be impartial, such a committee would find it very difficult to adopt a critical attitude toward the past actions or present position of the Mayos. Nevertheless, the committee noted that the Mayo affiliation had produced a division among members of the medical faculty, administrative officers, and alumni. "Some honestly thought," observed the committee, as if describing the beliefs of some peculiar religious sect, "that it was not the part of wisdom for a state institution to affiliate with a privately organized institution."[26]

Some persons interviewed by the committee criticized the continuance of William J. Mayo as a member of the Board of Regents because as a regent he would have to deal with the affairs of the Mayo Foundation with which he was closely connected. The committee stared Dr. Mayo's position of conflict of interest squarely in the face, and asserted it was not there. They were convinced that Dr. Mayo's presence on the Board of Regents "has not been and is not now characterized by any action on his part derogatory to the development of the Medical School of the University . . . ." The committee evidently dismissed the failure for ten years to expand the university hospital, the deeply destructive reorganization of the medical faculty in 1913, the years of controversy over the Mayo affiliation accompanied by the resignations of six members of the Department of Medicine, and the most recent loss of two department heads to Rochester, all events in which Dr. Mayo was involved, as doing no harm to the medical school. When, for instance, Dr. Mayo invited Dr. Rowntree to come to the Mayo Clinic, was he acting in the interest of the medical school or of the Mayo Clinic? The committee did not ask such questions.

As to the Mayo Foundation, the committee thought that it was to the University of Minnesota " . . . an asset which is not equaled in any other university in the world."[27] As a center of graduate medical education, they considered the Mayo Foundation unparalleled, which at the time it was. But the committee also went on to suggest that the Mayo Foundation was of benefit to the medical school—a much more doubtful proposition. They suggested that Mayo Foundation fellows who lacked adequate preparation in one of the basic medical sciences might come to the medical school to work in its laboratories. Although the possibility existed it was used rarely, primarily because Mayo Foundation fellows were a select group of young doctors who as graduates of leading medical schools usually already possessed excellent training in the medical sciences. The committee also said that Mayo Foundation fellows might " . . . be used as teaching assistants in the undergraduate Medical School."[28] The latter statement was untrue. In 1918 Dr. Mayo had refused to allow a teaching fellow in physiology at the medical school to be charged to the Mayo Foundation, and did so to establish the principle that Mayo Foundation funds should not be used to support teaching at the university.[29]

The committee argued at some length that it was the function of a state medical school to supply competent physicians to serve *all* citizens of the state. To do its work a state medical school needed well-equipped laboratories, staffed with full-time workers, adequately paid. At Minnesota the two laboratory buildings completed in 1912 remained after nine years with wings yet to be added. The delay, they noted, had created "a sense of disappointment" among the laboratory workers. Similarly the university hospital and the outpatient department were too small to provide adequate clinical training for the medical students. The university hospital needed to be enlarged to four to five hundred beds. Because a hospital was expensive to maintain, the university hospital could easily become a burden to the university. Indigent patients should be paid for by the state or by the county from which they came. On the awkward question whether the university hospital should admit private patients, the committee hesitated to express an opinion. Any physician in the state should have the privilege of sending a patient to the hospital for diagnosis, or for diagnosis and treatment, but the patients should remain patients of the physician sending them to the hospital. The fees charged to paying patients should correspond to those charged by consulting physicians in Minneapolis and St. Paul. "In no case and under no circumstances," said the committee, "should the salary of a teacher in the Medical School be determined by the consultation or other fees that patients coming under his charge may pay."[30] That sounded very well, but the committee left unasked and unanswered the delicate question of how to determine the salaries of full-time clinical faculty members.

When the committee visited the Minneapolis General Hospital they were told that members of the hospital staff had no definite hours for teaching medical students, and they concluded that the clinical instruction provided there was of little value. At the St. Paul City and County Hospital clinical teaching seemed to be much better organized. The committee thought that if the two city hospitals were used fully for clinical teaching, together with the proposed 500-bed university hospital, the three hospitals should provide ample clinical material for the teaching needs of the medical school.

Finally, the committee recommended that the medical school should concentrate on training general medical practitioners for the state and should not attempt to develop graduate medical education, because the University of Minnesota already possessed at Rochester "the greatest graduate school in the world."[31]

Of particular interest were the committee's recommendations concerning the dean of the medical school. No one, the committee said, questioned Dean Lyon's ability, honesty, or devotion to his work. Some individuals thought that the dean of a medical school should be a physician, but the committee disagreed. They recommended that a medical faculty should nominate its own dean, and recommended, therefore, that " . . . while Dean Lyon is able, honest, and conscientious in his dealings . . . the faculty should be asked to nominate its own dean."[32] In September 1921 when the Survey Committee Report was published in the *Journal-Lancet,* the editor, Dr. W. A. Jones, commented on the recommendation concerning Dean Lyon: " . . . it [the Committee] patted him affectionately on the back and placed a cake of ice on his chest, leaving him in a somewhat dazed condition and not knowing what they actually thought of him . . . ."[33]

President Coffman received the report of the Survey Committee early in July 1921, and immediately had copies made for the Board of Regents. During the second week in July when the members of the board with the exception of Pierce Butler accompanied President Coffman on a trip to visit the various agricultural schools of the university, he presented each member of the board, including Dr. William Mayo, with a copy of the report and they discussed it in considerable detail. The discussion of the report by the Board of Regents must have been curious in view of the immediate relation of one member of the board, Dr. Mayo, to the contents of the report. How did Dr. Mayo discuss with detachment a report that dealt with his own role as a regent, with the controversy over the Mayo affiliation, with the work of the the Mayo Foundation, and with the Mayo Foundation in relation to the medical school? True, he could take personal satisfaction in the committee's judgment on points in relation to himself and to the Mayo Foundation, but how could he view critically the opinions of a committee so favorably disposed toward himself? Evidently, Dr. Mayo wasn't critical of the report, and neither were other members of the board. While at Morris, Minnesota, the board agreed upon a resolution adopting the principles set forth in the report "as the general policy it would follow hereafter in the conduct and internal administration of the Medical School."[34] The board withheld the addition of the resolution to their official minutes until they could get the opinions of Dean Lyon and the absent Regent Butler on the report. It was well they hesitated. When the report was published, some of its findings were challenged as inaccurate and its principal recommendations criticized as impracticable.

On 3 August Dr. William Mayo expressed his own favorable opinion of the report in a letter to Pierce Butler. Dr. Mayo thought that the report would become classic and would serve as a basis for the organization of other American medical schools. He urged that the report be circulated widely, and that it be used as the basis for the Board of Regents' policy in relation to the medical school. The administrative board of the medical school should use the report to reply to the medical alumni while pointing out the large number of applications for admission to the medical school and the success of graduates in obtaining intern positions in hospitals all over the country so as " . . . to stop the miserable bickering that has been carried on by the malcontents."[35] Dr. Mayo was not about to allow any but petty motives to his critics.

A few days later President Coffman had begun to have doubts about the report, possibly as a result of a very clear analysis of it that had been prepared by his administrative assistant, John J. Pettijohn. President Coffman was worried particularly by the committee's recommendation that all medical graduate work should be done at Rochester because he had come to see that such a policy would be fatal to the medical school. He convinced himself that the committee intended to say " . . . that the Mayo Foundation will devote itself primarily to graduate work in medicine and surgery; the School of Medicine at Minneapolis will devote itself primarily to under-graduate instruction in medicine and surgery."[36] Meanwhile Dr. Mayo was urging that the report be printed and distributed widely, and President Coffman had arranged for its printing.[37]

On Saturday, 20 August, the committee's report was released to the press, and on 15 September the complete report appeared in the *Journal-Lancet*.[38] In an editorial in the same issue of the *Journal-Lancet*, Dr. W. A. Jones commented on the report: "Although this committee may have intended to pour oil on the troubled waters, in doing it they evidently spilled a couple of gallons of gasoline, for it produced a different reaction from what they manifestly expected."[39] He regretted the "stirring up of old memories" of the controversy over the Mayo affiliation. So far as the positive recommendations of the committee were concerned, apart from that concerning the election of the dean, which was impossible, he observed that they contained nothing new. For years the medical faculty had been trying to complete the laboratory buildings and to obtain more adequate salaries. From the time that the Elliot Hospital was built in 1911, the medical faculty had planned to enlarge it to a hospital of 500 to 1,000 beds. Similarly, since its founding in 1888, the medical school had cooperated with the medical profession and had been training practitioners for the state. The Minneapolis physicians, Dr. Jones noted, were angered by the committee's comments on the Minneapolis General Hospital, because not only were they inaccurate, but the committee had not attempted seriously to learn the truth. After a telephone call late the evening before, the committee had arrived at the Minneapolis General Hospital between 8:15 and 8:30 a.m. and spent about half an hour talking to the superintendent of the hospital. The committee had not asked why clinics were not given at the hospital. "If the medical students are not given advantages in the Minneapolis General Hospital," said Dr. Jones, "it is not because there are not enough teaching men in the Faculty who are in attendance at the Minneapolis General Hospital. They offer all kinds of courses and have submitted their offers to the Administrative Board of the Medical Faculty, yet students are not assigned to the General Hospital clinics."[40] Later Dean Lyon confirmed that the committee had been misinformed about the conduct of clinics at the Minneapolis General Hospital, where, he said, the instructors were as regular in meeting their classes as instructors at the university hospital.[41]

In his private memorandum to President Coffman, John Pettijohn noted that the two recommendations of the Survey Committee, namely, the election of the dean and the transfer of all graduate clinical work to Rochester, were both impracticable. The transfer of all graduate clinical education to the Mayo Foundation would make it impossible to have any full-time clinical faculty on the Minneapolis campus, and would prevent the development of clinical research here. The medical school would, in effect, become a half medical school, offering instruction only in the basic sciences.[42]

In the wake of two reports on the medical school, the capacity of the school to react to further criticism or recommendations, or to do much of anything except carry on its routine teaching, seems temporarily to have been exhausted. The year 1921–22 was very quiet. At the semiannual meeting of the general faculty on 19 May 1922, there was no business to conduct. Dean Lyon reported on two meetings that he had attended, one at Chicago on medical education and another at Washington on public health education, while Jennings Litzenberg added his impressions of the Chicago meeting, and there was some discussion—nothing more. Yet beneath the surface changes were occurring. At the meeting of the Minnesota State Medical Association held at Minneapolis in October 1922, the association's Committee on Medical Education, chaired by George Douglas Head of Minneapolis, presented a report which was inevitably also a report on the medical school. Since Dr. Head had also chaired the committee of the Medical Alumni Association, whose report on the medical school two years before had evoked so much controversy, a second report on the medical school might have been expected to stir up a new controversy. Strangely, it did not. Instead the medical school's reaction to the report was welcoming and appreciative.

Dr. Head's Committee on Medical Education began by asserting the need for practicing physicians to express their ideas on medical education because in medical practice they saw the end results of training received at the medical school, from a practical standpoint. The practicing physician was also aware of the demands made upon the medical profession by the public. Because the primary function of a state medical school was to train physicians for practice, the committee requested the medical school to develop more fully courses " . . . in those finer personal qualities of heart and mind so essential to the management of the sick, and . . . in the treatment of disease and symptoms," including various special forms of therapy.

Although the medical school should not sacrifice quality for quantity, the committee regretted that the medical school had had to limit the size of its classes because it was the only complete medical school in the Northwest. They regretted any limitation of the school to Minnesota residents as tending " . . . toward provincialism, inbreeding and mediocrity," and pointed out that medical students who came to Minnesota from outside the state were as liable to remain in Minnesota after graduation as those who were born and raised there. At present, said the committee, the medical school could not even admit all of the students from Minnesota who wished to study medicine.

When the committee considered the medical school itself, they found its needs acute. Millard Hall and the Institute of Anatomy were both crowded. There was not sufficient room for the medical library. The Department of Pharmacology was in temporary quarters lent by the Department of Physiology. There was no laboratory space for the Department of Preventive Medicine and Public Health. The splendid museum collection of the Department of Pathology could not be displayed or used. The dispensary had outgrown its quarters; another lecture room was needed. To meet such needs the committee recommended that the missing south wings be added to the Institute of Anatomy and Millard Hall as soon as possible.

In caring for the sick poor from throughout the state, the university hospital served a public purpose entirely apart from its use for medical education; the committee, therefore, recommended that Minnesota should adopt the plan used in Iowa for funding its teaching hospital. At Iowa the state treasury paid the university month by month for the cost of maintaining its hospital so that the hospital was not a drain on the educational funds of the university.

The committee recommended that, because knowledge in the basic medical sciences had expanded greatly, the medical school should attempt to teach these subjects not as pure subjects, but as they might be applied to the practice of medicine. The committee urged also that the medical school should continue to offer the review courses for practicing physicians that had been given during the summers of 1921 and 1922, and likewise urged the members of the State Medical Association to attend such courses. The committee recommended that the state enlarge the university hospital to a capacity of 600 *free* beds. They congratulated the university on the creation of the new Department of Preventive Medicine and Public Health. They noted the need for a nurses' residence, because when the hospital was enlarged the various old houses — always makeshift — would become completely inadequate to house the nurses. To use the city hospitals of Minneapolis and St. Paul more effectively for clinical instruction, the committee recommended that all members of the clinical staff of these hospitals be given teaching appointments in the medical school. The committee endorsed the proposal for a state psychopathic hospital on the campus, and urged the addition to the university hospital of a tuberculosis pavilion which might serve as a clearing house for patients with symptoms suggestive of early tuberculosis.[43]

The whole tone of the committee's report was sympathetic to the medical school and well informed about its needs. When it was read to the meeting of the State Medical Association, Jennings Litzenberg, professor of obstetrics and gynecology in the medical school, rose to say that the report was "so constructive and its intent so helpful" that he wished to have the honor of moving its adoption. Dr. Litzenberg moved also that copies of the report be sent to the Board of Regents and to the dean of the medical school. Later, under new business, Dr. Litzenberg moved that the Committee on Medical Education be made a standing committee of the State Medical Association. The motion was seconded and carried.[44] In his report on the medical school for 1922-23, Dean Lyon mentioned the "constructive report upon medical education by a committee of Minnesota State Medical Association," as "a significant event of the year," and said that its recommendations were being followed as fast as possible—a far cry from Dr. Mayo's dismissal of "the miserable bickering . . . carried on by the malcontents" of the year before.[45]

Nevertheless, the medical school continued to struggle along, crowded into cramped buildings with a hospital about one-third the size needed. When in the summer of 1923 Dean Lyon succeeded in persuading Clemens von Pirquet, head of the department of pediatrics at the University of Vienna, to come to Minneapolis from Vienna to become chief of the Department of Pediatrics, Dr. Pirquet remained only two weeks. Although various explanations have been offered for Dr. Pirquet's abrupt departure, the very small number of beds reserved for pediatric patients in the Elliot Memorial Hospital was the factor that discouraged him most. The most urgent problem confronting the medical school was clearly to find means to enlarge the university hospital.

NOTES

1. University of Minnesota, *President's report for 1917-18*, pp. 9-18.
2. University of Minnesota, *President's report for . . . 1918-19*, pp. 7-8.
3. University of Minnesota, *President's report . . . 1920-21*, pp. 62-64.
4. School of Medicine, Administrative Board, Minutes, 7 August 1919; and 3 November 1919.
5. Coffman to Lyon, 6 September 1919, President's Office, Papers.
6. Leonard G. Rowntree, *Amid masters of twentieth century medicine*, pp. 201-202. Dr. Rowntree wrote (p. 253) that after Dr. Marion Burton became president of the University of Michigan, Burton invited him to succeed Victor Vaughan as dean of the University of Michigan Medical School, and that it was the Michigan offer that caused Dr. W. J. Mayo to invite him to become chief of medicine at the Mayo Clinic. Nevertheless, Mayo first invited Rowntree to come to Rochester during the summer of 1919 before Burton went to Michigan.
7. Burton to Flexner, 9 December 1919, General Education Board, Box 707, Folder no. 7267.
8. Vincent diary entries, 4-5 March 1920, General Education Board, Box 707, Folder no. 7267.
9. Ibid.
10. Lyon to Pearce, 11 March 1920, General Education Board, Box 707, Folder no. 7267.
11. Pearce to Flexner, 16 March 1920; Rowntree to Pearce, 9 March 1920, both in General Education Board, Box 707, Folder no. 7267.
12. School of Medicine, Administrative Board, Minutes, 16 September 1920.
13. Ibid., 7 April 1920.
14. Helen Clapesattle, *The Doctors Mayo*, pp. 603-604.
15. Head to Coffman, 21 December 1920, President's Office, Papers.

16. George D. Head et al., "Report of the special committee of the Medical Alumni Association appointed to inquire into conditions in the Medical School," *Minn. Med.*, 1920, *3*, 597–600, p. 597.

17. [Editorial], "The Minnesota State Medical Association," *J.-Lancet*, 1920, *40*, 581–582, p. 582. In writing to President Coffman on 11 October, Louis Wilson said that he had attacked the report at the luncheon meeting on 1 October. See Wilson to Coffman, 11 October 1920, President's Office, Papers.

18. Wilson to Head, 2 October 1920 [copy], Medical School [papers], Miscellaneous Correspondence, 1883–1948.

19. Head to Coffman, 19 October 1920, President's Office, Papers. President Coffman sent copies of the report to members of the Board of Regents on 4 November.

20. "Editorial comment . . . . The medical school, the University battle ground . . . ," *Minn. Alumni Wkly*, 1920–21, *20* (no. 11), 3–4, p. 3.

21. Head et al. (n. 16).

22. "The facts from both sides on the Medical School controversy," *Minn. Alumni Wkly*, 1920–21, *20* (no. 13), 9–12.

23. Ibid., p. 11.

24. Lyon to Coffman, 11 November 1920, President's Office, Papers.

25. Coffman to Billings, 18 January 1921 [copy], President's Office, Papers.

26. Frank Billings, J. M. T. Finney, and Victor C. Vaughan, "Survey committee report on the Medical School of the University of Minnesota," *J.-Lancet*, 1921, *41*, 501–506, p. 503.

27. Ibid.

28. Ibid.

29. Wrote Dr. Mayo: "It is the duty of the State Legislature to appropriate money for teaching purposes at the University and for us to lift such just burdens from them to the Foundation would quickly defeat the good that the Foundation might do by advancing research which the Legislature might not be expected to do." Mayo to Burton, 31 January 1918, President's Office, Papers.

30. Ibid., p. 505.

31. Ibid., p. 506.

32. Ibid., p. 503.

33. [Editorial], "Pouring oil on the troubled medical waters," *J.-Lancet*, 1921, *41*, 498–499.

34. Coffman to Butler, 16 July 1921 [copy], President's Office, Papers, 1911–1945. Apart from a reservation as to the legal power of the Board of Regents to delegate the appointment of a dean, Pierce Butler also approved of the report. See Butler to Coffman, 29 July 1921, President's Office, Papers.

35. Mayo to Butler, 3 August 1921 [copy], President's Office, Papers.

36. Coffman to Butler, 6 August 1921, President's Office, Papers.

37. Ibid.

38. "Issue raised on status of Medical Dean," *Minneapolis Tribune*, 21 August 1921; "Survey Committee report on the Medical School, the University of Minnesota," *J.-Lancet*, 1921, *41*, 501–506.

39. "Survey Committee" (n. 39), p. 498.

40. Ibid., p. 499. In October 1921 the staff of the Minneapolis General Hospital wrote to the administrative board to protest the portion of the Survey Committee Report relating to the Minneapolis General Hospital, and the administrative board forwarded their protest to the Board of Regents, saying that the Board was " . . . assured of the incorrectness of the statement in the Report of the Survey Committee . . . ." School of Medicine, Administrative Board, Minutes, 2 November 1921.

41. E. P. Lyon, "Clinical teaching at the Medical School of the University of Minnesota," *J.-Lancet,* 1921, *41,* 622–624.

42. J. J. Pettijohn, "Memorandum to President Coffman," President's Office, Papers.

43. George Douglas Head (Chairman), John T. Rogers, and Charles Erdmann [Committee], "Report of the Committee on Medical Education of the Minnesota State Medical Association," in "Minnesota State Medical Association Minutes - . . . 1922," *Minn. Med.,* 1923, *6,* Appendix [following p. 126] pp. ix-xi.

44. Ibid., p. xvi.

45. E. P. Lyon, "The Medical School," in University of Minnesota, *The President's report for the year 1922–23,* pp. 164–166. Cf. Mayo to Butler, 3 August 1921 [copy], President's Office, Papers.

CHAPTER 12

"Hope resurgent": Expansion of the University Hospitals, 1923–1929[1]

In November 1918, several months after the death of Dr. Frank Todd at Chicago, Mrs. Todd informed the administrative board that she wished to donate funds to help provide a hospital building in memory of her husband.[2] Before his death, Dr. Todd had drawn up a plan for an eye, ear, nose, and throat hospital to be established near the university campus. He proposed that the medical school should create separate departments or divisions of ophthalmology and otolaryngology, and that they should be placed in charge of the best men available. The heads of such departments or divisions should be permitted to carry on private practice, and a private clinic should be established in connection with the proposed hospital. The earnings of the clinic should be used not only to pay the salaries of the two chiefs of service, but also to pay assistants and to develop research and teaching in connection with the hospital. Dr. Todd envisioned that his proposed hospital should be self-supporting, with most of its space devoted to private rooms and not more than a third of the beds in large wards. The hospital would not have any free beds, but ward patients might pay only the per diem hospital charges. To create such a hospital Dr. Todd intended to leave $20,000 in his will, but at the time of his death he had not signed a will containing such a provision.[3] In May 1917, more than a year before his death, Dr. Todd obtained from Mrs. Edward Gale of Minneapolis, a daughter of John Sargent Pillsbury, a promise to give an additional $20,000 for the proposed hospital.[4] Dr. Todd thought that the hospital would cost more than $100,000 for land and buildings, and he had planned to seek additional gifts to raise the sum required.

Mrs. Todd's proposal to carry out her husband's plan for a special eye, ear, nose, and throat hospital seems to have remained in abeyance until the autumn of 1919 when, as a result of the threatened departure of Dr. Rowntree, President Burton became keenly aware of the urgent need to enlarge the university hospital. In December 1919 Mrs. Edward Gale renewed her offer to contribute $20,000 toward the hospital envisioned by Dr. Todd, and President Burton met with Mrs. Todd to assure her of the university's interest in the proposed memorial to her hus-

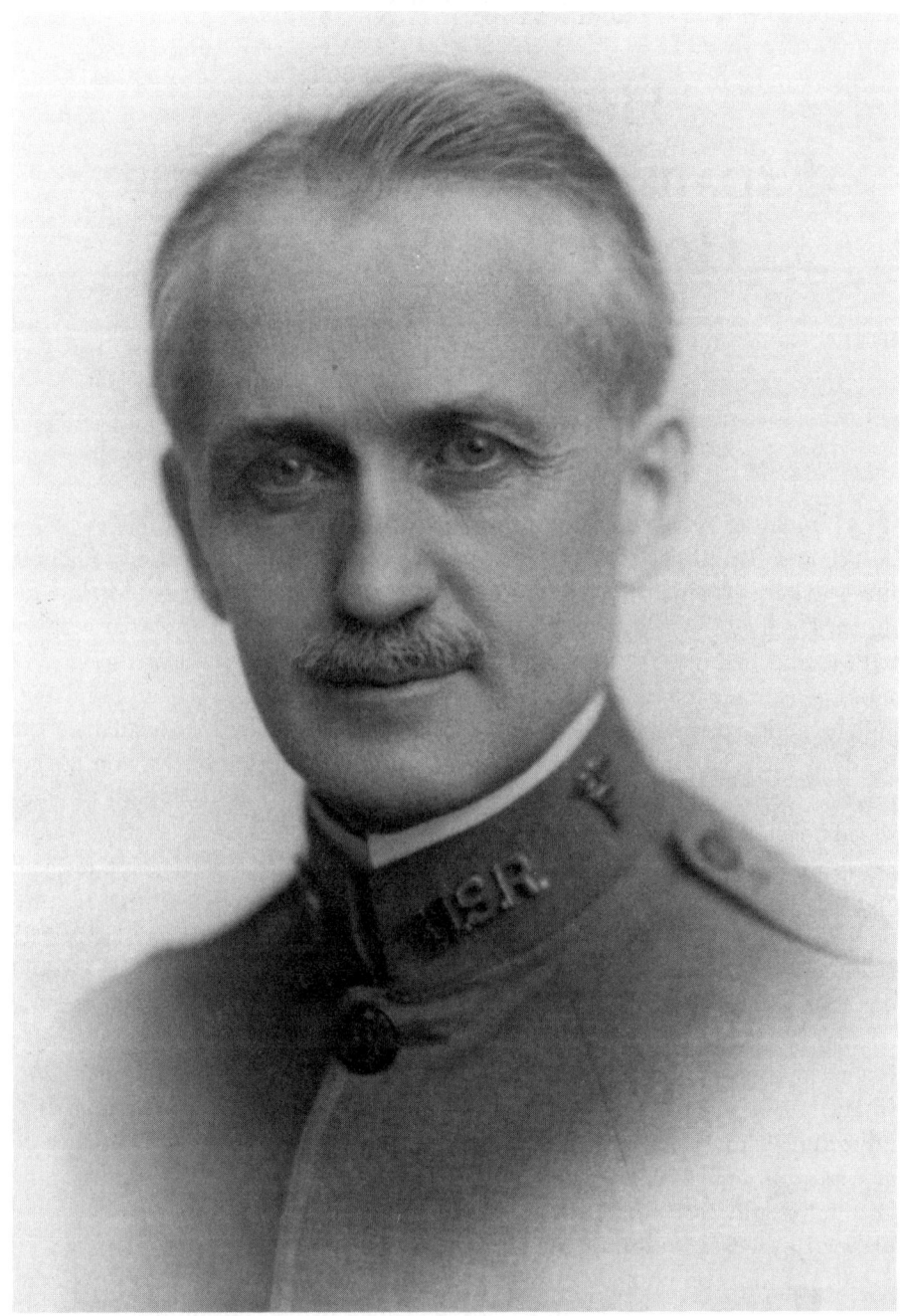

FIGURE 12:1 Major Frank Todd, 1917. Courtesy Mn U Archives.

band and to discuss other possible donors.[5] Early in the following year, President Burton presented the proposal for the Todd memorial to the Board of Regents, and wrote to Mrs. Todd that he was going to seek the help of friends and former patients of Dr. Todd to carry out the plan.[6] Fred B. Snyder, president of the Board of Regents, raised the question whether the proposed hospital should be located on or off the university campus, a delicate point because, as a hospital primarily for private patients, the Todd Memorial Clinic must be operated differently from the Elliot Memorial Hospital which served charity patients almost entirely.[7] In 1919 the university had set aside a number of beds in the Elliot Hospital as per diem beds, for which patients would pay a daily rate for hospital charges but not fees to the physicians for their medical or surgical care. Nevertheless, the per diem beds often remained unoccupied, apparently because physicians throughout the state were reluctant to refer patients who could pay hospital charges to the Elliot Hospital. As the controversy over the Mayo affiliation had brought out so clearly, the medical profession was deeply opposed to the medical school's engaging in private medical practice because the school then competed directly with physicians in practice. As a hospital primarily for private patients, the proposed Todd Memorial Clinic would involve the medical school in private medical practice, but Frank Todd had thought that such involvement was necessary to the effective training of specialists in ophthalmology and otolaryngology.

In May 1920 S. Marx White, while on a trip to medical centers in the East, wrote to President Burton from New York City to ask him to see Mrs. Todd concerning the proposed Todd memorial. Since President Burton was to leave Minnesota at the end of June to assume the presidency of the University of Michigan, Dr. White asked him to imbue incoming President Coffman " . . . with a knowledge of our needs and of our present pitiable state so far as Hospital at least is concerned." He added: "One needs only see what is being done in this part of the country to know how far short we are of fulfilling our needs — bare necessities even, and I hope Mr. Coffman will start his administration with some knowledge of how great both our need and our opportunities are."[8]

President Burton replied that his hands were absolutely tied on the question of the proposed Todd memorial because it involved " . . . a serious issue of whether we shall have pay patients on the campus of the University," an issue that, in view of his departure, he did not want to force. In the same letter President Burton reported that the Board of Regents had decided not to build an east wing to the Elliot Hospital with funds from the Comprehensive Building Program — a strange inconsistency with the admitted urgent needs of the university hospital.[9]

The same day President Burton wrote to President-elect Coffman to describe the proposed Todd memorial hospital. He was sending the various documents to Dr. William Mayo and hoped that the matter would be considered at the next meeting of the Board of Regents.[10] Burton said that the issue involved was whether a hospital for paying patients should be located on the university campus or not. He himself thought it ought to be possible to have on the campus all three kinds of patients — charity patients, per diem patients, and wholly private patients, who paid both hospital charges and professional fees—but he confessed that the issues were complex.[11] On 17 May, after Dr. Mayo had returned the Todd documents, Burton sent them to Coffman.[12] Although the Board of Regents presumably discussed the Todd proposal at their meeting on 24 May, they took no action at that time. Dr. Mayo thought that since the $20,000, which Mrs. Todd proposed to give in memory of Dr. Todd, would deprive her of a large portion of her husband's estate, possibly the Board of Regents should not accept her gift. However, S. Marx White reported, after a number of talks with Mrs. Todd, that she was chiefly anxious that a memorial be established to Dr. Todd before his memory faded and that her gift " . . . would mean very much more to her as a part of a memorial to him than it would mean to her as an income bearing principal."[13] Mrs. Todd was willing to give up certain of Dr. Todd's proposals and to entrust the character and use of the clinic to the Board of Regents. In view of Mrs. Todd's feelings, Dr. Mayo withdrew his objections to the acceptance of her gift.[14]

Although in December 1920 the hospital extension committee of the medical school appointed a subcommittee to seek additional gifts for the Todd memorial, little was accomplished perhaps because both faculty and administration were preoccupied with the controversy over the report of the Medical Alumni Association committee on the medical school, and the resultant study by an external survey committee. During the fall and winter of 1920–21, the university was also seeking legislation to establish a psychopathic hospital on the campus in cooperation with the State Board of Control, which was responsible for the state hospitals for the insane. In June 1922 Mrs. Todd informed Dean Lyon that she and Mrs. Gale would each pay their respective pledges of $20,000 on 1 January 1923.[15]

Also in June 1922, Dr. Mayo wrote to Dean Lyon to protest the medical school's policy of limiting the size of medical school classes to approximately eighty students, although more than two hundred students applied to enter.[16] In reply Dean Lyon said that the administrative board regretted as much as Dr. Mayo the need to restrict admission to the medical school, but the reason for the limited registration was the inadequate facilities of the school which the administrative board had repeatedly called to the attention of the Board of Regents. The laboratories would hold no more than eighty to ninety students. Especially in anatomy more students could not be crowded in. "It is an interesting fact," said Dean Lyon, "that, although the Medical School has doubled in attendance during the last 9 years, it has less space at its command today than it had at that time, having given up the Pathology building on the old campus and received nothing in place of it."[17] In the Elliot Hospital they could not provide clinical instruction to more than forty students at a time, or eighty in the course of the year. Nothing of what Dean Lyon said should have been news to Dr. Mayo, who was surely familiar with medical school affairs. The one bright spot to which Dean Lyon could point was the proposed Todd memorial building which might add eighty to one hundred beds to the university hospital.

The raising of funds for the Todd building went on slowly. S. Marx White obtained a donation of $5,000, but few other gifts were obtained.[18] Meanwhile the

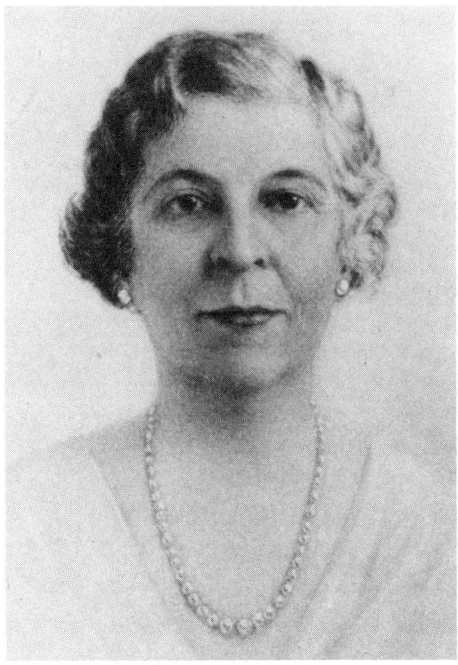

FIGURE 12:2 Mrs. George Chase Christian. Courtesy Mn U Archives.

Board of Regents decided to appropriate $110,000 from the Comprehensive Building Program allotment to add to the $45,000 privately donated for the construction of the Todd memorial hospital. The medical school hoped to raise an additional $100,000 to carry out all that Dr. Todd planned.[19] In December 1922, Dr. Mayo wrote to President Coffman to ask him to seek assurances from the medical faculty that the Todd Memorial Clinic would be self-supporting, a status which it could maintain only by taking private paying patients. Dr. Mayo anticipated "a good deal of disturbance with regard to the question of pay patients."[20]

A few weeks into the new year, the university was offered an additional opportunity to expand the university hospital when Mrs. George Chase Christian called on President Coffman to say that the Citizens Aid Society of Minneapolis, a private charitable corporation established in 1916 by George H. Christian, a pioneer miller of Minneapolis, would offer $250,000 to build a fifty-bed hospital for the care and treatment of cancer patients. The hospital building was to cost not more than $200,000, and the additional $50,000 was to provide radium and special x-ray equipment for the radiation treatment of cancers.[21] The cancer hospital was to be a memorial to Mrs. Christian's husband, and only son of George H. Christian, who died of cancer in January 1919 while still quite young.

In accepting the gift of the Citizens Aid Society, the Board of Regents was concerned that the proposed cancer hospital should be self-supporting, which meant that it must be able to take paying patients. The regents were particularly reluc-

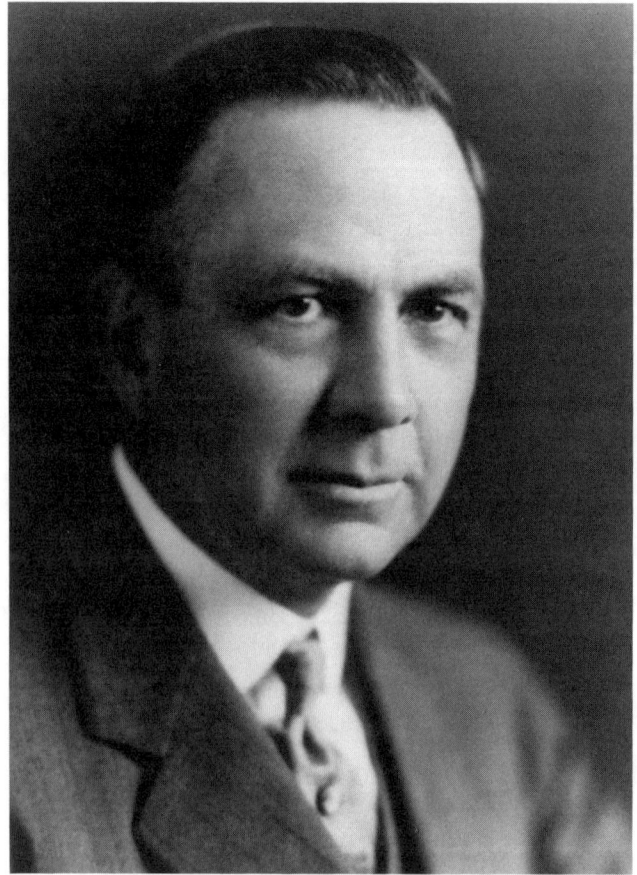

FIGURE 12:3 Lotus Delta Coffman, 1926. Courtesy Mn U Archives.

tant to expand the university hospital as a charity hospital, and Dr. Mayo suggested that they should ask the legislature to remove the legal restrictions that required the Elliot Hospital to receive only charity patients.[22] President Coffman demurred because in 1923 the legislature was sufficiently hostile to the university that he did not think they would be willing to remove the restrictive clauses in the Elliot Hospital Act.[23] In March negotiations between the Citizens Aid Society and the university concerning the proposed cancer hospital were completed. On 11 April 1923 the gift of $250,000 was formally accepted by the Board of Regents and announced to the public.[24]

Meanwhile, early in February 1923 yet a third dazzling possibility for the expansion of facilities for clinical teaching at the university appeared. The previous autumn, an article appeared in one of the Minneapolis newspapers calling attention to the inadequate facilities of the Minneapolis General Hospital. The Minneapolis Board of Public Welfare had announced that they were thinking of building a new city hospital. During a visit to New York City, President Coffman learned from a conversation with George Edgar Vincent, president of the Rockefeller Foundation, that the Rockefeller General Education Board, which was helping to finance expansion of the University of Iowa hospital, might also be willing to consider a major gift to the University of Minnesota hospital. In the course of a second visit to New York City in late February, President Coffman joined President Vincent and Abraham Flexner for luncheon at the Yale Club to discuss further the possibility of a Rockefeller gift for Minnesota.[25]

President Coffman hoped that the General Education Board would give a large sum, perhaps $1 million, to enable the university to purchase a block of land adjacent to the medical school and university hospital as a site for a new Minneapolis General Hospital. The difficulty in such a plan was that the General Education Board customarily required that its gifts be matched by an equal sum raised by the recipient institution. In the case of the Rockefeller gift to the University of Iowa, the Iowa State Legislature provided an appropriation equal to that of the General Education Board for building the Iowa University Hospital. President Coffman knew that the Minnesota legislature would not be willing to appropriate funds to help provide a hospital for the city of Minneapolis, so he hoped that the General Education Board would provide the entire amount to purchase a hospital site immediately, leaving the matching funds to be provided later. Vincent and Flexner evidently viewed Coffman's tentative proposals with considerable reserve, but they encouraged him to pursue the possibility of moving the Minneapolis General Hospital to the university campus to see whether he could devise a request that the Rockefeller board might consider. During succeeding months President Coffman pursued negotiations with the Minneapolis Board of Public Welfare, which was responsible for the city hospital, in an effort to interest them in moving the hospital to the university.

On 25 February 1923 Julius Parker Sedgwick, professor and chief of pediatrics from the time of its creation as a separate department of the medical school in 1915, died at his home in Minneapolis after a prolonged illness from progressive cerebrovascular disease. Dr. Sedgwick was a highly respected pediatrician who inspired others in his field to excel. His pediatric clinic at Northwestern Hospital in Minneapolis attracted many patients, and he created a distinguished part-time clinical faculty from among pediatricians practicing in the Twin Cities. In addition, Sedgwick was an active clinical investigator with particular interest in gastric acidity, blood sugar, and uric acid levels in newborns, and he introduced the use of restricted diets for the control of diabetes in children. In 1918 Sedgwick led a Red Cross Mission to France to study the effects of nutritional deficiencies and a chaotic environment on children living in the war zone. Appalled by the high death rates from infantile diarrhea that he found in France, which he realized were merely an extreme development of conditions that also existed commonly in the United States, Sedgwick became a strong advocate of breast feeding of children. At his lectures on pediatrics to medical students, Sedgwick is said to have passed around a beaker containing fresh human breast milk for them to taste.

"HOPE RESURGENT"

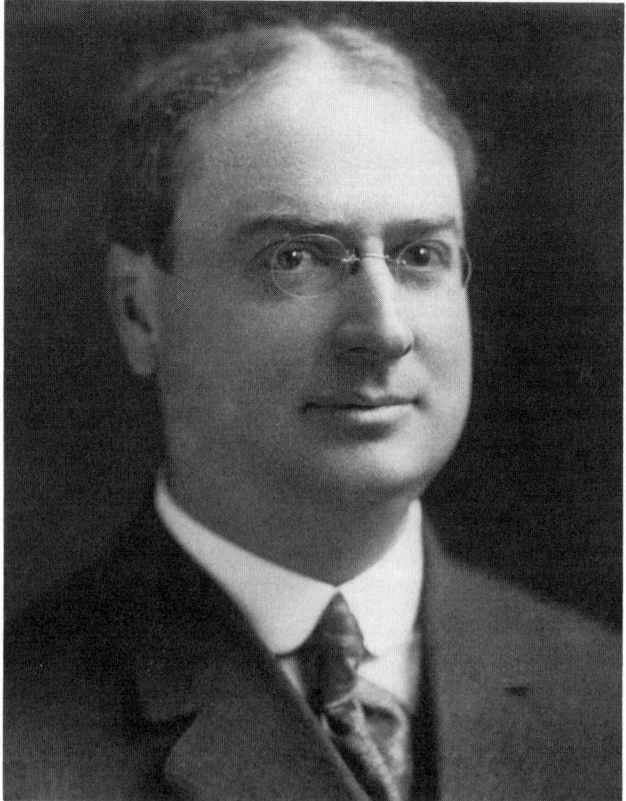

FIGURE 12:4   Julius Parker Sedgwick, circa 1915. Courtesy Mn U Archives.

At the university hospital Sedgwick was able to transfer the care of the newborn child from the obstetric to the pediatric service. He also developed a graduate program in pediatrics with emphasis on both clinical investigation and research in the basic sciences, and arranged exchanges of both fellows and faculty members with the Mayo Foundation at Rochester. In his laboratory research, Sedgwick was ably assisted by a young woman chemist, Mildred R. Ziegler, who joined the department in 1914 and in 1918 was appointed an instructor in pediatrics.

During the spring of 1923, when Dean Lyon was considering possible candidates to succeed the late Dr. Sedgwick as head of pediatrics in the medical school, he learned from Dr. Samuel Amberg of the Mayo Clinic and Woodard L. Colby, assistant in the Department of Pediatrics, that Clemens von Pirquet, professor of pediatrics in the University of Vienna and director of a large children's hospital there, might be interested in the Minnesota position. Dr. Pirquet was known internationally for his pioneer work in the study of allergy, for his description of serum sickness, and in 1923 most especially for his development of the skin tuberculin test. Pirquet found that a local inflammatory reaction of the skin following scarification and inoculation with tuberculin was much more pronounced in tuberculous individuals than in healthy ones, and was therefore valuable in diagnosis. From 1909 to 1910 Pirquet had been professor of pediatrics at Johns Hopkins so that he was acquainted with America, and at the Hopkins he had met Dr. Amberg who was also there at that time. In 1910 Pirquet left Johns Hopkins to accept a call to the University of Breslau in Germany, but with the agreement of the Hopkins authorities did not resign his Hopkins chair. In January 1911 Johns Hopkins offered Dr. Pirquet a full-time clinical appointment as professor of pediatrics, but Pirquet declined in order to succeed his former chief, Theodor Escherich, as professor of pediatrics in the University of Vienna.[26] Later in 1911, the Johns Hopkins authorities made a second effort to bring Pirquet to Baltimore as director of the Harriet Lane Home for Invalid Children, but failed.[27]

On 7 April 1923 Dean Lyon wrote to Dr. Pirquet to inquire informally whether he might consider the professorship of pediatrics at Minnesota. After characterizing briefly the University of Minnesota, which with slight exaggeration he said was "well supported by the people," Dean Lyon described the medical school in some detail, outlining the existing facilities of the Elliot Hospital where there were sixteen beds reserved for pediatrics. He described also the school's plans and hopes for future expansion.[28] Dean Lyon went on to describe the relationship of the medical school to the Minneapolis General Hospital, and the possibility, still uncertain, that the city hospital would be relocated across the street from the medical school, to mention salaries, graduate work, and the laboratories of the pediatrics department, staffed by "a competent chemist." He tried to describe the situation of pediatrics at Minnesota fully and fairly, although minimizing, as was natural, the difficulties and frustrations of the medical school.

On 3 May 1923 Dr. Pirquet replied from Vienna. He thanked Dean Lyon " . . . for the open way you explain the conditions of the Medical Department of the University of Minnesota," and said that the idea of building up a pediatric department at Minnesota appealed to him. "I would try of course," wrote Dr. Pirquet, "to get as soon as possible a children's hospital of the same kind and rank as I have here, with a staff of assistants and nurses . . . . " He asked for an annual salary of $6,000 and $1,000 to pay his expenses of moving to Minneapolis, and asked Dean Lyon to reply by cable, because Dean Lyon's letter of 7 April had taken nearly a month to reach him.[29]

When Dean Lyon received Dr. Pirquet's letter he called a special meeting of the administrative board which voted unanimously to recommend that Dr. Pirquet be elected professor of pediatrics.[30] After conferring with President Coffman, Dean Lyon cabled Dr. Pirquet to inform him of his appointment, and on 28 May wrote to confirm the cable.[31] After dealing with formal details, Dean Lyon wrote: " . . . You will find here old friends, such as Hirschfelder and Rowntree (the latter at Rochester). You will find several old pupils and a group of pediatrists who are enthusiastic and harmonious and ready to back you up in all your endeavors."[32] In a postscript Dean Lyon added that since he had dictated the letter (which he probably did on Friday, 25 May) the university had been promised a gift of about one and a quarter million dollars to be used for the benefit of crippled children, and that a portion of the gift could be used to build a children's hospital as part of the university hospital.

At the end of May, William Henry Eustis, a businessman and former mayor of Minneapolis, announced that he would entrust to the University of Minnesota money and property to the value of $1.3 million that he intended to give to build and endow a hospital and convalescent home for crippled children. Although Mr. Eustis had purchased a forty-four acre tract of land along the west bank of the Mississippi River in south Minneapolis, which he had at first intended as the site for the hospital and convalescent home, he was willing that the children's hospital should be built as part of the university hospital.[33] On 14 June Mr. Eustis confirmed his gift.[34] The Eustis gift ensured that the university hospital would shortly acquire a pediatric clinic sufficiently large for teaching and research purposes, and made the Minnesota appointment even more attractive for Clemens von Pirquet. The medical faculty, and especially pediatricians in the Twin Cities, were very pleased at the prospect of having such an internationally known authority on children's diseases at the university. During the summer of 1923, Dean Lyon sailed to Europe to attend the International Physiological Congress at Edinburgh, where he met and talked with Dr. Pirquet.

Dr. Pirquet arrived in Minneapolis on Saturday, 6 October 1923, with a certain amount of fanfare. He stated to the press that he was delighted with the opportunities afforded at the University of Minnesota to carry on his work, and added that he hoped to create at the university the most complete institution in the United States for the study of children's diseases. On Thursday and Friday of the next week, he attended the annual meeting of the Minnesota State Medical Association at St. Paul where he received an enthusiastic welcome, especially from the pediatricians of the Twin Cities. Then on the following Tuesday, at a meeting of the committee on hospital extension which Dean Lyon had called to acquaint Dr. Pirquet with plans for the new additions to the university hospital contemplated under the Todd, Christian, and Eustis gifts, Dr. Pirquet rose and began to read a statement intended to be his official resignation. He said that because the plans for hospital development provided for by the Eustis gift would require considerable time to complete, and because he was engaged in research which required a large group of patients and a fully organized hospital, he asked to be relieved of his duties so that he might return to his hospital in Vienna. He congratulated the medical school on the splendid outlook for pediatrics at Minnesota as a result of Mr. Eustis's gift, and thanked the medical faculty for inviting him to the chair.

Dean Lyon and the members of the committee were stunned by Dr. Pirquet's resignation barely ten days after he arrived at the university, but they immediately entered into a discussion with him of his reasons for his abrupt decision. Dean Lyon later summarized what they learned:

> Like most great scientists [said Dr. Lyon], Dr. Pirquet is a man of imagination and temperament. When he arrived here the task which, from the distance, had seemed alluring and immediate, began to look remote and difficult. He saw the important researches on which he had been engaged delayed not only by building operations, but by the necessity of making a new organization. He is 49 years old, and his thoughts turned to the limited years of activity which he may hope to enjoy.
>
> All these things came out in the very friendly conference we had with him, and I am sure all of us felt sorry for him.[35]

Dr. Pirquet's wife had been ill from the time that they arrived in the Twin Cities, and the combination of her illness, the strangeness of her surroundings, and the magnitude of the task that confronted him had discouraged him deeply. With tears in his eyes, Dr. Pirquet confessed to the committee that he was homesick. "Homesick not for Vienna," said Dean Lyon, "but for his hospital, 'his child,' the pride of his life. What was there for us to do but to sympathize with him and let him go?"[36] Despite the keen disappointment that he must have felt at Dr. Pirquet's departure, Dean Lyon was too generous spirited to complain.

Outside the committee nothing was said about Dr. Pirquet's impending departure during the next few days. On the morning of Friday, 19 October, Dr. Pirquet delivered a lecture to the medical students at which he demonstrated the scarification technique used in the Pirquet tuberculin test. For the demonstration Dr. Lawrence Richdorf, who was then the teaching fellow in pediatrics, carried the patient, a tuberculous child, from the Elliot Hospital to the lecture room in the Biology Building. After the lecture when he was about to carry the child back to the hospital, Dr. Pirquet told him to give the child to the nurse because he wanted to talk to him. They went to Pirquet's office where, to Richdorf's astonishment, Pirquet said that he was leaving for Vienna that evening. In explanation he said: "At Vienna I was the conductor of a symphony orchestra; here I am expected to play flute and fiddle."[37] He then offered Richdorf anything he wanted from among the books in his office.

Meanwhile, President Coffman renewed his efforts to interest the Rockefeller Foundation and General Education Board in helping to locate the Minneapolis General Hospital on a site next to the university hospital. He engaged in repeated consultations with the Board of Regents, the medical faculty, the Minneapolis Board of Public Welfare, and the Hennepin County Medical Society concerning the proposed relocation of the Minneapolis General Hospital. He was at the same time corresponding regularly with Abraham Flexner and George Edgar Vincent in New York City.

In late November 1923, George Edgar Vincent came to Minneapolis to speak at a luncheon celebrating the fiftieth anniversary of the *Northwestern Miller*. While at Minneapolis he conferred with President Coffman, Dean Lyon, and Fred B. Snyder, president of the Board of Regents, on the details of the plan, and during a tour of the campus visited the proposed hospital site.[38] On his return to New York, Vincent conferred with Abraham Flexner and Richard Pearce about the Minnesota proposals. President Coffman invited Abraham Flexner to come to

Minneapolis to look over the situation, but Flexner thought that he could not spare the time to come so far, so Coffman arranged to meet him at Chicago on Sunday morning, 9 December.[39] Following their meeting, Flexner nevertheless decided to come to Minneapolis to observe conditions for himself. When Flexner visited the medical school the next day he was shocked to find that it had developed hardly at all during the fourteen years since his previous visit in 1909. "As a matter of fact," wrote Flexner, "the institution by virtue of vigorous leadership, viz., a stand for a state medical school with high entrance and practice requirements, was in a leading position fifteen years ago. Since that date it has stood absolutely still, which means that it has gone back."[40] In 1923 Flexner thought that Minnesota no longer deserved to be considered an A grade school. He was disturbed by the failure of the university to allocate any of the Comprehensive Building Fund to the medical school, and its devotion of more than a million and a half dollars raised by public subscription to the building of a football stadium and a war memorial. Flexner thought that the proposal to build a new Minneapolis city hospital adjacent to the medical school was sound, but would probably have the effect of inhibiting the further development of the university hospital. He discussed the state of the medical school frankly with Dean Lyon, who agreed entirely with Flexner's pessimistic conclusions, but pinned his hopes on obtaining the Minneapolis city hospital because he despaired of ever enlarging the university hospital sufficiently to meet the needs of the medical school. Flexner also spoke to President Coffman and talked at some length with Dr. William Mayo, who was in Minneapolis for a meeting of the Board of Regents. "Nobody disputed the correctness of the facts," said Flexner, " . . . or the fairness of the conclusions, though there was some effort made to extenuate them, but when compared with what has been done by other state universities I do not see that any extenuation amounts to much." Flexner added: "The truth is that the Mayo Clinic has been allowed to run away with the whole medical show and men have been so interested in developing the Mayo Clinic that they have paid no attention to the medical department of the university, which is educationally of far greater importance."[41]

When Dr. Mayo and President Coffman spoke to Flexner of what the General Education Board had given the University of Iowa, Flexner said that their interest in Iowa arose from the great progress that had been made at the Iowa medical school during the previous ten years, up to the time they sought Rockefeller help. The situation of Iowa was, therefore, very different from that of Minnesota. That evening Dean Lyon visited Flexner at his hotel in Minneapolis to thank him for having, as Lyon said, "wrested the thing open." Dean Lyon said that he himself had tried, and failed, to point out the same things to the president and regents. Similarly, the superintendent of the university hospital, Dr. Louis Baldwin, described the inadequate and antiquated equipment of the hospital, " . . . though of course in confidence."[42] Flexner thought that conditions at the Elliot Hospital were prohibitive of good clinical work. Rowntree had been right to leave, and although Clemens von Pirquet had behaved badly, his abrupt departure was equally understandable. "He was undoubtedly told the truth before he came," wrote Flexner, "but I am not surprised that he failed to realize what the words written and said to him meant, for I myself was shocked when I came to the realization of how little progress had taken place in Minnesota in a dozen years."[43]

Despite Flexner's scathing analysis of the Minnesota situation, President Coffman decided to request from the General Education Board the sum of $2 million to help finance expenditures of $4 million for the expansion of the medical school and the university hospital, and for the relocation of the Minneapolis General Hospital. He planned to use about $1 million of the Rockefeller money to purchase a site for the Minneapolis General Hospital.[44] On 26 February 1924 the Minneapolis Board of Public Welfare held a special meeting to consider a possible joint request with the university to the Rockefeller Foundation and General Education Board to be used in part to purchase a site for the Minneapolis General Hospital.[45] At the meeting a committee of the Board of Public Welfare reported that the Minneapolis General Hospital was currently working to capacity with no extra beds available for emergencies, and that for some time they had been considering possible sites for a new hospital. They also noted that the existing relationship between the university and the General Hospital was particularly good, and that there were no conditions attached to the university's proposal except that when the city of Minneapolis was ready to build a new hospital, it should be built on the site that the university would provide. As a result of that meeting, the Minneapolis Board of Public Welfare on 4 March passed a resolution that it would join with the university in a request to the Rockefeller Foundation to provide land on which a new hospital might be built.[46] On 22 March 1924, President Coffman sent Abraham Flexner the joint petition of the University of Minnesota and the Minneapolis Department of Public Welfare for $2 million to be matched by an equal sum to be used in building laboratories and hospitals for the medical school and the college of dentistry, and to buy land adjacent to the campus on which to build a new Minneapolis General Hospital. The funds requested were to form part of a total expenditure of $4 million projected by the university to be spent in the next several years on new buildings for the medical school, the dental college, and the university hospital, and on land for the Minneapolis General Hospital. The request was accompanied by a detailed description of the medical school and its relationship with the Minneapolis General Hospital.

At its meeting at New York City on 20 November 1924, the General Education Board formally considered the Minnesota request. Because they did not make grants in the field of dentistry, the General Education Board eliminated the portion of the request relating to dentistry, thereby reducing the expenditures proposed from $4 million to $3.5 million. Of the latter sum the board authorized its executive committee to appropriate $1,250,000 for the University of Minnesota if such a grant would enable the university to carry through its entire program.[47] President Coffman was at New York when the General Education Board acted. From New York he wrote to his secretary, Miss Gregory, to advise her that in a few days a letter would come from Abraham Flexner to announce the proposed grant. Vincent and Flexner had told Coffman that if the legislature would extend the university's Comprehensive Building Program beyond 1929 to provide matching funds for the General Education Board grant, the grant funds would become available immediately and they could go ahead with the purchase of the land. Coffman added that Vincent thought that the whole project would be assured if the Mayos gave a gift of $500,000 for medical education at the university, and that Vincent was willing to help seek such a gift.[48]

After his return to Minneapolis, President Coffman wrote to Dr. Mayo on 10 December to inform him that if the medical program, which depended on the General Education Board grant, succeeded, they would have more than $3 million to spend on new buildings for the medical school and university hospital. He included a list of the proposed new buildings with their estimated costs.[49] Two days later, on 12 December, President Coffman made a public announcement of the General Education Board offer.

On 17 December in a memorandum to the Board of Regents, President Coffman set forth for the regents the points he had mentioned in his letter to Miss Gregory on 20 November. President Coffman told the regents: "When we have secured pledges and legislative action providing for $2,350,000 [*sic*], the entire sum offered by the General Education Board will be available at once."[50] Pledges might be payable over a period as long as six years. President Coffman thought it urgent to raise the matching funds because if they failed to do so, the university would have difficulty in making a new request to the General Education Board.

In allowing a broad latitude of time in which to make the matching funds available, the General Education Board was making allowance for the agricultural depression which was very severe in Minnesota during the early 1920s. What they were asking for was not cash, but commitments for the future, to match the General Education Board grant. Curiously, such commitments were not forthcoming, although in 1924 a grant of $1,250,000 represented a large sum of money of great potential benefit to the university. The gifts for the Todd Clinic, the Christian gift, and the Eustis gift could not be used to help match the General Education Board grant because they represented funds obtained before the grant was made and therefore were not new gifts or appropriations called forth by the grant. In a letter to Abraham Flexner on 13 December 1924 President Coffman suggested two sources of difficulty in raising the matching funds: " . . . one is that we propose to purchase land for the location of the Minneapolis General Hospital thereon, and the other is our proximity to the state of Iowa, where the gifts of the various [Rockefeller] foundations for medical education were on a fifty-fifty basis."[51] A few days later one of the regents, George H. Partridge, suggested that the response of private donors might depend on what the legislature would do to provide matching funds.[52] In response President Coffman said that the university could not launch a public drive for the matching funds, because they had not yet completed one to raise funds for the Northrop Memorial Auditorium and the football stadium. If the university asked the legislature for the matching money, they must ask for the whole amount and Coffman did not think that the state would be willing to appropriate that much money by extending the Comprehensive Building Program. On the other hand, if the university could obtain private gifts or pledges for half the total amount to be raised, or $1.8 million they could more easily persuade the legislature to extend the Comprehensive Building Program to provide the other $1.8 million, because then every dollar that the legislature appropriated would be matched by a dollar either from the General Education Board or from an individual donor. He ended by asking for Mr. Partridge's help " . . . in presenting the matter to the right people."[53]

In a press release to the Twin Cities Sunday newspapers for 21 December 1924, President Coffman and Dean Lyon announced that the medical school of the University of Minnesota, which ten years before had been far ahead of the medical schools of the Universities of Illinois, Iowa, Michigan, and Wisconsin, was in danger of falling behind them unless Minnesota could raise the funds required to match the $1,250,000 offered by the General Education Board. The University of Iowa was spending $4,500,000 on its medical school and hospital; Michigan had just completed a hospital at Ann Arbor that had cost more than $5 million; and so forth.[54] The next day that great-hearted man, William Henry Eustis, responded to their appeal. In a letter to Fred B. Snyder, president of the Board of Regents, Mr. Eustis said that that day he had completed the transfer to the university of income-bearing property in fulfillment of his pledge of 14 June 1923 to give $1 million for the benefit of crippled children, but that the said property together with the income accruing from it until 1 July 1927 would on the latter date have a value of $1.5 million. He wished, therefore, that the additional $500,000 which would become available in July 1927 and which would be over and above his pledge of June 23, should be used as matching funds to help secure the General Education Board gift.[55]

Apart from the press release in December, President Coffman appears to have been relatively inactive in the face of the need to raise funds to match the General Education Board grant. The University of Minnesota seemed tied down by invisible threads. It could not launch a public drive for contributions, and it could not ask the legislature to provide funds through extension of the Comprehensive Building Program past 1929 because the legislature might refuse. In the latter case, if the Board of Regents had made the request, and had it been denied, the burden of failure to obtain the General Education Board grant would rest with the legislature. As it was, failure remained the responsibility of the Board of Regents. As a result of Abraham Flexner's visit to Minnesota in December 1923, the General Education Board and the Rockefeller Foundation people suspected that a fundamental obstacle to the development of the university hospital and medical school was the rivalry of the Mayo Clinic exerted through Dr. William Mayo's membership on the Board of Regents. In the summer of 1924 in an interoffice memorandum on the Minnesota problem, Dr. Richard M. Pearce questioned whether funds were deflected from the medical school or building retarded by emphasis on the Mayo Clinic, and wondered what the attitude of the Mayo brothers toward the medical school really was. George Edgar Vincent thought that the

Minnesota medical school gained rather than suffered from the Mayo connection, but he also thought it important to get William J. Mayo to define his attitude.[56] Vincent thought that a substantial gift from the Mayos to be used on the Minneapolis campus, besides being valuable in itself, would provide the clearest evidence of Dr. Mayo's commitment to the development of the medical school. Early in December 1924 Vincent wrote to Mayo. He said that the willingness of the General Education Board to provide $1,250,000 " . . . ought to provide some inducement to the Legislature and to friends of the University to provide the remainder, but there is no disguising the fact that the project hangs in the balance." Vincent then said that one thing that would safely turn the scale would be a large gift at this time from the Mayo brothers to the University of Minnesota. He urged that because the Mayos were concerned chiefly for the graduate medical teaching carried on by the Mayo Foundation and the medical school they must realize " . . . that the proper development of the university medical equipment and clinical resources has a vital bearing upon the future growth and permanent prosperity of the joint undertaking." Urging that "Now is the critical hour . . . ," Vincent continued, "So out of my interest in Minnesota, my faith in you, my deep concern for the progress of scientific medicine, I am making bold to urge as earnestly as I know how that you and your brother make a handsome gift of say half a million to some unit of the building program on the Minneapolis campus. By doing this you would insure the success of the whole undertaking . . . ."[57]

To Vincent's eloquent pleas, Dr. Mayo said no. Mayo said that because he and his brother had turned over almost all their wealth to the Mayo Properties Association they were unable to make a large gift to the university, even if they wished to do so.[58] Unaware that Vincent had already tried and failed, President Coffman also attempted to obtain a gift from the Mayo brothers, which privately he had for some time hoped to do. That hope was promptly to be dashed. Early in the new year of 1925, Dr. William Mayo replied to President Coffman to say that he and his brother wished that they were in a position to make a gift, but that in 1919 all the property of the Mayo Clinic was transferred to trustees known as the Mayo Properties Association. Ultimately, said Mayo, the funds were to come to the university to support medical education and research. In addition to the endowment of the Mayo Foundation, the Mayo Properties Association then held, according to Dr. Mayo, some $5,250,000 worth of income-producing securities in addition to land and buildings worth perhaps $3 million. Nevertheless, the trustees of the Mayo Properties Association were prevented from using either income or principal for any purpose outside the terms of the gift, which was intended to endow the Mayo Clinic. The university, therefore, could hope for no gift from the Mayos in its immediate campaign.[59]

It was perhaps thoughtlessly cruel of Dr. Mayo to tantalize President Coffman with the prospect of so much wealth being hoarded for the future in the Mayo Properties Association, when the university needed urgently a much smaller sum to help provide matching funds. President Coffman may also have doubted that the funds were so completely inaccessible, if the Mayos wished to use them. At any rate when he received Dr. Mayo's letter written on 4 January, President Coffman replied immediately on 5 January to ask Dr. Mayo directly whether he and his brother might make a gift of $200,000 to the university for the medical school. Again Dr. Mayo replied that he and his brother did not have the means personally to make a gift of $200,000 to the university no matter how much they might wish to do so. In 1924 they had transferred to the Mayo Properties Association a considerable portion of their personal savings, retaining only the income during their lives so that they would not become pensioners on the Mayo Properties Association.[60] Lest President Coffman harbor any residual doubts concerning the ability of the Mayos to make a gift to the university, Dr. Mayo asked the two trustees of the Mayo Properties Association who were lawyers, Judge George W. Granger and Burt W. Eaton, for a legal opinion, and forwarded the opinion to President Coffman.[61] Judge Granger and Mr. Eaton wrote to Dr. Mayo that the powers of the Mayo Properties Association were limited to those stated in the deed of gift, and that it could not dispose of property for any purpose not authorized by the deed of gift.[62] Judge Granger and Mr. Eaton did not mention whether the donors might possess the power to alter the deed of gift to the Mayo Properties Association, nor does Dr. Mayo appear to have asked them to entertain such a possibility. President Coffman accepted their legal opinion as final.[63]

The refusal of the Mayos to make even a gift of $200,000 to help with the matching funds, as Abraham Flexner and George Edgar Vincent seem to have expected them to do, may have cast doubt on the feasibility of obtaining the funds to match the General Education Board grant.[64] A further difficulty was that some members of the Minneapolis Board of Public Welfare were interested in expanding the Minneapolis General Hospital on a site just across the street from where it was then located.[65]

During the winter of 1925, the medical school faculty formed a committee under Richard Olding Beard as chairman to seek building funds. When members of Dr. Beard's committee approached potential donors they were frequently confronted with two questions: "What is the University doing about it?" and "How much is the legislature asked to provide?" When the committee asked Dean Lyon how to answer such questions, he suggested that the university would request no building funds from the legislature because it was now doubtful whether the Minneapolis Board of Public Welfare would adhere to the plan to relocate the Minneapolis General Hospital, and referred them to President Coffman for further information. The committee then wrote to President Coffman that such wavering on the part of the Minneapolis Board of Public Welfare did not appear to be an adequate reason to halt the progress of the medical school and frustrate its efforts to secure funds.[66] The committee proposed that the university should immediately seek permission from the General Education Board to separate the question of the relocation of the Minneapolis General Hospital from the university's program and to divide the proposed fund into two parts, $2,800,000 for the university building program and $800,000 for future use to help in relocating the Minneapolis General Hospital. They would ask the General Education Board to apportion $1 million of its proposed gift to the first fund and $250,000 to the second fund. The committee recommended that the Board of Regents ask the legislature to extend the Comprehensive Building Program beyond 1929 and to seek private gifts to provide the matching funds required for the General Education Board grant.[67] The clarion call for action from Dr. Beard and his committee exerted no perceptible effect upon President Coffman or the Board of Regents. On 1 April President Coffman wrote to the committee concerning a possible request to the appropriation committees of the Minnesota State Legislature ". . . that it was the opinion of the members of the Board of Regents that it would be impossible to secure favorable action by either of the appropriation committees or by the legislature upon this request, and, as a matter of fact, it might tend to defeat any future consideration of the plan in case we wish to submit it to these houses two years hence."[68]

While President Coffman and the Board of Regents remained in a state of administrative paralysis, in New York Abraham Flexner was becoming restive. On 4 May he wrote to President Coffman to ask whether " . . . the project of rebuilding the municipal hospital on the University site, towards which our Board has made an appropriation, has fallen through?"[69] Although in May President Coffman remained hopeful that the Minneapolis Board of Public Welfare would decide ultimately to move the General Hospital to the university, by September he and the Board of Regents concluded that such hopes were vain. President Coffman then wrote to Abraham Flexner to ask the General Education Board to reduce the program by $750,000 from the original overall amount of $3.6 million to $2,850,000 of which he asked the General Education Board to provide $950,000, while the University of Minnesota would raise $1.9 million in matching funds.[70] In response to Coffman's proposal Flexner suggested that in the new situation " . . . I think you ought to work out a plan of development and once more submit your project to us."[71] Two days later he wrote that on 17 October he and Dr. Pearce expected to be in Minneapolis, when they hoped to see President Coffman and Dean Lyon. In fact they appear not to have made the trip, but that Flexner intended to do so suggests the seriousness with which he viewed the change in the Minnesota situation. On 31 October President Coffman wrote to Abraham Flexner that the proposal outlined briefly in his letter of 4 October *was* the new proposal of the University of Minnesota. He added that a number of beneficial results had already occurred as a result of the 1924 offer from the General Education Board. Two persons had made wills in favor of the medical school, and the prospective bequests would provide funds for new buildings and endowment. Also since the General Education Board had made their offer to Minnesota, William Henry Eustis, who had already given more than $1 million to the university for a hospital and convalescent home for crippled children, had offered a new gift of money and income-yielding property to a value of between a half million and three quarters of a million dollars which would become available in 1927, and could be used to match the General Education Board offer. President Coffman did not mention any request to the Minnesota State Legislature for matching funds (and the Board of Regents had made none), so he left unstated where the remainder of the matching funds were to come from. After repeating his request to reduce the Minnesota program by $750,000 to $2,850,000 of which the General Education Board would be asked to contribute $950,000, President Coffman offered to come to New York City to discuss the matter, if that should be necessary.[72] Abraham Flexner replied immediately that the Minnesota proposal was still too indefinite to be used as a basis for negotiation. Flexner asked Coffman to specify in detail what the money in the new request would be for. Flexner offered to see Coffman in New York at any time and also suggested that he might be able to meet him at Chicago in late November, but said that an interview would not be a substitute for a written statement of the Minnesota proposal.

On 16 November President Coffman sent Abraham Flexner an amended petition that had been approved by the Board of Regents at their meeting two days before. The amended petition listed uses for the $2,850,000 in the proposed program:

Additional Wing to Millard Hall	$300,000
Additional Wing to the Institute of Anatomy	450,000
Nurses building	450,000
Additions to the University Hospital:	
Psychopathic Unit	200,000
Children's Unit (Eustis gift)	400,000
Women's Hospital unit	350,000
General medicine and surgery	300,000
Hospital laboratories	150,000
Outpatient buildings	250,000
Total	$2,850,000

The Board of Regents asked that Mr. Eustis's new gift, valued at $500,000 or more, be permitted to count toward the matching funds for the $950,000 requested from the General Education Board. They also hoped to obtain additional private gifts, but would request the legislature to provide whatever additional matching funds might be needed.[73]

When Abraham Flexner received the amended Minnesota petition, he was making preparations to leave New York to be gone for several months, and would be abroad when the General Education Board met in late February 1926. On 5 December Flexner wrote to Coffman that he could do nothing then concerning the amended petition, but would take it up promptly on his return.[74] When Flexner's letter arrived in Minneapolis, President Coffman had himself left for a trip to Honolulu, not to return until mid-February 1926.[75] It is difficult to conjecture what may have been Abraham Flexner's reaction when he learned that President Coffman had left Minneapolis for an ocean voyage to Hawaii to be gone more than two months. At least it must have removed from his mind any sense of urgency about the Minnesota request. It may also have caused him to doubt whether the

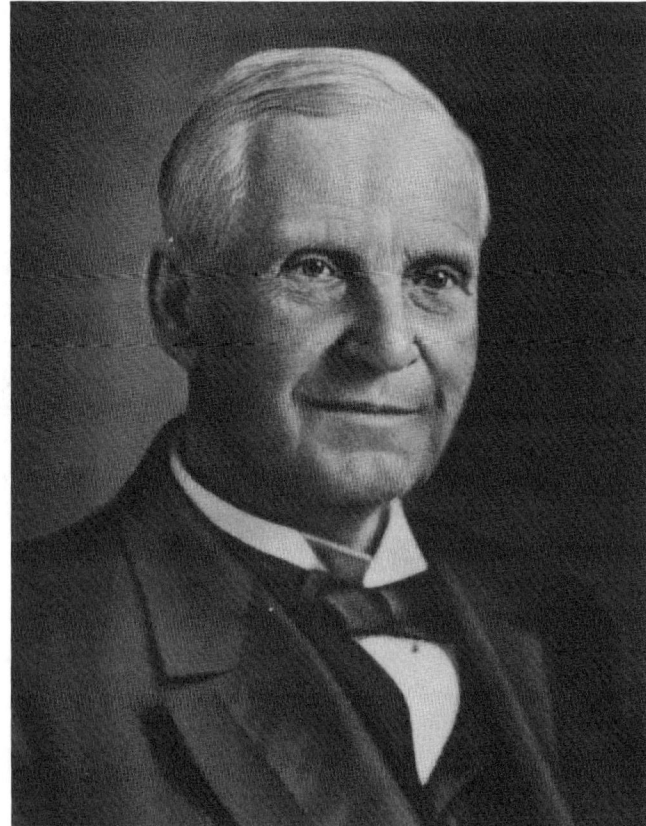

FIGURE 12:5 William Henry Eustis, circa 1925. Courtesy Minnesota Historical Society.

Board of Regents were in earnest in attempting to seek funds to match a General Education Board grant.

Despite the torpor of the Board of Regents, nothing seemed to discourage the generous spirit of William Henry Eustis. Mr. Eustis's pocket seemed bottomless. Having already given to the university his four-fifths interest in the Flour and Corn Exchange Building in Minneapolis, he decided in March 1926 to buy from his brother Gardner T. Eustis the remaining one-fifth interest in the building, and to give it also to the university to help match the General Education Board offer. Said Mr. Eustis to the regents:

> The time is ripe under your guidance to establish here one of the great medical centers of the World. The helpful generosity of the Rockefeller Foundation, the genius of the University, and the old time spirit of Minneapolis united and working in closest accord, bearing aloft the banner of Excelsior would establish here a beacon light of medical science and research that shall for all ages resound to the glory of man's genius and the highest welfare of his being.

He concluded: "The tide is at its flood. The golden opportunity is here, and I cannot believe that the heroic, civic spirit that once dominated Minneapolis will now be weighed in the balance and found wanting."[76] Well, when the civic spirit of Minneapolis was weighed in the balance, it was found wanting. Mean and petty calculations triumphed over the vision of a great united medical center. Yet it was no shame to Mr. Eustis that he thought better of his fellow citizens than they deserved. Through his own generosity, he, himself a citizen of Minneapolis, redeemed their shortcomings. Ultimately, he would achieve the fulfillment of his dream at the university.

In February 1926 a committee of the Minneapolis City Council attempted to revive the plan to relocate the Minneapolis General Hospital at the university and President Coffman sent a telegram to Abraham Flexner asking him to delay consideration of the modified request sent to the General Education Board the previous November.[77] In April President Coffman was still hopeful that the original plan might be rescued. On 6 April the Minneapolis City Council demanded that the university present its proposals "in proper written and definite form."[78] In reply President Coffman sent copies of all correspondence between the Board of Public Welfare and the Board of Regents and reviewed the history of negotiations on the question of relocation of the Minneapolis General Hospital.[79] Thereafter nothing happened. At the end of July President Coffman sent a polite inquiry as to what the city intended to do. The President of the Minneapolis City Council, O. J. Turner, replied that he hoped to have a decision in late August or early September.[80] Nevertheless, the Minneapolis City Council reached no decision. President Coffman and the Board of Regents continued to wait with folded hands. More than a year later, at the end of November 1927, Dean Lyon wrote to President Coffman to inquire about the status of negotiations, and to state that it was the unanimous opinion of the administrative committee of the medical school that the proposal was already dead.[81] Finally in December 1927 the Board of Regents decided to abandon further negotiations with the city of Minneapolis.[82] Meanwhile, the University of Minnesota had forfeited the possibility of obtaining a grant from the General Education Board. At President Coffman's request the General Education Board had not considered the university's modified petition sent in November 1925, and a year later without informing the University of Minnesota, which they evidently considered to be a body too incapable of action to respond, the General Education Board withdrew the authorization to its Executive Committee to make a grant of $1,250,000 on the basis of the petition submitted in 1924.

Although the possibility of obtaining a General Education Board gift died in 1925, and the General Education Board itself merely recognized the fact on 18 November 1926, various persons in Minnesota, including President Coffman, kept poking at the corpse. In January 1928 the Minneapolis City Council took the seemingly superfluous action of declining to continue negotiations with the university for acceptance of the General Education Board gift, an action that was condemned by vigorous editorials in the Minneapolis newspapers. President Coffman thought that the university was not free to pursue its own course for the development of the medical school, and in his innocence he thought " . . . that the General Education Board would be willing to modify its offer to the University in accordance with almost any reasonable proposal which we may submit."[83] But if the university were to obtain a General Education Board gift it would have to raise matching funds, and although Coffman thought that the Eustis gift and other smaller gifts would be allowed to count toward the matching money, additional gifts would be needed. He turned to Dr. Mayo for help.

> Frankly [Coffman wrote to Mayo], I think there is only one man who can do this, and you are that man. If you would take a month or two to confer with just the right persons in Minneapolis and St. Paul, you could, in my opinion, easily raise any sum which may be necessary to match the General Education Board gift. No one else could do it. Activity on your part among the right persons would arouse interest and confidence among all; the project would succeed. I wish you would think it over and let me know if you would be willing to undertake it with such cooperation, of course, as Mr. Snyder and I can give you.[84]

Dr. Mayo declined: "While I should be glad to talk to certain people I know and to do whatever I could," wrote Mayo, "in consideration of the load I am carrying and the engagements I have made, it would be impossible for me to give the length of time you suggest for a drive."[85] President Coffman was still insistent. "In case it seems necessary or advisable for us to attempt to raise a considerable sum of money locally," he wrote, "I am still certain that there is no one who can do it half so well as you."[86]

In May 1928 Dean Lyon sent to George Edgar Vincent a proposal for the university to take over the Minneapolis General Hospital on a long term agreement. In reply Vincent cautioned Lyon that Minnesota must not count on a gift from the General Education Board. The money set aside for the University of Minnesota in 1924 had now been appropriated for other institutions.[87] Dean Lyon was taken aback. "What you say in regard to the General Education Board is disquieting," he wrote to Vincent. "I did not think they would divert funds previously voted for use here without some notice to this institution and so far as I know none has ever been given."[88] George Vincent then consulted Abraham Flexner who confirmed that on 18 November 1926 the General Education Board had withdrawn authority to conduct negotiations with the University of Minnesota concerning a gift, and that he regarded the negotiations as then having been formally terminated. Undaunted President Coffman wrote to President Vincent at the Rockefeller Foundation the following October to say that he thought the Minneapolis Board of Public Welfare and City Council now recognized the mistake they had made earlier and to ask that he might have lunch with Vincent when he came to New York in late November. In reply Vincent wrote formally to say that the former application was dead, and that a new application from the University of Minnesota could not now be considered. He added: "I am sorry that things have turned out this way. Personally, as you know, I was much interested in this plan and did everything I could to promote it. You will, I know, agree that a Board cannot be expected to maintain outstanding offers indefinitely."[89] Persistent, now when persistence had become pointless, President Coffman called to see the president of the General Education Board, Trevor Arnett, on 21 November, during a visit to New York City, but again received a definite no.[90] So far as the General Education Board and the Rockefeller Foundation were concerned, the subject was closed and could not be reopened.

Although the effort to obtain the General Education Board grant failed, other parts of the plan to expand the university hospital moved forward during the 1920s. To the gifts given in memory of Dr. Todd, the Board of Regents added $117,500 from the Comprehensive Building Fund to provide a total of $162,500 for the Todd Memorial Clinic, intended to provide forty beds for eye, ear, nose, and throat patients. During the summer and fall of 1923 the architects prepared preliminary plans for the Todd Memorial Clinic and the George Chase Christian Cancer Hospital. In the fall the heads of the clinical departments of the medical school decided that the new wings to be added to the university hospital must contain a completely equipped lecture room capable of seating 125 to 150 persons. Although such a lecture room could not be fitted within the walls of the Christian and Todd buildings, as they had been first laid out, the architect was able to do it by widening the Todd building where it turned off from the Christian.[91] Thus was created the Todd amphitheater which has been used for grand rounds in medicine and surgery at Minnesota ever since the buildings were completed.

On 1 October 1924, in formal ceremonies, the cornerstones of the Todd and Christian units were laid, and a year later on 19 October 1925 they opened, their 120 beds bringing the total capacity of the university hospital to more than 300 beds.[92] They were the first significant additions to the Elliot Memorial Hospital since the latter had opened fourteen years earlier in 1911. The George Chase Christian Cancer Hospital was also planned to contain x-ray and radium laboratories, and a cancer outpatient department, but these facilities were not completed for another fifteen months, opening finally in February 1927. The x-ray room, behind its walls of greenish tile, was sheathed completely by a layer of lead more than half an inch thick, intended to prevent the escape of the radiation used in cancer treatment. With the help of a bequest from the Howard Baker estate, the cancer hospital also purchased a half gram of radium, costing more than $30,000, which was kept within a lead sphere and stored in a large iron safe.[93] When the cancer clinic opened in 1927, its facilities for the radiation treatment of cancer represented the most modern then available, and provided means of radiation therapy far more powerful than at any other medical center in the Northwest, including the Mayo Clinic. The equipment was selected and its installation supervised by a radiation physicist, Karl Wilhelm Stenstrom, who was invited to Minnesota from the New York State Institute of Malignant Disease at Buffalo, together with his wife, Dr. Annette Stenstrom, who was a radiation therapist. On 1 July 1927 Dr. Leo G. Rigler returned from a year of advanced study in radiology with Dr. Gösta Forssell at Stockholm, Sweden to become associate professor in the Depart-

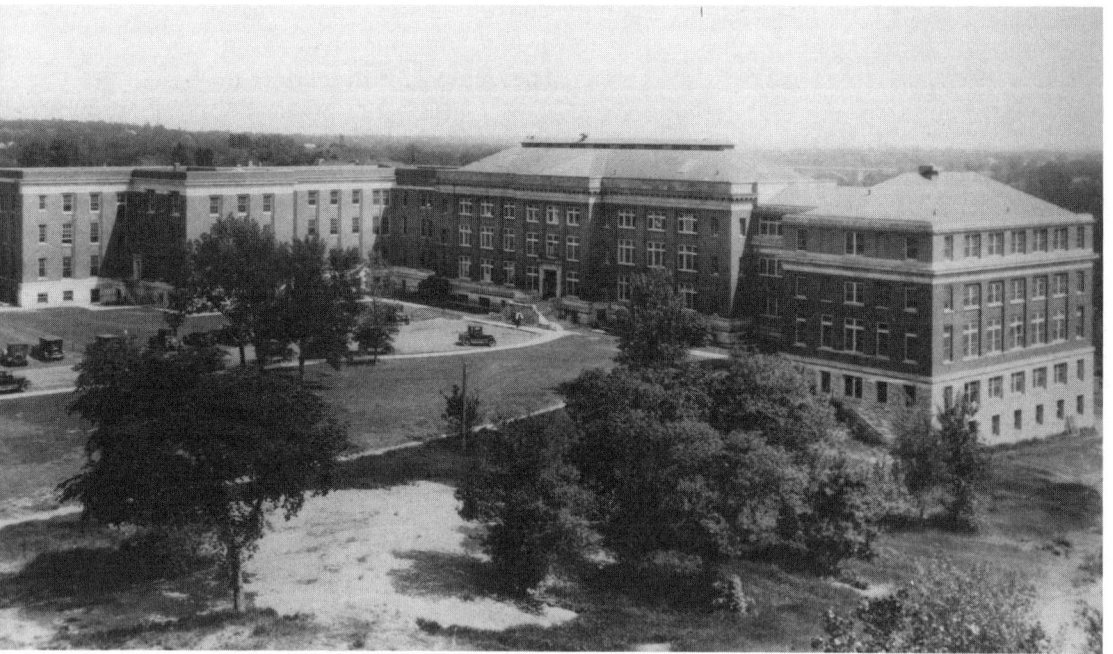

FIGURE 12:6 Elliot Hospital, center, with the new Christian and Todd wings on the left, circa 1926. Courtesy Mn U Archives.

ment of Medicine and chief of the Division of Radiology in the university hospital.[94] At the Christian Cancer Hospital Dr. Rigler assumed charge of diagnostic radiology while the Stenstroms supervised radiation therapy.

By the autumn of 1927 the trust fund, consisting of property and securities given by William Henry Eustis at various times since 1923, had accumulated sufficient income that the university could begin construction of the hospital for diseased and crippled children that was to form part of the university hospital.[95] The new Eustis children's hospital was to be connected to the Elliot Memorial Hospital as a three-story wing at right angles to the west end just as the Christian Cancer Hospital and Todd Memorial Clinic formed an extended wing at right angles to the east end of the hospital. In 1927 the Board of Regents also decided to build a new outpatient department as an extension of the wing to contain the Eustis children's hospital, the additional building to be paid for from the Comprehensive Building Fund. In July 1927 Dean Lyon recommended that a new building for the students' health service and a roof house to provide a residence for interns be included in the plans, and in September the Board of Regents approved Dean Lyon's recommendations.[96] The Eustis children's hospital, the outpatient department, and the students' health service would together add 148 beds to the university hospital and the whole building program would cost approximately $900,000, of which $250,000 would come from the Eustis fund and the remainder from the Comprehensive Building Program, provided by the Minnesota legislature.

The Eustis children's hospital was to include on the ground floor a lecture amphitheater and space for the Department of Pathology. On the main floor was to be a children's outpatient department and offices for the Department of Pediatrics, while the two upper floors would contain the hospital for crippled or sick children and would include a school for crippled children who had to be hospitalized for extended periods of time.

The new building for the outpatient department was to include on the ground floor the admission office for the whole group of university hospitals, a central pharmacy, the outpatient department with specially equipped examination rooms, and the social service department. The upper two floors of the outpatient building were to be hospital floors containing seventy-eight beds in two- and four-bed wards. In a roof house was to be a residence for the interns.[97]

The students' health service was founded by President Burton in 1918 with Dr. John Sundwall as director. During the period of the First World War it was located in two fraternity houses on University Avenue with two other locations on the St. Paul campus in the men's and women's dormitories, and was hardly opened when it had to deal with the devastating influenza epidemic of the fall of 1918. On 1 February 1919 the health service moved into the first floor of Pillsbury Hall, which was remodeled to accommodate it. During 1919–20 the health service had to deal with a second serious influenza epidemic with more than five thousand cases. In 1920–21 there was an epidemic of smallpox among the students with forty-three cases, and to prevent the spread of the epidemic the health service vaccinated more than three thousand students. During the same year the health service carried out an epidemiological study of a paratyphoid epidemic involving about a hundred students, and located its cause in a paratyphoid carrier, who was infecting the milk as he dipped it out of ten-gallon cans into glasses. As a result of the investigation the university began to serve milk sealed in individual bottles at the time of pasteurizing.

When Dr. Sundwall left the university in 1921, President Coffman appointed Harold S. Diehl director of the students' health service, and under Dr. Diehl the health service developed rapidly through the 1920s. During the winter of 1924–25 when an epidemic of malignant smallpox occurred in the Twin Cities, the health service vaccinated some eight thousand students within a month's time. Seven students, who had not been vaccinated, contracted smallpox and two of them died, but such numbers were very small when compared with 1,000 cases and 300 deaths from smallpox in Minneapolis. As a result of the epidemic the health service began to make vaccination part of the physical examination of each student upon admission to the university. The health service was also concerned with the early diagnosis and treatment of tuberculosis among students to restrict communication of the disease, but within the cramped confines of the first floor of Pillsbury Hall it was limited in what it could do. Although the health service gave every student a complete physical examination on admission, it did not require later ex-

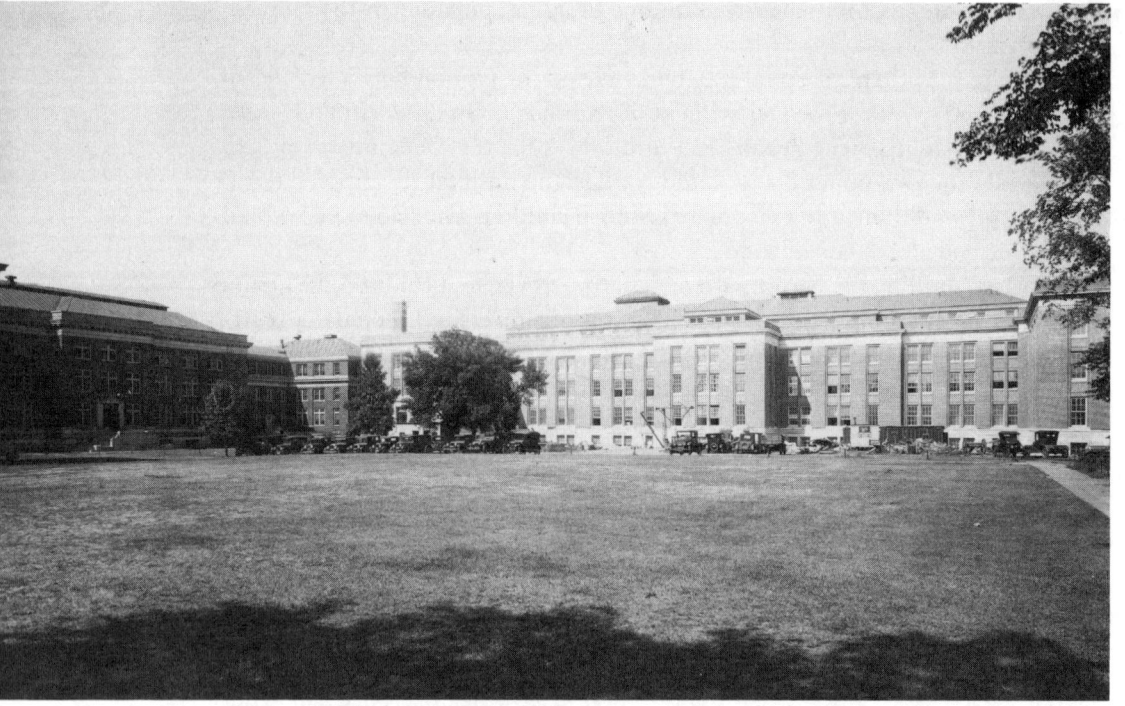

FIGURE 12:7 Eustis Hospital on completion in 1929. Outpatient department and Students' Health Service were in wings on the right. Courtesy Mn U Archives.

amination of students, except for medical students, members of the Reserve Officers Training Corps, and candidates for athletic teams. Medical students especially were at risk of contracting tuberculosis through their contacts with patients in hospital and dispensary, but in the 1920s all students were at some risk of contracting tuberculosis during the university years, so in 1926–27 the health service began to offer periodic health examinations to medical, dental, and law students and to seniors in other colleges. In the new building the health service planned to extend its offer of periodic health examinations to a still larger portion of the student population.

The cornerstone of the Eustis Hospital was laid on 10 November 1928 in a formal ceremony at which Dr. Charles H. Mayo was the principal speaker. Mr. Eustis, then eighty-three years of age, was at home ill, but listened to the speeches as they were broadcast over the radio, his brother acting for him in laying the cornerstone. Less than three weeks later on Friday, 29 November, Mr. Eustis died. At two o'clock the following Monday afternoon, the day of his funeral and at the time he was being buried, all classes of the medical school observed two minutes of silence. Although it had been suggested that the medical school should dismiss classes for the afternoon in honor of Mr. Eustis, Dean Lyon, who had come to know him quite well since Mr. Eustis made his first gift to the university in 1923, decided not. Dean Lyon said that all his life Mr. Eustis had been a hard worker, and if his burial were made an occasion to dismiss classes, Dean Lyon thought that Mr. Eustis would have resented it.

Born the son of a wagon maker at Exbow in northern New York State in 1845, at the age of fifteen William Eustis had suffered a fall from a horse which resulted in a hip ailment that left him permanently crippled. For three years he could only hobble about on crutches, but throughout his illness he continued to study. At the age of twenty he began to teach school, and later entered Wesleyan College where he was graduated in 1873. He then studied law at Columbia University and began to practice law, first in New York City and after 1881 in Minneapolis. He also invested in real estate with remarkable success. A lifelong Republican, Eustis became active in politics and in 1892 was elected mayor of Minneapolis. As mayor he was confronted almost immediately with the massive unemployment that accompanied the severe economic depression of 1893. He organized relief to provide food, clothing, and fuel for the poor. Eustis reorganized the Minneapolis police department. In response to complaints that customers were being robbed in saloons, Eustis acted to make saloon-keepers responsible for crimes committed on their premises, enforcing the law fearlessly. At the time of the great Hinckley fire in northern Minnesota, Mayor Eustis organized relief for those whom the fire had left destitute. Fierce but kind, William Eustis was a lonely man, who endured much pain throughout his life. Now at the end of his life he gave his fortune to help those who were crippled as he had been.

Mr. Eustis had not wished the hospital that he gave to bear his name, lest the fact that it was named for him should deter others from making gifts to it. Nevertheless, Dean Lyon and the superintendent of the university hospital, Paul Fesler, both thought that the children's hospital should be called the Eustis Hospital, as did also the state architect, Clarence Johnson. When they discussed the question with Mr. Eustis, he refused. "Finally," wrote Dean Lyon, "Mr. Fesler took a set of the plans to him; on the outside view the name Eustis had been put in. Mr. Eustis laughingly concurred."[98] From a practical point of view, Dean Lyon knew that they must call the building by some name so that patients, their families, and other visitors could find it, and *Eustis* was the only fitting name for it.

When the Eustis Hospital opened in 1929, the Board of Regents assigned $40,000 annually of the income from the Eustis endowment to support twenty beds for children's orthopedics in the hospital.[99] Other child patients in the Eustis Hospital were either to be paid for from county-state funds or might be per diem patients or private patients.[100]

The addition of the three new units to the university hospitals in 1929, an addition which increased their total capacity to 400 beds, was a major expansion that affected every service. In its larger, better-equipped, and more cheerful quarters, the outpatient department began to receive an increasing flow of patients. During the first year the number of patient visits grew from fewer than 61,000 to more than 65,000. Patients who needed hospital care were referred from the outpatient

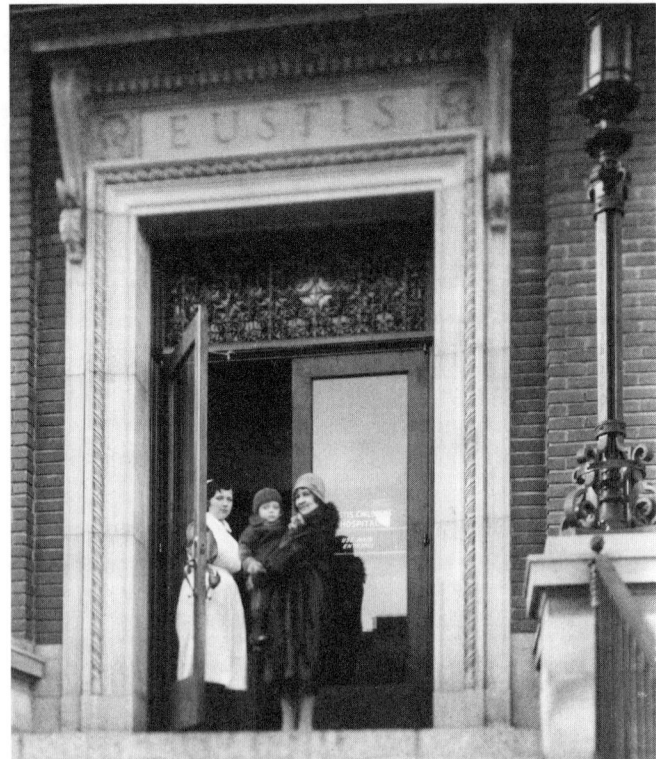

FIGURE 12:8   Entrance, Eustis Children's Hospital, 1930. Courtesy Mn U Archives.

department to the university hospital so that the daily average number of patients in the hospital also increased some 27 percent during the first year.[101] The enlarged hospital, with its greater population of patients offered new opportunities for clinical investigation in medicine, surgery, pediatrics, and radiology, which a young and vigorous group of full-time clinicians at Minnesota began eagerly to exploit.

NOTES

1. " 'Hope deferred maketh the heart sick,' and conversely, hope resurgent means the uplift of the spirit." Editorial [W. A. Jones], "A greater medical school in Minnesota," *J.-Lancet,* 1924, *44,* 520–521, p. 520.

2. School of Medicine, Administrative Board, Minutes, 12 November 1918.

3. Frank C. Todd, draft of will and accompanying document, "The Eye, Ear, Nose and Throat Hospital to be established near the University Campus thru funds provided in the will of Frank C. Todd, M.D.," President's Office, Papers.

4. Sara Pillsbury Gale, promise to pay $20,000 "to Dr. Todd or those whom he may designate," dated 22 May 1917 [copy], President's Office, Papers.

5. "Excerpt from the Minutes of the Committee on Hospital Extension, December 17, 1919," President's Office, Papers.
6. Burton to Mrs. Frank C. Todd, 19 January 1920, President's Office, Papers.
7. Snyder to Burton, 21 January 1920, President's Office, Papers.
8. White to Burton, 8 May 1920, President's Office, Papers.
9. Burton to White, 11 May 1920, President's Office, Papers.
10. Ibid. Cf. Burton to Mayo, 12 May 1920 [copy], President's Office, Papers.
11. Burton to Coffman, 11 May 1920, President's Office, Papers.
12. Burton to Coffman, 17 May 1920, President's Office, Papers.
13. White to Mayo, 30 November 1920 [copy]; cf. Coffman to Mayo, 30 November 1920 [copy], President's Office, Papers.
14. Mayo to Coffman, 3 December 1920, President's Office, Papers.
15. Lyon to Coffman, 20 June 1922, President's Office, Papers.
16. Mayo to Lyon, 21 June 1922 [copy], President's Office, Papers.
17. Lyon to Mayo, 30 June 1922 [copy], President's Office, Papers. Dr. Mayo, undeterred by the considerations noted by Dean Lyon, suggested at a meeting of the Board of Regents in July that the medical school should go on double shift. The *Journal-Lancet* commented: "Physicians do this stunt in emergencies but can teachers do it continually?" *J.-Lancet,* 1922, *42,* 373.
18. Lyon to Coffman, 30 June 1922, President's Office, Papers.
19. Lyon, "The medical school, the medical profession, and the public welfare," *J.-Lancet,* 1922, *42,* 275–380, p. 328.
20. Mayo to Coffman, 19 December 1922, President's Office, Papers.
21. Coffman to Snyder, 7 February 1923 [copy], President's Office, Papers . The Board of Regents voted to accept the gift at their meeting the following day, Tuesday, 6 February 1923, and appointed a committee to confer with a committee of the Citizen's Aid Society on the details of the gift. Coffman to Mrs. George C. Christian, 8 February 1923 [copy], President's Office, Papers.
22. Mayo to Coffman, 9 February 1923, President's Office, Papers.
23. Coffman to Mayo, 13 February 1923 [copy], President's Office, Papers.
24. Coffman to Mrs. George C. Christian, 17 April 1923 [copy], President's Office, Papers.
25. Coffman to Vincent, 19 February 1923 [copy], President's Office, Papers.
26. Alan M. Chesney, *The Johns Hopkins Hospital and the Johns Hopkins University School of Medicine,* III, 78–79, 106, 122–127.
27. Ibid., pp. 194–202.
28. Lyon to Pirquet, 7 April 1923 [copy], President's Office, Papers.
29. Pirquet to Lyon, 3 May 1923, printed in "Why did Dr. Pirquet leave Minnesota . . . ?" *Minn. Alumni Wkly,* 1923, *23,* 93–96, p. 95.
30. School of Medicine, Administrative Board, Minutes, 23 May 1923.
31. Lyon to Pirquet, 28 May 1923, printed in "Why did Dr. Pirquet leave Minnesota . . . ?" *Minn. Alumni Wkly,* 1923, *23,* 93–96, p. 95.
32. Ibid.
33. Coffman to Flexner, 31 May 1923 [copy]; Coffman to Vincent, 31 May 1923 [copy], President's Office, Papers.
34. William H. Eustis to Fred B. Snyder, 14 June 1923 in Board of Regents, Minutes, 19 June 1923.
35. Dean Lyon's statement on Dr. Pirquet's departure in "Why did Dr. Pirquet leave Minnesota . . . ?" *Minn. Alumni Wkly,* 1923, *23,* 93–96, p. 96.
36. Ibid.

37. Tape recorded interview with Dr. Lawrence Richdorf by Dr. Stuart Lane Arey, 1984, Mn U Archives.
38. "Excerpts from G.E.V.'s diary, Saturday, November 24, 1923," General Education Board, Box 7078, Folder no. 7267.
39. Coffman to Flexner, 5 November 1923 [copy]; Flexner to Coffman, 20 November 1923, President's Office, Papers.
40. Flexner, "University of Minnesota, Minneapolis, Minnesota, December 10, 1923," General Education Board, Box 707, Folder no. 7267.
41. Flexner, "Memorandum for Dr. Vincent, December 15, 1923," General Education Board, Box 707, Folder no. 7267.
42. Ibid.
43. Ibid.
44. Coffman to Richard Tattersfield, 21 February 1924 [copy], President's Office, Papers.
45. Tattersfield to Coffman, 19 February 1924, President's Office, Papers.
46. Tattersfield to Albert J. Lobb, 4 March 1924, President's Office, Papers.
47. Flexner to Coffman, 25 November 1924, President's Office, Papers.
48. Coffman to Miss Gregory [20 November 1924], President's Office, Papers.
49. Coffman to Mayo, 10 December 1924 [copy], President's Office, Papers.
50. Coffman to members of the Board of Regents, 17 December 1924, President's Office, Papers, 1911–1945.
51. Coffman to Flexner, 13 December 1924 [copy], President's Office, Papers.
52. George H. Partridge to Coffman, 18 December 1924, President's Office, Papers.
53. Coffman to Partridge, 19 December 1924, President's Office, Papers.
54. "Sunday Papers, December 21 [1924]," President's Office, Papers.
55. Eustis to Snyder, 22 December 1924, Board of Regents, Minutes, 23 January 1925.
56. Richard M. Pearce, "The Minnesota problem;" Vincent, "Memorandum of comments on R.M.P.'s analysis," General Education Board, Box 707, Folder no. 7268.
57. Vincent to Mayo, 4 December 1924 [copy], General Education Board, Box 707, Folder no. 7268.
58. Mayo to Vincent, 10 December 1924, General Education Board, Box 707, Folder no. 7268.
59. Mayo to Coffman, 4 January 1925, President's Office, Papers, 1911–1945.
60. Mayo to Coffman, 6 January 1925, President's Office, Papers.
61. Mayo to Coffman, 8 January 1925, President's Office, Papers.
62. George W. Granger and Burt W. Eaton to Mayo, 7 January 1925, President's Office, Papers.
63. Coffman to Mayo, 19 January 1925, President's Office, Papers.
64. When George H. Partridge happened to meet George Edgar Vincent on the train from Chicago to New York on 25 January, Partridge told him that there was much doubt whether the city hospital and university plan would go through. Vincent to Coffman, 26 January 1925, President's Office, Papers.
65. Coffman to Vincent, 29 January 1925 [copy], President's Office, Papers.
66. Richard Olding Beard and members of the committee to Coffman, 4 March 1925, President's Office, Papers.
67. Ibid.
68. Coffman to Beard, 1 April 1925 [copy], President's Office, Papers.
69. Flexner to Coffman, 4 May 1925, President's Office, Papers.
70. Coffman to Flexner, 24 September 1925 [copy], President's Office, Papers.
71. Flexner to Coffman, 7 October 1925, President's Office, Papers.

72. Coffman to Flexner, 31 October 1925 [copy], President's Office, Papers. Coffman sent Flexner two letters dated 31 October 1925. In the second letter he enclosed a copy of a letter from George Leach, Mayor of Minneapolis, in which Mr. Leach asked that, although the university should proceed with its development without waiting for the city of Minneapolis, he hoped that it might be possible to renew the request for funds to relocate the Minneapolis General Hospital at a future time.

73. Coffman to Flexner, 16 November 1925 [copy], President's Office, Papers.

74. Flexner to Coffman, 5 December 1925, President's Office, Papers.

75. President Coffman's secretary to Flexner, 12 December 1925 [copy], President's Office, Papers.

76. Eustis to Snyder, 29 March 1926, Board of Regents, Minutes, 1 April 1926.

77. Coffman to Flexner, 5 April 1926 [copy], President's Office, Papers.

78. O. J. Turner [Chairman, Special Committee on Public Welfare, Minneapolis City Council] to Coffman, 6 April 1926, President's Office, Papers.

79. Coffman to Turner, 9 April 1926 [copy], President's Office, Papers.

80. Coffman to Turner, 31 July 1926 [copy], Turner to Coffman, 11 August 1926, President's Office, Papers.

81. Lyon to Coffman, 29 November 1927, President's Office, Papers.

82. Coffman to John Ryan [President, Minneapolis City Council], 20 December 1927 [copy], President's Office, Papers.

83. Coffman to Mayo, 16 January 1928 [copy], President's Office, Papers.

84. Ibid.

85. Mayo to Coffman, 28 January 1928. President's Office, Papers.

86. Coffman to Mayo, 31 January 1928 [copy]., President's Office, Papers.

87. Vincent to Lyon, 22 May 1928 [copy], President's Office Papers.

88. Lyon to Vincent, 26 May 1928 [copy], President's Office, Papers.

89. Vincent to Coffman, 12 November 1928, President's Office, Papers.

90. Trevor Arnett to Coffman, 7 December 1928, President's Office, Papers. In his history of the university, James Gray states inaccurately that in January 1928 the university notified the Rockefeller Foundation that the Board of Regents were unable to take advantage of its offer. See Gray, *The University of Minnesota 1851-1951*, p. 292.

91. Lyon to Coffman, 26 November 1923. President's Office, Papers.

92. "Todd, Cancer Institutes opened," *Minn. Alumni Wkly,* 1915-26, 25 (no. 5), 96.

93. "Cancer clinic opens to public this week," *Minn. Alumni Wkly,* 1926-27 , 26 (no. 19), 316.

94. Leo G. Rigler, "Learning and teaching under Dean Lyon," in Owen H. Wangensteen, ed., *Elias Potter Lyon,* pp. 121-141.

95. Board of Regents, Minutes, 19 July 1927; Coffman to Eustis, 21 July 1927 [copy], President's Office, Papers.

96. Lyon to Coffman, 28 July 1927, Coffman to Lyon, Diehl, and Fesler, 28 September 1927 [copy], President's Office, Papers; Board of Regents, Minutes, 28 September 1927.

97. "University Hospital adds three important units. Eustis Children's Hospital, Outpatient Department, and Students' Health Service will be housed in a new wing now to be built," *Minnesota Chats,* 1927, 8, 3-7.

98. Lyon to Coffman, 30 April 1929, President's Office, Papers.

99. School of Medicine, Administrative Committee, Minutes, 24 April 1929. Cf. Coffman to Lyon, 28 May 1929 [copy], President's Office, Papers.

100. Lyon to Coffman, 31 May 1929, President's Office, Papers.

101. Paul H. Fesler, "University Hospitals" in University of Minnesota, *President's report for . . . 1928-30,* pp. 299-302.

CHAPTER 13

The Development of a Full-time Clinical Faculty 1925–1930

The abrupt departure of Clemens von Pirquet in October 1923 after only twelve days as head of the Department of Pediatrics at Minnesota raised in sharp relief all the difficult questions surrounding clinical appointments in the medical school—questions that had haunted the administrative board since the reorganization of the school ten years before. The swift coming and going of Dr. Pirquet was merely an unusually striking episode in a continuing procession of clinical teachers to and then away from the medical school. In 1916 Leonard Rowntree had come from Johns Hopkins to head the Department of Medicine only to depart in 1920, attracted by the golden lure of the Mayo Clinic, but frustrated also by the lack of clinical facilities at the university hospital. Francis Blake came with Dr. Rowntree from Johns Hopkins as assistant professor of medicine, but left three years later for Yale. In 1925 the heads of the Departments of Medicine and Surgery, S. Marx White and Arthur Strachauer, both resigned to devote themselves to private practice at the Nicollet Clinic in Minneapolis. Both had been members of the medical school faculty for many years. No one could question either their loyalty to the school or their personal generosity. Yet they left. Although any medical school will have regularly a certain proportion of turnover in the faculty, at Minnesota from 1915 to 1930 the heads of clinical departments changed so frequently as to inhibit the development of clinical teaching and residency training.

Before 1930 all of the clinicians who continued to teach in the medical school over a long period of time were part-time teachers who maintained their own private medical practice either in Minneapolis or St. Paul. For such men their medical practice provided them with an income comparable to that of other members of the medical profession of similar skill and experience. Any stipend that they received from the university was usually only a minor supplement to their income from practice. From their practices such part-time clinical teachers gained also both clinical experience and familiarity with the realities of medical practice—a familiarity that was especially important in the preparation of medical students to become practitioners.

The inauguration of full-time clinical appointments at Johns Hopkins University in 1914 made full-time appointments a seemingly desirable goal for any medical school, but Johns Hopkins had only been able to make such full-time appointments with the aid of a very large grant of $1,500,000 from the Rockefeller General Education Board to endow clinical chairs. By contrast the University of Minnesota did not have sufficient money to pay more than small stipends to some of its part-time clinical faculty, and occasionally had to withdraw even such nominal stipends to use the money for other and more urgent purposes. Nevertheless, in September 1915, following Charles Lyman Greene's forced resignation, the committee appointed to make recommendations concerning a professor of medicine to succeed Dr. Greene recommended that the professor of medicine should be " . . . practically a full-time man," but should be allowed a limited consultation practice so as not to separate him from the medical profession of the state and its problems.[1]

S. Marx White offered to become acting chief of medicine, and proposed to eliminate his office in downtown Minneapolis, to restrict his practice to consultation and hospital practice, and to limit all outside practice to not more than two hours of the working day.[2] Although the administrative board did not accept Dr. White's offer at the time, the terms he suggested probably corresponded closely to what the committee had in mind when they referred to "practically full-time." After further deliberation, the administrative board decided that a limited consultation practice not to consume more than ten hours per week should be made part of the basis of negotiations with any candidate for the professorship of medicine.[3] When later that month Leonard Rowntree came out from Baltimore to look over the Minnesota situation, such a limited consultation practice was made one of the conditions of his appointment. On his part, in accepting the appointment, Dr. Rowntree stipulated that his university offices should be available for consultation work.[4]

Nevertheless, when Dr. Rowntree arrived in Minneapolis in January 1916 to assume his duties as chief of medicine in the lonely little Elliot Memorial Hospital perched on its bluff above the frozen waters of the Mississippi River, he soon began to chafe at the restrictions imposed upon him. Because the Elliot Hospital received charity patients only, Dr. Rowntree could not admit to the Elliot Hospital any private patients referred to him. In order to conduct a consultation practice, he therefore had to go to other hospitals in the Twin Cities, which he found a serious waste of time and energy.[5] By the spring of 1918 Rowntree had to undergo surgery at the Mayo Clinic for a perforating duodenal ulcer.[6]

On 7 March 1918 a committee of the administrative board appointed to report on the relations of "practically full-time clinical chiefs" to the medical school recommended that the clinical chiefs should be permitted to have offices and to treat private patients (presumably no longer necessarily referred patients) in a private hospital to be built adjacent to the university campus. In the meantime, and until such a private hospital could be brought into being, the "practically full-time" clinical chiefs should be permitted "to see and to treat patients at certain designated points," and should be allowed to devote up to fifteen hours a week to private practice.[7] The committee recommended further that clinical chiefs should be permitted to retain their private practice income until their total income including salary reached $10,000, but should donate a substantial portion of their income above $10,000 annually to a clinical research fund. They were to be permitted to provide consultation outside the Twin Cities only when patients could not be brought to Minneapolis, and then only with permission of the dean.

At a meeting of the general faculty on 19 March, with President Burton present, the chairman of the committee on the relations of clinical chiefs to the medical school, Dr. Arthur Hirschfelder, reviewed the committee's recommendations. Dr. Fred Adair pointed out that the income limits proposed would be very high for the Twin Cities. He said that only 7.5 percent of medical men in Minneapolis received gross incomes of more than $15,000 per year, and their net income was usually only half the gross. Dr. Adair said that local physicians with such incomes were " . . . first: very few in number; second, very busy men; third, unable to give much of their time to other than their private work." Such men could not undertake the administrative, research and teaching work required of department heads. Adair thought it impractical to restrict a physician to set hours for medical practice, because practice imposed obligations which had to be fulfilled. If instead a limit were placed on the amount of income that a clinical chief could receive, there would be no need to place restrictions on the use of his time.[8] The income limit would remove the incentive to develop a large private practice. The committee's report and Dr. Adair's proposals were approved by the general faculty.

On 9 April 1918 Dr. Hirschfelder's committee recommended to the administrative board that the work of clinical chiefs, apart from consultations, should be done in a designated hospital, and that a clinical chief should not maintain a downtown office. In contrast to Dr. Adair, the committee recommended that a full-time clinical chief should devote thirty-three hours a week to university work and not more than fifteen hours a week to private practice. The administrative board then accepted the comittee's recommendations, ignoring the financial restrictions proposed by Dr. Adair and recommended by the general faculty on 19 March.[9] There was some disagreement between members of the scientific and clinical departments. The basic scientists supported the upper limit on the incomes of clinical chiefs, proposed by Dr. Adair, and also restriction on the hours that clinical chiefs might devote to private practice. Dr. Rowntree's salary soon rose above the level of $5,000 mentioned in the 1918 discussion, because when he went to Rochester in 1920, his university salary for 1920–21 was to have been $8,000.[10] Nevertheless, when S. Marx White was appointed chief of the Department of Medicine in 1921, his salary was set at $5,000.[11] Also in 1921 George Fahr was appointed assistant professor in the Department of Medicine at a salary of $3,500 per year. Such salaries presupposed that both Dr. Fahr and Dr. White would earn a significant portion of additional income through private practice.

FULL-TIME CLINICAL CHIEFS

In November 1923, in the wake of the departure of Clemens von Pirquet, when the administrative board considered the question of filling the vacant chiefship of pediatrics, the question arose whether the appointment should be full-time or part-time, and if it were to be full-time, what were to be the conditions of such a full-time appointment. After extended discussion the administrative board appointed a committee, under Dean Lyon as chairman, " . . . to clearly define the conditions of a full-time appointment as chief of a department."[12] As was true at Johns Hopkins, where the pressure for full-time clinical appointments came not from clinicians but from the professor of anatomy, Franklin P. Mall, so at Minnesota the head of the Department of Pathology, E. T. Bell, moved that the administrative board " . . . endorse the plan of a full-time man for chief of the Department of Pediatrics." To deflect Dr. Bell's motion, with its implied rigidity, the chief of surgery, Arthur Strachauer, offered a substitute motion, " . . . that the consensus of opinion of the Administrative Board favors the full-time principle in filling the Chair of Pediatrics," and Dr. Strachauer's motion was passed.[13]

On 25 January 1924 Dean Lyon's committee to study the conditions that should govern full-time appointments offered its report, and after extensive discussion and various amendments the administrative board adopted the following regulations.

1. In general, the full-time members of the Medical School Faculty will conform with the present regulations for outside work as outlined in the University rules and regulations.

2. The full-time medical teacher shall not maintain an outside office; he shall have no affiliation with any partner, clinic or group; he shall not be on the active staff of any private hospital.

3. The outside work of a full-time clinical teacher shall be limited to consultation work with other members of the profession.

4. The full-time medical teacher will keep a record of all outside work, which shall include,
   a. Date and time of work
   b. Physician calling consultation or person for whom laboratory work is done.
      The Dean of the Medical School shall be furnished monthly with a copy of the record.

5. The Dean of the Medical School, the President of the University and the University Comptroller shall constitute a Board to pass upon the extent of outside work which any full-time member of the Medical School may carry and the decision of the Board shall be final.[14]

At the same meeting the administrative board recommended Frederic W. M. Schlutz to be appointed as chief of the Department of Pediatrics, under the rules thus established.

There are several striking features to the administrative board's regulations governing full-time appointments. They separated the full-time clinical professor from any participation in private practice away from the university hospital, which in 1924 still consisted only of the Elliot Memorial Hospital with fewer than 200 beds. The regulations subjected the full-time clinical professor to constant and close supervision by the dean of the medical school of any outside practice. If applied to all clinical departments, the regulations would require several of the clinical chiefs either to alter drastically their modes of practice or resign their university appointments.

On 10 April 1924 the administrative board decided " . . . that all full time men are under the rules which were formulated in the case of the headship in Pediatrics and entitled to the same privileges."[15] The privileges were not specified. At the meeting of the general faculty on 23 April, both Dr. Strachauer and Dr. White emphasized that full-time faculty should receive preference in both promotion and salary over part-time teachers.[16]

In the fall of 1924 in submitting the proposed budget for the medical school for the 1925–27 biennium, Dean Lyon planned to use most of any additional funds, together with a large part of the funds then used to pay part-time clinical teachers, to provide salaries for full-time teachers in the clinical departments. To President Coffman, Dean Lyon wrote: " . . . that only by a corps of competent teachers devoting their thought and time to the work of the University can the clinical departments be made of the same excellence in undergraduate instruction and strength in graduate teaching and research as the fundamental departments in medicine, or any other departments of the University."[17] Yet Dean Lyon did not wish to dispense entirely with the part-time faculty. He requested a free hand to recommend changes in salaries then paid to part-time clinical teachers, saying that there was no system in the level of part-time salaries paid, and that in many cases such salaries could be reduced or abolished.[18]

In November 1924 Dean Lyon again outlined to the general faculty his plans to reduce the number of part-time faculty. He " . . . referred to differences of opinion and judgment among the members of the faculty and pleaded for a unity of feeling in the interests of the School and the dismissal of personal suspicions of other's motives." He emphasized the value of that type of medical school in which scholarship is an ideal and research is promoted. Clarence M. Jackson spoke, referring to " . . . the fitness of discussion of clinical problems by the laboratory men," and discussing " . . . the difficulties involving the part-time teacher." Dean Lyon was a physiologist, Dr. Jackson an anatomist. Their pronouncements on clinical teaching, of which they had no experience, and in which they took no part, were deeply resented by the clinicians. When the professor of nervous mental diseases, Arthur S. Hamilton, rose to speak, he " . . . acknowledged his deeply hurt feelings, in which he believed many others present shared, by certain references in the Dean's remarks concerning part-time teachers," and expressed the hope that " . . . the Administration would most carefully consider the experiences of other schools in the matter of full-time or

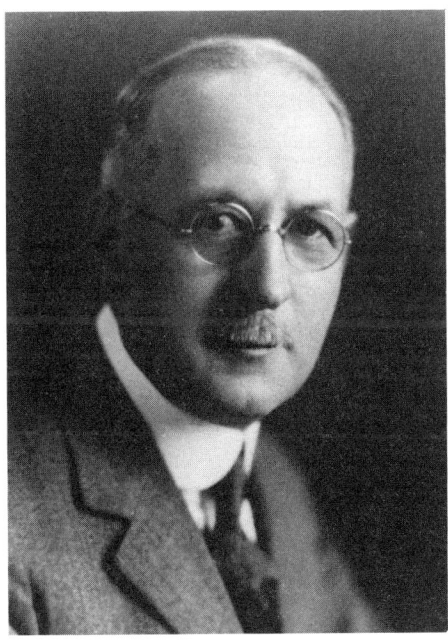

FIGURE 13:1   Arthur S. Hamilton, 1926. Courtesy Mn U Archives.

part-time teachers before it embarked upon new policies."[19] Dean Lyon then expressed regret that he had hurt the feelings of any member of the faculty and expressed his high regard for the services of the part-time teachers.

Charles B. Wright, assistant professor of medicine, described the difficulties that other medical schools had experienced in finding suitable candidates for full-time clinical positions. Franklin R. Wright, chief of the Division of Urology, noted that Johns Hopkins University with $45,000 income annually from the Rockefeller endowment had been able to provide only three full-time clinical chiefships, which they had difficulty in getting candidates to accept. Fred L. Adair noted that the so-called full-time plan varied in different places, and asked Dean Lyon to define the Minnesota plan. In reply Dean Lyon said that he " . . . favored an elastic system meeting so far as possible the desires of the candidate for a particular position."[20] In other words, at Minnesota there was no consistent plan for full-time clinical positions.

The discussion at the November 1924 faculty meeting must have impressed Dean Lyon with the complexity and sensitivity of the issues involved in full-time clinical appointments. The advocacy of full-time clinical positions by anatomists and physiologists, expressed in high-minded terms of the need to promote research, were inspired in large measure by simple envy of the larger incomes obtained by clinicians from practice. Nevertheless, no matter how much the laboratory scientists might affect to despise the part-time clinical teachers, the medical school could not do without them if it were to continue to train students to become medical practitioners.

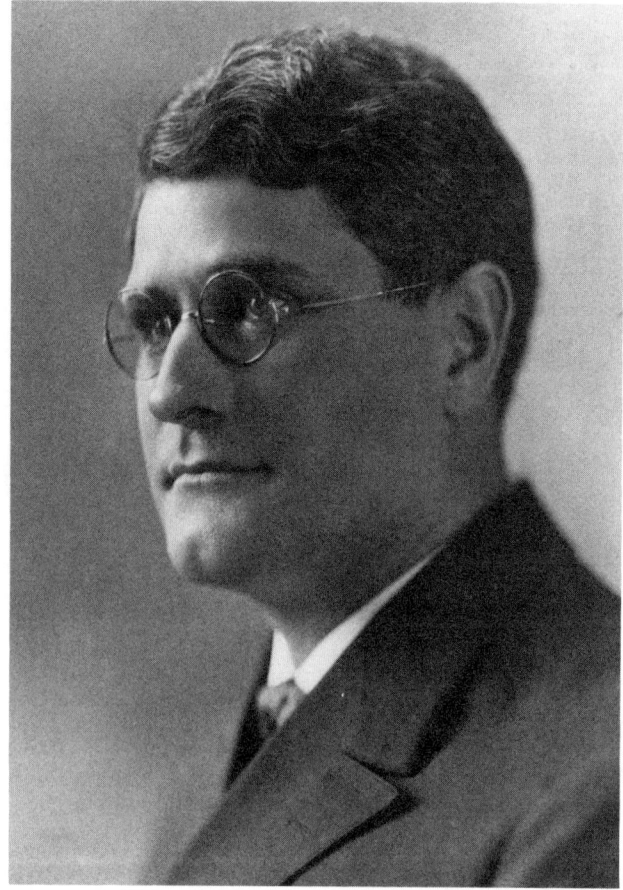

FIGURE 13:2 Arthur C. Strachauer, 1925. Courtesy Mn U Archives.

Within a few months, the medical school's difficulties in keeping clinical teachers became acute. In March 1925 Arthur Strachauer resigned as chief of the Department of Surgery to become director of the new George Chase Christian Cancer Hospital. Dr. Strachauer's new appointment was, like his former chiefship, part-time, with a salary of $2,400.[21] Dean Lyon approached Mont R. Reid of Cincinnati, a former student of William Stuart Halsted at Johns Hopkins, to offer him the chiefship of the Department of Surgery, but Dr. Reid declined the offer. In June, because of the failure to find a new chief of surgery, the administrative board asked Dr. Strachauer to continue for another three months.

At the beginning of the year, before either Dr. Strachauer or Dr. White had resigned, but when Dean Lyon probably knew that their resignations were pending and that he would shortly have to try to replace them with full-time appointees, he had written to the deans of medical schools in the East to ask what arrangements they used for appointments in their clinical departments. Dean William Darrach of the College of Physicians and Surgeons at Columbia University replied with an account of Columbia's experience. Until 1921 all the clinical departments at Columbia had been on a part-time basis with the department heads receiving only nominal salaries. Then in 1921 Columbia had placed its departments of medicine and surgery on a strict full-time basis, paying the two department chiefs salaries, which were very large in comparison with other university salaries, but small when compared with the incomes of physicians or surgeons in private practice. The full-time professors were allowed to have private patients in the Presbyterian Hospital, but no charges were made to such patients by anyone. The system quickly proved impossible. The hospital then began to make charges to the private patients and to turn over to Columbia University part of the money, which was then used to pay additional salaries to the full-time clinical professors. After two years' experience of the latter plan, Columbia began to allow the full-time clinicians to select their private patients, to make their own charges directly, and to collect the money. "This means," wrote Dean Darrach, "that we tried out and practically gave up the plan which, by legislative methods, endeavored to create an academic atmosphere. These men are now all working on the basis that is covered by an old statute of the University, which states: No officer of instruction shall be employed in any occupation which interferes with the thorough, efficient and earnest performance of the duties of his office." Darrach added: "We believe that far greater progress can be made . . . if the right type of individual is selected and the responsibility then placed on him, together with full opportunities for developing academic Medicine, than if an attempt is made by rules and regulations to compel him to do or not do certain things."[22] Dean Lyon immediately sent a copy of Dean Darrach's letter to President Coffman, saying: "The Columbia plan is exactly my 'geographical full-time' idea and what I advocate for Minnesota."[23]

During the summer of 1925 the medical school renewed its search for a chief of surgery, and in September invited Francis Newton, who had trained as a resident in surgery at the Peter Bent Brigham Hospital in Boston, to come out to Minnesota to be interviewed and look the situation over. Dr. Newton created a favorable impression on Dean Lyon who described him in glowing terms to President Coffman.[24] Nevertheless, in the course of his visit to Minnesota, Dr. Newton decided not to accept the chiefship in surgery. Before he left, Newton remarked to Owen Wangensteen, then the resident in the Department of Surgery, who had shown him around the Elliot Memorial Hospital: "Well, there isn't anything here, nor will there ever be."[25] Dr. Newton's pessimism about surgery at Minnesota was based probably on the pathetic smallness of the Elliot Memorial Hospital and the stranglehold with which he knew that William Mayo prevented its development. After his return to Boston, Newton wrote to decline the chiefship of surgery.

In January 1926, when the surgery department still had no chief, Dean Lyon was obliged to develop a temporary plan for conducting the work of the department by a supervisory committee, until a new chief could be appointed. Three

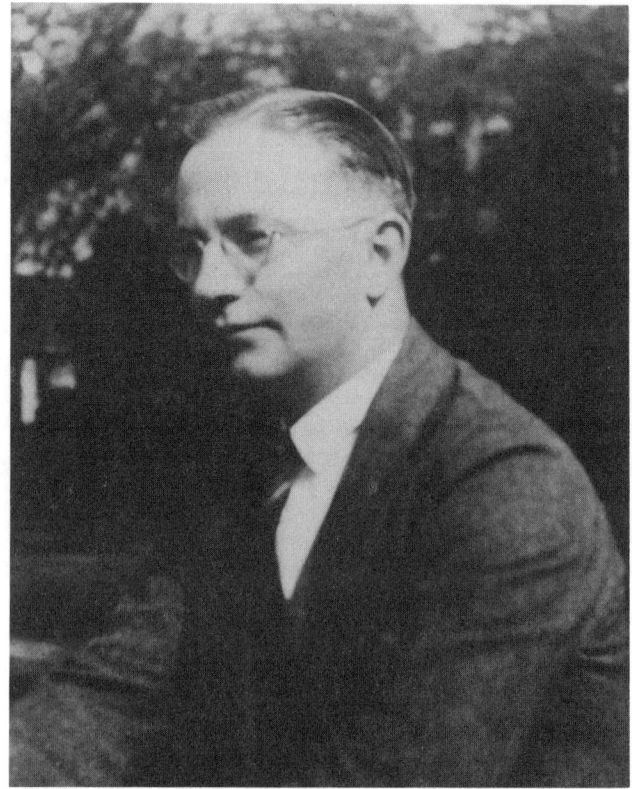

FIGURE 13:3 Owen H. Wangensteen, circa 1926. Courtesy Mn U Archives.

months later, when surgery still had no chief, the administrative committee (as the former administrative board was now termed) decided that ample time should be taken to find one.

Dean Lyon reopened negotiation concerning the chiefship of surgery with Mont Reid, who was then in China at Peking Union Medical College. On 24 May 1926, in response to a cablegram from Dr. Reid, the administrative committee decided to await his decision whether he would accept the chair of surgery.[26] The following November, after an interval of almost six months, a letter from Dr. Reid concerning the chiefship of surgery was read and discussed at a meeting of the administrative committee.[27] Evidently Dr. Reid either turned down the surgery professorship, or imposed conditions that the administrative committee was unwilling to accept.

Meanwhile, the work of the Department of Surgery was going on under the temporary committee arrangement. On 17 November 1926 Owen H. Wangensteen, who had been appointed an instructor in the Department of Surgery the previous July after completing his surgical residency at the university hospital, described to the executive faculty the organization of the work in the courses offered to the medical students in surgery.[28] Dean Lyon and the members of the executive faculty were very favorably impressed by their new instructor in surgery, then twenty-eight years old, and Dean Lyon together with senior members of the faculty decided that if they could not attract a chief of surgery from outside the school, they had best try to develop one from one of their own promising young surgeons. Dean Lyon then approached Arthur Strachauer to ask him to reassume the chiefship of surgery for a two-year period, during which Dr. Wangensteen might go abroad to prepare himself for that position. Dr. Strachauer agreed to do so, but thought that a three-year period was necessary both for his own work and for the proper preparation of Dr. Wangensteen.[29] Strachauer's willingness once again to become chief of surgery, simply as a caretaker of the department for three years, was a demonstration both of his loyalty to the medical school and his generosity to his young colleague and former student, Owen Wangensteen. Arthur Strachauer was carrying a heavy burden. He was director of the Christian Cancer Hospital, he had a large private surgical practice, and now once again he was chief of surgery, with the teaching and administrative duties that that position imposed. Yet like Dean Lyon, Dr. Strachauer also believed in the future promise of Dr. Wangensteen.

Owen H. Wangensteen stood out already as a remarkable young man. He was born at Lake Park, Minnesota, where his father, an immigrant from Norway, was a merchant and farmer. Owen Wangensteen grew up on his father's farm where he helped to care for horses, cows, and pigs, and where, while still quite young, he helped to supervise the work of the hired men while his father was running the store in the town of Lake Park. In 1914, during his junior year in high school, the herd of fifty sows on the Wangensteen farm were unable to farrow their young and the local veterinarian recommended that they be sent to slaughter. After the death of two sows because they couldn't deliver, Owen succeeded in delivering a litter of live piglets from the third sow by using his hand to assist delivery, and during the next three weeks he delivered more than 300 piglets in the same manner. This success convinced Owen Wangensteen's father that his son should study medicine, although Owen himself wished to become a farmer. In 1915 Owen Wangensteen entered the College of Science, Literature and the Arts at the University of Minnesota. As a student he lived in a fraternity house in southeast Minneapolis close to the home of former President Folwell, and occasionally walked to the university with Dr. Folwell, who was then about eighty. In the fall of 1918 Owen Wangensteen entered the medical school. Although Wangensteen intended at first to go into internal medicine, when he heard his first lecture in surgery from Arthur Strachauer, on the subject of appendicitis, he decided to become a surgeon, and never departed from that decision.

In the fall of 1921, during Owen Wangensteen's senior year, George Fahr came to the medical school as associate professor of medicine, and began a course of lectures on medicine for the senior class in the small lecture room on the second floor of the Elliot Memorial Hospital. Then at the age of thirty-nine, George Fahr had had an unusually varied career. Born at Meadville, Pennsylvania, where his father was a successful banker, George Fahr had begun to learn German at the age of nine, and when he was eleven accompanied his father, who had been born at Ulm in Würtemberg, on a three-month trip to Europe. At that time he could read and write German almost as well as English. In 1901, after one year at Allegheny College, George Fahr entered the University of Chicago where he studied physics and chemistry. His adviser was the physicist Robert A. Millikan, who later won a Nobel prize, and the dean of Chicago's undergraduate college was George Edgar Vincent. Fahr graduated from Chicago in 1904 and then spent a year at Cornell University doing graduate work in physical chemistry and organic chemistry. In addition to chemistry, Fahr must also have been interested in biology because he spent the summer of 1905 at Woods Hole, Massachusetts, where many of the leading American biologists and physiologists were accustomed to spend the summer in research. In the fall of 1905 George Fahr entered the Johns Hopkins School of Medicine where he was befriended by the professor of anatomy, Franklin P. Mall, who gave him a place in the research laboratory next to a young Californian, Herbert M. Evans, who as a senior medical student at the Hopkins, was already engaged in anatomical research. Later, as professor of anatomy at the University of California, Evans would become famous for his discovery of the pituitary growth hormone, Vitamin E, and other investigations in endocrinology. When Professor Mall learned that Fahr planned to go to Germany for postgraduate study, Mall arranged for him to meet Professor Max von Frey of the University of Würzburg who came to the United States in June 1906 to deliver a lecture to the meeting of the American Medical Association. Mall suggested that Fahr should go to Würzburg to complete his medical studies. Accordingly, in the summer of 1906 Fahr went to Würzburg to begin his second year of medical study and to start research in Max von Frey's laboratory. During the next three and a half years at Würzburg, Fahr published three papers, one on the effect of potassium chloride on muscle contraction, a second on the sodium content of skeletal muscle, and a third on electrical changes in damaged muscles. Because of his interest in electrophysiology George Fahr went in July 1909 to the laboratory of Professor Willem Einthoven at the University of Leiden in Holland, which then possessed the best electrophysiological equipment in the world. In 1901 Einthoven had developed a new string galvanometer to record electromotive changes in the heartbeat. At Leiden during the summer of 1909 Fahr completed the experimental work for two outstanding papers. One, on the simultaneous recording of the heart sounds and the electrocardiogram, Fahr published by himself. The second paper, published with Einthoven and de Waart, contained the classic description of the Einthoven triangle and the electrical axis of the heart.[30]

In the autumn of 1909 George Fahr left Leiden for Copenhagen where he intended to work with Christian Bohr on experiments to test Bohr's theory of the secretion of oxygen by the alveolar cells of the lung, but the work was cut short by Bohr's unexpected death from a heart attack a few weeks after Fahr arrived. Nevertheless, while working in Bohr's laboratory at Copenhagen, Fahr met Bohr's younger son, Nils Bohr, who was then working on his paper—for which he was to win a Nobel prize—on the structure of the atom.

Early in 1910 Fahr returned to Einthoven's laboratory at Leiden, where he remained until the summer of 1913 when he went to Giessen to work in Siegfried Garten's laboratory. He was still at Giessen when the First World War broke out in August 1914. With the outbreak of war, Dr. Garten and his staff left for the front. Fahr, who had been mountain climbing in the Berchtesgaden when war broke out, served through September 1914 on the hospital staff at Giessen, helping to care for wounded French soldiers sent from the western front, and doing experiments in Adolph Weber's laboratory at Bad Nauheim near Giessen. He had an opportunity to observe also various forms of heart failure among hundreds of German soldiers sent back from the front. The exhaustion and stress of battle had evoked heart failure in some soldiers with preexisting, but previously undiagnosed, heart disease. In other soldiers with symptoms of heart failure, the heart was healthy. The German physicians called the condition *cardiac neurosis;* it was later described in England as soldier's heart. In October 1914 Fahr left Germany for neutral Switzerland, settling at the University of Bern where Leon Asher had just become head of the department of physiology. At Asher's request Fahr set up an electrophysiological laboratory, helping to design and construct a string galvanometer. In 1916 Fahr left Bern for Basel in order to spend some time working in Rudolph Staehelin's clinic in internal medicine. In the fall of 1916, when it began to seem probable that the United States would enter the war, Dr. Fahr returned home after ten years in Europe to become a resident at the Montefiore Hospital in New York City, where he was in charge of the electrocardiographic laboratory. After being turned down initially when he volunteered to join the army because he had no license to practice medicine in the United States, George Fahr entered the United States Army in April 1918 and spent the remainder of the war at San Antonio, Texas. In 1921 he accepted an invitation from S. Marx White to come to Minnesota as associate professor of medicine.[31]

Thus it was that in the fall of 1921 George Fahr, rich with the experience of ten years of medical study and research in Europe during which he had met and worked with some of the greatest clinicians and investigators in the world, began to lecture to the small class of senior medical students in the lecture room on the second floor of the Elliot Memorial Hospital. In his first lecture Fahr astonished the students with the extent of his knowledge, and his complete absorption in the subject. He was so brilliant and interesting that they did not think that he could continue at that rate. Yet Fahr did. Owen Wangensteen recalled that " . . . week after week, on unrelated subjects in the general field of medicine, George Fahr returned with fresh information, tracing the historic development of the field under review, pointing out the important contributors, and often adding much of interest about the men themselves."[32] Owen Wangensteen was astonished and fascinated. George Fahr opened for him a new vision of clinical medicine, and of what a medical teacher might be. Owen Wangensteen was impressed particularly by Fahr's view, gained from Rudolf Krehl, professor of pathol-

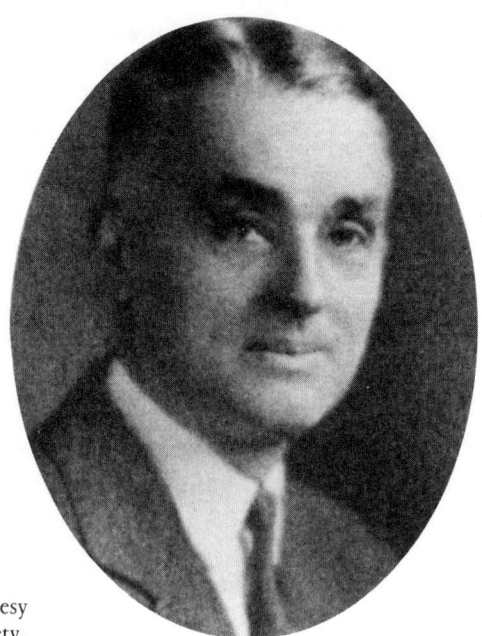

FIGURE 13:4 George Fahr. Courtesy Minnesota Historical Society.

ogy at Heidelberg, that the signs and symptoms of disease reflected internal changes in function. "Disturbances in function and alterations of physiology in disease," Dr. Wangensteen recalled, "—these were terms on George Fahr's lips in every lecture."[33]

In December 1921, when Dr. Fahr's series of lectures was over, Owen Wangensteen had also completed his medical courses. For the next twelve months he held a rotating internship at the Elliot Memorial Hospital. In January 1923, because there was no surgical residency available for him, Dr. Wangensteen was appointed a teaching fellow in the Department of Medicine and spent the year at the Minneapolis General Hospital, where George Fahr had been appointed to the medical service. For Dr. Wangensteen, 1923 was an extremely stimulating year because as he worked in close association with George Fahr, Dr. Fahr opened to him an ever broader picture of the problems that awaited investigation in medical research.[34] In September 1923, while Dr. Fahr was on vacation, a forty-six-year-old woman entered the Minneapolis General Hospital suffering from symptoms of heart failure: shortness of breath, swelling of the ankles, legs, and abdomen, palpitation of the heart, and great weakness. She said that for eleven years she had suffered such symptoms of heart disease, but along with them other signs and symptoms, such as loss of hair, dry skin, puffy eyes, and cold extremities, which indicated myxedema. She was diagnosed as suffering from both heart disease and myxedema and was treated with bed rest and digitalis, but when Dr. Fahr returned from vacation three weeks after her admission, she had shown little improvement. Fahr immediately diagnosed her condition as *myxedema heart,* a condition which had been described in 1918 by Bernard Zondek at Munich. X-rays of the patient's chest showed that her heart was enormously dilated. Fahr ceased the treatment with digitalis and ordered thyroid extract to be administered daily. Four weeks later the symptoms of heart failure had disappeared, the dilatation of the heart was reduced, and the patient was up and moving actively about the wards. During the following year, two more patients with well-defined myxedema heart came into the Minneapolis General Hospital, but Fahr concluded that all patients with myxedema showed some degree of heart failure, although in many cases it could be detected only from the slight dilatation of the heart revealed by x-rays.[35]

George Fahr's work on myxedema heart was the kind of contribution which could be made only by a clinician deeply familiar with the European, and particularly the German, medical literature, who also worked in a large hospital where he saw many patients and had the help of an experienced diagnostic radiologist, and who devoted himself to medical investigation instead of private practice. It was exactly the kind of contribution that Owen Wangensteen wished himself to make in clinical surgery.

At the conclusion of his year in medicine at the Minneapolis General Hospital, Dr. Wangensteen went to the Mayo Clinic as a fellow in the Department of Surgery. In 1925 he returned to Minneapolis to become surgical resident in the university hospital where he completed the requirements for a Ph.D. in surgery with a dissertation on the problem of the undescended testis. In 1926 Dr. Wangensteen was appointed an instructor in surgery, and at the end of that year, faced with the failure of their other efforts to find a chief of surgery, Dean Lyon and the administrative committee looked to Owen Wangensteen to become the future chief of surgery. In the *President's Report* for 1926–27, Dean Lyon mentioned the difficulty that the medical school had experienced in obtaining a professor of surgery fully prepared for teaching and research, and added that the university had come to recognize that it possessed in one of their own assistant professors of surgery, Owen H. Wangensteen, a young man whose scholarship, teaching ability, and growing experience suggested that he would make a future professor of surgery. They had, therefore, decided to raise their own professor of surgery. Accordingly, the university would send Dr. Wangensteen abroad in 1927 for a year of study. On his return he would continue in the surgery department until 1 January 1930 when he would assume the headship. In the meantime, Arthur Strachauer had agreed to continue as chief of surgery for the three years from 1927 to 1930.[36]

On 13 September 1927 Dr. and Mrs. Wangensteen and their two-year-old daughter, Mary, sailed from New York for Copenhagen. Dr. Wangensteen's friend and fellow student, Dr. George Eitel, and his wife sailed on the same ship as did Dr. and Mrs. George Fahr with their son and daughter. From Copenhagen the party of Minnesotans traveled by train to Hamburg, then south through Germany stopping at Frankfort-on-Main, Mannheim, and Basel. From Basel they proceeded to Bern, where they arrived at the beginning of October. Dr. Wangen-

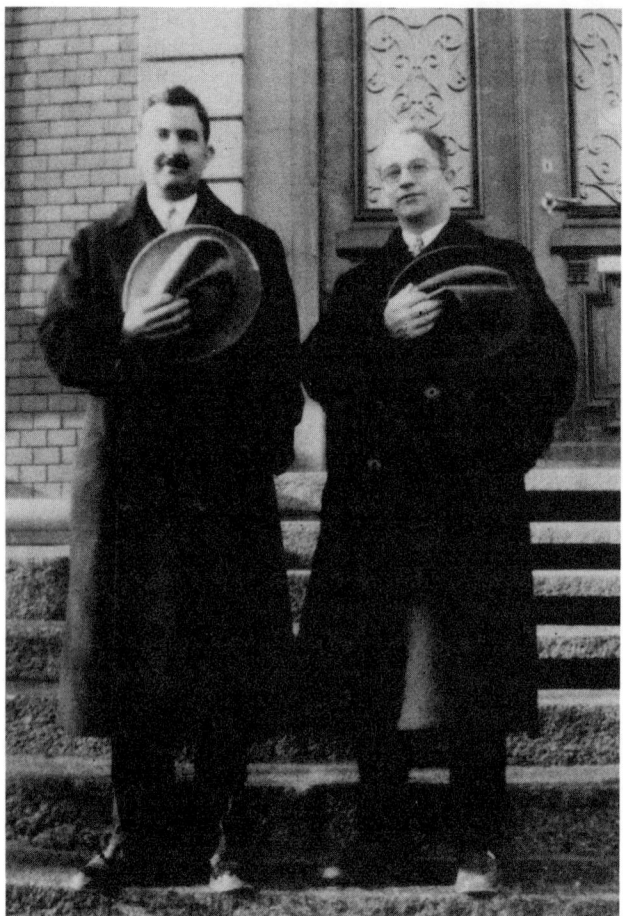

FIGURE 13:5 George D. Eitel and Owen H. Wangensteen in front of the Physiological Institute, Berne, Switzerland, 21 November 1927. Photograph by Leon Asher. Courtesy Mn U Archives.

steen carried with him letters of introduction from Dr. William Mayo, which he found produced an immediate warm welcome at every surgical clinic he visited. On the recommendation of George Fahr, Owen Wangensteen and George Eitel began to attend the surgical clinic of Fritz de Quervain. Then at the age of sixty, Professor Quervain was a dignified, courteous, and good-humored surgeon, particularly expert in surgical diagnosis, and well known throughout the United States for his excellent textbook on diagnosis.[37]

Under Professor Quervain's direction, Dr. Wangensteen began a study of the blood supply of the normal thyroid gland and the thyroid enlarged in goiter, for which he was given access to Quervain's personal library. He learned that Quervain was not only a skilled surgeon, but also widely read in the medical literature, skilled in the use of apparatus, the preparation of microscopic sections, photography, and other techniques used in medical research. Nevertheless, Dr. Wangensteen found the routine work of Quervain's clinic insufficient to occupy him; after a couple of months he went to see the professor of physiology, Leon Asher, a former student of Carl Ludwig, who gave Dr. Wangensteen laboratory space to study liver autolysis in rats.[38] Professor Asher was friendly and helpful to Dr. Wangensteen; as their friendship developed they went together on long walks through the countryside.

From Bern Dr. Wangensteen also visited Lausanne, Zurich, and Heidelberg. At the end of February 1928 he was at Rome.[39] In March Wangensteen visited Ferdinand Sauerbruch's clinic at Berlin, and then spent some time at Freiburg in Ludwig Aschoff's laboratory. In the fall of 1928 he visited surgical clinics at London and Edinburgh. At Edinburgh, Wangensteen was impressed favorably by the professor of surgery, David Wilkie, who maintained an active research laboratory, with numerous workers, in connection with his surgical clinic. When Wilkie was appointed at Edinburgh in 1924, the conditions of the surgical chair were modified to make it practically a full-time academic appointment and to enable Wilkie to develop a research group. Late in 1928 Dr. Wangensteen returned to Minneapolis, where during his absence he had been promoted to associate professor. With the varied experiences of his year in Europe fresh in his mind, he took up his surgical work at the university hospital and plunged immediately into research, choosing for investigation the difficult question of intestinal obstruction. In January 1930, at the age of thirty-two, Owen Wangensteen became chief of the Department of Surgery.

Five years earlier, when the position of chief of the Department of Medicine also became vacant, Dean Lyon was able immediately to appoint Hilding Berglund to a full-time position as chief of medicine, replacing S. Marx White who left for private practice. A native of Sweden, Dr. Berglund had worked with Otto Folin at Harvard University and had then gone to China to teach at Peking Union Medical College. Berglund's appointment at Minnesota proved unfortunate because he quickly became embroiled in quarrels with the hospital administration, the nursing staff, and his medical colleagues. A brilliant man with a hot temper and deeply suspicious of his coworkers, Berglund's career at Minnesota was extraordinarily stormy. One morning in the autumn of 1925, and shortly after Dr. Berglund's arrival, Owen Wangensteen, then senior surgical resident at the university hospital, happened to see the new professor just leaving his house, and stopped to offer him a ride to the hospital in his Model T Ford. When Dr. Wangensteen introduced himself, Dr. Berglund said that he was just the person he needed to see. Berglund explained that he had recommended open rib resection for a student suffering from empyema of the lungs, but the physicians in the students' health service " . . . know nothing of the treatment of empyema and have never heard of Hippocrates, who insisted that wherever pus is present, it must be completely evacuated." Dr. Wangensteen reminded Dr. Berglund that Hippocrates had also urged the need for cautious delay in opening the pleural cavity to drain pus. "What began as a friendly discussion of the surgical management of acute empyema, less than a mile distant from the hospital," said Dr. Wangensteen, "had become a controversy of some proportions as we neared the hospital." Berglund cursed Wangensteen in Norwegian, saying, when translated, ". . . may the devil cut, whip and burn you," which Wangensteen understood perfectly. Nevertheless, when Dr. Wangensteen mentioned Evarts Graham's work on the management of empyema, Dr. Berglund responded, "I now see a dim light on your mental horizon," and when Wangensteen gave him two recent references to Graham's work, Berglund later admitted that they were "not half bad."[40] Dr. Berglund remained only until 1932 when he returned to Sweden, but during his seven years at the medical school Berglund carried out much research. In 1930 he organized a very successful symposium on kidney physiology and pathology in which leading medical investigators from the United States, Canada, and various European countries participated. When the proceedings of the kidney symposium were published in 1935, they became a classic.[41]

When Hilding Berglund came to the medical school in 1925, he soon expressed dissatisfaction with the radiology service at the university hospital which was provided by a part-time member of the clinical faculty, Robert G. Allison. Dr. Allison was director of the Division of Radiology within the Department of Surgery. He had a flourishing medical practice in Minneapolis, but since 1920 he had given a required course in radiology, including lectures, demonstrations, and plate reading, for the medical students. He also offered three elective courses in plate reading, x-ray technique, and x-ray therapy, but the limited amount of time that he could spare for teaching probably made such courses quite sketchy. Certainly the need to carry on his practice meant that much of the time Dr. Allison was not at the university hospital and was consequently unavailable for consultation. By contrast, Hilding Berglund had been accustomed to the excellent department of radiology at the university hospital in Stockholm where the chief, Gösta Forssell, one of the outstanding radiologists in the world, offered a complete teaching program in both x-ray diagnosis and in radiation therapy. At Minnesota, Hilding Berglund was eager to obtain the appointment of a full-time chief for the Division of Radiology, a radiologist who would be available for consultation on a daily basis at the university hospital. Dean Lyon was equally eager to appoint a full-time chief for radiology because he was working steadily to appoint full-time chiefs for all the clinical departments and divisions of the medical school. Since Dr. Allison was unwilling to give up his medical practice to accept a full-time appointment, Dean Lyon and Dr. Berglund realized that they must look elsewhere for a full-time chief of radiology. The medical school did not have the means to search the nation for an established radiologist, so Dean Lyon decided that Minnesota must in effect grow its own; the school must select a young physician interested in radiology and encourage him to develop into a full-fledged radiologist.

Early in 1926 Dean Lyon and Dr. Berglund went to call on Leo Rigler, who served part-time as radiologist at the Minneapolis General Hospital. Dean Lyon knew Dr. Rigler well from his days as a medical student. In fact, during Rigler's senior year, Dean Lyon saved him from summary dismissal as an intern at the City and County Hospital in St. Paul when Rigler was reported returning late to the hospital on the evening that he became engaged to be married. After an internship during 1919–20 at the St. Louis City Hospital, where he spent much time working in the x-ray department with the hospital radiologist, Dr. Rigler entered general practice in a small village in North Dakota, with the idea of earning money to enable him to pursue further medical training. Mrs. Rigler taught high school while Leo Rigler practiced medicine, but the agricultural depression of 1921 was particularly severe in North Dakota and few of his patients could pay him. In 1922 Rigler borrowed money to return to the University of Minnesota as a fellow in internal medicine at the Minneapolis General Hospital. He also took a minor in pathology under E. T. Bell. At the Minneapolis General Hospital, radiology had been the responsibility of the hospital pathologist, Kano Ikeda, but in 1923 the chief of medicine, Henry Ulrich, and the head of pathology, E. T. Bell, decided that Dr. Ikeda should devote his full time to pathology and the clinical laboratory. They appointed Leo Rigler as the hospital radiologist because, recalled Dr. Rigler, "I knew more radiology than anyone around — little as it was . . . ."[42] Leo Rigler thus began his career as a radiologist in 1923 with almost no training. During 1924 he went to study radiology with Dr. J. T. Case at Battle Creek, Michigan and with Dr. P. J. Hickey, at the University of Michigan at Ann Arbor. In 1925 Rigler reduced his appointment at the Minneapolis General Hospital to half-time in order to begin private medical practice in Minneapolis. Immediately successful in practice, he soon earned enough money to pay his debts and to provide a better living for his family.

When Dean Lyon and Dr. Berglund discussed with Dr. Rigler the possibility of his becoming chief of radiology at the university, Dean Lyon proposed that Rigler go to Europe to spend a year at Stockholm with Gösta Forssell in order to acquire a thorough training in radiological diagnosis. Dean Lyon offered $1,000 to help pay the Riglers' travel and living expenses while they were abroad. On his return from Europe, Leo Rigler would be appointed associate professor and chief of the Division of Radiology in the medical school at an annual salary of $5,000, an amount less than half what Rigler was then earning in practice. Although they would have to go into debt again to pay for the year in Europe, and faced the prospect of a smaller income into the indefinite future, Dr. and Mrs. Rigler decided that he should accept Dean Lyon's offer. They never regretted it. Sweden was then the foremost center of radiology in the world, and Gösta Forssell the outstanding Swedish radiologist. Leo Rigler was Gösta Forssell's first American student, and they became personal friends. Forssell was active not only in the use of x-rays for diagnosis, but was also chief of a center for radiation therapy in which both x-rays and radium treatments were used. Rigler thus gained experience in radiation therapy as well as in diagnosis. Near the end of the year in Europe, Rigler visited clinics at various cities in Germany and at Vienna before returning to the United States. On 1 July 1927 he took up his duties as associate professor and chief of the Division of Radiology which, with Rigler's appointment, became a division within the Department of Medicine instead of Surgery.

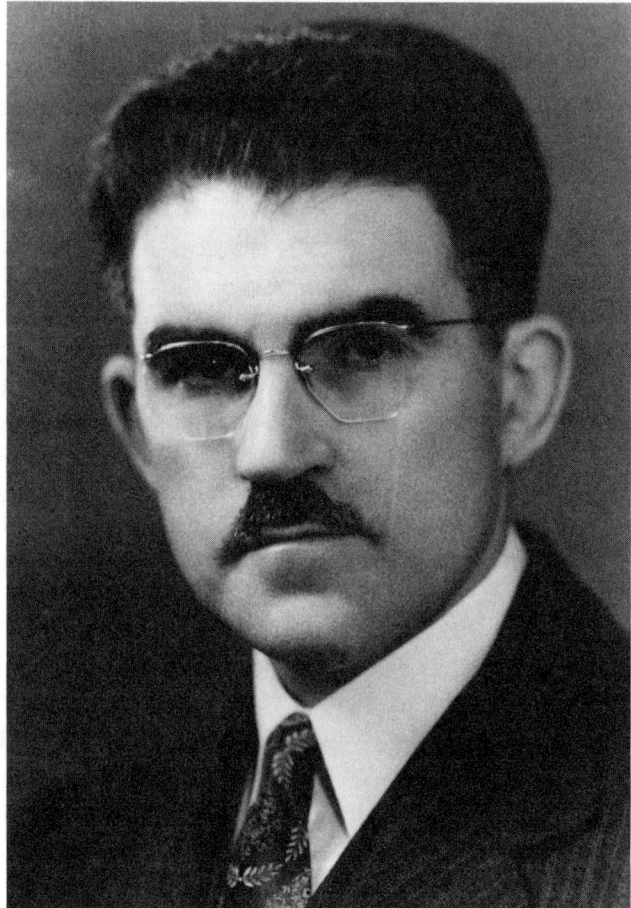

FIGURE 13:6   Leo Rigler, circa 1926. Courtesy Mn U Archives.

In 1927 the Division of Radiology at the university hospital consisted of one large room, which served the various functions of reception room for patients, film conference room for the staff, and office. In addition there was a small darkroom for processing x-ray films and two small rooms for fluoroscopic examinations. When the new Eustis Hospital and outpatient department were completed in 1929, the Division of Radiology moved to the fifth floor of the hospital where it remained until 1954. In their new and larger quarters, Dr. Rigler created a wet film viewing room so that x-ray films might be examined while they were still in the clearing solution so as to gain information from them more rapidly in urgent cases. The technique also enabled the staff to make sure that the films were satisfactory before the patient left. Simultaneously with the move to the fifth floor of the hospital, Leo Rigler, at the age of thirty-three, was promoted to the rank of

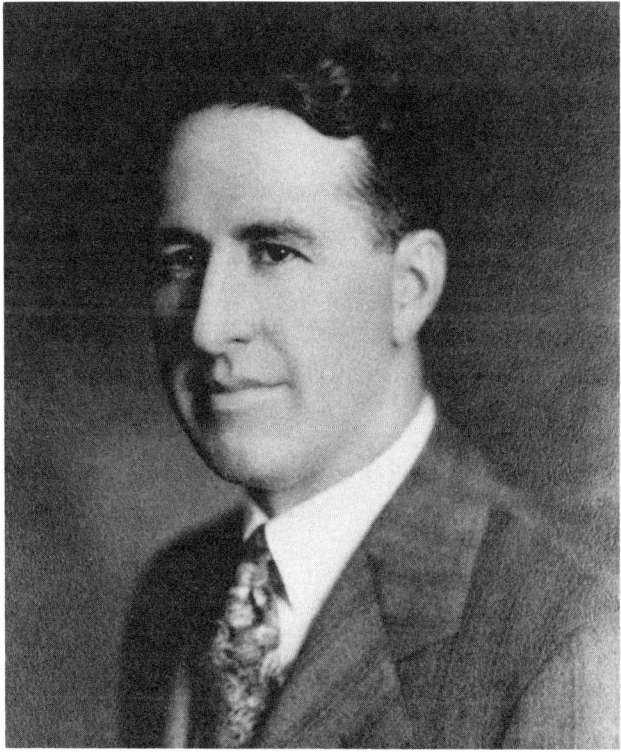

FIGURE 13:7   Irvine McQuarrie, circa 1920. Courtesy Mn U Archives.

full professor. He now had the organization and the facilities to carry on an active program of clinical investigation in radiology.

In 1930 with clinicians working on a geographic full-time basis in medicine, radiology, and surgery, Dean Lyon had an opportunity to appoint a fourth full-time clinical chief when the part-time chief of pediatrics, Frederic W. M. Schlutz, resigned to go to the University of Chicago. Since his appointment in 1924, Dr. Schlutz had developed further the part-time clinical faculty in pediatrics and enlarged both the house staff in the university hospital and the departmental budget. On 28 February 1930 Dean Lyon reported to the administrative committee that he had obtained memoranda on various potential candidates for the headship of pediatrics from Milton Winternitz, dean of the Yale medical school.[43] Dean Lyon and two members of the faculty were elected a committee to search for a new chief of pediatrics. The result of their search was the selection of Irvine McQuarrie, then associate professor of pediatrics at the University of Rochester School of Medicine at Rochester, New York.

At age thirty-nine when he came to Minnesota in 1930, Irvine McQuarrie was a native of Silver Reef, Utah, where his father operated a silver mine. Irvine McQuarrie first studied mining engineering at the University of Utah, where in

1912, at the end of his freshman year, he married a fellow student, Vera Perkins. During his senior year at Utah, Vera McQuarrie taught school to provide them with an income. When he was graduated from the University of Utah in 1915, Irvine McQuarrie decided to switch from mining engineering to medicine, influenced by the example of a maternal uncle who was a physician and by the prolonged sufferings of his mother from arthritis. He succeeded in winning a scholarship for Utah students at the University of California, and in the fall of 1915 went to Berkeley, California to begin the study of medicine. At the University of California the preclinical subjects were taught on the Berkeley campus during the first two years of the medical course, while clinical training in the junior and senior years was given ten miles away in San Francisco. When Irvine McQuarrie arrived at Berkeley in 1915, Herbert M. Evans had just returned from Johns Hopkins to head the department of anatomy and was organizing a very active program of research, particularly in pituitary and reproductive physiology. From Johns Hopkins Dr. Evans had brought George W. Corner, who at Berkeley began to study ovulation in hogs, while Evans himself with Joseph A. Long studied the estrus cycle in the rat.[44] Evans also recognized the research ability of a young anatomy instructor already at Berkeley, Philip E. Smith, and reduced Smith's teaching load so that he could carry on research. At Berkeley the head of the department of pathology and bacteriology, Frederick P. Gay was, like Evans, a graduate of the Johns Hopkins Medical School and similarly imbued with the spirit of research, as was also his colleague, the Swiss pathologist Karl F. Meyer. In the lively atmosphere of the Berkeley classrooms and laboratories, Irvine McQuarrie could hardly fail to become interested in research, and in 1917 he published his first paper, on a pharmacological subject. The same year McQuarrie was appointed to a student fellowship at the Hooper Foundation for Medical Research in San Francisco, a research laboratory of the University of California established in 1914 under the directorship of George Hoyt Whipple, who, like Evans and Gay, came to California from Johns Hopkins. At the Hooper Foundation, Irvine McQuarrie carried out investigations of the effects on kidney function of intestinal obstruction and proteose intoxication. In 1919 he received a Ph.D. degree from the University of California in experimental pathology and biochemistry, and at the urging of George Whipple and Herbert Evans, went for the last two years of his medical course to the Johns Hopkins where in 1921 he received the M.D. degree. At Johns Hopkins, McQuarrie's interest in pediatrics was aroused by weekly grand rounds with Edwards A. Park and Grover F. Powers. After graduation from the Hopkins, McQuarrie became a house officer at the Henry Ford Hospital at Detroit, Michigan, where in 1923 he was appointed director of the section on endocrinology and metabolism. In 1924 he went for a year as an instructor in pediatrics to Yale where his former teacher at Johns Hopkins, Edwards Park, was now head of pediatrics. After another year at the Henry Ford Hospital as director of pediatrics, Dr. McQuarrie went in 1926 to the then recently opened medical school of the University of Rochester at Rochester, New York, where his former chief at the Hooper Foundation in San Francisco, George Hoyt Whipple, was now dean. At Rochester

Irvine McQuarrie became assistant professor and then associate professor of pediatrics under Samuel W. Clausen, who had, like McQuarrie and so many of his teachers, studied medicine at Johns Hopkins.[45]

With the arrival of Irvine McQuarrie at Minnesota in July 1930, Dean Lyon had achieved the appointment of full-time chiefs for medicine, surgery and pediatrics. In addition, Leo Rigler was working full-time in diagnostic radiology, and George Fahr full-time in medicine at the Minneapolis General Hospital. The fruits of such full-time clinical appointments were soon to appear in an accelerated pace of clinical research at Minnesota marked by striking discoveries of far-reaching importance.

NOTES

1. School of Medicine, Administrative Board, Minutes, 13 September 1915.
2. Ibid.
3. School of Medicine, Administrative Board, Minutes, 7 October 1915.
4. School of Medicine, Administrative Board, Minutes, 1 November 1915.
5. Leonard G. Rowntree, *Amid masters of twentieth century medicine*, p. 201.
6. Moore to Law, 3 April 1918, Moore papers.
7. School of Medicine, Administrative Board, Minutes, 7 March 1918.
8. School of Medicine, General Faculty, Minutes, 19 March 1918.
9. School of Medicine, Administrative Board, Minutes, 9 April 1918.
10. School of Medicine, Administrative Board, Minutes, 3 November 1918.
11. School of Medicine, Administrative Board, Minutes, 12 January 1921.
12. School of Medicine, Administrative Board, Minutes, 6 November 1923.
13. Ibid.
14. School of Medicine, Administrative Board, Minutes, 26 January 1924.
15. School of Medicine, Administrative Board, Minutes, 10 April 1924.
16. School of Medicine, General Faculty, Minutes, 23 April 1924.
17. Angus L. Cameron, M.D., Ph.D., was assistant professor of surgery; George E. Fahr, M.D., was assistant professor of medicine; J. Charnley McKinley, M.D., Ph.D., was assistant professor of neurology.
18. School of Medicine, Administrative Board, Minutes, 27 October 1924.
19. School of Medicine, General Faculty, Minutes, 25 November 1924.
20. Ibid.
21. School of Medicine, Administrative Board, Minutes, 18 March 1925; 14 May 1925.
22. Darrach to Lyon, 20 February 1925 [copy], President's Office, Papers.
23. Lyon to Coffman et al., 24 February 1925. President's Office, Papers.
24. Lyon to Coffman, 21 September 1925, President's Office, Papers.
25. Owen H. Wangensteen, *Owen H. Wangensteen,* p. 25.
26. School of Medicine, Administrative Committee, Minutes, 24 May 1926.
27. School of Medicine, Administrative Committee, Minutes, 15 November 1926.
28. School of Medicine, Executive Faculty, Minutes, 17 November 1926.
29. School of Medicine, Administrative Board, Minutes, 13 December 1926.
30. George Fahr, "On simultaneous records of the heart sounds and electrocardiogram," *Heart,* 1912, *4,* 147–170.
31. Details of George Fahr's education and years in Europe were derived chiefly from

George E. Fahr, "Memoirs of a scientist," in Arthur C. Kerkhof, ed., *Festschrift, George E. Fahr, M.D.*, pp. 3-12.

32. Owen H. Wangensteen, "Our teachers," *J. med. Educ.*, 1962, *37*, 698-703, p. 699. This essay was published also in Kerkhof, ed., *Festschrift* (n. 31), pp. 26-29.

33. Ibid., p. 700.

34. Wangensteen, *Owen H. Wangensteen* (n. 25), p. 16.

35. George Fahr, "Myxedema heart," *J. Am. med. Ass.*, 1925, *84*, 345-349.

36. E. P. Lyon, "The Medical School," in University of Minnesota, *The President's report for the year 1926-27*, pp. 135-138, p. 136.

37. Fritz de Quervain, *Clinical surgical diagnosis for students and practitioner*.

38. O. H. Wangensteen, "Untersuchungen Über die Autolyse der Leber: die Implantation der Leber in die Bauchhöhle der Ratte," *Endokrinologie*, 1928, *2*, 170-181.

39. Ms. note by Owen H. Wangensteen on a reprint of Raffaele Bastianelli, "Operative treatment of malignant disease of the large intestine," in Intestinal Medical Congress, XVII, London, 1913, *Proceedings* (London, 1913), "Owen H. Wangensteen, Rome, Feb. 27, 1928."

40. Owen H. Wangensteen, "Surgical reminiscences," *Minn. Med.*, 1978, *61*, 623-633, pp. 626-627.

41. Hilding Berglund et al., eds., *The kidney in health and disease*.

42. Leo G. Rigler, "Learning and teaching under Dean Lyon," in Owen H. Wangensteen, ed., *Elias Potter Lyon: Minnesota's leader in medical education*, pp. 121-141, p. 128. Biographical information on Rigler is drawn also from Owen H. Wangensteen, "Tribute to a wonderful colleague, teacher, scientist and humanist, Leo G. Rigler," *Minn. Med.*, 1980, *63*, 791-794.

43. School of Medicine, Administrative Committee, 28 February 1930.

44. George W. Corner, *The seven ages of a medical scientist*, pp. 124-127.

45. Biographical information about Irvine McQuarrie was derived from two obituary articles: Arild E. Hansen, "Irvine McQuarrie (1891-1961)," *J. Pediat.*, 1963, *62*, 448-454; J. Arthur Myers, "Irvine McQuarrie, M.D.," *J.-Lancet*, 1961, *81*, 552-560.

CHAPTER 14

The Clinical Renaissance of the Medical School, 1930–1941

In 1930 Professor Richard E. Scammon left the Department of Anatomy to become dean of the college of medical sciences at the University of Chicago. His going left a great gap in the life of the medical school. Since 1914 Scammon had taught embryology to successive medical classes. His lectures, delivered in the early morning, were very popular, the classroom always packed. "By 7 o'clock," wrote Edith Boyd, "every student was in his seat with his notebook open, colored pencils clutched in one hand, pen poised in the other, ready to go when Scammon ambled in and without fanfare started painting in colored chalk the diverse yet recurrent patterns of differentiation of all the tissues and structures of the body."[1] Born at Kansas City, Missouri, and educated at the University of Kansas, Scammon went for graduate study in anatomy to Harvard, where he received his Ph.D. in 1909. After two years of teaching anatomy at the University of Kansas, Scammon came in 1911 to the University of Minnesota as assistant professor of anatomy, and in 1914 took over from Thomas G. Lee the teaching of embryology and histology. A tall, massive man, Scammon possessed a vast knowledge of history and literature. He read Latin and Greek as well as English, and was deeply familiar with English history, politics, and economics. Scammon was interested in the history of medicine and encouraged medical students to study the history of their field.[2] He was an authority on the London plague. In science Scammon studied the phenomena of human growth, both the growth and development of the embryo and the growth of the child to adulthood. He was a scientist and teacher of such standing that both students and faculty considered his departure a real loss to the school.

Scammon's departure coincided with a renewed outburst of criticism of Dean Lyon from the medical alumni. Although in several conferences with representatives of the Medical Alumni Association President Coffman defended Dean Lyon vigorously, he decided that some attempt must be made to meet alumni criticisms. Although the alumni recognized Dean Lyon's honesty and fairness, they thought that because Dean Lyon was not a physician, he was insensitive to the in-

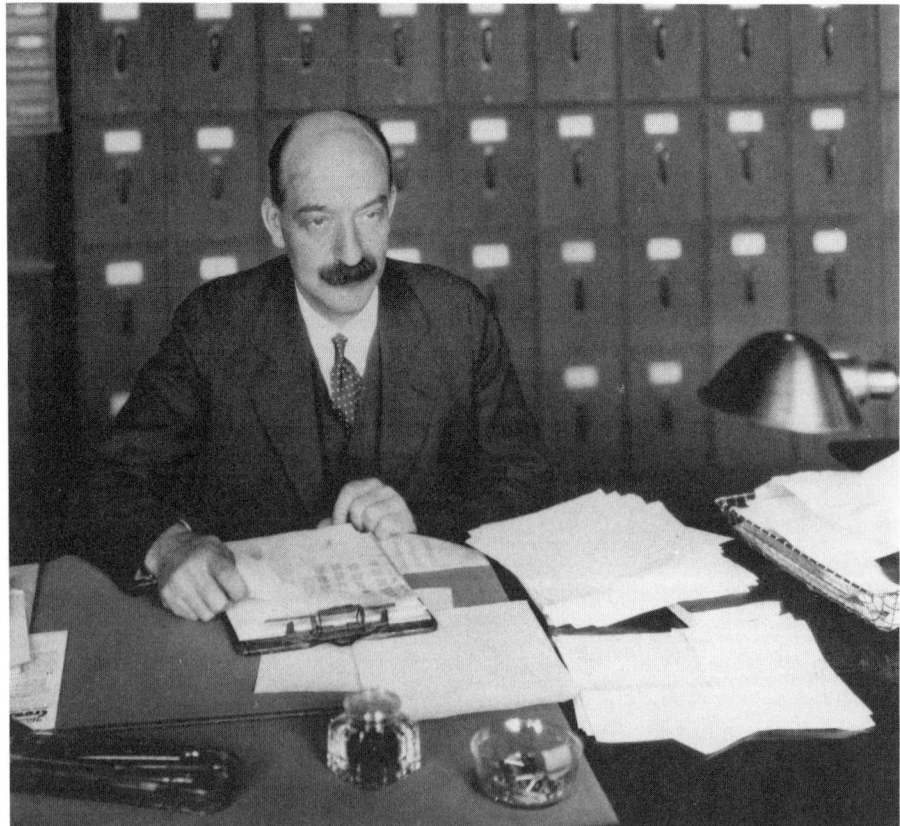

FIGURE 14:1   Richard E. Scammon, circa 1931. Courtesy Mn U Archives.

terests and feelings of the medical profession in the state. In 1931 President Coffman found what seemed a happy solution to the difficulty when he persuaded Richard Scammon to return to Minnesota to fill a new role as dean of a newly-created College of Medical Sciences. The College of Medical Sciences was to include the schools of medicine and nursing and the university hospital. Dean Lyon would continue as dean of the medical school, but as dean of medical sciences Dr. Scammon would be concerned with general policy, educational programs, faculty, and the relations of medicine to other branches of the university. The news of Scammon's return to Minnesota was greeted with enthusiasm among the medical alumni who retained from their student days delightful memories of his classes. Meanwhile, Dean Lyon's years of patient effort to expand the university hospital and appoint full-time chiefs of the clinical departments were beginning to yield their harvest.

Surgery

When Owen H. Wangensteen became chief of the Department of Surgery in January 1930, the department consisted of two other full-time clinical teachers: Dr. O. N. Campbell and Dr. William T. Peyton. Dr. C. Donald Creevy was a teaching fellow and there were seventeen part-time clinical teachers. The department budget was about $34,000 of which some $12,000 was devoted to salaries for the part-time clinical teachers. When he came to prepare his budget for the coming year 1930–31, Dr. Wangensteen wrote to Dean Lyon to define the aims of the Department of Surgery which he thought ought to include the training not only of good practical surgeons, but also of men who would contribute to the development of surgery, who would add "to the patrimony of knowledge . . . ." The existing budget was sufficient only for the training of practical surgeons. In order to train surgeons to become active investigators, the surgery supply budget needed to be sufficient to support a laboratory. Dr. Wangensteen urged that it be increased from the current $2,100 to at least $5,000. He asked that the surgery department again be given the full-time stenographer and the laboratory technician that it had before he went abroad in 1927. Dr. Wangensteen urged also that the number of surgical teaching fellows at the university be increased so that the time of teaching fellows would not be taken up entirely with the routine care of patients. He hoped that most of the surgical teaching fellows would go on to pursue academic careers in surgery, but if loaded with routine hospital duties, no matter what their abilities might be, they would never develop into more than "bread and butter" surgeons. Dr. Wangensteen hoped to establish in the near future an instructorship in surgery for the man of unusual promise who, after four or five years as a teaching fellow, wished to remain at the university pursuing his investigations while waiting for a surgical teaching appointment to open at some other university.[3]

In his request for a larger budget for the Department of Surgery, Dr. Wangensteen emphasized the need for a larger supply budget to support research and for stipends to support additional teaching fellows. Evidently Dean Lyon was unable to provide the additional funds requested, because in order to find funds for additional teaching fellows, Dr. Wangensteen was obliged to take away from the part-time clinical teachers the salaries previously paid to them. Dean Lyon advised Dr. Wangensteen to go slowly in depriving the part-time teachers of their salaries, but Wangensteen went ahead and did it anyway. He recognized that the part-time teachers probably didn't like to lose their salaries but, since they were among the best surgeons in the Twin Cities, he thought that they would not suffer too much. At any rate Dr. Wangensteen said that they did not complain to him.[4] A factor in their acceptance of the sacrifice of their salaries may have been the respect which the surgeons had already gained for their young chief because of his intense efforts to develop research in the department.

When Dr. Wangensteen took up his duties as associate professor of surgery in the fall of 1928, he found that frequently he was called upon to close intestinal fistulas on patients who had undergone enterostomy to relieve intestinal obstruction. About 80 percent of patients who suffered from acute obstruction of the small intestine had previously undergone abdominal surgery, so that in the great majority of patients intestinal obstruction occurred as a complication of an earlier surgical operation. Consequently as the number of surgical operations increased rapidly after 1900, the number of patients with acute intestinal obstruction grew apace. The only effective treatment for acute intestinal obstruction was surgical intervention. Without operation patients with acute intestinal obstruction would almost invariably die. Even with surgical operation, the chances of death for patients operated upon for intestinal obstruction at the beginning of the century was over 60 percent, and in the 1920s it was still 44 percent; that is, almost half of patients operated on for intestinal obstruction died.[5] The longer the time that had elapsed between the onset of obstruction and the operation, the more frequently the patients died. Surgeons were generally agreed that early diagnosis of intestinal obstruction was the critical factor in saving the life of the patient.

When a surgeon operated to relieve intestinal obstruction, he might seek to relieve the obstruction by separating the bands or adhesions within the abdomen that caused it. He might in addition perform an enterostomy, that is, create an opening from the intestine to the exterior in order to drain the intestine above the obstruction. Surgeons had found that an enterostomy by itself frequently was able to relieve intestinal obstruction, because when the intestine was no longer distended with gas and fluid above the obstruction, the intestinal canal reestablished its natural continuity. The early technique of enterostomy, and the method commonly used by American surgeons in the 1920s, was to bring a loop of intestine to the surface in order to create a fistula from the intestinal canal to the exterior. While in Europe during 1927–28, Dr. Wangensteen learned of a much better technique of enterostomy developed in 1891 by a German surgeon, Oscar Witzel, of Bonn. Witzel made an oblique enterostomy over a catheter so that only the catheter passed through the wall of the intestine and out through the abdominal wall, but in the 1920s few American surgeons knew of Witzel's technique. Dr. Wangensteen's realization of the relatively crude methods of enterostomy used by American surgeons aroused his interest in intestinal obstruction as a field for investigation in which few other surgeons were working.

In 1928 the explanation usually given for the high mortality from intestinal obstruction was that the contents of the obstructed intestine became extremely toxic, causing the patients to die of toxemia resulting from the absorption of toxins. In 1913 at Johns Hopkins, George Hoyt Whipple and his colleagues discovered a toxic substance in a loop of duodenum tied off at both ends, and had suggested that the toxin was produced by the mucosa of the isolated loop.[6] In 1916 Whipple and his colleagues, by then at the Hooper Institute at San Francisco, identified the toxin as a proteose, and showed that when it was injected into the circulation of a healthy dog it produced severe illness and death. For nine years, first at Baltimore and then at San Francisco, Whipple and his colleagues performed experiments and assembled evidence tending to show that death in intestinal obstruction resulted from the production of a toxic proteose by the mucosa of the obstructed intestine.[7] Nevertheless in 1912 at Cornell University Medical College in New York City, John A. Hartwell and J. P. Hoguet had shown that experimental obstruction of the upper portion of the small intestine in dogs resulted in severe dehydration.[8] Hartwell and Hoguet showed that injections of saline could prolong the life of a dog with experimental intestinal obstruction, and suggested that death from intestinal obstruction occurred as a result of dehydration.

When Dr. Wangensteen began to study intestinal obstruction in 1928, most clinicians and investigators accepted the toxic theory of death from intestinal obstruction, although some investigators had shown that dehydration and loss of electrolytes were probably decisive in causing death. In 1923 at the University of Kansas, Russell L. Haden and Thomas G. Orr had found that following experimental intestinal obstruction in dogs there was a fall in the concentration of chlorides and a rise in the level of sodium carbonate in the blood plasma, the latter reflected in a rise in the carbon dioxide-combining power of the plasma.[9] As Dr. Wangensteen surveyed the literature on intestinal obstruction, he became skeptical of the toxic theory of mortality in intestinal obstruction. Together with a senior medical student, Stanley S. Chunn, Dr. Wangensteen compared the toxicity of the contents of obstructed bowel with those of normal bowel in dogs and rabbits. Both proved toxic, but the contents of normal bowel were just as toxic as those of obstructed bowel.[10] Once he had demonstrated that death from intestinal obstruction was probably unrelated to the toxicity of intestinal contents, Dr. Wangensteen proceeded to carry out a systematic series of experiments on dogs to study the various physiological consequences of intestinal obstruction. Together with another medical student, Milo Loucks, Dr. Wangensteen showed that the obstructed intestine was no more permeable to dissolved substances than normal intestine, so that the obstructed intestine was no more liable than the normal to permit the absorption of toxic substances.[11] Then he and Stanley Chunn studied the effect of intestinal obstruction on the blood chemistry, confirming the fall in chlorides and the rise in sodium carbonate and nonprotein nitrogen observed by other investigators. As Hartwell and Hoguet had shown in 1912, Wangensteen and Chunn found that the administration of saline to a dog with experimental intestinal obstruction would prolong its life for three weeks. Even if they gave the dog saline for only one week, it still lived for three weeks, an observation which suggested that the saline was not acting to detoxify an absorbed poisonous substance. In 1928 Dr. Wangensteen had helped to remove the basis for the toxicity theory of death from intestinal obstruction. The same year at the Harvard medical school, Monroe A. McIver and James L. Gamble argued that death from intestinal obstruction was due to the loss of chloride and sodium ions, with a resultant inability of the tissue cells to maintain their normal fluid content.[12] In 1930, also at the Harvard medical school, Drs. J. C. White and F. A. Fender provided further dramatic experimental evidence that death in high intestinal obstruction was due to a loss of digestive fluids and salts. From a dog in which they had produced an

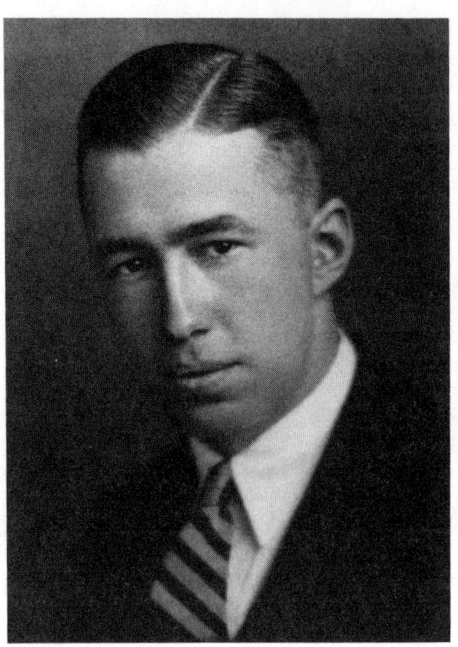

FIGURE 14:2 N. Logan Leven, 1927.
Courtesy Mn U Archives.

experimental intestinal obstruction, they collected the vomitus, and after diluting it with water, injected it through a catheter into the unobstructed lower intestine. Under these conditions the dog remained alert and active throughout the entire month of the experiment, with little change in its blood chemistry except for a slow decline in the level of chloride ion because the daily recovery of vomitus could not be perfectly complete. White and Fender demonstrated that an animal with a complete obstruction of the small intestine could be kept alive and in good health so long as the loss of digestive secretions was prevented and the animal remained adequately nourished. They observed no toxemia as a result of the obstruction, and noted that there could be no absorbable toxic substance in the gastrointestinal contents because it was through reinjection of those same contents into the intestine below the obstruction that the dog's life and health was maintained.[13]

In 1930, working with a newly-appointed surgical teaching fellow, N. Logan Leven, Dr. Wangensteen studied the effects of experimental intestinal obstruction at various levels in dogs. When the obstruction was in the duodenum, the animal soon had a high blood urea, low blood chloride, and alkalosis as a result of vomiting a large volume of gastric juice, bile, pancreatic juice, and intestinal secretion. The lost fluid and electrolytes could be replaced by injections of saline. If the obstruction were made low in the ileum, no significant loss of fluid or change in blood chemistry occurred, but still the dog died. If the obstruction were made in the colon, the dog lived much longer, but died finally of starvation or of acute distention of the colon with feces. Wangensteen and Leven distinguished

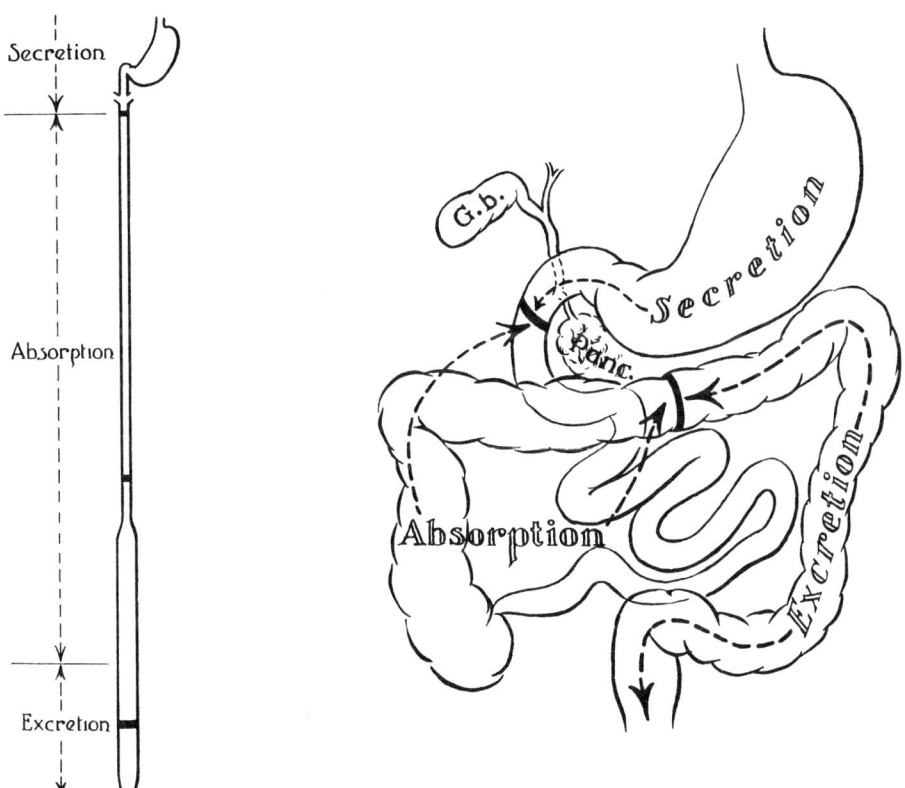

FIGURE 14:3 Wangensteen's and Leven's diagrams of functional zones in the alimentary canal. Courtesy *Archives of Surgery*.

three functional zones along the length of the alimentary canal. The stomach and the upper part of the duodenum, where several litres daily of gastric juice, bile, pancreatic juice, and intestinal juice were secreted, was a zone of *secretion*. The remainder of the small intestine and the upper part of the large intestine formed a zone of *absorption*. The lower part of the large intestine and rectum were a zone of *excretion*.[14]

The originality and force of the short paper by Owen Wangensteen and Logan Leven, published in 1931, can only be appreciated fully when it is compared with a paper published two years earlier by John J. Morton, professor of surgery in the University of Rochester School of Medicine. Influenced perhaps by George Hoyt Whipple, then dean of the Rochester medical school, Dr. Morton adhered to the toxic theory of intestinal obstruction. In an experimental study of the differences between high and low intestinal obstructions in the dog, Morton showed that high intestinal obstruction was more *toxic* than low intestinal obstruction because of anatomical and physiological differences, but he argued that such differences existed because the wall of the duodenum was able to absorb more toxin than the wall of the intestine lower down. Dr. Morton assumed, and cited many distinguished investigators who likewise assumed, that death in intestinal obstruction resulted from the absorption of toxins from the obstructed intestine.[15] In 1931, following the line of research begun by Hartwell and Hoguet in 1912, Wangensteen and Leven came to radically different conclusions. Death from intestinal obstruction was a consequence of dehydration and loss of electrolytes resulting from the vomiting of gastrointestinal secretions.

The same year, 1931, Dr. Wangensteen elaborated new criteria for the early diagnosis of intestinal obstruction. Although surgeons had long known that surgical intervention for intestinal obstruction was much more effective when undertaken at an early stage, they were frustrated by the lack of physical signs to confirm the presence of intestinal obstruction. Such symptoms as pain, vomiting, and constipation suggested intestinal obstruction, but they might also indicate other abdominal conditions. By themselves they did not justify surgical operation at an early stage. In 1929 Owen Wangensteen with the help of a third-year medical student, Francis Lynch, introduced the use of x-ray photographs for the early detection of intestinal obstruction. Wangensteen and Lynch noted that, although gas was normally present throughout the gastrointestinal tract, in the small intestine it usually occurred as small bubbles in fluid so that it did not appear in an x-ray photograph. If, however, a portion of small intestine were distended with gas, the distention would appear as a shadow on an x-ray film. When Wangensteen and Lynch created intestinal obstructions experimentally in dogs, they found that within four to five hours x-rays would provide a clear picture of the presence of loops of small intestine distended with gas. After twenty-four hours the whole of the small intestine above the point of obstruction became distended with gas. Nevertheless, despite the distention of the intestine, there was no measurable external distention of the abdomen until much later, at a time when the dog was close to death. When barium was given it took twenty hours to reach the site of obstruction and barium was really not needed to detect the presence of obstruction because the shadows produced on an x-ray by gas-distended intestines could reveal obstruction so much earlier.[16]

In 1931 Dr. Wangensteen suggested that when a patient complained of intermittent, crampy, colicky pain accompanied by nausea and vomiting, but without local physical signs, the absence of local physical signs should suggest intestinal obstruction. He emphasized that a physician should not be misled by the passage of gas and feces, when an enema was administered, into thinking that no intestinal obstruction was present. Dr. Wangensteen cited the case of a patient, an eight-year-old boy, whom he had lost because a bowel movement had led him to think that there was no obstruction in the child's intestine. He found that a most useful diagnostic tool was the stethoscope. If intermittent abdominal cramps were accompanied by loud gurgling noises, heard most intensely through the stethoscope at the height of the pain, the patient probably had acute intestinal obstruction. In peritonitis, by contrast, the abdomen was as still as the grave. The x-ray photograph was particularly valuable for diagnosis because visible accumulations of gas appeared a few hours after onset of obstruction. Later a characteristic *ladder pattern* of gas shadows appeared, but the physician did not need to wait for it to make a diagnosis. The x-ray could confirm the existence of intestinal stasis while the stethoscope could be used to determine whether the obstruction were mechanical or the result of paralysis caused by peritonitis.[17]

In December 1931 Dr. Wangensteen noted that the presence of gas in the colon might also be used to rule out intestinal obstruction. After the administration of several enemas, if an intestinal obstruction existed, the colon would become empty of gas, so that if gas continued to appear in the colon, the small intestine could not be obstructed. In the emergency treatment of intestinal obstruction, Dr. Wangensteen used enterostomy. He inserted a catheter into the intestine and buried a short length of the catheter in the body wall by Oscar Witzel's technique. Gas and fluid could then drain out through the catheter to relieve the distention of the small intestine above the obstruction. In keeping with his physiological approach to surgery, Dr. Wangensteen regularly measured the quantities of fluid released from the obstructed intestine and found that after the first twenty-four hours, the amount of fluid escaping became very small. In most patients the relief of distention had the happy effect of permitting the intestine to restore its natural continuity. If the obstruction were caused by adhesions, nothing more than enterostomy was required to relieve it.

Most of the gas distending the obstructed intestine was known to be swallowed air. Sometime during 1931 Dr. Wangensteen decided that, if the chief value of enterostomy were to relieve the distention of the obstructed intestine by gas that consisted mostly of swallowed air, it might be possible to intercept the swallowed air in the stomach before it entered the intestine. Any gas already in the intestine could then dissipate gradually, either by regurgitation through the pylorus or by absorption into the circulating blood. Late in the summer he had an opportunity to test the hypothesis.

In August 1931 a seventy-two-year-old woman was admitted to the university hospital, gravely ill. For three days she had been suffering from intestinal obstruction thought to be caused by a carcinoma of the caecum. Because of the patient's age, her feeble condition, and state of severe dehydration, Dr. Wangensteen judged that she could not stand a surgical operation to create an enterostomy. Unable to operate, Dr. Wangensteen passed a tube through the patient's nose down into the stomach and applied moderate, continuous suction to it. The results were dramatic. The patient's cramps ceased immediately. After eight hours, when some 200 cc. of fluid and 800 cc. of gas had been withdrawn, her condition was much improved, and after forty hours all signs of gaseous distention had disappeared. When Dr. Wangensteen then operated, he found not a carcinoma, but a stricture of the ileum, which he was able to release.

In October 1931 Dr. Wangensteen used suction on a second patient with intestinal obstruction, a nine-year-old boy, who three years before had undergone an operation for appendicitis. Again suction relieved the child's intestinal cramps immediately, and after a period of time not only relieved the distention of the

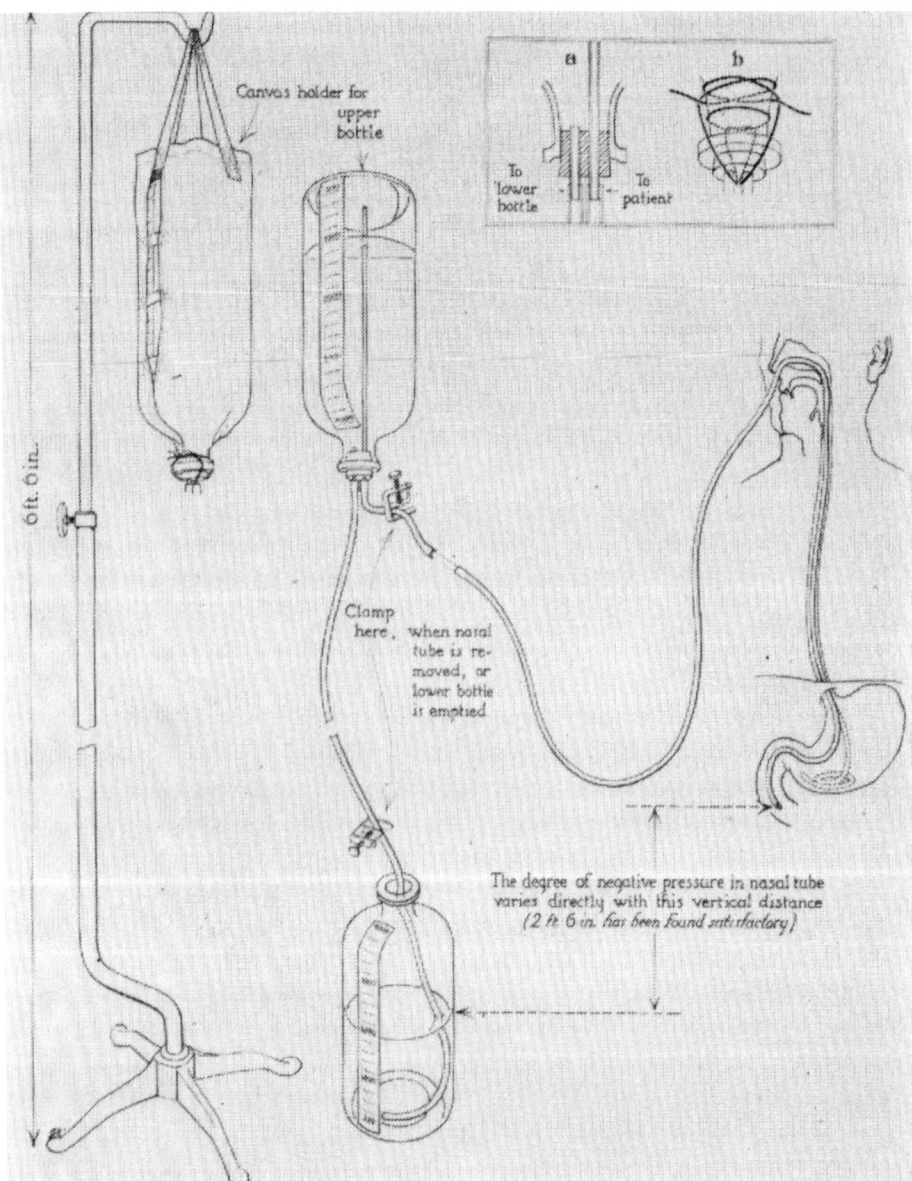

FIGURE 14:4 Diagram of Wangensteen suction apparatus; bottle is inverted so that gas, as well as fluid, may be collected and measured. Courtesy *Western Journal of Surgery, Obstetrics and Gynecology*.

intestines, but the intestinal obstruction itself. Only because the child had suffered several attacks, did Dr. Wangensteen operate fifteen days later to release the band that had caused the obstruction.

The third patient, a twenty-six-year old man, developed intestinal obstruction seven days after an appendectomy. For him seventy-two hours' suction was sufficient to decompress the intestine and to remove the obstruction so that he could be discharged without further surgery.[18] By May 1932 Dr. Wangensteen had used suction through a nasal catheter on seven patients suffering from intestinal obstruction, with excellent results. In some patients the tube made its way from the stomach into the duodenum so that suction was applied directly to the small intestine. In successive patients the application of suction served both to relieve the pain and distention caused by obstruction and to restore the functional continuity of the intestine. The first sign that the intestine was again working normally was the appearance of gas in the colon, a sign, said Dr. Wangensteen, that " . . . has in a manner the same significance for patient and physician as the exultation and delight experienced by a shipwrecked mariner on the sight of another sail" — a novel view of intestinal gas, but perhaps an analogy natural to a physician with Viking ancestors.[19]

By 1931 the torrent of research which Dr. Wangensteen had carried on, in collaboration with surgical fellows and medical students since the fall of 1928, had brought him to the verge of revolutionary developments in abdominal surgery. Dr. Wangensteen had defined the criteria for early diagnosis of intestinal obstruction with the aid of x-rays and stethoscope, and he had discovered that suction through a nasal catheter extended into the stomach or even the duodenum could relieve the distention by gas as effectively as enterostomy. Nevertheless, Dr. Wangensteen's work on intestinal obstruction was only part of his work as a surgeon, and as a professor of surgery. He also did many operations for cancer. Frequently he operated on patients on whom other surgeons had refused to operate because they considered such patients poor risks. Many surgeons did not wish to endanger their record of successes by operating upon patients who had only slight hope of obtaining a successful result. Undaunted by such fears, Dr. Wangensteen was willing to operate whenever there was any reasonable chance of saving the life of a patient.

On 7 April 1932 the Department of Surgery provided the program for a meeting of the Minneapolis Surgical Society held in the Eustis Amphitheater at the university hospital. Dr. Wangensteen presided. Among the papers delivered by the surgical faculty and teaching fellows, Dr. John R. Paine described the use of suction on a nasal catheter to relieve postoperative discomfort in patients who had undergone abdominal surgery. Suction through a nasal catheter was able to relieve nausea, vomiting, and distention with gas, especially in those who had undergone opertations on the stomach or biliary tract.[20]

In June 1932 Paul Fesler resigned as superintendent of the hospital to become director of the Wesley Hospital connected with the Northwestern University School of Medicine at Evanston, Illinois. During the five and a half years that he

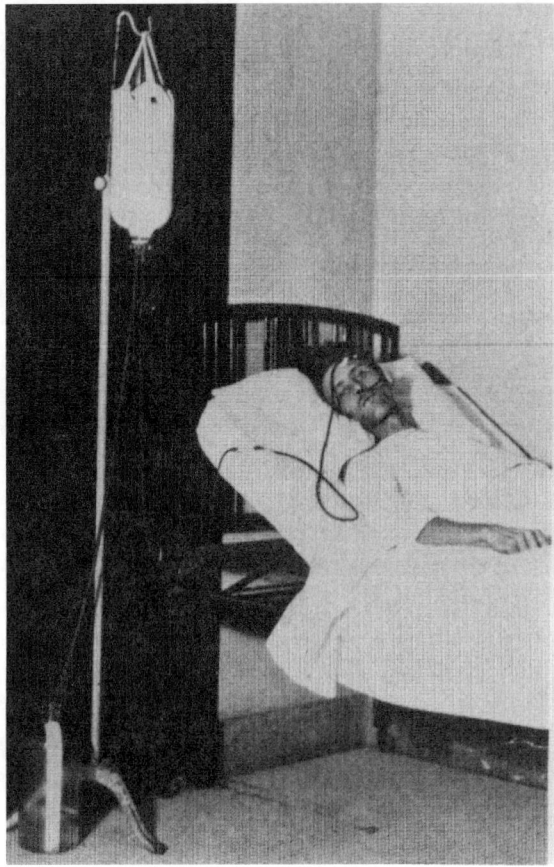

FIGURE 14:5   An early patient for whom suction relieved and removed acute intestinal obstruction. Courtesy *Western Journal of Surgery, Obstetrics and Gynecology*.

had been at Minnesota, Mr. Fesler had guided the university hospital through a major expansion, marked by the addition of the Eustis hospital, the new outpatient department, and students' health service, which increased the capacity of the hospital by 200 beds. Mr. Fesler had organized a social service department, and had enlarged and developed the nursing service. The clinical departments had moved their offices from Millard Hall into the enlarged hospital and had begun to hold weekly departmental seminars. A weekly hospital staff meeting was organized. Mr. Fesler supervised the steady development of the former small university hospital into a still small, but increasingly complex, medical center with research and diagnostic laboratories, operating rooms, a physiotherapy department, and other special services. "Newcomers in our group fail to realize this remarkable evolution," noted one observer, "so smoothly have these innovations been put into effect."[21] Also during Mr. Fesler's tenure the medical profession throughout Minnesota had gained increasing confidence in the university hospital. Paul Fesler

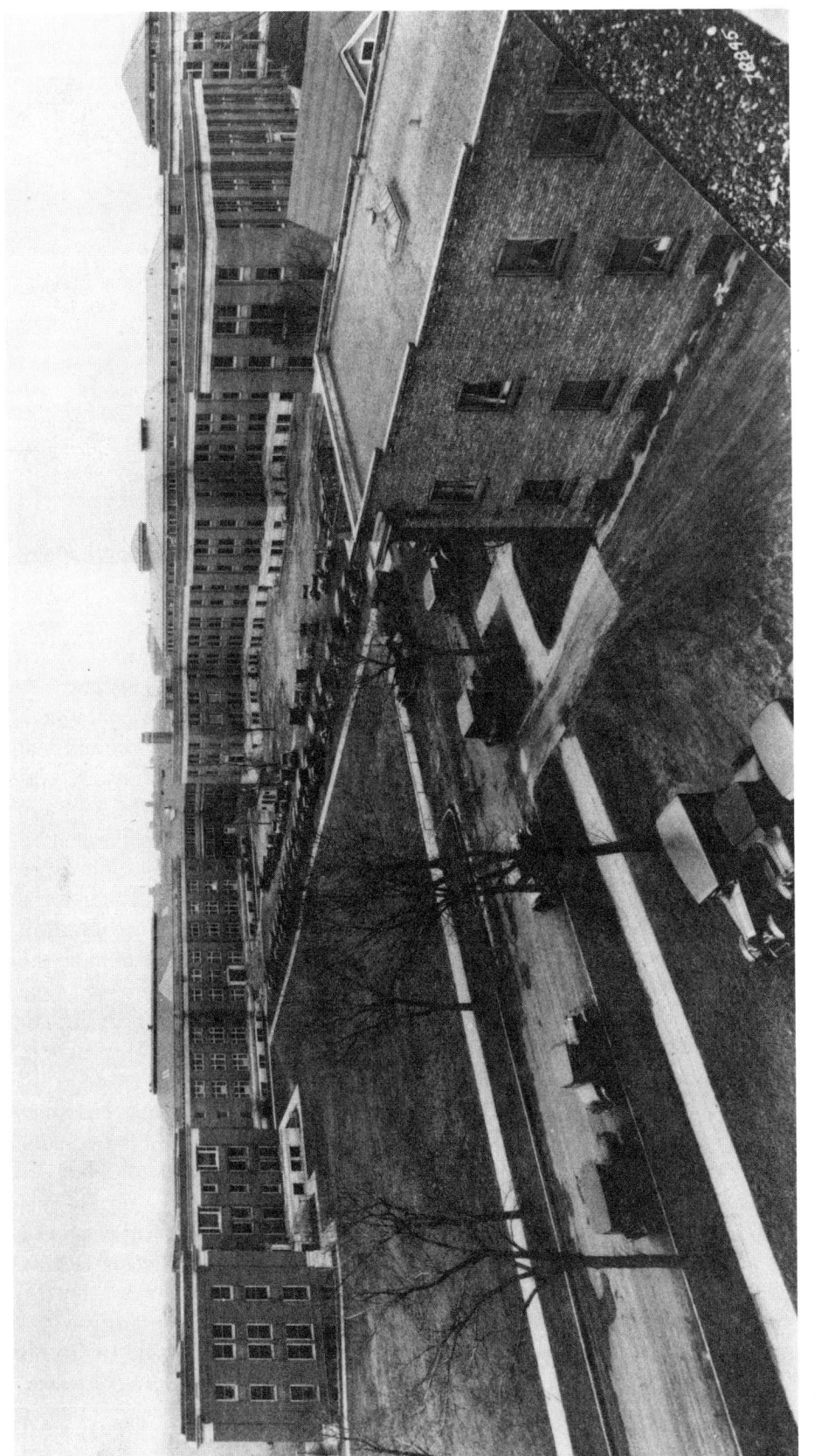

FIGURE 14:6 University hospital buildings, circa 1930; side wall of Madsen flats in foreground. Courtesy Mn U Archives.

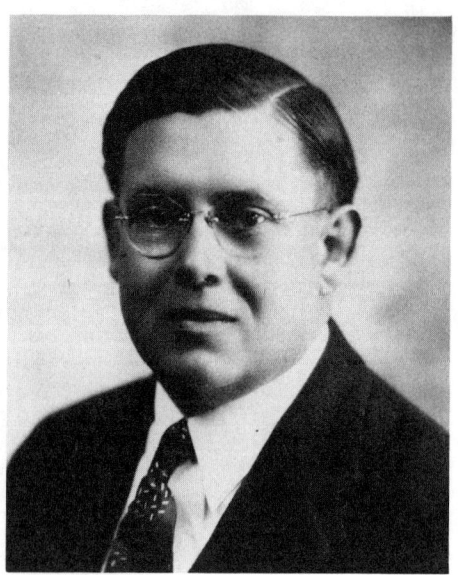

FIGURE 14:7 Paul Fesler, circa 1930.
Courtesy Mn U Archives.

had provided the stable sustaining institutional environment in which Owen Wangensteen and other clinical chiefs did their work at the university hospital.

In July 1932 Dr. Halbert L. Dunn became director of the university hospital. The son of a Minneapolis surgeon, Dr. Dunn was educated at the University of Minnesota where he was graduated B.A. in 1917 and M.D. in 1922. After a year of internship at Presbyterian Hospital in New York City and another year as a Mayo Foundation fellow at Rochester, Dr. Dunn became associate professor of biometry and vital statistics at Johns Hopkins in 1925. From 1930 until his return to Minneapolis in 1932, he was the director of the statistical department at the Mayo Clinic. In his research Dr. Dunn had studied the mathematics of human growth and development, an interest that he shared with Richard Scammon, the new dean of the College of Medical Sciences. Possibly their shared interest in the mathematical analysis of growth was a factor in Dunn's appointment as director of the university hospital. Certainly from the time of his arrival at Minnesota in July 1932, Dr. Dunn was close to Dean Scammon.

On Thursday, 4 May 1933, when Dr. Wangensteen was planning to leave that evening by train to attend a medical meeting at Washington, D.C., Dean Scammon summoned him to his office and presented him with a long letter from Dr. Dunn containing complaints about his actions as chief of the Department of Surgery. Dr. Dunn wrote that during the whole time that he had been director of the hospital he had received complaints, either against Dr. Wangensteen or against the activities of the Department of Surgery from interns, fellows, nurses, and members of the clinical staff. In November 1932 six of the seven surgical interns complained about the surgical teaching they were receiving, and Dr. Dunn suggested that they should present their complaints in writing to Dean Scammon,

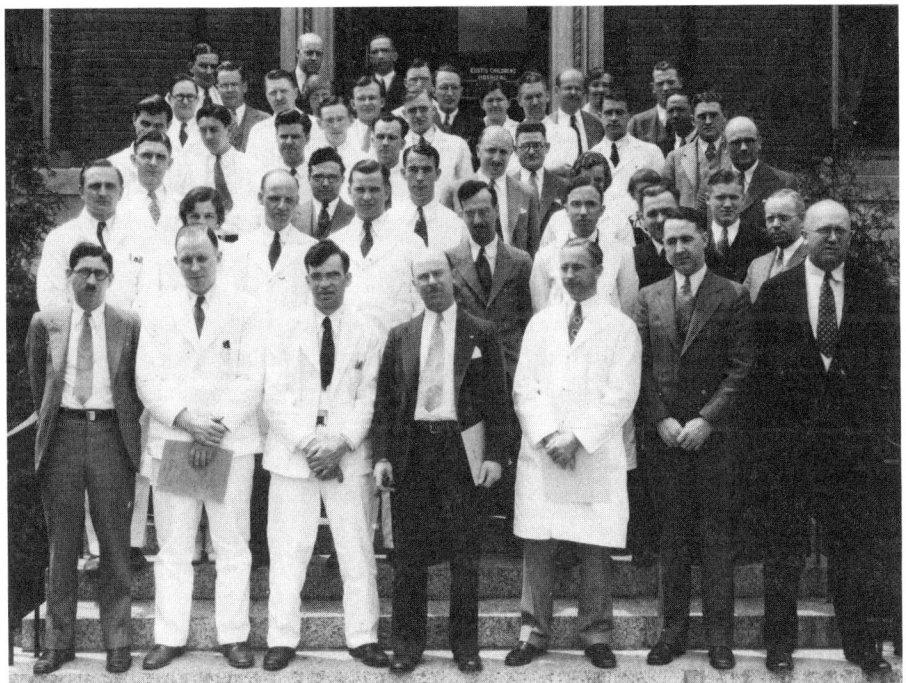

FIGURE 14:8 University hospital staff group, circa 1932. Front row from right: Hilding Berglund, Irvine McQuarrie, Owen Wangensteen, Halbert Dunn. Back row, left: Chester Stewart and Harold Diehl (in doorway). Others unidentified. Courtesy Mn U Archives.

which they did. The complaints of the interns were that they had little opportunity to perform surgical diagnosis because surgical cases were worked up either in the outpatient department or on the medical service and were sent to surgery merely for operation. They thought there was a lack of staff instruction with little explanation of surgical procedure during operations. General rounds were unwieldy and hasty, with cursory discussion of too many cases. The service on dressings was of little value, and the surgical dispensary was poorly organized.[22] In December 1932 one intern, Dr. E. V. Speckman, resigned his internship to return to Lethbridge, Alberta, Canada, because he was dissatisfied with Dr. Wangensteen's attitude toward teaching. In March 1933 the surgical interns began to show their discontent by breaking hospital regulations so that Dr. Dunn was forced to tell them that if they did not obey the rules of the hospital he would dismiss all of them. At the same time he promised that he would, in due course, ask Dean Scammon to review their complaints.

Dr. Dunn said that he had been told by various persons that many of the patients upon whom Dr. Wangensteen operated for stomach cancer died. Among thirty-one patients on whom Dr. Wangensteen had performed abdominal operations in 1932, fourteen had died in hospital. Although Dr. Dunn said that he did not feel qualified to judge the meaning of such data, he thought they raised the question whether the patients had died because of Dr. Wangensteen's lack of ability as a surgeon, and the subject required investigation. Dr. Dunn said also that in casual conversations with Dr. Irvine McQuarrie, chief of pediatrics, and Dr. Hilleboe, fellow in pediatrics, he had learned that the pediatrics staff continually had to urge the surgical staff to give smaller doses of drugs and smaller volumes of intravenous saline and transfused blood when surgery was performed on children.

Nevertheless, the immediate occasion for Dr. Dunn's letter were events that had occurred in surgery on Monday, 24 April 1933. According to Dr. Dunn, Dr. Wangensteen had been scheduled to operate on a patient for stomach cancer, but when the abdomen was opened the cancer was found to be inoperable because of metastases in the liver, and Dr. Wangensteen ordered the abdomen closed. Dr. Wangensteen then ordered that another patient, who was in the hospital awaiting operation for stomach cancer but who had not been scheduled for operation that morning, be brought up for operation, but the patient refused operation because his wife could not be notified. Dr. Wangensteen then ordered up for operation four other patients, none of whom had been scheduled or prepared for operation, and operated on three of them. All of the patients operated upon had had breakfast that morning. On 1 May, a week after operation, all three patients were recovering, but one of the patients had vomited food while under anesthesia, and all had been subjected unnecessarily to the risk of aspiration pneumonia, which could easily have been fatal. Dr. Dunn concluded his letter by stating: "I feel that an impartial investigation of Dr. Wangensteen and his administration of the Department of Surgery, which will either prove or disprove this evidence, must be made or the effectiveness of the Minnesota General Hospitals will be definitely impaired."[23]

Dr. Dunn's letter contained a curious mixture of grave charges with vague complaints based on hearsay evidence gathered in casual conversations. When Dr. Wangensteen first read the letter in Dean Scammon's office, he told Scammon, "This is a bunch of trivial drivel."[24] He and Dean Scammon talked for several hours on that Thursday afternoon until after the train, on which Dr. Wangensteen was to have left for Washington, had pulled out of the station. At the end Scammon asked Wangensteen to bring him next morning a letter containing his reply to the various criticisms.

If Dr. Dunn and Dean Scammon had anticipated that Dr. Wangensteen would resign quietly to avoid further criticism, they had mistaken their man. The following day Dr. Wangensteen sent Dean Scammon a five page letter, containing his detailed response to the complaints mentioned by Dr. Dunn. He sent copies of the letter to President Coffman and to Dr. Dunn.

Dr. Wangensteen said that when he had received the interns' complaints he had called the surgical staff together to discuss them. They concluded that for the most part the complaints were those commonly expressed by groups of interns. Dr. Wangensteen thought that one complaint, namely, that they could not see undiagnosed cases, was just. Nevertheless, when he discussed the matter with Dr. Dunn, Dr. Dunn explained that it was not feasible to give the surgical interns a service in the outpatient admitting department. To deal with one complaint about the surgical dressing service, Dr. Wangensteen changed the intern assignments so that each intern could do his own dressings, but on the general surgical service the interns had chosen to continue to do group dressings.[25]

So far as his ability as a surgeon was concerned, Dr. Wangensteen requested a review of the patients who had come under his care at the university hospital, and that his work be compared with that of other surgeons. He added that in 1932 he had performed gastric resections on three elderly patients, aged seventy-three, seventy-nine, and eighty-one respectively.

Dr. Wangensteen said that Dr. Dunn's account of events on Monday, 24 April, was only partially correct. A Dr. Gunnar Redell of Upsala, Sweden was visiting his clinic that day, and Dr. Wangensteen said " . . . I felt obliged (perhaps more than necessary) to try to show him some of my own surgery in which he was interested."[26] Nevertheless, he had not urged operation upon any patient and added: " . . . I have ever and always will respect the patient's wishes and interests as paramount." The patients upon whom he did operate on 24 April were thoracic cases, whom he had told the day before that he would operate on them in a day or two. They gave their consent willingly on 24 April; their families or friends were notified. The first operation did not begin until 10:41 a.m., and the patients had had breakfast at 7:30 a.m. "None of the patients had an unusual reaction to operation," said Dr. Wangensteen; "all have continued to do well and are very well satisfied."

Dr. Wangensteen considered that the details in Dr. Dunn's letter were " . . . largely matters of idle gossip which have been given undue credence," but they needed to be cleared up. "I earnestly insist, Dean Scammon," he wrote, "that you investigate searchingly any of their ramifications and I pledge you my whole-hearted support in the inquiry." He added: "I appreciate that the University has extended me unusual opportunities and I have sincerely tried to prove worthy of that trust . . . ." If he had made any mistake, he said, it was in the acquisition of too large a junior staff. In his final paragraph Dr. Wangensteen wrote: "If, however, the interests of the School are better served by my stepping aside for some one more capable to take up these burdens, I shall gladly do so, with some regrets, but without resentment or remorse."[27]

When Dr. Wangensteen presented the complaints against him to the other clinical chiefs, Dr. J. Charnley McKinley, professor of neurology and acting chief of the Department of Medicine, agreed to defend him at a meeting with Dean Scammon.[28] Meanwhile, until the question was settled, Dr. Wangensteen told Dean Scammon that he would stay away from the university hospital. Others also came to his support. On the morning of Saturday, 6 May, President Coffman held a conference in his office with Dean Scammon and others to discuss the situation in the Department of Surgery. Scammon proposed to make an inquiry, which would be restricted to a determination of the facts of the case, without attempting

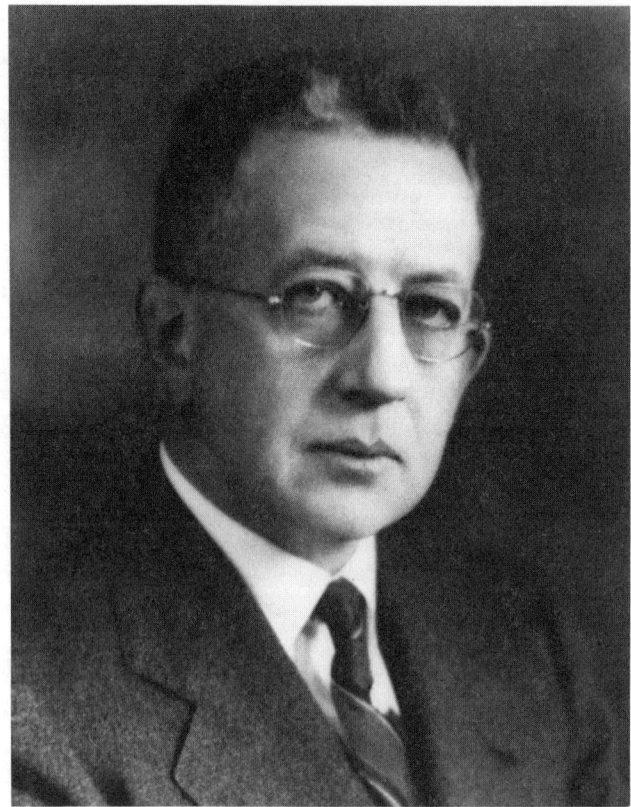

FIGURE 14:9 John Charnley McKinley, circa 1933. Courtesy Mn U Archives.

to pass judgment on them. Later that morning President Coffman telephoned Dean Scammon to direct him not to proceed with the proposed inquiry, and at Scammon's request confirmed the instruction by a letter written shortly after the telephone call. In a medical matter, and especially a surgical matter, President Coffman very probably consulted Dr. William Mayo by telephone after that Saturday morning conference, and Dr. Mayo may have seen the potential harm to the university of such an inquiry. It would be impossible to separate a determination of facts from the conclusions to be drawn from them because the selection of facts to be determined implied a judgment of their significance. Scammon was not satisfied to drop the inquiry. The next day (Sunday, 7 May) he wrote to President Coffman to urge " . . . an early and complete determination of the facts in this situation," which he considered " . . . imperative both as a matter of Medical School and Hospital policy, and as an act of justice to all persons involved."[29]

President Coffman did not yield; no inquiry was held. Dean Lyon, who had remained in the background after Scammon's appointment as dean of the college of medical sciences, was still dean of the medical school, and exerted considerable influence with President Coffman. Lyon now came to Owen Wangensteen's support as did his old teacher Arthur Strachauer. But Wangensteen's most powerful defender was William Mayo. In the Board of Regents William Mayo's word was law on medical matters, and Mayo felt a ready sympathy for a young surgeon under fire for the operations he performed. Moreover, Mayo liked Wangensteen, and respected the research he was doing.

During the two or three weeks in May 1933 that his fate was being determined, Dr. Wangensteen remained at home, away from the turmoil of the university hospital. The unaccustomed leisure gave him time to reflect both on the research of the previous four years and the general direction of his career. During this period in May 1933 he read proofs for a detailed paper on the use of the suction tube on some twenty patients suffering from intestinal obstruction.[30] The suction tube was also proving increasingly valuable to relieve the nausea, pain, and vomiting that followed abdominal operations so frequently even when there was no intestinal obstruction. Patients treated with suction felt almost no nausea. One patient, who had part of his stomach removed for a recurrent peptic ulcer, had undergone three previous operations at another hospital without suction. When on the third day after his operation he was asked what he thought of the suction tube, the patient replied, "I never knew anyone could have an operation on his stomach and be so comfortable." By June 1933 Dr. Wangensteen and his colleagues had used nasal catheter suction in the postoperative treatment of more than 500 patients with remarkably uniform success.[31]

Two years later, in July 1935, Owen Wangensteen received the Samuel D. Gross Prize, awarded by the Philadelphia Academy of Surgery, for his essay "The therapeutic problem in bowel obstructions." The award of the Gross Prize, which was given only every five years, was one of the highest honors open to American surgeons, and represented national recognition of Dr. Wangensteen's years of work on intestinal obstruction. When he published the essay as a monograph in 1937, it quickly became the standard work on intestinal obstruction.[32] In 1938 Dr. Wangensteen was invited to address the members of the Massachusetts Medical Society on the subject of bowel obstruction. He felt keenly the honor of being asked to address this, the oldest state medical society in the country. After describing the various methods used to achieve the prompt diagnosis of intestinal obstruction, Dr. Wangensteen recommended conservative treatment by suction except when there were signs of strangulation. During the discussion that followed, a distinguished Boston surgeon said that suction was so simple and so satisfactory "that one wonders how we ever practiced surgery before the Wangensteen method was devised."[33] But perhaps the most satisfactory evidence of the value of Dr. Wangensteen's work came from the records of the Massachusetts General Hospital where for the decade 1928 to 1937 the mortality among patients treated for intestinal obstruction had declined to 20 percent, less than half the mortality rate of 44 percent for the preceding decade 1917 to 1928. It was the first real decline in deaths from intestinal obstruction in the forty-year period for which the hospital

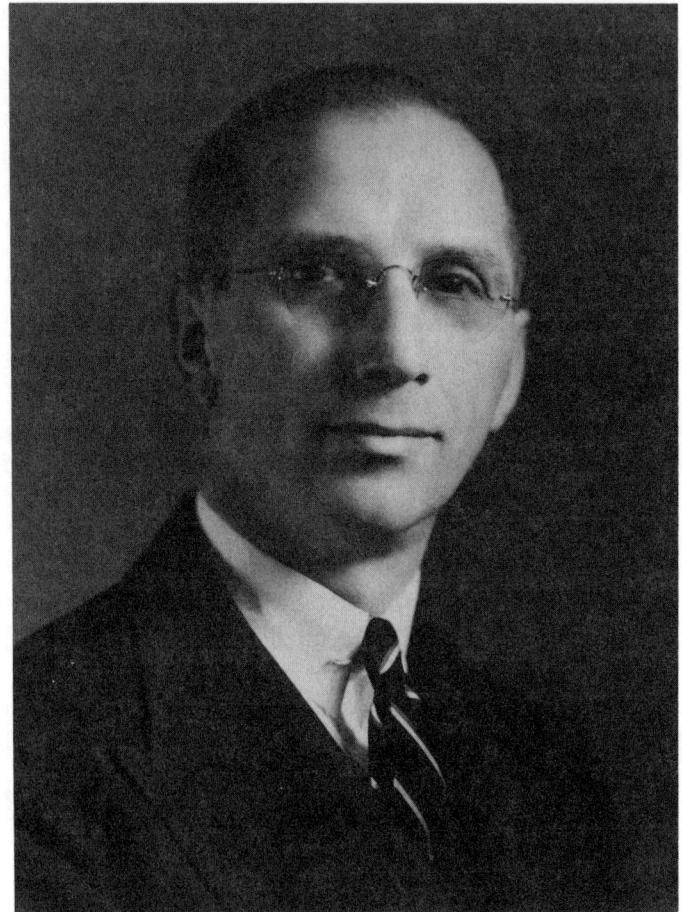

FIGURE 14:10   Harold S. Diehl, circa 1937. Courtesy Mn U Archives.

possessed comparable statistics.³⁴ To paraphrase words that Dr. Wangensteen had used often: Minnesota had made a solid contribution to the patrimony of surgical learning.

Change in the Deanship

In 1935 Dr. Richard Scammon resigned as dean of the College of Medical Sciences, and the Board of Regents created for him a distinguished service professorship in the graduate school. The regents had come sadly to the realization that despite his brilliance as a scientist and teacher, or perhaps because of it, Dr. Scammon was not well suited to administration. The turmoil in surgery two years earlier was only part of the difficulty. At the commencement ceremonies in June 1935, when President Coffman called on Dean Scammon to present the graduates in medicine for their degrees, Scammon was unable to reply—a very public loss of speech that some persons attributed to the effects of alcohol. Meanwhile the duties of administration prevented Scammon from making progress with his great study of human growth, on which he had been at work for many years.

To replace Scammon as dean of the College of Medical Sciences, the Board of Regents appointed Harold S. Diehl. Then forty-four years old, Dr. Diehl had been director of the students' health service at Minnesota since 1921, and under his direction the health service had grown from cramped quarters in the basement of Pillsbury Hall to occupy an entire wing of the university hospital, while the staff had grown to nine full-time and thirty part-time physicians. Under Dr. Diehl the students' health service had introduced compulsory vaccination and tuberculin tests for all incoming students and had developed a tuberculosis-prevention program. Diehl's very successful administration of the students' health service had fulfilled the promise that he had shown during his service as a senior medical student with Base Hospital No. 26 and after the war with the American Red Cross Commission in Poland.

When Harold Diehl became dean of the College of Medical Sciences in 1935, Dean Lyon was still dean of the medical school. In 1933, frustrated by the fact that the real responsibilities of his office had been removed, Dean Lyon suggested that the separate position of dean of the medical school be abolished. When Dean Lyon retired in 1936, Harold Diehl became both dean of the medical school and the medical sciences. To replace Diehl at the students' health service, the Board of Regents appointed his assistant, Dr. Ruth Boynton. In 1935 the director of the university hospital, Dr. Halbert Dunn, resigned to become chief statistician of the Bureau of the Census in Washington, D.C. and Ray Amberg, assistant director of the hospital and business manager of the students' health services, was appointed to succeed him.

Medicine

When Hilding Berglund took over the Department of Medicine in 1925, he moved quickly to develop a faculty who were interested in the pursuit of research. In 1927 George Fahr was promoted to become chief of the medical service at the Minneapolis General Hospital. S. Marx White and Moses Barron continued to be especially active as part-time clinical teachers. Dr. Barron's early training and extensive experience as a pathologist made his class clinics especially valuable to the medical students. The department contained three divisions: general medicine, directed by Dr. Berglund; nervous and mental diseases, directed by Arthur S. Hamilton; and dermatology, directed by Henry E. Michelson.

In 1930 Dr. Berglund brought Hobart A. Reimann to Minnesota from the Peking Union Medical College where Dr. Reimann had been since 1927 as associate professor of medicine. Then thirty-three years of age, Dr. Reimann was a native of Buffalo, New York, and had studied medicine at the University of Buffalo where he was graduated M.D. in 1921. During the three years from 1923 to 1926, he had become interested in pneumonia through his research on the pneumococcus carried out with Oswald Avery at the Rockefeller Institute for Medical Research in New York City. At Minnesota Dr. Reimann continued to pursue research on the diagnosis and treatment of pulmonary infections. When Hilding Berglund resigned as chief of the Department of Medicine in 1932, Dr. Reimann was appointed director of the Division of Internal Medicine while J. Charnley McKinley became chief of the department. Dr. Reimann remained at Minnesota until 1936 when he left to become professor of medicine at Jefferson Medical College in Philadelphia. Two years later, when Reimann published his classic monograph on pneumonias, it included a number of beautifully clear x-ray photographs provided by Leo Rigler, Reimann's colleague in radiology during his six years at Minnesota.[35]

In 1932, when Hobart Reimann became director of the Division of Internal Medicine, Cecil Watson returned to Minnesota as a teaching fellow and resident in medicine at the Minneapolis General Hospital. Then thirty-one years old, Dr. Watson had just spent two years in research in Hans Fischer's laboratory at Munich, Germany. A native of Minneapolis, Cecil Watson had studied medicine at Minnesota where he was graduated M.D. in 1926. He then spent two years as a fellow in pathology at the Minneapolis General Hospital where he became interested in the bile pigments and attempted the isolation of urobilin and stercobilin from urine and feces. In 1928 he had received his Ph.D. in pathology and had gone to Minot, North Dakota, to become pathologist in a clinic founded there by Angus Cameron, a former member of the surgery department at Minnesota. In 1930 Dr. Watson decided that he wanted to do further work on the chemistry of bile pigments and that, if he were to do so, he wanted to work with the world authority on the bile pigments, Hans Fischer. Fischer had been working on the bile pigments since 1910. He had shown that bilirubin consisted of four pyrrole rings, and that it was a degradation product of hemin, the active part of the hemoglobin molecule. In 1926 Fischer had achieved the first synthesis of a pyrrole and in 1929 he synthesized hemin, the feat which may have especially aroused Cecil Watson's interest and for which in 1930 Fischer received the Nobel Prize in chemistry.[36] To obtain an introduction to Fischer, Watson sought the help of his former teacher, George Fahr, who, from his early years in Germany, retained many friends among German physicians and scientists. Fahr gave Watson a letter of introduction to Friedrich Mueller, professor of medicine at Munich, and when Watson arrived at Munich in the autumn of 1930, Mueller introduced him to Hans Fischer. Fischer immediately offered Watson a place to work in his laboratory at the Technische Hochschule, and Cecil Watson set to work to isolate stercobilinogen from feces. Part of the research required the collection of stools from patients with hemolytic anemia in a hospital several miles from the Technische Hochschule. Dr. Watson then carried the feces in a small milk can across the city on the handlebars of his bicycle. Presently, from a violet solution extracted from feces, Watson obtained orange crystals which proved to be pure *stercobilin*.[37] When later he succeeded in crystallizing the substance giving the violet color to the solution, he identified it as a *mesobiliviolin*, a substance related to stercoblin.[38]

On his return to Minneapolis, Cecil Watson was eager to continue his research on the bile pigments and porphyrins and to apply such knowledge to clinical medicine. He began a residency in medicine at the Minneapolis General Hospital under George Fahr and then moved to the university hospital under Hobart Reimann. Dr. Watson also began to teach the medical school course in clinical chemistry and microscopy. At Minneapolis Watson continued his research on the porphyrins excreted in the urine and feces of patients suffering from such diseases as hemolytic anemia, pernicious anemia, liver disease, and lead poisoning.

In 1933, a fifty-two-year-old man came into the university hospital gravely ill and severely jaundiced. His stools were clay-colored while his urine was dark brown in color. The patient rapidly sank into a coma, and after a few days died. At autopsy he was found to be suffering from advanced cirrhosis of the liver, which had been caused by cincophen in a patent medicine that he had taken for arthritis for several months. During his illness part of the liver tissue was still forming bile pigments, but the liver was completely unable to secrete bile. From the urine of this patient, Cecil Watson isolated coproporphyrin. It was the first time that a porphyrin had been isolated from the urine of a patient suffering from jaundice or liver disease.[39]

From the feces of another patient suffering from a familial hemolytic jaundice, Cecil Watson isolated a previously undescribed porphyrin, which occurred together with greatly increased amounts of coproporphyrin excreted because of the heightened destruction of red blood cells.[40] Watson next isolated coproporphyrin I from the feces of two women patients with pernicious anemia. After one of the patients had been treated for ten months with liver therapy, the coproporphyrin disappeared from her feces, showing that the coproporphyrin had appeared in the feces as a consequence of the pernicious anemia.[41]

In July 1936, when Hobart Reimann departed, Cecil Watson was appointed director of the Division of Internal Medicine. Despite the burden of administrative and teaching duties, he continued his research, often returning to work in his laboratory in the evening. He studied particularly the biochemistry of the porphyrins, the group of compounds to which hemoglobin and the bile pigments belong. He became interested particularly in the disease porphyria. With one of his residents, William Clarke, Dr. Watson detected protoporphyrin in the reticulocytes.[42] From a study of the uroporphyrins in acute porphyria he determined that both Uroporphyrin I and Uroporphyrin III were present in Waldenström porphyria. In 1950 with his colleagues Rudi Schmid and Samuel P. Schwartz, Dr. Watson showed that in certain types of acute porphyria, porphyrin occurred abundantly

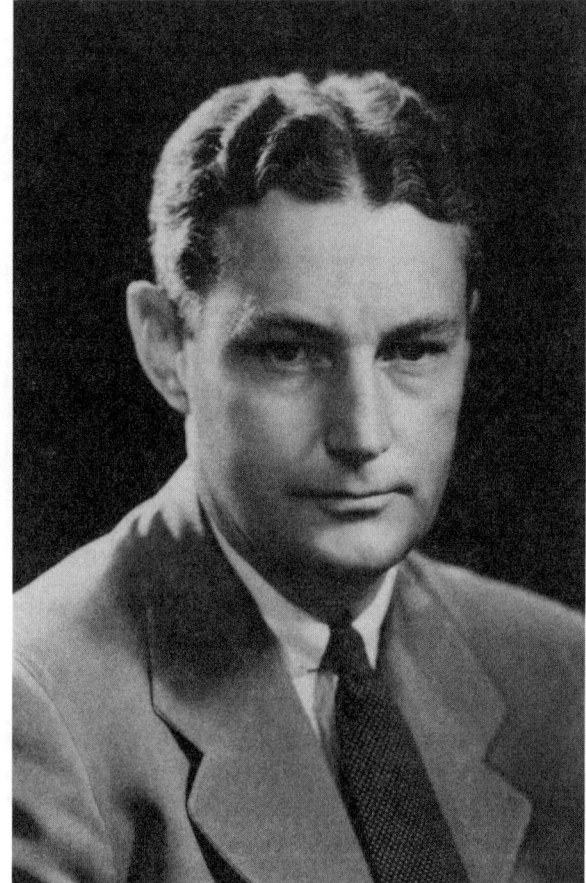

FIGURE 14:11   Cecil Watson, 1944. Courtesy Mn U Archives.

in the liver cells, whereas in classic congenital porphyria, porphyrin was present in the circulating red blood cells, a discovery that permitted the differentiation of the porphyrias into hepatic and erythropoietic types.[43] The work of Watson and his colleagues laid the basis for laboratory tests to diagnose not only the various forms of porphyria but also the various forms of liver and gall bladder disease.

In 1937 Wesley W. Spink came to the medical school as assistant professor of medicine. A native Minnesotan, Dr. Spink was born at Duluth and attended Carleton College at Northfield, Minnesota, where he was graduated A.B. in 1926. After two years of teaching at Doane College in Nebraska where he also coached football and track, Wesley Spink entered the Harvard medical school where he was graduated M.D. in 1932. During his senior year, when he was a clinical clerk at the Boston City Hospital, Spink presented a patient suffering from trichinosis to Dr. George Minot during rounds. When the rounds were over Dr. Minot invited Spink to his office to discuss the significance of eosinophilia in trichinosis, and suggested that Spink use the three-month elective period in his senior year to work on trichinosis in the department of parasitology at Harvard. The preliminary results proved so interesting that Dr. Minot obtained a scholarship for Spink to spend an additional six months in trichinosis research. Ultimately Dr. Spink published five papers on the results of the research. In January 1933 Wesley Spink began an internship on the Fourth Medical Service at the Boston City Hospital, and in 1934 continued as a resident physician at the Thorndike Memorial Laboratory attached to the Boston City Hospital, where he worked with Dr. Chester S. Keefer in research on infectious diseases. Then at the age of thirty-six, Dr. Keefer had been since 1930 associate physician at the Thorndike Laboratory. A graduate of the Johns Hopkins Medical School, he had in 1926 published an account of a case of brucellosis in Baltimore, the first of his many publications on infectious disease.[44] Together with Dr. Keefer, Dr. Spink studied gonococcal infections and the arthritis so frequently caused by gonococcal infection. When sulfanilamide became available in 1935, they began studies of the effect of sulfanilamide on gonococcal, streptococcal, and other infections.[45] In 1937, his residency at the Thorndike completed, Wesley Spink came to Minnesota, where he began work at the university hospital on 1 August.

About six weeks after Dr. Spink's arrival, a twenty-nine year old farmer was brought into the university hospital suffering from weakness, loss of weight, and fever. He had become ill seven months earlier when he developed a swelling of his right big toe, and began to suffer from loss of appetite and to cough up blood-stained sputum. He had been chronically ill ever since. In June 1937 an agglutination test of his blood gave an intense reaction for *Brucella abortus,* but despite treatment with sulfanilamide and with blood from a donor who had recovered from brucellosis, he had grown worse. When examined on admission to the hospital, the patient was running a fever and had heart murmurs. He was diagnosed as suffering from chronic brucellosis accompanied by rheumatic heart disease. Twenty-seven days after he entered the university hospital, the patient died. Postmortem examination, four hours after death, revealed on the aortic valve large vegetative lesions containing masses of coccus-like microorganisms. At this point Dr. Spink obtained the help of Dr. Orianna McDaniel at the Minnesota State Department of Health, who with her staff made cultures from the aortic-valve vegetations from which they obtained pure growths of *Brucella abortus.* They obtained cultures of *Brucella* also from the kidney, spleen, heart's blood, and lung. The patient had, therefore, died from an endocarditis caused by Brucella infection, not by a streptococcus. Half of the patient's herd of milk cows, which he had handled daily, were later found to be infected with brucellosis, and he had been accustomed to drink raw milk from his cows.[46] The case was unusual because few instances of Brucella endocarditis had been described previously. Commonly when a patient who died from brucellosis also suffered from endocarditis, the endocarditis resulted from a concurrent infection with *Streptococcus viridans.*[47]

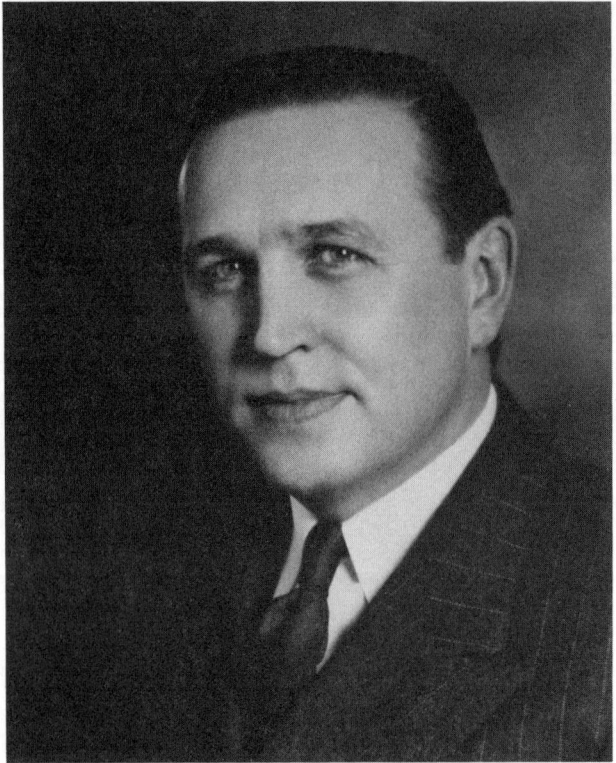

FIGURE 14:12 Wesley W. Spink, 1940. Courtesy Mn U Archives.

The case of brucellosis that Dr. Spink studied at the university hospital during the fall of 1937 was the first of a series. During the summer of 1940 three more patients with brucellosis entered the university hospital. One of them, a thirty-six-year-old farmer, died of Brucella endocarditis; like the young farmer who died of Brucella endocarditis in 1937, the 1941 patient owned a herd of cattle infected with *Brucella abortus,* and in the course of his work had handled aborted material. By the fall of 1941, Dr. Spink had cared for seven patients with brucellosis, among whom two with Brucella endocarditis had died. All seven patients had either drunk unpasteurized milk from cows infected with brucellosis (Bang's disease), or, in the case of the two dead young farmers, had been involved in the care of such infected cattle.

Although the seven cases of brucellosis that Dr. Spink saw in his first four years at the university hospital was not a large number, it was sufficient to demonstrate that brucellosis was a much more common disease in Minnesota than had been realized previously. Furthermore, each of the seven cases had been identified with certainty on the basis of culture of *Brucella abortus* taken from the blood or other tissues. Because few medical practitioners in Minnesota, or elsewhere in the United States, possessed the laboratory equipment and skill required to grow cultures of *Brucella abortus,* many cases of brucellosis went undiagnosed. Brucellosis was a protean disease, extremely variable in its manifestations, that frequently mimicked those of other infectious diseases. At the University of Minnesota the proximity of the laboratories of the State Department of Health (formerly the State Board of Health), where by 1940 Dr. Orianna McDaniel had been working on the bacteriology of disease problems for nearly half a century, to the university hospital, made frequent bacteriological tests for brucellosis feasible.

In 1896 the Danish veterinary pathologist and bacteriologist Bernhard Bang isolated a microorganism that he proved was the specific cause of contagious abortion in cattle, and which he named *Bacillus abortus.*[48] Although Bang's work was confirmed in England, for more than ten years American bacteriologists were unsuccessful in isolating Bang's organism from cattle suffering contagious abortion in the United States. They had begun to believe that in the United States contagious abortion in cattle was a disease different from that in Europe, but at the University of Minnesota in 1911, Winford P. Larson obtained a culture of *Bacillus abortus* from the Royal Veterinary Laboratory at Copenhagen and, using the *Bacillus abortus* as antigen, found that it gave the same complement fixation reaction as the sera of American cattle suffering from contagious abortion. Dr. Larson also succeeded in isolating from American cattle an organism identical in every respect with Bang's *Bacillus abortus.*[49] Dr. Larson and Julius P. Sedgwick, then clinical instructor in pediatrics at Minnesota, used the complement fixation reaction to test some 425 children of whom 73 (17 percent) reacted positively to *Bacillus abortus antigen,* indicating that they had been exposed to the organism.[50] Since the most probable means of exposure was through the drinking of unpasteurized milk from infected cows, Larson and Sedgwick's results suggested a further danger to children from unpasteurized milk. That danger was emphasized by Schroeder and Cotton's discovery in 1911 that *Bacillus abortus* was shed in the milk from infected cows.[51] In 1918 at the Dairy Division of the Bureau of Animal Industry in Washington, D.C., Alice C. Evans, proceeding from the knowledge that the organism causing Malta fever was a common infection of goat's milk on the island of Malta and that *Bacillus abortus* was a common infection of cow's milk in the United States, decided to compare them to learn whether the two organisms might be related. Dr. Evans found that the biochemical characteristics of *Bacillus abortus* were exactly the same as those of the Malta fever organism. Even more significant, the two organisms possessed the same agglutination reactions and the same ability to produce abortions when inoculated into pregnant guinea pigs. The only distinction between them was that the Malta fever organism produced more brown pigmentation when grown in culture. She concluded that the two organisms were closely related and emphasized that milk from cows infected with *Bacillus abortus* might easily transmit the infection to humans.[52] In 1920 at Berkeley, California, Karl Meyer and E. B. Shaw confirmed Evans's conclusions and suggested the generic name *Brucella* for the two organisms previously known as *Bacillus* or *Bacterium abortus* and *Micrococcus melitensis*. They became known as *Brucella abortus* and *Brucella melitensis*.[53]

At Salisbury, Rhodesia, in 1924 L. J. Orpen provided undeniable proof of cases of undulant fever caused by *Brucella abortus*. Orpen's patients had never drunk goat's milk but had worked with cattle suffering from contagious abortion.[54] In 1927 the first human case of brucellosis was recognized in Minnesota, but by 1929 some thirty cases had been reported.[55] Thus by 1930 American physicians realized that contagious abortion, or Bang's disease, was widespread among cattle herds in the United States and that the infection could be communicated to people either by drinking unpasteurized milk or by physical contact with infected cattle.

The distinctive feature of the seven cases of brucellosis that Wesley Spink and his colleagues had described by 1941 was that each was proven bacteriologically to be brucellosis. Such cases showed that brucellosis infection originating from the large reservoir of *Brucella abortus* existing in the cattle herds of the United States represented a widespread and serious threat to human health. At that point the entrance of the United States into World War II in December 1941 suspended further research on brucellosis at the medical school. Nevertheless, a breakdown in the control of brucellosis brought about by wartime conditions made the disease a serious public health problem — a problem which Dr. Spink and his colleagues would help to solve.

Research on Tuberculosis: the Lymanhurst School

On a winter's day early in January 1920, Mrs. Laura Dickson was relieving the information clerk in the front office of the Minneapolis Public Health Division when a tall, handsome man in the dress uniform of an officer of the United States Public Health Service, including spurs, appeared at the counter. He waited his turn and then said, "I am Dr. Harrington, your new Health Commissioner." A few months earlier the Minneapolis Board of Public Welfare had appealed to the United States Public Health Service for help in reorganizing the Division of Public Health in Minneapolis, and the Public Health Service had assigned Francis Edward Harrington to the task. Then at the age of forty, Francis Harrington was born at Norfolk, Virginia, the son of a brigadier general in the United States Marine Corps, and had studied medicine at Columbian University, later George Washington University, where he worked under Major Walter Reed and Captain James Carroll, who were investigating yellow fever. In 1914 Dr. Harrington joined the United States Public Health Service as an assistant epidemiologist and in the course of his work had been involved in the reorganization of health departments in several states.

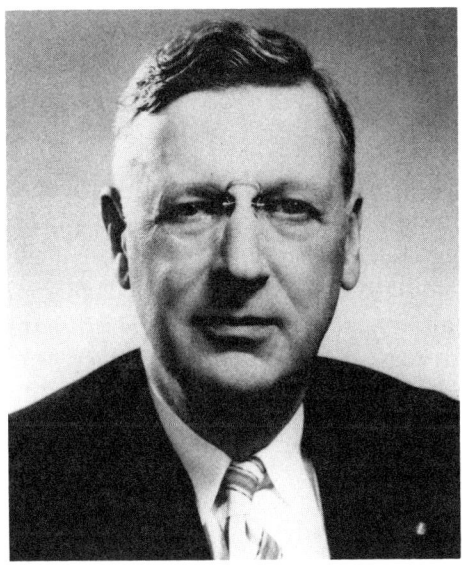
FIGURE 14:13 Francis E. Harrington, n.d. Courtesy Mn U Archives.

Dr. Harrington's initial appointment as commissioner of public health for Minneapolis was for one year, for the purpose of reorganizing the public health work of the city, but at the end of the year the Minneapolis Board of Public Welfare asked him to remain permanently as commissioner of public health. He was also appointed director of school hygiene for Minneapolis.[56]

In his survey of the public health of Minneapolis, Dr. Harrington became convinced that one of the serious health problems in the city was tuberculosis. Because it was known that persons with active tuberculosis could easily communicate the disease to others, Minnesota state law prohibited children with tuberculosis from attending the public schools. Dr. Harrington found that in Minneapolis there were 123 children who could not attend school because they had been diagnosed as having tuberculosis. Nevertheless, many such children were well enough to pursue school work, if they had an opportunity to do so. He, therefore, conceived the idea of creating a special school for tuberculous children where they might study without danger of communicating their disease to healthy children, and where they might also receive treatment that would promote their recovery and enable them to grow into healthy adulthood.[57]

In February 1921 Dr. Harrington was enabled to realize his plan through the circumstance that in 1912 two Minneapolis citizens, George and Frederick Lyman, had given to the city the site of their family homestead, at Chicago Avenue and Eighteenth Street, for a children's hospital. The Minneapolis Board of Public Welfare was in the process of erecting on the Lyman land a hospital building to be named Lymanhurst, intended to serve as the children's department of the Minneapolis General Hospital. The flaw in the plan was that Lymanhurst was about a mile from the main Minneapolis General Hospital so that it would be impracticable to conduct it as part of that hospital. Dr. Harrington, therefore, persuaded the Board of Public Welfare to use Lymanhurst as a school for tuberculous children.

Once he had gained the board's approval to establish such a school, Dr. Harrington sought to create a medical staff to provide the medical examinations and treatment that the tuberculous children at Lymanhurst would need. He thought also that such a school should pursue an organized study of tuberculosis among children to determine what proportion of children were infected with tubercle bacilli, how children became infected, and what happened to infected children as they grew to adulthood. Dr. Harrington wondered also what happened to individuals who did not become infected with tubercle bacilli until they were adults. In 1921 physicians commonly assumed that infection with tubercle bacilli occurred almost universally among children, and conferred an immunity that would help to protect them against tuberculosis later in life, but no controlled studies had been carried out to prove or disprove such assumptions. In February 1921, with such ideas and plans for the long term study of tuberculosis in mind, Dr. Harrington went to call on a young physician, Dr. J. Arthur Myers, who had begun practice in Minneapolis only the previous summer after spending a couple of months at the Trudeau School for Tuberculosis at Saranac Lake, New York. Dr. Myers was also an instructor, part-time, in the Department of Medicine at the medical school, where he participated in the tuberculosis clinic and taught physical diagnosis.

Then at the age of thirty-two, Jay Arthur Myers had a deep personal interest in tuberculosis. He was born on a farm near Hartford, Ohio; the physician who delivered him died a few months afterward from consumption. In 1908 he entered the University of Ohio, and in a biology class taught by W. F. Mercer, he learned to stain and identify tubercle bacilli. After graduating from Ohio in 1912, Myers went to Cornell University for graduate study in anatomy. After one year at Cornell and another at the University of Missouri, Myers came in 1914 to the University of Minnesota as an instructor in anatomy. While at Minnesota in the fall of 1915, he developed symptoms that aroused the concern of his supervisor, Dr. Charles Erdmann, who arranged for him to see a Minneapolis physician with a special interest in tuberculosis, Dr. George Douglas Head. A few months earlier Dr. Head had resigned from the department of medicine in protest against the Mayo affiliation. In 1898 Dr. Head had introduced the teaching of clinical microscopy to the medical school, and he had also begun to use the tuberculin test for the diagnosis of tuberculosis. When Dr. Head gave Myers a tuberculin test, Myers developed a strongly positive reaction, and Head recommended that he seek immediate treatment for pulmonary tuberculosis. Dr. Clarence Jackson then arranged a leave of absence for him. The fact that Drs. Head and Jackson were on opposite sides of the bitter quarrel over the Mayo affiliation that divided the medical school in 1915 seems not to have had any influence on their actions concerning Jay Myers. Myers went first for several months to a sanatorium in Ohio and then to one at Denver, Colorado, where in 1916 he for the first time received

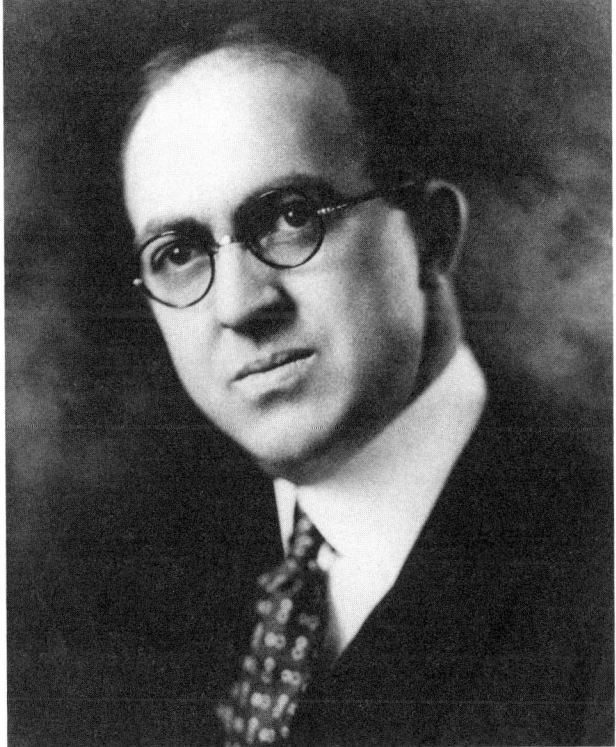

FIGURE 14:14 Jay Arthur Myers, circa 1930. Courtesy Mn U Archives.

an x-ray examination of his chest.[58] When he returned to Minnesota in the fall of 1916 to resume the teaching of anatomy, Myers began to take a few medical subjects until in 1920 he completed the medical course and received the M.D. degree.

When Francis Harrington called on Jay Myers at his office in February 1921, he said that he wanted at Lymanhurst a medical staff with sufficient interest, vision, and persistence to carry out long-term studies on tuberculosis. He had no funds to pay physicians, but if Dr. Myers were willing to undertake the task, he would appoint him medical director at Lymanhurst. Dr. Myers accepted and began to recruit other physicians and medical scientists from the university to form a medical staff. Everyone he approached responded with enthusiasm. Among those who joined the first staff was a young pediatrician, Chester Stewart, whom Dr. Myers had known first at the University of Missouri and with whom he had shared an office when they were both teaching anatomy at the medical school.[59] Owen Wangensteen joined the staff while he was a resident in internal medicine at the Minneapolis General Hospital.

On 31 May 1921 the Lymanhurst School for Tuberculous Children was dedicated in a formal ceremony attended by the Lieutenant Governor of Minnesota,

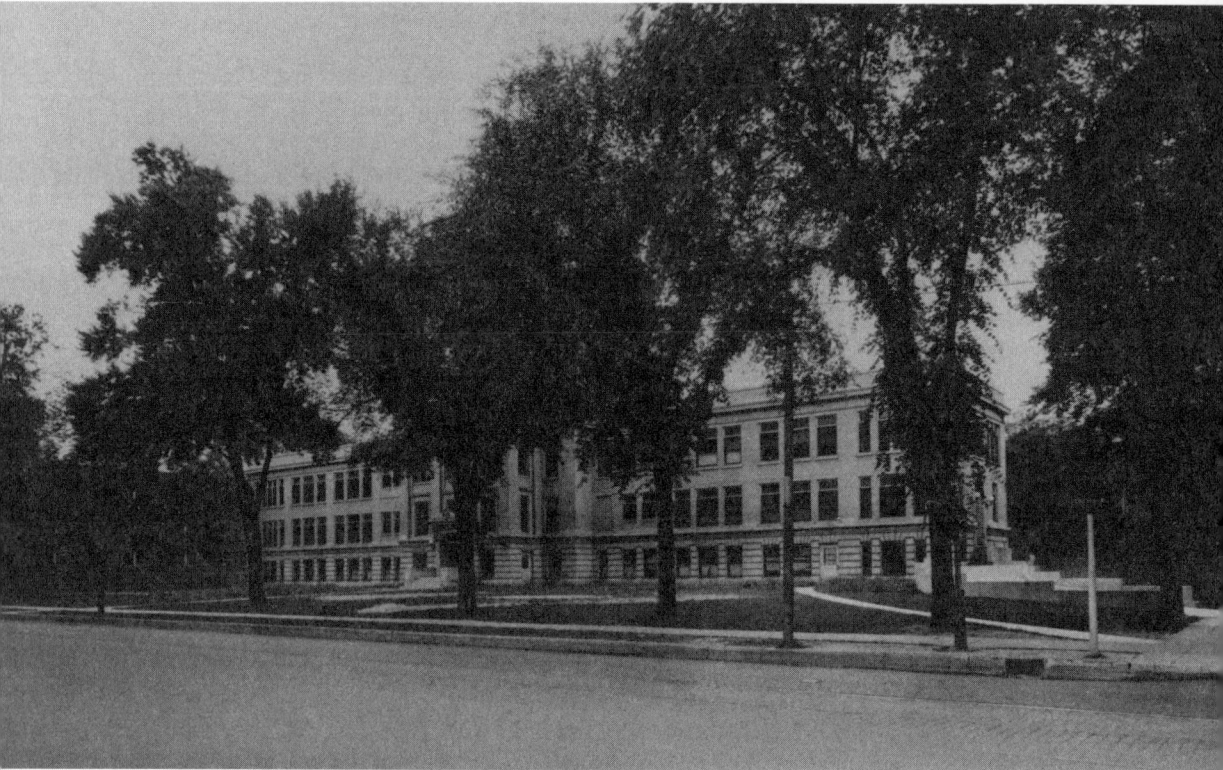

FIGURE 14:15   Lymanhurst, 1921. Courtesy Mn U Archives.

various Minneapolis officials, and many members of the public. Before the assembled crowd a thin pale boy—who was on that day the first and only pupil of Lymanhurst—unfurled the United States flag.[60] The second day 25 children came, and enrollment soon rose to 160. Each child had been diagnosed as tuberculous and was therefore unable to attend the ordinary public schools.

At Lymanhurst the children were fed nourishing meals. During the day they were given rest periods in rooms furnished with cots. Sunlight was thought to be beneficial for tuberculous children, and Lymanhurst was provided with rooms equipped with sun lamps. To ensure an abundance of fresh air, the windows were kept open in the coldest weather, and during the frigid Minnesota winter the children were provided with Eskimo suits to protect them from the cold.

In addition to children who were admitted with a definite diagnosis of tuberculosis, school physicians, nurses, and teachers were soon referring to the medical staff at Lymanhurst many other children suspected of being tuberculous. In January 1922, seven months after Lymanhurst opened, Dr. Myers organized an outpatient clinic to examine children suspected of having tuberculosis or known to have been exposed to a case of active tuberculosis. Each child was given a thorough medical examination, including, when needed, examinations by specialists. By 1923 the medical staff had grown to thirty volunteer physicians and medical scientists among whom were many members of the medical school faculty. In addition to internists and pediatricians, there were surgeons, bronchoscopists, hematologists, neurologists, otolaryngologists, and ophthalmologists. The neurologists found one twelve-year-old boy, who for many months had been treated for tuberculosis, suffering from syphilis as well as tuberculosis. The university hematologist, Hal Downey, found a thirteen-year-old girl with enlarged lymph glands in the neck to be suffering not from tuberculosis but from Hodgkin's disease, a cancerous condition. Because Dr. Myers and his staff kept systematic records on every child examined, Lymanhurst soon began to accumulate data on the clinical characteristics and epidemiology of tuberculosis in children. "Without actually realizing it," Dr. Myers said, "we were pioneering in observing the course tuberculosis takes in the bodies of children, including those infected during the first year of life and those who become infected at different ages through high school and into adulthood."[61]

In March 1922 the medical staff at Lymanhurst opened, in addition to the day school, a small hospital section for children who were ill. As the Lymanhurst physicians studied such children they found that their illnesses resulted from causes other than tuberculosis. As their studies continued, the staff came to the startling conclusion that tuberculosis rarely caused significant illness in childhood. Only occasionally, and as a result of reinfection, did the tubercle bacilli attack bones and joints, lungs, or meninges to cause serious or fatal illness. In 1926, therefore, the medical staff recommended that the hospital section at Lymanhurst be closed. Thereafter the occasional child found to have active tuberculosis was sent to other hospitals or sanatoria for treatment.

When the Lymanhurst staff examined children for tuberculosis, they routinely performed on each child a Pirquet test for sensitivity to tuberculin. At Vienna in 1907 Clemens von Pirquet had introduced the test, which consisted of scratching the skin lightly and placing a drop of tuberculin on the scratched area. If the scratched area and surrounding skin became reddened, the child was hypersensitive to tuberculin. Such hypersensitivity (an allergic reaction) indicated that tubercular infection was present in the body. If the Pirquet test were negative, the child was considered free of tuberculosis, but if the test were positive the Lymanhurst staff proceeded to search for the site of possible tubercle infection in the child's body, using x-ray examination, detailed physical examination, and examination of stomach contents for tubercle bacilli. By April 1925 Dr. Myers and his colleagues had performed the Pirquet test on 2,000 children brought to Lymanhurst suspected of being tuberculous. The children fell into three groups: those with an established history of exposure to tuberculosis, those in which the history of exposure was uncertain, and those with no history of exposure. While 57 percent of children with a definite history of exposure gave a positive Pirquet test, only 27 percent of children with no known history of exposure gave positive Pirquet tests.[62] The Pirquet test, therefore, appeared to be an accurate indicator of exposure to tubercular infection. The Pirquet test did not tell where in the child's body the tubercular infection might be located. Since children who gave a positive reaction were usually to all appearance healthy, there was no illness with characteristics that might suggest the location of the infection.

In the beginning Dr. Myers and his colleagues assumed, in accord with then accepted medical opinion, that they would rely primarily on the physical examination of children — on percussion and auscultation with the stethoscope — to detect the early signs of tuberculosis. Nevertheless, the physical examination of most children with positive Pirquet tests yielded no evidence of tubercular infection. When the physical examination of a child did reveal tuberculosis, the tuberculosis was advanced, and usually too far advanced for any treatment to be effective. Although at first Dr. Myers and his staff expected to use x-ray examination only occasionally, after physical examination had revealed indications of tuberculosis, they soon found that they had to use x-ray examination immediately if they were to find any indications of tuberculosis in children with positive Pirquet tests. More and more in their search for the primary focus of tubercular infection, they resorted to stereoscopic x-ray plates of the chest. Soon they took stereoscopic x-ray plates routinely on admission of each child and made repeated plates at intervals of six months unless more frequent examinations were needed. In some children the x-ray plates revealed a primary tubercular infection in the lung parenchyma, but in many others the x-ray plates showed no lung infection. Instead, the child might have merely an enlargement of the lymph nodes in the neck and along the trachea and bronchi.[63] In more than a thousand children examined at the Lymanhurst School whose x-ray plates showed some calcification of the lymph nodes of the lungs, 45 percent gave positive Pirquet tests that indicated tuberculous infection.[64]

After the Pirquet test was introduced in 1907, tests on large numbers of children in European cities had revealed an incidence of tubercular infection as high as 60 to 90 percent, and because most such children were healthy, physicians assumed that they had become immune to tuberculosis through a slight initial infection. Pirquet tests on children in the United States revealed generally a smaller proportion of positive tests than in Europe, indicating a lower frequency of tubercular infection. In 1924 Dr. Sidney A. Slater found among children at Worthington, Minnesota, a prosperous farming community, that only about 10 percent of children gave a positive Pirquet test and that the percentage of positive reactors did not increase as the children grew older.[65] At Lymanhurst Dr. Myers and his staff concentrated their attention on children who gave a positive Pirquet test. They attempted by x-ray examination to locate the focus of primary infection, and then by successive x-ray examinations to follow over time any changes that occurred in the focus of primary infection. They hoped to trace the natural history of the stages through which foci of primary infection passed. Their preliminary studies suggested that some primary lesions in the lungs of children healed gradually, so as to leave no trace of their former presence.[66] By 1926 they found to their astonishment that in more than three-quarters of the children, the lesions produced by tubercular infection either shrank or disappeared completely with the passage of time.[67] The tendency of tubercular infection to heal and disappear in children was even greater, Dr. Myers realized, than their figures suggested, because the children brought to Lymanhurst were brought by reason of ill health. If the group had included a larger group of children who simply gave a positive Pirquet reaction, the proportion of healed or improved children would have been greater.

The evidence that tuberculosis infections might disappear as a child grew induced Dr. Myers and his staff to study a group of children from infancy to adulthood, giving each child a Pirquet test together with a complete medical examination at periodic intervals. In 1924 they had begun with a study of tuberculosis among infants under the age of two, impelled by their experience with a six-month-old baby boy whose parents had brought him to Lymanhurst for examination.

> The parents were well-to-do and intelligent, but the mother was crying. She stated that she had just been told that their baby would die within the next six months. A little questioning revealed the fact that the parents had taken the baby to a physician who, knowing that a near relative had recently died of tuberculosis, made no examination except a Pirquet test. This test proved positive and, without further examination, the physician told the parents that their baby could not live to its first birthday.[68]

Nevertheless, the child had never been ill, and appeared perfectly healthy; it continued to grow and develop without showing any sign of tuberculosis. Previously, physicians had assumed that tuberculosis in infants was extremely fatal, because the cases of tuberculosis that they observed were far advanced. The Pirquet test revealed tuberculosis infections in their earliest stages, but physicians did not realize that such early infections might have a fate very different from that of advanced tuberculous disease.

Among seventy-one infants with positive Pirquet tests, the Lymanhurst staff found that more than 95 percent had a history of exposure to a case of active tuberculosis, usually in one of the parents. They urged, therefore, that children should be separated promptly from any individual with active tuberculosis. Six of the seventy-one children died before the age of two, two of them from tuberculous meningitis and four from pulmonary tuberculosis. The death rate from tuberculosis among infants was thus much lower than many physicians had assumed, although it was higher than the tuberculosis death rate among children from two to fourteen years of age.

In 1930 Drs. J. Arthur Myers and Leila Kernkamp reported on an additional 532 infants examined for tuberculosis at the Lymanhurst Clinic since 1926.[69] Among the 532 children, 236 gave positive tuberculin reactions when first examined. Myers and Kernkamp had attempted to follow the children with positive tuberculin tests and had maintained complete histories for 172 of them. Only six had died, four from tuberculous meningitis. Most of the children infected with tuberculosis in infancy had remained healthy and developed normally.

In 1930 Myers and Kernkamp also reported on their study of tuberculosis among teenage boys and girls. Although by 1930 overall mortality from tuberculosis had declined sharply from its high levels in the nineteenth century, the tuberculosis death rate in the age group from fifteen to twenty- four years remained high in the United States. Dr. Myers had become interested in the occurrence of tuberculosis among teenagers because of a particular patient whom he had cared for, a young man thirty-three years of age, who, when first examined, was found to have advanced tuberculosis and soon died of it. On inquiry Myers learned that at the age of seventeen the young man had suffered a sudden sharp attack of pleurisy from which he recovered in a few days. Although thereafter the youth had remained well until his fatal illness began at the age of thirty-one, Myers thought that the attack of pleurisy fourteen years before was tuberculous in origin and indicated that at that time tuberculosis was already established in the youth's lungs. Dr. Myers' purpose, therefore, in examining teenagers was to discover any tuberculosis that might exist among them at a stage early enough to give effective treatment. The risk of fatal tuberculosis among teenagers was so high that Myers and Kernkamp urged prompt and drastic treatment, including artificial pneumothorax in addition to complete bed rest. The tragic consequences of tuberculosis among teenagers were reflected in the fact that when Myers and Kernkamp published their study in 1930, 47 of the 242 teenagers whom they had studied were already dead.[70]

In the fall of 1928 at the students' health service, H. D. Lees and J. Arthur Myers administered the Pirquet test to the freshman class entering the University of Minnesota. Among more than 2,000 students tested, only a third reacted positively to tuberculin, contrasted with 50 percent positive among 6,000 children examined at the Lymanhurst School.[71] Since more than two-thirds of students entering the university had not been exposed to tuberculosis, there was clearly advantage in protecting them, insofar as possible, from exposure. One of the most dangerous reservoirs of infection lay in elderly persons infected with tuberculosis, because in the elderly the disease might appear only as chronic bronchitis, emphysema, or asthma, and might go undetected for years. Among the elderly tuberculosis was usually of long standing and had originated in exposure to tuberculosis many years before.[72] It represented a source of disease, often hidden, that could infect large numbers of younger people, including young children. In 1930 Jay Arthur Myers suggested that because " . . . the tuberculosis in a community is reflected to a considerable extent in the children of that community," the study of tuberculosis among children, coupled with an effort to seek out the sources of infection in each child, was probably the best method of reducing the incidence of advanced tuberculosis among adults in whom the onset and progress of the disease was so often hidden.[73]

When the Lymanhurst School was founded in 1921, a positive Pirquet test in an otherwise healthy-appearing child was thought to confer a long lasting benefit by granting immunity to tuberculosis. The generally benign character of tuberculous infection among children, revealed by studies at the Lymanhurst School through the 1920s, strengthened the assumption that a positive tuberculin test represented immunity to tuberculosis. In the spring of 1931, Dr. Myers and his group received a rude shock. That pale, thin boy who had been Lymanhurst's first patient and pupil—he, who had unfurled the flag at the dedication in 1921—and who in 1922 had been discharged from Lymanhurst fully recovered and considered immune to tuberculosis—this patient, the symbol of the faith and hope on which Lymanhurst had been founded—and now a young man of twenty-two, walked into the free chest clinic at the Minneapolis General Hospital, where he was found to have advanced pulmonary tuberculosis. Within a few weeks he was dead. "Thus our first Lymanhurst case, about whom we had talked and written so much and for whom we had rendered such an excellent prognosis based upon opinion not fact," said J. Arthur Myers, "shattered our teachings."[74]

In his work on tuberculosis, Dr. Myers was repeatedly impelled to further efforts by the personal tragedies that he saw in his clinic and practice, especially among nurses and medical students. Traditionally tuberculosis was considered an occupational disease, thought to be connected with long hours, insufficient food, and loss of sleep, and for such reasons, especially common among nurses and physicians. From his studies at Lymanhurst and at the students' health service, Dr. Myers became convinced that the real reason for the prevalence of tuberculosis among nurses and physicians was their exposure in their work to patients with active tuberculosis. During the summer of 1932, Dr. Myers received a letter from a recent graduate of the medical school, who was pursuing an internship at a hospital in another city, who wrote that his Mantoux test (i.e., tuberculin test) had changed from negative to positive during his six weeks clerkship on a tuberculous service while he was a senior medical student in 1931, and two of his fellow students had the same experience. In the late 1920s the Mantoux test, in which a measured quantity of tuberculin was injected into (but not beneath) the skin, was substituted for the Pirquet test because it proved more reliable. X-ray examination of his chest in July 1931 was negative, but ten months later, in May 1932, he developed pain in the chest and an x-ray examination in June showed that a pleural effusion was present.[75] Similarly, among a class of twenty-one nurses graduating in 1927, seven, or one-third of the class, were already ill with tuberculosis. At the Ancker Hospital in St. Paul, Dr. E. K. Geer found that practically no student nurse graduated without a positive tuberculin reaction.[76]

In October 1933 the Lymanhurst School established a tuberculosis clinic for adults, partly because many of the children who had been studied by the medical staff during the 1920s had now become adults, and partly in order to examine the adult contacts of children who gave a positive reaction to tuberculin, in a search for the source of the tubercle bacilli that had infected the children.

By 1934 Dr. Myers and his medical colleagues at Lymanhurst concluded that there was no purpose to be served in continuing Lymanhurst as a school, because there was no need to separate children with tuberculosis from other children nor to give them any special care. Primary tuberculosis in children was benign; it produced no perceptible illness; and children with primary tuberculosis did not shed tubercle bacilli in sputum so that they did not communicate the disease to others. The primary lesions in their lungs healed, sometimes to leave small calcifications, other times to leave no trace.[77] The course of first-infection type tuberculosis was the same in Negro and Mexican children as in white children, thereby showing that among different races there was no discernable difference in susceptibility to tuberculosis. The terrible ravages of tuberculosis among American Indians and Negroes were the result of crowded living conditions and failure to separate tuberculous from healthy individuals, so that Indians and Negroes were frequently subjected to overwhelming doses of tuberculous infection.[78]

> When our work began [said Dr. Myers in 1935] we strongly recommended sanatorium care for every child who was found to have a focus of first-infection tuberculosis in the pneumonic stage. Many families refused to carry out our recommendations because there were no outward manifestations of tuberculosis. We then advised that their children who were old enough be admitted to the Lymanhurst School. Many even refused this for the same reason and insisted upon having their children remain at home with no treatment whatever. Thus our children were divided into three groups . . . .[79]

The course of tuberculous infection was the same in all three groups, and except for three who had developed reinfection tuberculosis, the 136 children from all three groups, who could be traced, were normal, healthy individuals in 1935. Nevertheless, from their experience with tuberculosis among teenagers, Dr. Myers and his colleagues thought that after the age of twelve about 20 percent of children with positive tuberculin tests would develop clinical pulmonary tuberculosis.

Since the school at Lymanhurst was unneeded, it was discontinued in 1935 on the recommendation of the medical staff, but the diagnostic and epidemiological work on tuberculosis continued there and the institution was renamed the Lymanhurst Health Center. The medical staff expanded the work of the outpatient department by performing tuberculin tests on larger numbers of children, and then seeking out the sources of infection of those children who gave positive reactions to tuberculin. They also sought to make periodic chest x-rays of children with positive Mantoux tests from the age of ten or twelve onward. If cases of reinfection tuberculosis were detected when they first appeared on a chest x-ray, they could usually be treated successfully by collapsing the infected lung or by rest. The essential thing in the treatment of the tuberculous child, Dr. Myers and his colleagues emphasized, was to separate the child from the sources of infection to which it had been exposed.

By 1935 the program of isolation of patients with active tuberculosis in sanatoria or hospitals, with the consequent protection of more and more children from exposure to tuberculosis, was showing ever greater results. From 1921 to 1934 the proportion of positive tuberculin reactors among children tested at Lymanhurst fell 18 percent.[80] The long-term studies carried on at Lymanhurst had demonstrated that children with a positive tuberculin reaction had a chance of developing clinical tuberculosis in early adulthood approximately nine times greater than children with a negative tuberculin reaction. The initial tuberculosis infection made the host tissue allergic to tuberculin so that reinfection produced a massive destruction of tissues and progressive clinical tuberculosis. Experimental studies on guinea pigs, carried out by others, showed that when the tissues of an animal had been rendered sensitive to tuberculin by a first infection, a second infection resulted in the formation of many tubercles and the development of progressive and fatal disease.[81] The declining death rate from tuberculosis among children in Minnesota was, Dr. Myers suggested, the result of fewer children being exposed to infection with tubercle bacilli, and those who were infected were receiving smaller doses of infection, and not repeated doses. When infants died from tuberculosis, they died from a reinfection type of disease, which implied repeated doses of infection.

When the students' health service opened at the University of Minnesota in the fall of 1920, the director, John Sundwall, included in it a clinic for the diagnosis and treatment of tuberculosis. At that time tuberculosis was very common among students, and a frequent cause of disabling illness and death. Entering students were given routine physical examinations, but such examinations could detect only the relatively few cases of advanced tuberculosis among the students, and the experience of Dr. Myers and his colleagues at the Lymanhurst School showed that patients with active tuberculosis were only a small fraction of those infected with tubercle bacilli. In 1927 Ivar Sivertsen, a surgeon on the staff of the Fairview Hospital in Minneapolis where tuberculosis was an especially severe problem among nurses and nursing students, returned from Europe with a report of his observations of Johannes Heimbeck's work on tuberculosis among nursing students at Oslo. Since 1924 Dr. Heimbeck had been administering Pirquet tests to nursing students when they entered the nursing school attached to the Oslo Municipal Hospital. Contrary to Heimbeck's expectations, 52 percent of the entering nursing students gave negative Pirquet tests. When Heimbeck turned to examine other groups of young adults, he found that 47 percent of entering medical students and 55 percent of military recruits gave a negative reaction to tuberculin.[82] Nevertheless, after one or two years in the Oslo Municipal Hospital, practically all of the student nurses who previously had negative Pirquet tests had turned positive.

In 1927 the medical school as an experiment required all medical students to have a physical examination, including a chest x-ray at the students' health service. Then in the fall of 1928 Harold Diehl, director of the students' health service, decided to administer tuberculin tests to all students entering the University of Minnesota. Previously occasional students had entered the university with contagious tuberculosis, sometimes in advanced stages, and had communicated the disease to others. When such students became ill, they often went to their family physician. Before 1928 the students' health service might remain unaware of a student's illness unless the student reported voluntarily for examination.[83] Dr. Diehl and Dr. Myers, who, in addition to his work at Lymanhurst, conducted the tuberculosis clinic at the students' health service, were also curious to see how the results of Pirquet tests at Minnesota would compare with Heimbeck's results in Norway.

To their astonishment, among more than 2,000 students only about a third gave positive Pirquet tests.[84] With such a low proportion of tuberculin reactors, the students' health service could concentrate its attention on them alone, and in the fall of 1931, with special financial support provided by President Coffman, began to give chest x-ray examinations to all students with a positive tuberculin reaction.

In 1928 medical students and nursing students were accustomed to have considerable contact with tuberculous patients. Myers and Diehl realized that if they periodically performed tuberculin tests on the nonreactors among nursing and medical students, they would have an unusual opportunity to observe the development of first-infection tuberculosis in previously healthy young adults. They could also determine what proportion of students who were negative to tuberculin became positive during their period of study. In the fall of 1928, they began to give tuberculin tests to all students entering the medical school and the nursing school and to repeat the tests for students negative to tuberculin until they turned positive. They also required all medical and nursing students to have chest x-rays annually, whether they were positive or negative to tuberculin. Of twenty-eight nursing students tested in 1929, eleven were positive, but by the time the class graduated all were positive to tuberculin. In 1930 only 14 percent of the entering nurses gave positive tuberculin reactions, whereas by the time of their graduation 87 per cent were positive. Thus during their period of study, most of the nurses became infected with tubercle bacilli. By contrast, in the school of education the proportion of students with positive tuberculin tests rose only from 23 percent in the first year to 27 percent in the fourth year. Clearly nursing students at Minnesota were acquiring tuberculosis infection to an extent far greater than other groups of university students.[85]

When a student previously negative to tuberculin gave a positive reaction, chest x-rays usually revealed no signs of disease. In a few students after several months, a small area of infiltration might appear in the lung without any physical signs or symptoms of disease. The pattern of first-infection tuberculosis in adults was exactly like that which Dr. Myers and his colleagues had observed among children at the Lymanhurst School. Initially in 1929, Myers and his colleagues observed the development of first-infection tuberculosis in a woman medical student who had remained negative to the tuberculin test until, as an intern, she was required to spend several weeks at a tuberculosis sanatorium. After studying her case, they found other instances of first-infection lesions in their records, which they had not previously recognized. When they first encountered students whose chest x-rays showed first-infection lesions, Dr. Myers and his colleagues recommended drastic treatment, such as strict bed rest, because they feared the development of rapidly progressive tuberculosis. They soon found such fears unjustified. With strict bed rest, tuberculous lesions resolved no more quickly than they did in students who went about their normal daily life. They soon learned to recommend only that such students follow ordinary rules for healthy living, avoid exposure to tuberculosis, and be examined periodically.

Although first-infection tuberculosis in adults appeared benign, Dr. Myers and his colleagues recognized that it posed two threats: first, from the continued presence in the body of living tubercle bacilli, and second, from the development of an allergy to tuberculin, which would make the individual liable to develop progressive tuberculosis from a second infection. Frequently medical or nursing students did become ill with tuberculosis, either while they were students or shortly after graduation.[86] To prevent the inadvertent exposure of students to tuberculosis, Dr. Myers recommended that general hospitals do a chest x-ray on every patient when admitted. In 1937 they recommended that medical and nursing students who gave a negative reaction to tuberculin should be retested with tuberculin at least every six months. Those with positive reactions should have periodic chest x-rays to detect any development of pulmonary tuberculosis as early as possible.

In the 1930s medical students at Minnesota remained seriously exposed to tuberculosis, not only while they took clerkships in a tuberculosis sanatorium, but also in general hospitals where little effort was made to determine whether contagious tuberculosis might exist in patients admitted for other conditions. Among medical students graduated from 1933 to 1936, the proportion of tuberculin reactors increased from 41 percent to 68 percent during their senior year. In 1936 when Harold Diehl became dean of the medical school, he ceased to require a tuberculosis clerkship in a sanatorium and permitted a student to substitute other work in tuberculosis. The incidence of new tuberculosis infection among medical students began to decline in 1937 and continued to decline through 1941.[87]

In 1939 Dr. Myers and his colleagues at the students' health service attempted to trace graduates of the medical school from 1919 through 1936. Among 1,304 physicians who had graduated from 1919 to 1932, 92 had developed clinical tuberculosis and 11 had died of the disease.[88] After 1929 all medical students had received tuberculin tests annually, and those with positive tuberculin reactions were given chest x-ray examinations. After medical students began to receive tuberculin tests in 1929, Dr. Myers found that almost half of physicians who were nonreactors to tuberculin when they graduated turned positive during their year of internship, and more turned positive later.[89]

Appalled by the great risks to which nurses and medical students were subjected when they worked in hospitals, Harold Diehl, when he became dean of the College of Medical Sciences in 1935, established a requirement that all patients admitted to the university hospital should be given a tuberculin test on admission. Patients with positive reactions were then given chest x-ray examinations. During the first year the hospital staff identified forty-eight patients with active tuberculosis, previously undiagnosed, who had been admitted for other conditions.[90] Such patients were then handled with special isolation techniques used for patients with tuberculosis. In 1932 in the small tuberculosis service at the university hospital, a nurse, Elisabeth Phillips, had developed communicable disease techniques designed to prevent the spread of tubercle bacilli from tuberculous patients. Behind Dean Diehl's new policy lay the grim fact that among graduates of the medical school from 1919 to 1936, tuberculosis was responsible for a quarter of the deaths and for more sickness than any other disease.[91] Among nurses tuberculosis was even more devastating because they were in contact with tuberculous patients more frequently, and for longer periods of time, than medical students. By 1941 Drs. Myers, Diehl, and their colleagues had learned so thoroughly how to locate the tubercle bacillus and prevent its spread that when the students entering the University of Minnesota School of Nursing that fall graduated in 1945, not one of the forty-four women who entered as nonreactors to tuberculin had turned positive.[92] Between 1942 and 1946 only one nursing student developed the reinfection type of tuberculosis; she was treated successfully by artificial pnemothorax and graduated with her class.[93]

Pediatrics

When Irvine McQuarrie arrived at the University of Minnesota in July 1930 as the new chief of pediatrics, the department consisted of one half-time assistant professor, two instructors, and the chemist, Dr. Mildred R. Ziegler, who had been with the department since 1915. The pediatric service was quite small, but it was located in the sparkling new Eustis Hospital and it could use the income of the William Eustis endowment to support the care of sick or crippled children.

While at the University of Rochester, Dr. McQuarrie had become interested in the control of seizures in epileptic children. In 1927 McQuarrie and Haddow M. Keith showed that a high fat diet, which resulted in the excretion of acetone and other ketone substances in the urine, could control convulsions, and in many epileptic children prevent them completely.[94] McQuarrie and Keith also found that the acid-base balance was a factor in epileptic seizures; administration of sodium bicarbonate, or even a diet with a slightly alkaline ash, could cancel the seizure-controlling effect of a high fat, ketogenic diet.[95] In 1929 Irvine McQuarrie showed that epileptic patients tended to retain water in their bodies, and when the accumulation of water reached a certain point, seizures followed. By contrast, if the retention of water were prevented by a restricted water intake coupled with the use of diuretics and a ketogenic diet, epileptic convulsions could be prevented.[96] A low carbohydrate, high fat diet, together with a restricted water intake seemed to offer a promising means to control seizures in an epileptic child, but from a nutritional standpoint such diets were seriously unbalanced and would produce harmful effects if continued for any length of time. A ketogenic diet tended to be particularly deficient in protein.[97]

At Minnesota Irvine McQuarrie continued his investigation of epilepsy. In 1931 McQuarrie and Peeler showed that by giving water, while at the same time suppressing the child's secretion of urine by means of the pituitary hormone *pitressin*, a seizure could be induced in twelve to forty-eight hours in an epileptic child, but not in the nonepileptic, and that the difference could be used in diagnosis.[98] Such relationships suggested to McQuarrie that in epileptics the semipermeability of the brain cell membranes was somehow defective. The following year McQuarrie showed that when epileptic patients were secreting abundant urine and were free from seizures, their urine tended to contain more sodium and chloride ions than potassium, but some hours before the onset of a seizure, an increased amount of potassium began to appear in the urine. Since most of the potassium in the body was known to be held inside cells, while most of the sodium was in the fluid bathing the tissue cells and in the circulating blood, McQuarrie suggested that an epileptic seizure was preceded by a leakage of potassium from the brain cells caused by some change in the semipermeability of the brain cell membranes.[99] In children suffering from a frequent recurrence of violent epileptic seizures, McQuarrie recommended a combination of a ketogenic diet with a restricted water intake and the use of sedative drugs, especially phenobarbitol. To protect the patient against bodily injury during a convulsion, he advocated ether or chloroform anaesthesia, to be followed by phenobarbitol and a strong diuretic, such as urea, to achieve dehydration.[100]

Irvine McQuarrie's interest in questions of water balance was stimulated further at Minnesota by a tragic but highly unusual patient, a two-year-old girl, who was admitted to the university hospital on 5 October 1931 suffering from a general edema of unknown origin, which could not be reduced by diuretics or any other medication. The child had been normal at birth, and during the first fifteen months of her life her growth and development remained essentially normal. In January 1931 she caught cold and shortly thereafter her face and limbs were noticeably swollen. In March the swelling appeared to subside during an attack of whooping cough, but presently it returned and by July was pronounced. In September her abdomen had become enlarged, the swelling of her face and limbs was more noticeable than ever, and she was uncomfortable and irritable. Nevertheless, the child did not show any sign of heart, liver, or kidney disease — the usual causes of edema.

At the university hospital McQuarrie assigned his assistant, Willis H. Thompson, to care for the child, but McQuarrie himself took a very active interest in her. Together with Mildred Ziegler, Thompson and McQuarrie examined the child's blood chemistry, which proved essentially normal except for one striking feature — a very low concentration of serum proteins in the blood plasma. Because the osmotic pressure of the plasma proteins normally acts to retain water, salts, and other dissolved substances in the circulating blood, a deficient concentration of plasma proteins permitted fluid to move from the circulating blood into the intercellular spaces of the tissues, thereby causing them to swell. Although the child had always been well fed, Thompson and McQuarrie placed her on a high protein diet in an effort to raise the level of her plasma proteins, but without effect. Nothing helped, but when, toward the end of February 1932, the child came down with bronchopneumonia, they gave her a rather large blood transfusion. For two days nothing happened, but then the child began to excrete large quantities of urine. As if by magic her swelling subsided, and her appearance changed to that of a normal two-year-old. Because the child's blood plasma had a very low protein content and the urine contained no protein, her disease was clearly caused by the inability of her body to produce plasma proteins. In April the child developed an ear infection, complicated by a mastoid infection, and on 29 April she died of pneumonia within a few days of having taken ill.

When the pathologist, E. T. Bell, performed the autopsy, he found no obvious signs of disease other than pus draining from the mastoid, which had been opened surgically during the child's illness. The heart, kidneys, and liver all appeared normal. But, although the liver looked normal, when Dr. Bell examined sections of it under the microscope, the tissue showed striking changes. The cells of the hepatic cords were atrophied and many had degenerated and disappeared completely. The child, therefore, had been suffering from a general atrophy of the liver, which differed from the usual forms of liver atrophy in that it involved no hardening or cirrhosis.

McQuarrie and his colleagues realized that the child's inability to produce plasma proteins must be connected with the peculiar atrophy of the liver cells, and, therefore, that the liver must be responsible for production of the plasma proteins.[101] They were enabled to draw that conclusion because of their sustained clinical observation and intensive laboratory study of a single patient for almost seven months. The endowment provided by William Henry Eustis worked, as he had intended it should, to pay the costs of the long period of hospitalization, and Irvine McQuarrie saw in that swollen, suffering two-year-old child a unique "experiment of nature," whose careful study might provide valuable medical knowledge.[102]

In another patient, a two-year-old boy, studied at the university hospital from September 1935 until his death from carcinoma of the liver in February 1937, McQuarrie and his colleagues showed that the liver cancer was accompanied by a severe and progressive degeneration of all the bones in the skeleton. By thorough metabolic studies, they found that the liver played a role in calcium and phosphorus metabolism necessary for bone formation throughout the body. Although many cases of liver carcinoma had been reported in the medical literature, most had been in adults, and none before had been accompanied by metabolic studies.[103]

Also in 1935 a four-year-old boy was brought to the university hospital suffering from an extremely rare disease in which all the fatty tissue had disappeared from his body so that his muscles stood out in such extraordinarily sharp relief that the hospital staff referred to him as "the little anatomical man." The child's liver was enlarged, and over the next four years grew ever larger, rougher, and harder as his disease progressed. The child's spleen also became enlarged, and he suffered from increasingly severe diabetes until his death in 1939 at the age of nine. The cause of his illness remained a mystery, but its connection with cirrhosis of the liver showed that the liver must also play an essential role in the normal deposition of body fat.[104]

In 1930 Irvine McQuarrie became interested in a possible connection between salts and carbohydrate metabolism when a diabetc child showed an abnormal craving for common salt and was able to control her blood sugar level better when she ate larger quantities of salt. In the fall of 1933 a fifteen-year-old boy with moderately severe diabetes came into the university hospital and attracted attention immediately by his ever greater craving for salt of which he ate sixty to ninety grains daily. When McQuarrie and his colleagues studied the boy together with other diabetic children, they found that large quantities of sodium chloride in the diet did reduce the blood sugar level, and that the effect was greatest on diets low in potassium. Sodium and potassium exerted antagonistic effects on blood sugar level and on blood pressure, sodium tending to raise the blood pressure, potassium to lower it.[105]

On 11 February 1935 a forty-four-year-old married woman was admitted to the Minneapolis General Hospital under the care of Henry L. Ulrich, professor of medicine, and R. M. Johnson, resident. For eight months she had been suffering from abnormally excessive thirst, with a correspondingly excessive production of urine, together with sugar in the urine, all indicative of diabetes mellitus. But, in addition to diabetes, for more than a year the woman had been embarrassed by an abnormal growth of beard on her face. She also complained of weakness, fatigue, and breathlessness on exertion. She was obese, yet her arms and legs remained thin. Her neck was unusually thick and her face round and florid. Her whole appearance and physical signs corresponded to those of a syndrome described in 1932 by Harvey Cushing, which Cushing attributed to pituitary basophilism.[106] The patient's blood was abnormally alkaline and showed an unusually high carbon dioxide-combining power; her blood pressure was elevated. The patient's abnormal electrolyte balance caused Dr. Ulrich to consult Irvine McQuarrie, who arranged to have Mildred Ziegler carry out studies on her blood chemistry. Patients with Cushing's syndrome were peculiarly susceptible to infections, and after ten weeks in the hospital, the patient developed pneumonia and septicemia following the extraction of an infected tooth and died on 26 April 1935. During the ten weeks of her life in hospital, Irvine McQuarrie and his colleagues found that her blood electrolytes remained consistently in imbalance in a pattern the exact opposite of the electrolyte imbalances that occurred in Addison's disease. Since Addison's disease was known to result from insufficient adrenal cortical secretion, a pattern opposite to that of Addison's disease probably was caused by excessive secretion by the adrenal cortex, and might be called *hypercorticoadrenalism*.[107]

Following the patient's death, the university neuroanatomist, A. T. Rasmussen, studied serial sections of her pituitary body and found in the basophil cells of the anterior lobe the characteristic changes of Cushing's syndrome.[108] The collaboration of members of the Departments of Medicine, Pediatrics, and Anatomy in the study of this one patient was not unusual at Minnesota in the 1930s and gave the medical school the ability to bring all of its slender resources to bear on questions of clinical and scientific medicine.

In 1935 in addition to the small full-time faculty in pediatrics at the university hospital, there was a part-time faculty of more than thirty associate and assistant professors, instructors, and assistants, who together were in charge of practically all of the pediatric hospital services in the Twin Cities. Such hospitals were available, therefore, for teaching purposes. Nevertheless, apart from the university hospital, the regular teaching of pediatrics was carried on at only two hospitals, the Minneapolis General Hospital where E. J. Huenekens was chief of the children's service, and at the Ancker Hospital (the city and county hospital) in St. Paul under Walter Ramsey. Both were part-time teachers. Dr. Huenekens was also in charge of clinics for the Infant Welfare Society of Minneapolis and held two clinics weekly at the university outpatient department for the purpose of teaching well-baby care to the medical students. The Department of Pediatrics was also responsible for the care of infants at the Saint Paul Salvation Army Home for illegitimate children and for medical care at the Shriners' Hospital for Crippled Children in Minneapolis, only two miles from the university.

In 1913 the chiefs of obstetrics and gynecology, Jennings Litzenberg, and of pediatrics, Julius P. Sedgwick, had agreed that the care of the newborn should be transferred from the obstetric to the pediatric service immediately after birth, and that policy was maintained thereafter. Whenever a birth occurred in the obstetric service, a member of the pediatric service was notified so that he might examine and care for the infant immediately. If a child required a major operation, it became the responsibility of the Department of Surgery, but its medical care remained a pediatric responsibility. Resident members of the pediatric staff performed all autopsies on children, under the supervision of the hospital pathologist. Such overlapping of responsibilities among various staffs might have created opportunities for rivalry and conflict, but the steady flow of clinical research from Minnesota suggests that it did not. "Due very largely to the generous attitude of the entire personnel on the associated services," said Irvine McQuarrie, "this plan of interdepartmental cooperation works very smoothly for all concerned."[109]

Obstetrics

When Jennings C. Litzenberg became professor of obstetrics and gynecology in 1913, the maternal mortality rate in Minnesota was almost 7 per 1000 live births. In teaching obstetrics to the medical students, Dr. Litzenberg sought to reduce the number of deaths of women in childbirth by advocating conservative obstetrics, with a minimum of intervention. He became interested in ectopic pregnancy, which he showed was analogous to a normal pregnancy within the uterus but wholly pathological in its results because the wall of the Fallopian tube was completely unsuited to the implantation of an ovum. He also studied the phenomenon of missed abortion in which a pregnancy terminates with the death

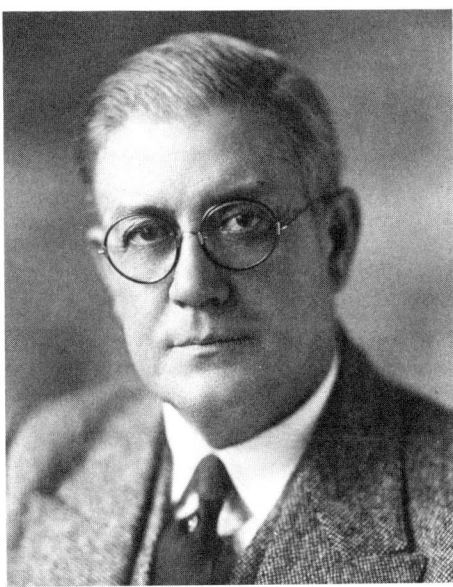

FIGURE 14:16 Jennings C. Litzenberg, circa 1925. Courtesy Mn U Archives.

of the fetus, but the fetus is not discharged and may remain within the uterus indefinitely.[110]

In 1922 Dr. Litzenberg found that an otherwise perfectly healthy young married woman, who came to him for relief from sterility, had a slightly subnormal metabolic rate. When he started her on small doses of thyroid extract she became pregnant. After she gave birth to a healthy child in October 1922, Litzenberg stopped the thyroid treatment. A year later she returned asking to have her basal metabolism measured because she wished to have another child but could not become pregnant. Although her basal metabolism was only very slightly below normal, Dr. Litzenberg again started her on small doses of thyroid extract, and again she became pregnant. After the patient's second successful pregnancy, Litzenberg began to think that a moderately low basal metabolic rate might be connected with sterility and began to take the basal metabolism in all women patients complaining of sterility. In 1926 he reported that about half of women seeking relief from sterility had subnormal basal metabolic rates, and when treated with thyroid extract a third of women with low basal metabolism became pregnant. He then investigated further the relationship between slightly subnormal basal metabolism and sterility in women, and he found that a normal basal metabolism rate was evidently necessary for conception and normal pregnancy.[111] In 1929, with James B. Carey, Dr. Litzenberg confirmed in a larger series of women the close relationship between a low metabolic rate, which served as an index of otherwise undetectable hypothyroidism, and sterility. In many women sterility caused by such slight hypothyroidism could not be overcome by administration of thyroid extract.[112] In 1935 at the Mayo Clinic, Haines and Mussey confirmed the value of thyroid extract for the treatment of menstrual disturbance in women. In 1937 Jennings Litzenberg reported on a series of more than 300 women with low basal metabolic rates that he had treated with thyroid extract and obtained a consistent 30 percent of conceptions.[113]

Jennings Litzenberg's influence on obstetrics and gynecology from 1913 when he assumed the leadership of the department in the medical school until his retirement in 1938 was founded upon his profoundly biological approach to the process of reproduction and his thorough knowledge of clinical obstetrics. In 1909 he took his family and went to Vienna to spend two years in the study of obstetrics with Friedrich Schauta, who contributed greatly to the development of gynecological surgery, especially for cancer.[114] During his second year at Vienna, Litzenberg worked as Schauta's voluntary assistant. After his appointment at Minnesota in 1913, Litzenberg organized a program of graduate training in obstetrics and gynecology that during the next twenty-five years produced about a dozen Ph.D. graduates, a number of whom became teachers of obstetrics and gynecology at other universities. Among obstetricians in the Twin Cities, Litzenberg enjoyed an extraordinary authority. It was said that if during labor an obstetrician encountered a hand presentation he "shook hands with the child, said a prayer, and sent for Jennings Litzenberg."

On Dr. Litzenberg's retirement in 1938, he was succeeded by John L. McKelvey, who, in contrast to Dr. Litzenberg, was appointed as a full-time chief of the department. A Canadian, McKelvey was born at Kingston, Ontario, and studied medicine at Queen's University where he was graduated in 1926. After internships in obstetrics at the Montreal General Hospital and Johns Hopkins Hospital, he went to Europe in 1930, first to spend a year at the University of Kiel, Germany, and then a second year with Dr. Robert Meyer at Berlin. By this time, Meyer was a world-renowned gynecological pathologist, having done extensive work on the various forms of tumors. In 1913, with Carl Ruge, Meyer had shown that the cyclical development of the corpus luteum coincided with that of the endometrium in the human menstrual cycle.

In 1932 Dr. McKelvey returned to Baltimore where he was successively resident and instructor in obstetrics at the Johns Hopkins Hospital. In 1934, his residency training completed, McKelvey went to China to become associate professor of obstetrics and gynecology at the Peking Union Medical College where his former teacher at the Hopkins, Nicholson J. Eastman, was head of the department. At Peking, McKelvey organized a system that enabled all mission hospitals in China (hospitals usually staffed with Western-trained physicians) to send unusual pathological specimens to the Peking Union Medical College for diagnosis. As a result some 1,500 specimens a year passed through the laboratory at Peking, providing it with the richest collection of pathological material in the world, and giving McKelvey unparalleled experience in gynecological pathology.

When Nicholson Eastman returned to Johns Hopkins in 1935, John McKelvey was appointed acting head of obstetrics and gynecology at the Peking Union Medical College, and in 1937 he became its permanent head. Although the Peking

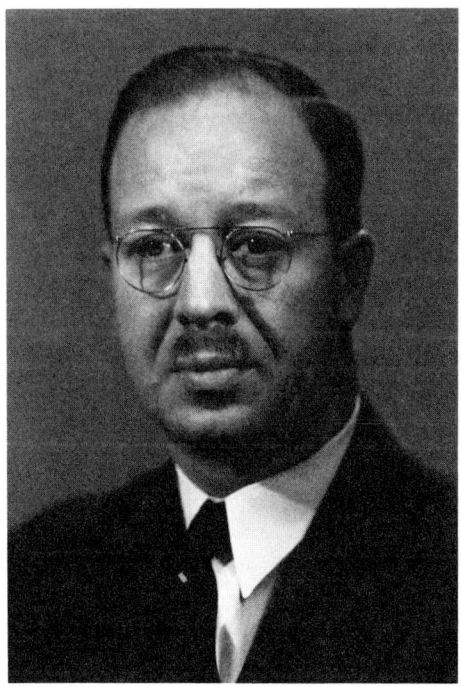

FIGURE 14:17 John L. McKelvey, 1941. Courtesy Mn U Archives.

Union Medical College continued to operate in a more or less normal way following the Japanese invasion of China in 1937, the future in China was ominous, and in the spring of 1938 McKelvey accepted the invitation to succeed Jennings Litzenberg at the University of Minnesota, where he was given a full-time clinical appointment, with the opportunity to do a small amount of private consultation work in the university hospital.

Early in 1939, McKelvey's former teacher at Berlin, Dr. Robert Meyer, wrote to say that Nazi authorities had declared that as a Jew he must leave Germany, and therefore he was seeking a position in the United States. McKelvey was able to offer Meyer an appointment at Minnesota, and in September 1939 Dr. and Mrs. Meyer arrived at Minneapolis.[115] Although then seventy-five years old, Dr. Meyer continued to work actively in the Department of Obstetrics and Gynecology until 1946. He died in 1947 of gastric cancer at the age of eighty-three. During his seven years at Minnesota, Dr. Meyer left a deep impression on the work in gynecology and obstetrics by showing how necessary an exact knowledge of histology was to the making of sound clinical decisions.

When John McKelvey came to Minnesota the largest and most serious problem in gynecology was how to deal with the various forms of cancer that occurred so commonly among women, especially in the reproductive organs, and were so frequently fatal. Two methods of treatment were then available: the surgical removal of malignant tissue, and the use of radiation, either in the form of x-rays

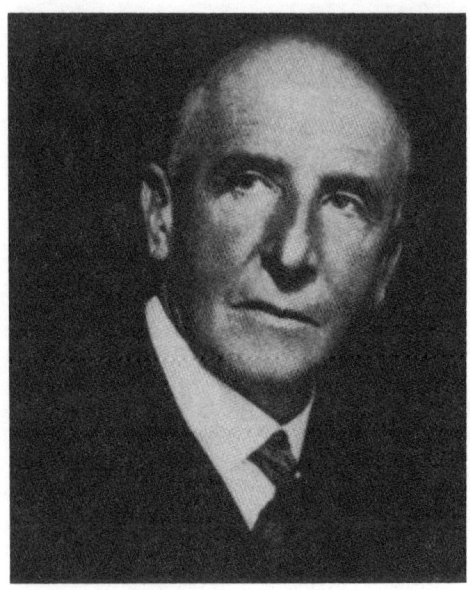

FIGURE 14:18 Robert Meyer. Courtesy *Journal of the History of Medicine and Allied Sciences.*

or by the use of radium. In order to be effective, both kinds of treatment had to be guided by a reliable differentiation of diseased from normal tissue and an exact determination of the location of the malignant tissue. Through his training at Berlin and his enormous pathological experience gained in China, McKelvey was prepared to recognize clinically the presence of cancer in women even in its more obscure and unusual manifestations. With the arrival of Robert Meyer in 1939, he had the benefit of the collaboration and stimulus of the foremost gynecological pathologist in the world. At Minnesota Robert Meyer demonstrated that carcinomas arose from the basal cells within a limited area of old squamous epithelium. The tumor grew from its point of origin by proliferation of cells, destroying the surrounding normal epithelium, and could be diagnosed before it had broken through the basement membrane into the deeper tissues. Meyer disproved the earlier opinion that the cells had to be shown to invade the underlying tissues before they could be diagnosed as malignant.[116]

At the beginning of 1939, John McKelvey and his colleagues began to treat patients suffering from carcinoma of the cervix with large, but carefully measured, doses of radiation, Karl Wilhelm Stenstrom supervising the administration of radiation. For twenty-eight days the patient received x-ray therapy followed by the insertion within the uterus of radium, which was left in place for 100 hours. During the whole period of treatment the patients remained in hospital where their condition, especially their blood cell levels, was watched carefully, and particular attention was paid to their nutrition. When in 1949 John McKelvey described the results of such therapy applied to 577 patients during the eight years 1939 through 1947, he was able to report an overall five-year survival rate of 53.6 percent, which

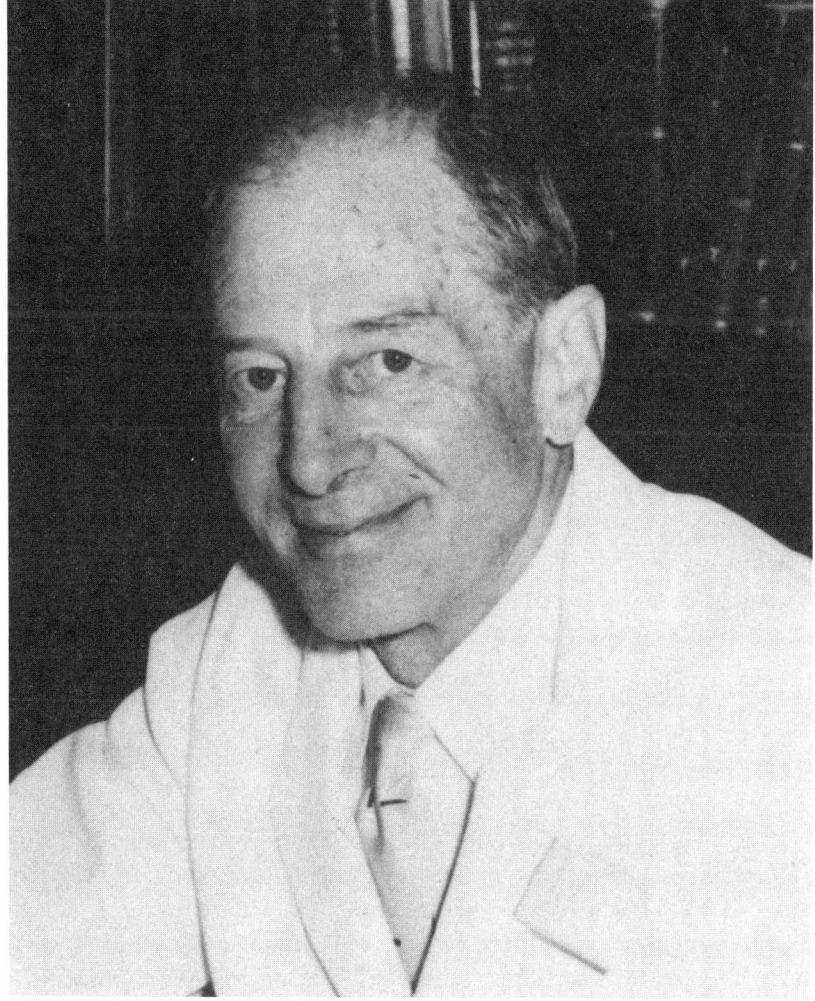

FIGURE 14:19   Karl Wilhelm Stenstrom. Courtesy Eleanor M. Larson.

was about double the world five-year survival rate reported in 1939 by the League of Nations Health Organization, and significantly above the survival rates reported by other leading medical centers in the United States. McKelvey and his colleagues were particularly successful in treating cervical carcinoma in its early stages where they achieved a five-year survival of over 81 percent. The detection of carcinoma depended on the identification of carcinoma cells in biopsies of the cervix. "For all those who have passed five years since treatment," said McKelvey, "the histologic material has been passed upon by the late Dr. Robert Meyer. There is no questionable carcinoma in the series."[117] Even past the age of eighty, Robert Meyer thus continued to contribute significantly to medical research.

The other factor in the successful experimental treatment of carcinoma of the cervix at Minnesota was the close cooperation between John McKelvey in obstetrics and gynecology and Karl Wilhelm Stenstrom in the Department of Radiology. Stenstrom was responsible for ensuring that each patient received the same uniform dose of radiation.

During the 1930s Karl Wilhelm Stenstrom also pioneered in the aggressive treatment of Hodgkin's disease (lymphoblastoma) by radiation therapy. His remarkable success with certain individual patients encouraged him to persist in a search for the most effective mode of radiation treatment. By 1940 it was clear that patients given radiation treatment survived for an average of more than four years, whereas patients without treatment had an average survival of less than seventeen months.[118] By 1947 Stenstrom had refined the radiation treatment of Hodgkin's disease sufficiently that he had achieved a five-year survival rate of 21 percent and ten-year survival of 8 percent. He gave a full course of radiation treatment to each area of lymph gland involvement and treated large masses with even greater intensity.[119] The aggressive radiation treatment of Hodgkin's disease has continued to evolve so that in 1985 Stenstrom's successor at Minnesota, Seymour Levitt, considered that, if treatment were begun early enough, the otherwise fatal disease could be effectively cured.[120]

Radiology

When Leo Rigler became director of the Division of Radiology in 1927, one of the more common and useful applications of roentgenology, apart from the examination of bone fractures, was the detection of pleural effusion in the chest. Pleural effusion was an early sign of tuberculosis that signaled a need for prompt treatment. Because tuberculosis was then such a common and serious disease of young adults, physicians were anxious to detect the occurrence of pleural effusion whenever it occurred in a patient, and at as early a stage as possible, but effusions into the pleural cavity of less than 400 cc. of fluid could not be detected either by auscultation and percussion, or by x-ray examination in the ordinary upright position. In 1930 Leo Rigler found from studies on a series of patients that if the x-ray plate were taken while the patient lay on his side with his head resting on one arm (the lateral decubitus position), any fluid in the pleural cavity shifted so as to create a sharply defined shadow. X-ray examination in this way could detect small effusions that were otherwise invisible.[121] When Dr. Rigler presented his results to the American Roentgen Ray Society in September 1930, one physician, after complimenting Rigler on the excellence of his x-ray plates, commented: "I think less of physical diagnosis the more I learn about roentgenology."[122]

In 1933 Leo Rigler and Lester Ericksen drew attention to an inferior accessory lobe present in almost half of lungs examined anatomically that created a faint linear shadow, observable in about 8 percent of patients. The identification of such an inferior accessory lobe, when present, was important in order that it should not be misinterpreted as representing some pathological change.[123] In 1936 Leo Rigler showed that when a patient with a pleural effusion lay in a horizontal position, the effusion might extend into the fissures between lobes of the lung so as to look like an encapsulated infusion on the x-ray plate. If adhesions formed while an effusion was present, the portions of effusion in the interlobar spaces might become isolated and encysted, and such encapsulations were frequent complications of pneumonia.[124] In 1939 Leo Rigler demonstrated that observation of the relative density of the right and left side of the heart in x-ray films of the chest might provide the earliest signs of lobar pneumonia, particularly in the left lower lobe, and might be used to diagnose other lung lesions such as lung abscess, tumors, or mediastinal pleural effusion.[125] Thus he showed how to reveal many lesions of the lung, previously hidden by the heavy shadow of the heart.

Leo Rigler's papers in the 1930s on the presence and location of pleural effusion and other lesions of the lungs rapidly became classics in the diagnostic radiology of the chest, but Rigler also described x-ray signs of various acute abdominal conditions, including strangulated intestinal obstruction. In 1938 he published his *Outline of Roentgen diagnosis* which quickly became a popular reference among medical students, residents, and practicing physicians.[126] By 1941 Leo Rigler was one of the outstanding radiologists in the United States, well prepared to deal with the new problems confronting radiology, particularly the early diagnosis of lung cancer, a disease that by 1941 was increasing ominously in its frequency among American adults.

Sister Kenny at the Medical School 1940–1941

During the 1930s, Americans became intensely aware of poliomyelitis as a disease that especially threatened children with death or lasting paralysis, but which could also attack adults, as it had done to Franklin D. Roosevelt at his summer home on Campobello Island in New Brunswick in August 1921. Crippled as he was by polio, Roosevelt remained keenly interested in the search for better treatment and prevention of the disease. In 1934, when Roosevelt was president of the United States, the first President's Birthday Ball was held in cities across the country to raise money to fight poliomyelitis, and in 1938 the National Foundation for Infantile Paralysis was established to organize the annual March of Dimes campaign to raise funds for research on poliomyelitis.

The first great polio epidemic in the United States occurred in 1916, but during the 1930s there were epidemics every summer and from year to year the annual epidemic of polio tended to grow. Polio struck fear into the hearts of parents and during epidemics fear often became panic.

In May 1940 an Australian nurse, Sister Elizabeth Kenny, with her adopted daughter Mary, arrived in Minneapolis, a few weeks after first landing at San Francisco. Sister Kenny had come to the United States because she believed that she possessed a method of treatment for victims of poliomyelitis that was far superior to the methods then used in the United States. She believed also that the success of her method was based upon her concept that poliomyelitis was not simply a disease of the anterior horn cells of the spinal cord, but that the virus attacked the muscles as well, throwing them into painful spasm. For several years she had been using her methods successfully in a clinic at Brisbane, Australia, and had gained the respect of a number of physicians who had observed her work closely. The government of Queensland paid for her trip to the United States.[127]

In 1940 American physicians were accustomed to immobilize the paralysed limbs of polio patients with splints or plaster casts in order to rest the limb completely and to prevent its distortion by unequal contractions of the muscles. They acted on the assumption that muscle paralysis occurred as a result of damage to the motor neurons in the spinal cord, and that opposite unparalysed muscles then pulled the skeleton into distorted positions. In Australia, Sister Kenny had found that the painful muscle contractions occurring in the acute state of polio could be eased with hot, moist compresses, and that the distortion of joints could be avoided by passive movement of the limbs. She believed that the disease caused not the paralysis of the flaccid muscles, but instead the spasm of the opposite, contracted muscles. The apparent paralysis was a reflex reaction to avoid the pain of pulling against the opposite muscles in spasm, a reaction that Elizabeth Kenny described as "mental alienation." After the disease subsided, the system of reflexes needed for coordinated movements had to be reestablished by a process of gradually educating the patient to use the required muscles. In Elizabeth Kenny's opinion the use of splints and plaster casts on polio patients was not only ineffective but downright harmful because it did nothing to relieve spasm in affected muscles. Yet, if muscles remained in spasm indefinitely they would become destroyed, and incapable of movement.

Sister Kenny brought with her to the United States letters of introduction to Basil O'Connor, president of the National Foundation for Infantile Paralysis at New York City, to the American Medical Association at Chicago, and to Dr. Melvin Henderson, orthopedic surgeon at the Mayo Clinic. At New York and Chicago Sister Kenny found no opportunity to demonstrate her methods. At the Mayo Clinic, Dr. Henderson talked to her and sent her to Dr. F. H. Krusen who frankly disbelieved her statement that she could cure "toe-drop" in poliomyelitis in twenty-four hours.[128] Nevertheless, Dr. Henderson suggested that since they saw very few cases of poliomyelitis at the Mayo Clinic, she should go to Minneapolis where polio epidemics occurred every summer.

On her arrival at Minneapolis, Sister Kenny went to see Sara Kollman, physical therapist at the university hospital, and Miss Kollman introduced her to Dean Diehl to whom Sister Kenny presented her letters of introduction and described her methods for the treatment of infantile paralysis.[129] In Harold Diehl, Elizabeth

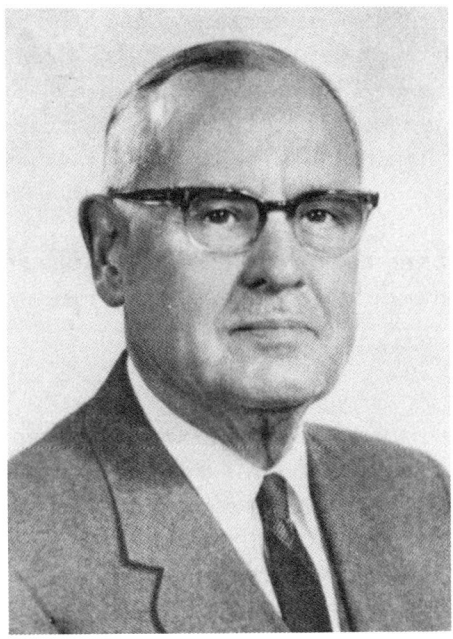

FIGURE 14:20 Wallace Cole, circa 1945. Courtesy Dr. Lyle O. Johnson.

Kenny found a sympathetic listener. Perhaps because of his experiences during and just after the First World War, Dean Diehl was remarkably open to new ideas, and he was a perceptive judge of character. He arranged for Sister Kenny to meet Dr. Wallace Cole, professor of orthopedic surgery, who already had read about her work in Australia and had heard of her from Dr. Henderson of the Mayo Clinic. A tall, stern figure of military bearing, Dr. Cole was himself dissatisfied with the results of the treatment of polio patients with splints and plaster casts. More than a third of the children in the Shriners Hospital for Crippled Children in Minneapolis were there because of the effects of polio and Dr. Cole had much experience in attempting to correct their deformities. He arranged for Sister Kenny to present her ideas and demonstrate her methods at the Shriners Hospital and in St. Paul at the St. Paul Children's Hospital and the Gillette Hospital for Crippled Children. Within three days at the St. Paul Children's Hospital, Sister Kenny corrected the distorted feet of a two-year-old boy, and in other instances she was able to correct deformities which, she said, had been caused by muscle spasm rather than by paralysis. As a result of her demonstrations, six days after Sister Kenny's arrival in the Twin Cities, Dr. George Williamson ordered frames, splints, and casts to be removed from all his polio patients at the St. Paul Children's Hospital and Gillette Hospital.

Sister Kenny's demonstrations impressed Wallace Cole sufficiently that he introduced her to Miland Knapp, a young surgeon who the year before had become director of a new Division of Physical Therapy at the university hospital and was also responsible for physical therapy at the Minneapolis General Hospital. Dr.

Knapp recalled later that after listening to Sister Kenny lecture for two hours on " . . . muscle spasm, mental alienation, incoordination, and the like, which I had never before heard associated with anterior poliomyelitis," he was thoroughly confused. Nevertheless, when she demonstrated in his own patients that muscle spasm existed even after eight months' treatment, and when she restored function in apparently paralysed muscles after a few minutes of reeducation, he thought that her procedures required thorough investigation.[130]

The polio victims in hospitals that spring were patients who had had polio the summer before. They showed the after effects of the disease rather than the disease itself. Since Elizabeth Kenny considered that her methods were most effective when administered during the acute phase of polio, Drs. Cole and Knapp thought she should remain in Minneapolis through the summer so that they might observe her treatment of acutely ill polio patients during the annual summer epidemic. Almost at the end of her funds, Sister Kenny was willing to remain if she could get sufficient money to pay living expenses for herself and her daughter. On 21 May Wallace Cole telephoned Basil O'Connor, president of the National Foundation for Infantile Paralysis, who promptly agreed to make a grant of $2,500 to the University of Minnesota so that Sister Kenny might demonstrate her ideas and methods of treatment of poliomyelitis to the medical faculty.[131] Dean Diehl arranged for her to work at the university hospital and the Minneapolis General Hospital, where later in the summer a ward was set aside for poliomyelitis patients. In the meantime Dr. Knapp invited Sister Kenny and her daughter to spend a week as guests in his home, and in conversations at mealtime and in the evening he struggled to learn what she meant by such terms as *spasm, incoordination,* and *mental alienation.*

Sister Kenny also won over a Minneapolis orthopedist, Dr. John Pohl, who had learned strict immobilization of polio patients at the Harvard Medical School and Boston Children's Hospital. She succeeded in enabling one of his patients, an eighteen-year-old youth who had been severely stricken by polio the year before, to recover movement in his legs and ultimately to walk.

In 1940 polio returned to Minneapolis in August, and during the next few months Sister Kenny treated twenty-six patients at the Minneapolis General Hospital and the university hospital. For twenty patients she was able to begin treatment within two weeks of the onset of polio, and eleven so treated were discharged within two months. Of the remaining nine patients, only one remained completely paralysed in both legs; the others continued to recover through the winter of 1940–41. In December 1940 Wallace Cole and Miland Knapp prepared a preliminary report on the results of the Kenny treatment that was published the following June. What impressed them about the Kenny treatment was that the polio patients were so much more comfortable and cheerful than those with immobilized limbs. Their bodies remained flexible and seemed to suffer less residual disability. Certainly none of Sister Kenny's patients had come to any harm.[132]

The experience with the Kenny treatment in 1940 was sufficiently encouraging that the medical school wished Sister Kenny to remain through another poliomye-

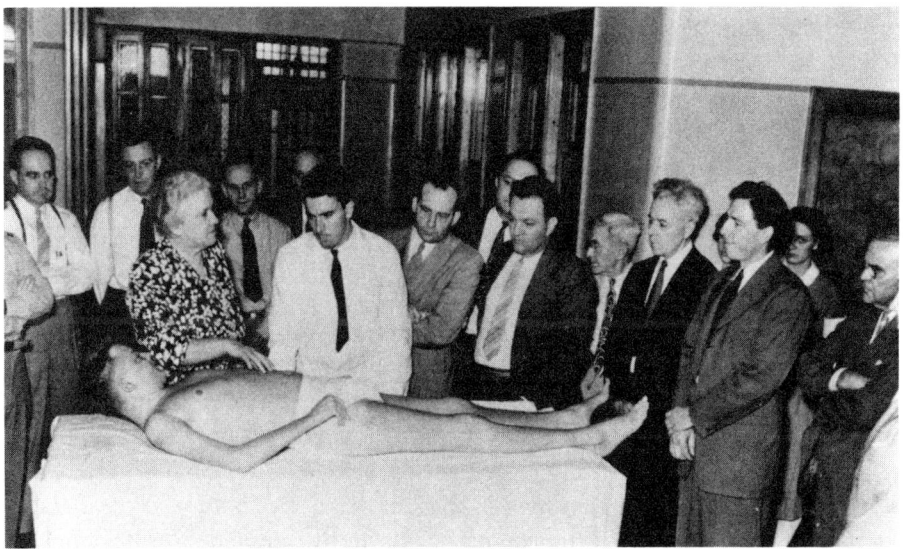

FIGURE 14:21 A Hippocratic physician teaching her students: Sister Kenny demonstrates her methods to physicians in the lobby of the Minneapolis General Hospital, 1941. Courtesy Minnesota Historical Society.

litis season in order to observe further the results of her treatment and in order to acquaint physical therapists and nurses at the university hospital and Minneapolis General Hospital with her methods. Sister Kenny agreed to stay if she could return to Australia for several months and bring back with her two technicians, trained and experienced in her methods. In January 1941 Sister Kenny returned to Australia, leaving her daughter, Mary, to continue the treatment of the remaining patients. In May she was back in Minneapolis accompanied by her two assistants, Valerie Harvey and William Bell. Meanwhile, in March the National Foundation for Infantile Paralysis had made a grant to the university of $11,250 to support the work of Sister Kenny and her group, and the university hospital set aside a seventeen-bed ward for poliomyelitis patients.

During the summer of 1941, the polio epidemic in Minneapolis was worse than the year before and children suffering from the high fever and excruciating pain of acute poliomyelitis began to fill the Kenny wards of the Minneapolis General Hospital and the university hospital. Sister Kenny objected to any polio patients being put into a respirator even when they had difficulty in breathing. She removed one ten-year-old boy from a respirator and within a day had him breathing normally and eating.[133] To prove her contention that respirators were harmful, when two patients were brought into hospitals to go into respirators she asked to treat the worst case, and the doctors assigned the patient to her. That patient recovered, while the other patient, placed in the respirator, died within twenty-four hours.[134] Drs. Cole and Knapp's account of the Kenny method published in the *Journal of the American Medical Association* in June aroused intense interest in the work of Sister Kenny, and during August and September of 1941 physicians and therapists began to come to Minneapolis to watch her at work. The National Foundation for Infantile Paralysis was glad to pay the travel expenses of several such observers, because they were somewhat uneasily providing financial support for Sister Kenny's work and were anxious to determine its value accurately. Among such visitors was Philip Lewin, an orthopedic surgeon at the Northwestern University Medical School at Chicago. Previously skeptical, Dr. Lewin became a convert. He saw that her treatment eliminated pain and stiffness and reduced any subsequent deformity to a minimum. When the Kenny treatment was carried out from the beginning, the muscles of the abdomen and back remained strong; there were no deformities; and the muscles were even more flexible than in an average normal child. "My observations of her personally treated patients," said Dr. Lewin, "revealed that they were in better condition than any similar group I have seen anywhere in the world."[135] By contrast, a comparable group of patients treated at Minneapolis by previously accepted measures, showed deformity, contractures, limitation of movement, and disability.[136]

On 23 September 1941, Dr. Mary Daly and her colleagues began to administer the Kenny treatment at the Willard Parker Hospital in New York City. They found that after one to three days of hot packs polio patients were completely comfortable at rest, and they became capable of unrestricted passive motion weeks and months earlier than polio patients treated with splints. They concluded that the patients given the Kenny treatment were more comfortable, suffered no atrophy or deformity, and recovered more rapidly and perhaps more completely than patients treated by previous methods.[137]

When the National Foundation for Infantile Paralysis began to support Sister Kenny's work at the University of Minnesota in 1940, Basil O'Connor appointed a medical committee to evaluate the results of the Kenny methods, including among its members highly skeptical physicians such as Dr. Frank H. Krusen of the Mayo Clinic. On 3 December 1941, the committee decided on the basis of reports from the University of Minnesota and other medical centers that the Kenny method should be adopted generally for the treatment of poliomyelitis, and they gave the widest publicity to their decision.[138] Thereupon followed a revolution in the treatment of poliomyelitis throughout the United States.

Even before the national foundation's decision, the medical school had realized the need to train nurses thoroughly in the proper administration of the Kenny methods, and Mr. C. C. Webber of Minneapolis gave $4,500 to provide scholarships for nurses in Minneapolis hospitals to be trained in the Kenny method. In February 1942 the medical school established a teaching program, funded by the National Foundation for Infantile Paralysis, to train doctors, nurses, and physical therapists in the Kenny method. The courses for physicians, intended simply to acquaint them with the Kenny method so that they might prescribe it and direct its use, lasted only a week; the courses for technicians and nurses, intended to train them to administer the Kenny treatment, extended from four to six

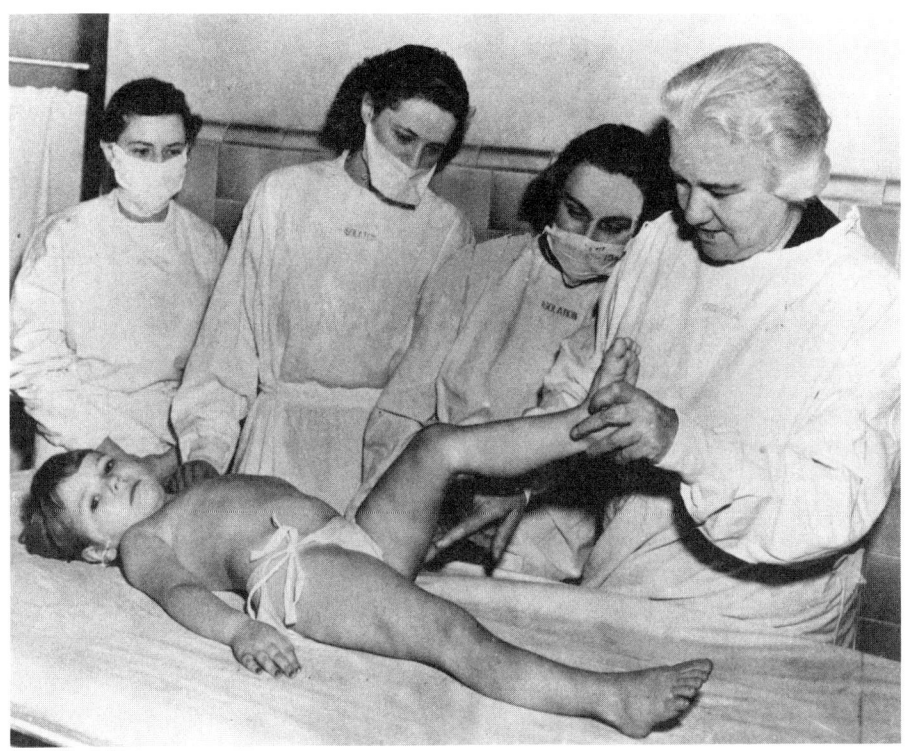

FIGURE 14:22 Sister Kenny demonstrates therapeutic techniques to nurses at the Minneapolis General Hospital, circa 1942. Courtesy Minnesota Historical Society.

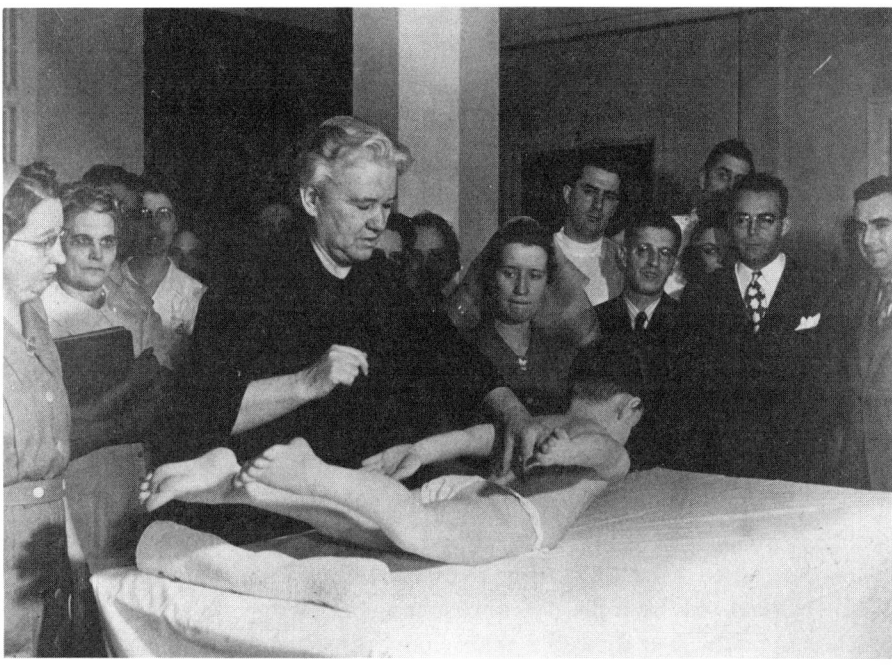

FIGURE 14:23 Sister Kenny demonstrates control of the extensor muscles of the back in a poliomyelitis patient to a class for technicians and doctors, February 1943. Courtesy Minnesota Historical Society.

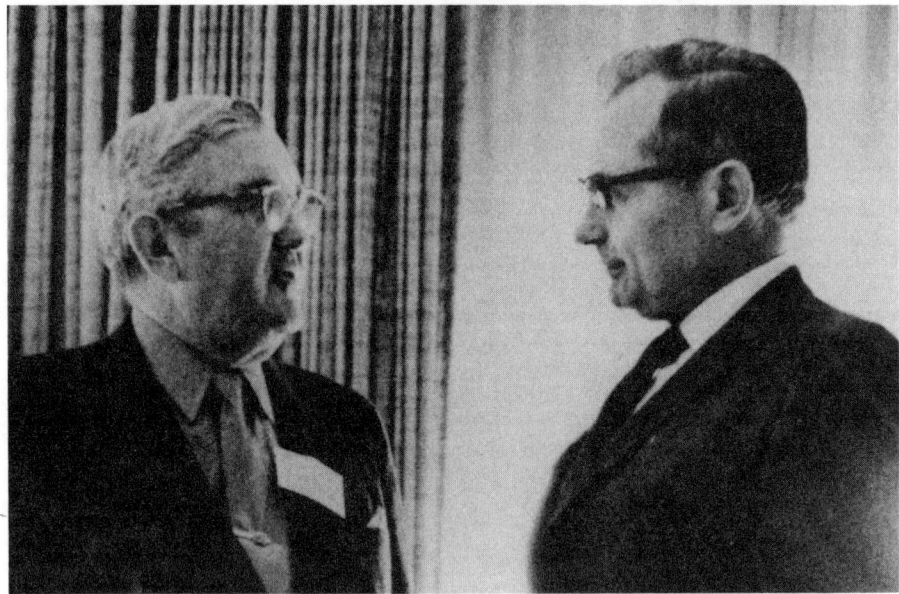

FIGURE 14:24 Miland E. Knapp (left) with Frederic J. Kottke, circa 1955. Courtesy Dr. Frederic J. Kottke.

months. The program was directed by Miland Knapp and trained doctors, nurses, and physical therapists from all over the United States and Canada. It was the first of six such training programs that the national foundation set up at medical centers in the United States.

In 1942 the Minneapolis Board of Public Welfare evicted the tuberculosis, rheumatic fever, and other child health clinics from the Lymanhurst Health Center and remodeled the building for poliomyelitis patients, naming it the Sister Kenny Institute. The loss of Lymanhurst, after twenty years of splendid work on tuberculosis and rheumatic fever, was a bitter blow to Drs. Jay Arthur Myers and Morse J. Shapiro, but it led to their later successful efforts to create the Variety Club Heart Hospital. Many medical men were never reconciled to Sister Kenny, and attacked her repeatedly, but the clinical value of her work was unquestionable. Although her training was that of a nurse, Sister Kenny acted toward poliomyelitis as a Hippocratic physician. By acute observation of the sick patient she saw the tightening and shortening of muscles, accompanied by pain; she discovered the relief offered by hot compresses. In later years Frederic J. Kottke, who in 1947 succeeded Miland E. Knapp as director of physical therapy in the medical school, worked with his colleagues to determine the changes in muscle and nerve function in polio. They showed that the muscle spasm and other phenomena described by Sister Kenny were real, and that the success of the Kenny method could be explained by a more accurate and complete knowledge of neuromuscular physiology.[139]

The University of Minnesota gave Elizabeth Kenny's methods a full and fair trial when no one else would, to the immeasurable benefit of poliomyelitis patients during the fifteen years or so before the introduction of polio vaccines eliminated poliomyelitis as a widespread and desperately serious disease.

NOTES

1. Edith Boyd, "Richard Everingham Scammon 1883–1952," *Anat. Rec.*, 1953, *116* 259–262, p.260.
2. E. T. Bell, "Students rose early to hear him: A colleague recalls Dr. Richard Scammon's early days at the University of Minnesota," *Minneapolis Star*, 22 September 1952.
3. Wangensteen to Lyon, ms draft [1930], Wangensteen papers.
4. Owen H. Wangensteen, *Owen H. Wangensteen*, p. 27.
5. Edward P. Richardson, "Acute intestinal obstruction: a study of a second series of cases from the Massachusetts General Hospital," *Boston med. surg. J.*, 1920, *183*, 288–298; Monroe A. McIver, "Acute intestinal obstruction. II. Acute mechanical obstructions exclusive of those due to neoplasms and strangulated external hernias," *Archs Surg., Chicago*, 1932, *25*, 1106–1124.
6. H. B. Stone, B. M. Bernheim, and G. H. Whipple, "Intestinal obstruction . . . . A study of a toxic substance produced in closed duodenal loops," *J. exp. Med.*, 1913, *17*, 286–306, 307–323.
7. In his biography of George Hoyt Whipple, George W. Corner discusses at some length Whipple's toxic theory of death from intestinal obstruction without stating, and evidently without realizing, that Whipple's theory later proved to be completely mistaken. See George W. Corner, *George Hoyt Whipple and his friends*, pp. 65, 77, 96–98.
8. J. A. Hartwell and J. P. Hoguet, "Experimental intestinal obstruction in dogs with special reference to the cause of death and treatment with large amounts of normal saline solution," *J. Am. med. Ass.*, 1912, *59*, 82–87.
9. Russell L. Haden and Thomas G. Orr, "Chemical changes in the blood of the dog after intestinal obstruction," *J. exp. Med.*, 1923, *37*, 365–375.
10. Owen H. Wangensteen and Stanley S. Chunn, "Studies in intestinal obstruction. I. A comparison of the toxicity of normal and obstructed intestinal content," *Archs Surg., Chicago*, 1928, *16*, 606–614.
11. Owen H. Wangensteen and Milo Loucks, "Studies in intestinal obstruction. II. The absorption of histamine from the obstructed bowel," *Archs Surg., Chicago*, 1928, *16*, 1089–1111.
12. Monroe A. McIver and James L. Gamble, "Body fluid changes due to upper intestinal obstruction," *J. Am. med. Ass.*, 1908, *91*, 1589–1594.
13. J. C. White and F. A. Fender, "The cause of death in uncomplicated high intestinal obstruction," *Archs Surg., Chicago*, 1930, *20*, 897–905.
14. Owen H. Wangensteen and N. Logan Leven, "Correlation of function with cause of death following experimental intestinal obstruction at varying levels," *Archs Surg., Chicago*, 1931, *22*, 658–665.
15. John J. Morton, "The differences between high and low intestinal obstruction in the dog, an anatomic and physiologic explanation," *Archs Surg., Chicago*, 1929, *18*, 1119–1139.
16. Owen H. Wangensteen and Francis W. Lynch, "Evaluation of x-ray evidence as criteria of intestinal obstruction," *Proc. Soc. exp. Biol. Med.*, 1929–30, *27*, 674–676.

17. Owen H. Wangensteen, "Elaboration of criteria upon which the early diagnosis of acute intestinal obstruction may be made with special consideration of the value of x-ray evidence," *Radiology*, 1931, *17*, 44–62.

18. Owen H. Wangensteen, "The early diagnosis of acute intestinal obstruction with comments on pathology and treatment, with a report of successful decompression of three cases of mechanical bowel obstruction by nasal catheter suction siphonage," *West. J. Surg. Obstet. Gynec.*, 1932, *40*, 1–17.

19. Owen H. Wangensteen, "Therapeutic considerations in the management of acute intestinal obstruction: Technic of enterostomy and a further account of decompression by the employment of suction siphonage by nasal catheter," *Archs Surg., Chicago*, 1933, *26*, 933–961, p. 944.

20. J. R. Paine, "Constant suction by nasal catheter as an adjunct in postoperative treatment," *Minn. Med.*, 1932, *15*, 444–446.

21. William A. O'Brien, "Paul Hill Fesler," *Univ. Minn. Hosp. staff Meet.*, 1932, *3*, 206–207.

22. Fred Jarvis, Robert Plant, Robert Holmen, E. Spackman [sic], De Remus, J. W. Tedder, and R. M. Cushing [surgical interns] "To whom it may concern," 25 November 1932 [copy], Medical School Papers.

23. Dunn to Scammon, 1 May 1933 [copy], Medical School Papers.

24. Wangensteen, *Wangensteen* (n. 4), p. 28.

25. Although Dr. Wangensteen did not mention the fact, one of the surgical interns, Dr. George S. Bergh, had not joined in the interns' petition because he did not think it was justified and was satisfied with his training.

26. Wangensteen to Scammon, 5 May 1933 [copy], Medical School Papers.

27. Ibid.

28. Wangensteen, *Wangensteen* (n. 4), p. 29.

29. Scammon to Coffman, 7 May 1933 [copy], Medical School papers.

30. Wangensteen (n. 19).

31. John R. Paine, Herbert A. Carlson, and Owen H. Wangensteen, "The postoperative control of distention, nausea and vomiting," *J. Am. med. Ass.*, 1933, *100*, 1910–1917.

32. Owen H. Wangensteen, *The therapeutic problem in bowel obstructions*.

33. Owen H. Wangensteen, "Acute bowel obstruction: its recognition and management," *New Engl. J. Med.*, 1938, *219*, 340–348, p. 348.

34. Leland S. McKittrick and S. Peter Sarris, "Acute mechanical obstruction of the small bowel," *New Engl. J. Med.*, 1940, *222*, 611–622.

35. Hobart A. Reimann, *The pneumonias*, see especially pp. 82–91.

36. *Dictionary of Scientific Biography, Supplement*, s.v. "Fischer, Hans."

37. C. J. Watson, "Über Stercobilin und Porphyrine aus Kot," *Hoppe-Seyler's z. physiol. Chem.*, 1932, *204*, 57–67; C. J. Watson, "An improved method for the isolation of crystalline stercobilin," *J. biol. Chem.*, 1934, *105*, 469–472.

38. C. J. Watson, "Über Stercobilin, Kopromesobiliviolin, Kopronigrin," *Hoppe-Seyler's z. physiol. Chem.*, 1932, *208*, 101–119.

39. Cecil James Watson, "Concerning the naturally occurring porphyrins. I. The isolation of coproporphyrin I from the urine in a case of cincophen cirrhosis," *J. clin. Invest.*, 1935, *14*, 106–109.

40. Cecil James Watson, "Concerning the naturally occurring porphyrins. II. The isolation of a hitherto undescribed porphyrin occurring with an increased amount of coproporphyrin I in the feces of a case of familial hemolytic jaundice," *J. clin. Invest.*, 1935, *14*, 110–115.

41. Cecil James Watson, "Concerning the naturally occurring porphyrins. III. The isolation of coproporphyrin I from the feces of untreated cases of pernicious anemia," *J. clin. Invest.*, 1935, *14*, 116–118.

42. Cecil James Watson and William O. Clarke, "The occurrence of protoporphyrin in the reticulocytes," *Proc. Soc. exp. Biol. Med.*, 1937, *36*, 65–70.

43. C. J. Watson, "The erythrocyte coproporphyrin: Variation with respect to erythrocyte protoporphyrin and reticulocytes in certain of the anemias," *Archs intern. Med.*, 1950, *86*, 797–809; Rudi Schmid, Samuel Schwartz, and C. J. Watson, "Porphyrins in the bone marrow and circulating erythrocytes in experimental anemias," *Proc. Soc. exp. Biol. Med.*, 1950, *75*, 705–708.

44. C. S. Keefer, "Report of a case of Malta fever originating in Baltimore, Maryland," *Johns Hopkins Hosp. Bull.*, 1924, *35*, 6–14.

45. Maxwell Finland, *The Harvard Medical Unit at Boston City Hospital*, I, 189–194.

46. Wesley W. Spink and Arthur A. Nelson, "Brucella endocarditis," *Ann. intern. Med.*, 1939, *13*, 721–728.

47. Wesley W. Spink et al., "A case of Brucella endocarditis with clinical, bacteriologic, and pathologic findings," *Am. J. med. Sci.*, 1942, *203*, 799–801. Cf. Wesley W. Spink, *The nature of brucellosis*, pp. 291–292.

48. Bernhard Bang, "Die Aetiologie des seuchenhaften (infectiosen) Verwerfens," *Z. Tiermed.*, 1897, *1*, 241–278.

49. W. P. Larson, "The complement fixation reaction in the diagnosis of contagious abortion of cattle," *J. infect. Dis.*, 1912, *10*, 178–185.

50. W. P. Larson and J. P. Sedgwick, "The complement fixation reaction of the blood of children and infants, using the Bacillus abortus as antigen," *Am. J. Dis. Child.*, 1913, *6*. 326–333.

51. E. C. Schroeder and W. E. Cotton, "[Infectious abortion of cattle and the occurrence of its bacterium in milk.] II. The bacillus of infectious abortion found in milk," in *U.S. Bureau of Animal Industry, Ann. Rep.*, 1911, *28*, 139–146.

52. Alice C. Evans, "Further studies on Bacillus abortus and related bacteria. II. A comparison of Bacterium abortus with Bacterium bronchisepticus and with the organism which causes Malta Fever," *J. infect. Dis.*, 1918, *22*, 580–593.

53. K. F. Meyer and E. B. Shaw, "A comparison of the morphologic; cultural and biochemical characteristics of B. abortus and B. melitensis: Studies on the genus Brucella nov. gen. I," *J. infect. Dis.*, 1920, *27*, 173–184.

54. L. J. Orpen, "The connection between undulant (Malta) fever and contagious abortion," *Trans. r. Soc. trop. Med. Hyg.*, 1924, *17*, 521–524.

55. Frank J. Hirschbock, "Undulant fever," *Minn. Med.*, 1929, *12*, 590–598.

56. J. Arthur Myers, "Francis Edward Harrington: physician, administrator and benefactor of man, a personal appreciation," *J.-Lancet*, 1947, *67*, 2–9.

57. F. E. Harrington, "Lymanhurst: the reason for and the establishment of the school," *J.-Lancet*, 1922, *42*, 237–239.

58. Biographical information about Dr. Myers is from his autobiography, J. Arthur Myers, *Tuberculosis, a half century of study and conquest*, pp. 3–7.

59. J. Arthur Myers, "Chester Arthur Stewart—physician, teacher, clinical investigator, organizer, and friend of man: a personal appreciation," *J.-Lancet*, 1946, *66*, 132–137.

60. J. Arthur Myers, *Lymanhurst, a report of ten years of activity*, pp. 133–134.

61. Myers, *Tuberculosis* (n. 58), p. 31.

62. J. A. Myers and Estella Magiera, "The relation of exposure to infection in 2,000 children examined for tuberculosis," *Am. Rev. Tuberc. pulm. Dis.*, 1925, *11*, 375–385.

63. J. A. Myers and E. O. Lodmell, "Studies on tuberculosis in infancy and childhood.

II. The detection of the primary lesion in a group of children examined for tuberculosis," *Am. Rev. Tuberc. pulm. Dis.*, 1925, *11*, 386-392.

64. J. A. Myers and Kuen Tsiang, "Studies on tuberculosis in infancy and childhhood. V. The relation of tuberculous infection to calcification of the hilum lymph nodes of the lung," *Am. Rev. Tuberc. pulm. Dis.*, 1925, *11*, 403-406.

65. S. A. Slater, "The results of Pirquet tuberculin tests on 1,654 children in a rural community in Minnesota," *Am. Rev. Tuberc. pulm. Dis.*, 1924-25, *10*, 299-305. Cf. J. Arthur Myers, "Sidney A. Slater, M.D.," *J.- Lancet*, 1959, *79*, 372-375.

66. E. Leggett, Dorothy Hutchinson, and J. A. Myers, "Studies on tuberculosis in infancy and childhood. VII. Serial examinations of children with evidence of primary foci," *Am. Rev. Tuberc. pulm. Dis.*, 1926, *14*, 428-436, p. 434.

67. Dorothy Hutchinson and J. A. Myers, "Studies on tuberculosis in infancy and childhood. VII. Serial examinations of children with pulmonary lesions," *Am. Rev. Tuberc. pulm. Dis.*, 1926, *14*, 437-447.

68. H. F. Wahlquist and J. A. Myers, "Studies on tuberculosis in infancy and childhood. XI. Serial examinations of infants showing positive tuberculin skin reactions while under two years of age," *Am. Rev. Tuberc. pulm. Dis.*, 1926, *14*, 461-467, p. 463.

69. J. A. Myers and L. M. Kernkamp, "Tuberculous infection in infancy," *Am. Rev. Tuberc. pulm. Dis.*, 1930, *21*, 423-478.

70. J. A. Myers and L. M. Kernkamp, "Tuberculosis among girls and boys in their teens," *Am. Rev. Tuberc. pulm. Dis.*, 1930, *21*, 509-531. In 1930 Dr. Myers also described the distinguishing characteristics of the childhood and adult forms of tuberculosis in a monograph on tuberculosis among children.

71. H. D. Lees and J. A. Myers, "Tuberculous infection among adults," *Am. Rev. Tuberc. pulm. Dis.*, 1930, *21*, 532-540. Cf. Myers, *Tuberculosis among children*, pp. 72-73.

72. J. A. Myers and H. R. Anderson, "The significance of tuberculosis among the aged," *Am. Rev. Tuberc. pulm. Dis.*, 1930, *21*, 541-556.

73. J. A. Myers, "Some dangers of insidious and acute onsets in pulmonary tuberculosis," *Am. Rev. Tuberc. pulm. Dis.*, 1930, *21*, 557-567.

74. J. Arthur Myers, "Ten years at the Lymanhurst School for Tuberculous Children," *Ann. intern. Med.*, 1932, *6*, 672-688.

75. Quoted in J. Arthur Myers, "Types of tuberculous lesions found in the chests of students of nursing and medicine," *Am. Rev. Tuberc. pulm. Dis.*, 1933, *28*, 93-117, p. 94.

76. E. K. Geer, "Tuberculosis among nurses," *Archs intern. Med.*, 1932, *49*, 77-87; idem, "Primary tuberculosis among nurses," *Trans. natn Tuberc. Ass., N.Y.*, 1932, *28*, 118-128.

77. J. Arthur Myers et al., "First-infection-type tuberculosis, its treatment and prognosis," *Am. Rev. Tuberc. pulm. Dis.*, 1935, *32*, 631-643.

78. Wathena Myers Johnson and J. A. Myers, "Tuberculosis in infants and primitive races," *Am. Rev. Tuberc. pulm. Dis.*, 1933, *28*, 381-409.

79. Myers et al. (n. 77), p. 637.

80. J. Arthur Myers and Francis E. Harrington, "The effect of initial tuberculosis infection on subsequent tuberculous lesions," *J. Am. med. Ass.*, 1934, *103*, 1530-1536.

81. J. Arthur Myers, "The first-infection type of tuberculosis," *Am. Rev. Tuberc. pulm. Dis.*, 1936, *34*, 317-339.

82. Johannes Heimbeck, "Immunity to tuberculosis," *Archs intern. Med.*, 1928, *41*, 336-342.

83. Harold S. Diehl, "Tuberculosis control in University of Minnesota students," *J.- Lancet*, 1932, *52*, 224-225.

84. Lees and Myers (n. 71).

85. J. Arthur Myers et al., "The evolution of tuberculosis in students of nursing and medicine," *Trans. natn. Tuberc. Ass., N.Y.*, 1934, *30*, 345–365.

86. In 1933 Dr. Myers summed up what they had learned about tuberculosis over the preceding twelve years. See J. Arthur Myers, "Some drastic changes in our conception of tuberculosis," *J.-Lancet*, 1933, *53*, 457–463.

87. J. Arthur Myers, et al., "Tuberculosis among students and graduates of schools of law and medicine," *Yale J. Biol. Med.*, 1942–43, *15*, 390–451.

88. J. Arthur Myers et al., "Tuberculosis among students and graduates of medicine." *Ann. intern. Med.*, 1941, *14*, 1575–1594, p. 1580.

89. Ibid., p. 1583. By 1940 more than three quarters of physicians who had graduated from 1933 to 1936 were positive reactors to tuberculin.

90. J. Arthur Myers, Ruth E. Boynton, and Harold S. Diehl, "Tuberculosis among nurses," *Dis. Chest*, 1955, *28*, 610–637, p. 612.

91. Harold S. Diehl and Jay Arthur Myers, "Tuberculosis prevention, immunization and periodic health examinations among medical students," *J. Ass. Am. med. Coll.*, 1940, *15*, 104–116.

92. J. A. Myers, Ruth E. Boynton, and Harold S. Diehl, "Prevention of tuberculosis among students of nursing," *Am. J. Nurs.*, 1947, *47*, 661–666, p.663.

93. Ibid., p. 664.

94. Irvine McQuarrie and Haddow M. Keith, "Epilepsy in children: Relationship of variations in the degree of ketonuria to occurrence of convulsions in epileptic children on ketogenic diets," *Am. J. Dis. Child.*, 1927, *34*, 1013-1029.

95. Irvine McQuarrie and Haddow M. Keith, "Influence of acid-forming and base-forming constituents of ketogenic diet used in treatment of idiopathic epilepsy," *Proc. Soc. exp. Biol. Med.*, 1928, *25*, 418–420.

96. Irvine McQuarrie, "Epilepsy in children: the relationship of water balance to the occurrence of seizures," *Am. J. Dis. Child.*, 1929, *38*, 418–420.

97. Irvine McQuarrie, "Protein metabolism of children on diets extremely low in carbohydrates," *J. Nutr.*, 1929, *2*, 31–47.

98. Irvine McQuarrie and D. B. Peeler, "The effects of sustained pituitary antidiuresis and forced water drinking in epileptic children. A diagnostic and etiologic study," *J. clin. Invest.*, 1931, *10*, 915–940.

99. Irvine McQuarrie, "Some recent observations regarding the nature of epilepsy," *Ann. intern. Med.*, 1932, *6*, 497–505.

100. Irvine McQuarrie, R. C. Manchester, and Clara Husted, "Study of the water and mineral balances in epileptic children: I. Effects of diuresis, catharsis, phenobarbitol therapy and water storage," *Am. J. Dis. Child.*, 1932, *43*, 1519–1543.

101. W. H. Thompson, Irvine McQuarrie, and E. T. Bell, "Edema associated with hypogenesis of serum proteins and atrophic changes in the liver, with studies of the water and mineral exchanges," *J. Pediat.*, 1936, *9*, 604–619.

102. In his book *The experiments of nature and other essays* (Lawrence, Kansas: University of Kansas, 1944), Irvine McQuarrie discussed the case of the child whose body was unable to synthesize plasma proteins (pp. 3–8). McQuarrie used the phrase "experiments of nature" from William Osler who, in one of his early addresses, said: "The facts obtained by precise anatomical investigation, from experiments on animals in the laboratory, from the study of nature's experiments upon us in disease . . . have brought order out of the chaos of fifty years ago," from "The leaven of science" in Osler, *Aequanimitas with other addresses* . . . (Philadelphia, 1905) pp. 79–101, p. 92.

103. Arild Hansen, Mildred R. Ziegler, and Irvine McQuarrie, "Disturbance of osseous

and lipid metabolism in a child with primary carcinoma of the liver," *J. Pediat.*, 1940, *17*, 9–30.

104. McQuarrie, *Experiments of nature* (n. 102), pp. 15–21. Cf. Arild E. Hansen and Irvine McQuarrie, "Study of certain tissue lipids in generalized lipodystrophy ('lipohistodiaresis')," *Proc. Soc. exp. Biol. Med.*, 1940, *44*, 611–613.

105. Irvine McQuarrie, Willis H. Thompson, and John A. Anderson, "Effects of excessive ingestion of sodium and potassium salts on carbohydrate metabolism and blood pressure in diabetic children," *J. Nutr.*, 1936, *11*, 77–101.

106. Harvey Cushing, "The basophil adenomas of the pituitary body and their clinical manifestations (pituitary basophilism)," *Johns Hopkins Hosp. Bull.*, 1932, *50*, 137–195.

107. Irvine McQuarrie, R. M. Johnson, and M. R. Ziegler, "Plasma electrolyte disturbance in patient with hypercorticoadrenal syndrome contrasted with that found in Addison's disease," *Endocrinology*, 1937, *21*, 762–772.

108. A. T. Rasmussen, "The relation of the basophilic cells of the human hypophysis to blood pressure," *Endocrinology*, 1936, *20*, 673–678.

109. Irvine McQuarrie, "The Department of Pediatrics, University of Minnesota," *J. Pediat.*, 1934, *5*, 365–369, p. 367.

110. In 1936 Dr. Litzenberg discussed both subjects in his Porter lectures at the University of Kansas School of Medicine, Kansas City, Kansas. See Jennings C. Litzenberg, *Contributions to the pathology of pregnancy*.

111. Jennings C. Litzenberg, "The relation of basal metabolism to sterility," *Am. J. Obstet. Gynec.*, 1926, *12*, 706–709.

112. Jennings C. Litzenberg and James B. Carey, "The relation of basal metabolism to gestation," *Am. J. Obstet. Gynec.*, 1929, *17*, 550–552.

113. Samuel F. Haines and Robert D. Mussey, "Certain menstrual disturbances associated with low basal metabolic rates without myxedema," *J. Am. med. Ass.*, 1935, *105*, 557–560; Jennings C. Litzenberg, "The endocrines in relation to sterility and abortion," *J. Am. med. Ass.*, 1937, *109*, 1871–1873.

114. Erna Lesky, *The Vienna Medical School of the 19th century*, p. 431–434.

115. Robert Meyer, *Autobiography*, pp. 92–95.

116. Robert Meyer, "The basis of the histological diagnosis of carcinoma with special reference to carcinoma of the cervix and similar lesions," *Surg. Gynec. Obstet.*, 1941, *73*, 14–20; idem, "The histological diagnosis of early carcinoma," *Surg. Gynec. Obstet.*, 1941, *73*, 129–139.

117. J. L. McKelvey, K. W. Stenstrom, and J. S. Gillam, "Results of an experimental therapy of carcinoma of the cervix," *Am. J. Obstet. Gynec.*, 1949, *58*, 896–907, p. 898.

118. Charles B. Craft, "Results with Roentgen ray therapy in Hodgkin's disease," *Bull. Univ. Minn. Hosp.*, 1940, *11*, 391–409.

119. T. B. Merner and K. W. Stenstrom, "Roentgen therapy in Hodgkin's disease," *Radiology*, 1947, *48*, 355–368.

120. Seymour H. Levitt et al., "Radical treatment of Hodgkin disease with radiation therapy: Results of a 15-year clinical trial [The 1985 Erskine Lecture]," *Radiology*, 1987, *162*, 623–630.

121. Leo G. Rigler, "Roentgenologic observations on the movement of pleural effusions," *Am. J. Roentg.*, 1931, *25*, 220–230.

122. Ibid., p. 229.

123. Leo G. Rigler and Lester G. Ericksen, "The inferior accessory lobe of the lung," *Am. J. Roentg.*, 1933, *29*, 384–392.

124. Leo G. Rigler, "A Roentgen study of the mode of development of encapsulated lobar infusions," *J. thorac. Surg.*, 1936, *5*, 295–305.

125. Leo G. Rigler, "The density of the central shadow in the diagnosis of intrathoracic lesions," *Radiology*, 1939, *32*, 316–324.

126. Leo G. Rigler, *Outline of Roentgen diagnosis*.

127. The chief source of biographical information about Sister Kenny is the work by Victor Cohn, *Sister Kenny: the woman who challenged the doctors*.

128. F. H. Krusen, "Observations on the Kenny treatment of poliomyelitis," *Proc. staff Meet. Mayo Clinic*, 1942, *17*, 449–460, p. 450.

129. Harold Diehl, "Summary of the relationship of the medical school of the University of Minnesota to the work of Sister Elizabeth Kenny" [report to President Coffey, 31 March 1944], Snyder papers.

130. Miland E. Knapp, "Commentary" in John F. Pohl and Elizabeth Kenny, *The Kenny concept of infantile paralysis and its treatment*, pp. 343–355, p. 343.

131. Diehl (n. 129).

132. Wallace H. Cole and Miland E. Knapp, "The Kenny treatment of infantile paralysis. A preliminary report," *J. Am. med. Ass.*, 1941, *116*, 2577–2580. In 1942 John Pohl published a complete account of the first twenty-six patients treated in America by Elizabeth Kenny and concluded: "At the end of eighteen months . . . it can be stated that these patients have all made a far more satisfactory recovery than they would have made by any previously known method. No deformities have occurred in spite of the complete omission of splinting." John F. Pohl, "The Kenny treatment of anterior poliomyelitis (infantile paralysis). Report of the first cases treated in America," *J. Am. med. Ass.*, 1942, *118*, 1428–1433.

133. Cohn, *Sister Kenny* (n. 127), p. 145.

134. Philip Lewin, "The Kenny treatment of infantile paralysis during the acute stage," *Illinois med. J.*, 1942, *81*, 281–296, p. 294.

135. Ibid., p. 293.

136. Ibid., p. 294.

137. Mary M. I. Daly et al., "The early treatment of poliomyelitis, with an evaluation of the Sister Kenny treatment," *J. Am. med. Ass.*, 1942, *118*, 1433–1443.

138. "Medical committees' statements on Kenny method," *Natn Fdn News*, 1941, *1* (no.2), pp. 1, 6. Cf. [Morris Fishbein, editorial] "The Kenny method of treatment in the acute peripheral manifestations of infantile paralysis," *J. Am. med. Ass.*, 1941, *117*, 2171–2172.

139. See Cohn, *Sister Kenny* (n. 127), pp. 253–258.

CHAPTER 15

Research in the Basic Sciences 1913 to 1941

Anatomy

In the Department of Anatomy under Clarence Jackson, every staff member was given an opportunity to do the kind of work he liked best. Those who wished to teach were assigned heavy teaching schedules while those who desired to do investigative work were given every facility for research. Jackson possessed an almost uncanny knowledge of each investigator's work, and he was able to make constructive suggestions without creating antagonism. Whenever Jackson believed research was ready for publication, he read the manuscript with meticulous care, making valuable corrections and criticisms. He even corrected punctuation, but always indicated his reasons for change.[1] Among the hundreds of scientific articles published from the Department of Anatomy, those by Andrew T. Rasmussen, Richard Scammon, Hal Downey, and Edward A. Boyden were especially noteworthy.

Andrew T. Rasmussen, a Cornell physiologist, came to the Department of Anatomy in 1916 to teach neuroanatomy.[2] In his research, Rasmussen was concerned primarily with the pituitary gland and its relation to the nervous system. When Rasmussen began his research on the hypophysis, or pituitary gland, both its structure and function were poorly understood. As part of a systematic effort to learn more about the pituitary, Rasmussen completed an extensive series of microscopic measurements of that gland in male and female humans, establishing for the first time the norms of pituitary structure.[3] In animal studies, Rasmussen showed that hibernation is probably a result of pituitary inactivity.[4] Rasmussen's contributions to neuroanatomy included more precise determinations of the course and connections of various fiber tracts.[5] His investigation of the central vestibular pathways, which appeared in 1932, was for decades afterwards regarded as the most accurate and comprehensive treatment of that difficult subject.[6] In collaboration with the neurosurgeon William T. Peyton, Rasmussen produced

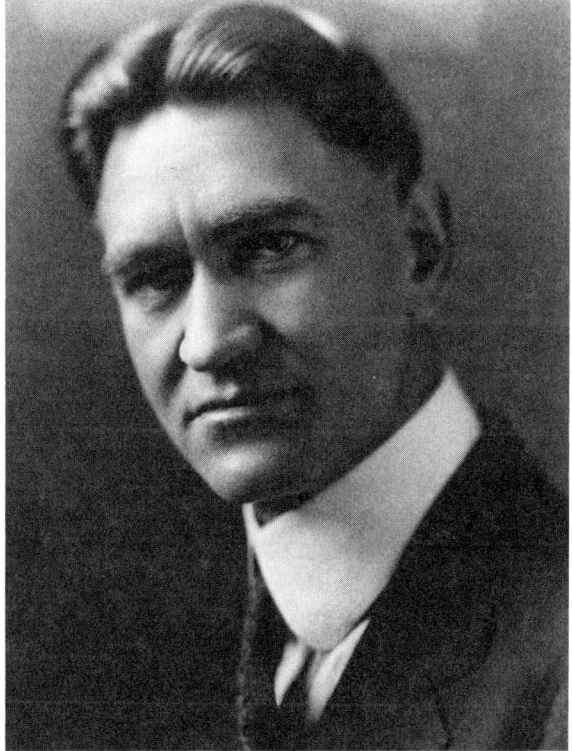

FIGURE 15:1   Andrew T. Rasmussen, 1921. Courtesy Mn U Archives.

studies on various human fiber tracts which proved extremely useful to neurosurgeons.[7]

Richard E. Scammon, a member of the anatomy department since 1911, studied human growth from the embryonic state through adulthood. His extensive application of biometrical and statistical methods to these studies made his data useful to investigators in a variety of disciplines.[8] Scammon's results were published in a larger series of articles and monographs, including two books.[9]

On the retirement of Thomas G. Lee from the Department of Anatomy in 1929, Hal Downey was transferred from the Department of Zoology to anatomy to fill Lee's position. Then at the age of fifty-one, Hal Downey, although not a physician, was an authority on hematology consulted by physicians throughout Minnesota for the diagnosis of blood diseases, particularly for the discrimination of mononucleosis from the various forms of leukemia. Son of the mathematician John Downey, who had served for many years as dean of the College of Science, Literature, and the Arts at the University of Minnesota, Hal Downey was educated at Minnesota where he was graduated in 1903 and took a master's degree in zoology in 1904. For his doctoral dissertation, Downey studied the process of blood formation in the Mississippi paddlefish, *Polyodon spathula*. From his observations on *Polyodon spathula,* Downey became convinced of the common origin of the various types of blood cells, and he made the study of blood cells his life work. After a year in Europe during 1910–11, he taught in the Department of Animal Biology at Minnesota. He continued his studies of blood cells and served as American editor of the journal *Folia Haematologica.* In 1921 Dr. C. A. McKinlay consulted Downey about a patient whom he thought to be suffering from acute leukemia, but which Downey recognized as a different and benign condition. After a study of nine such patients, Downey and McKinlay published in 1923 their classic description of infectious mononucleosis.[10] From the hematological features of mononucleosis, Downey was able to establish criteria by which it might be distinguished clearly from the leukemias. In 1938 Downey edited a monumental four-volume *Handbook of Hematology,* which was for many years the standard work on the subject.[11] In his later years Downey was regarded as the father of hematology in the United States.[12]

In 1931 Edward Allen Boyden came to Minnesota from the University of Alabama where he had spent two years reorganizing their department of anatomy. A native of Bridgewater, Massachusetts, Boyden was educated at Harvard University where he was graduated B.S. in 1908 and M.S. in zoology in 1911. On completion of his master's work, he went to Freiburg, Germany, in order to spend a year at the anatomical institute. Although he went to the institute to pursue zoology, he left with a keen interest in human anatomy. When he returned to Harvard in 1912 Boyden began graduate study in anatomy, and in 1916 received his Ph.D. degree. For the next ten years Boyden taught anatomy at Harvard. In 1922, as the result of a chance observation of an accessory pancreatic bladder alongside the gall bladder in a cat, Boyden began to compare biliary with pancreatic secretion. In dissecting a large number of cats, he found their gall bladders in all stages from fullness to complete emptiness. By experiment he then found that in cats the gall bladder could be emptied completely by a fatty meal of egg yolk and cream.[13]

In 1924 Evarts Graham and Warren Cole announced that when certain x-ray opaque substances, such as the calcium salt of tetrabromphenolphthalein, were injected intravenously, they were excreted in the bile and caused the outline of the gall bladder to emerge clearly in x-ray photographs.[14] Boyden then began to use the Graham and Cole method in combination with his egg yolks and cream meal to study the action of the gall bladder through the successive phases of digestion in man, and he found that the functional cycle of the gall bladder was essentially in man as it was in cats.[15] The gall bladder appeared to collapse passively as it emptied, the discharge of bile being controlled by the sphincter of Oddi and intra-abdominal pressure on the surface of the gall bladder. Nevertheless, Boyden thought that the gall bladder itself was not wholly inactive. In 1926 he showed that the gall bladder of a fasting cat could be activated by injection of blood from a cat which was digesting egg yolk, an observation that led within two years to the discovery by Ivy and Oldberg of the hormone cholecystokinin, secreted by the mucosa of the duodenum.[16]

After Boyden came to Minnesota in 1931, he continued his studies of the function of the gall bladder, doing the x-ray work needed for his research in the early hours of the morning because the equipment of the radiology department was needed during the day for the care of patients. The chief of radiology, Leo Rigler, collaborated with Boyden on several investigations of gall bladder function, using medical students as experimental subjects.[17] In 1935 Dr. Boyden showed that congenital anomalies of the gall bladder, such as the "Phrygian cap" described by German pathologists, had no connection with gall bladder disease.[18] He also reviewed the historical descriptions of the junction of the common bile duct with the duodenum.[19]

In the 1940s with the introduction of sulpha drugs and penicillin, improvements in anesthesiology, and the more extensive use of blood transfusions, thoracic surgery was practiced increasingly. In February 1945, Owen Wangensteen asked Dr. Boyden to speak to a surgery staff conference on the segmental anatomy of the lungs as a basis for segmental pneumonectomy. When Boyden came to prepare his talk, he was astonished to discover that the literature contained no adequate account of the anatomy of the lungs.

In 1889 in England, William Ewart had described the general topography of the lungs, tracing out the main branches of the bronchi and the pulmonary blood vessels for the purpose of more exact diagnosis and treatment of lung diseases, especially of tuberculous cavities in the lungs. Ewart realized that the lung must be divided into smaller regions than the lobes in order to achieve an adequately simple description. In 1932 at Mt. Sinai Hospital in New York, Rudolph Kramer and Ameil Glass introduced the term *bronchopulmonary segment* to describe anatomic units of the lung.[20] During the 1930s the surgical treatment of pulmonary tuberculosis had advanced to a point that surgeons wished not merely to collapse the tuberculous lung to promote healing, but to remove the tuberculous portion of the lung completely. Surgeons also needed to know the segmental anatomy of the lung in order to operate effectively for bronchiectasis, or lung abscess. Similarly, the growing frequency of lung cancer made it desirable for surgeons to be able to remove the cancerous portion of a lung without removing the whole. Ewart described nine primary branches of the bronchus.[21] In 1938 at Harvard, Edward Churchill and Ronald Belsey pointed out that the brochopulmonary segment, formed by a single branch of the bronchial tree, could serve also as a surgical unit important in operations for bronchiectasis.[22] Churchill and others had also written on the surgical anatomy of the hilum, including the distribution of the blood vessels. Nevertheless, it remained difficult for a surgeon to identify structures in the hilum unless he knew how they were distributed. In 1942 Russell Brock, thoracic surgeon at Guy's Hospital, London, began a series of studies on the anatomy of the bronchial tree in connection with the surgery of lung abscess.[23]

To provide a more adequate knowledge of the distribution of bronchi and blood vessels, Edward Boyden dissected lungs, while the medical school artist, Jean Hirsch, made detailed drawings of the various stages of dissection. In 1945

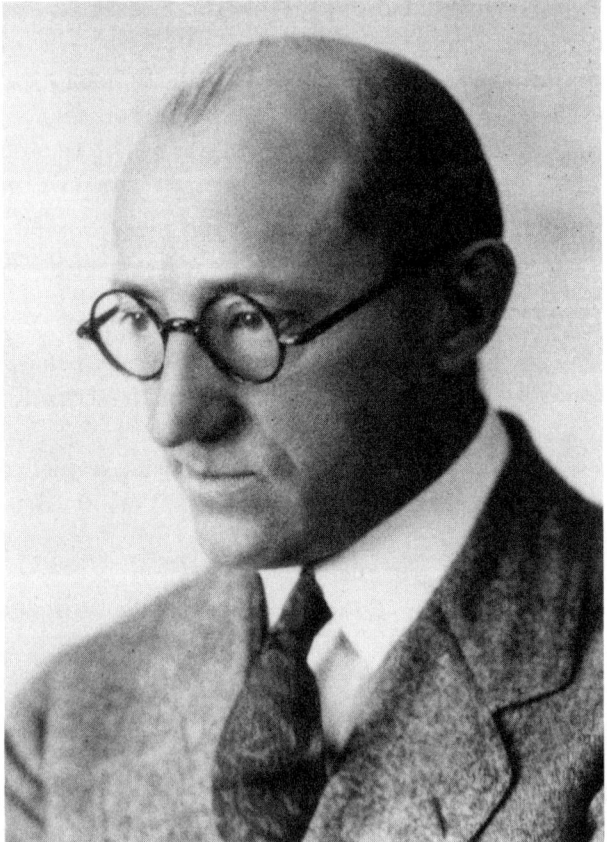

FIGURE 15:2 Edward Allen Boyden, circa 1945. Courtesy Mn U Archives.

Boyden published seven plates with supplementary figures showing the distribution of the segmental bronchi with their associated blood vessels in each of the lobes of the lung. He emphasized that although the bronchopulmonary segment was a convenient unit for surgical resection, it was not a morphologic unit. It might be crossed by arteries from adjacent segments and usually contained veins that drained neighboring segments.[24]

From 1945 to 1951, Boyden published a series of papers in which he analyzed the variations in arrangement of the structures of the lung so as to establish the prevailing patterns. In 1955 he published the cumulative results of his and his colleagues' nine years' study of the anatomy of the lungs in a masterly monograph.[25] It provided the first adequate maps of the distribution of the bronchioles, arteries, and veins within the various lobes of the lung, and thereby laid a solid foundation for precise lung surgery.

Physiology

Elias P. Lyon's administrative duties as dean left him little time to devote to teaching or research in physiology. He entrusted the operation of the department largely to Frederick Scott, who consequently was so burdened with teaching that he could accomplish little research, despite great ability demonstrated early in his career. Frederick Hughes Scott was born at Toronto, Canada, in 1876, and educated at the University of Toronto where he was graduated M.D. in 1904. While a graduate student in physiology at Toronto under Professor A. B. MacCallum, Scott studied the chemical nature of the Nissl substance in nerve cells, which he believed to be a nucleoprotein. In 1905 he announced that a substance identical with the Nissl substance occurred also in secretory cells, such as the exocrine cells of the pancreas and the gland cells of the fundus of the stomach, both of which secreted proteolytic enzymes. Scott decided that since the cells of the pancreas and the stomach secreted enzymes, the nerve cells might also secrete an active substance. "I formed the hypothesis," wrote Scott, "that nerve cells are true secreting cells, and act upon one another, and upon the cells of other organs by the passage of a chemical substance . . . from the first cell into the second . . . ."[26] He suggested that there was probably a difference between conduction of the nerve impulse and excitation of the next cell, based upon his clear understanding that while nerve cell endings might touch processes of other cells, the boundaries of the two cells remained distinct. The excitation of a neuron involved, Scott believed, the discharge at the synapse, and, because a discharge into other cells meant the using up of the substance discharged, the nerve cell would become exhausted, resulting in fatigue.[27]

About 1905 Scott went to Europe where he worked first in the physiological laboratories of the *Thierärztliche Hochschule* (veterinary school) at Berlin. In 1906 he moved to Ernest Starling's laboratory at University College London, where he worked with Starling and had the opportunity to attend meetings of the Physiological Society. Professor John Newport Langley of Cambridge University provided him with valuable help in the preparation of his second paper which dealt with the relation of nerve cells to fatigue.[28] Scott showed that when the dorsal roots of a frog's spinal nerve were stimulated, they became fatigued much sooner if the nerve fibres were separated from the bodies of their neurons in the dorsal root ganglion. Scott postulated that each neuron produced a substance which passed out along the axon of the nerve fiber to the nerve ending where it was secreted to stimulate, for instance, the contraction of a muscle. Scott attributed fatigue to the exhaustion of the supply of the stimulating substance at the nerve endings. The inability of frog nerves to recover after prolonged stimulation in his experiments was because all of the stimulating substance in the nerve fibers had been used up, and the fibers were unable to make more when separated from the bodies of their neurons.[29] In 1906 Frederick Scott thus foresaw the secretory function of neurons, which was demonstrated in 1921 by Otto Loewi.[30]

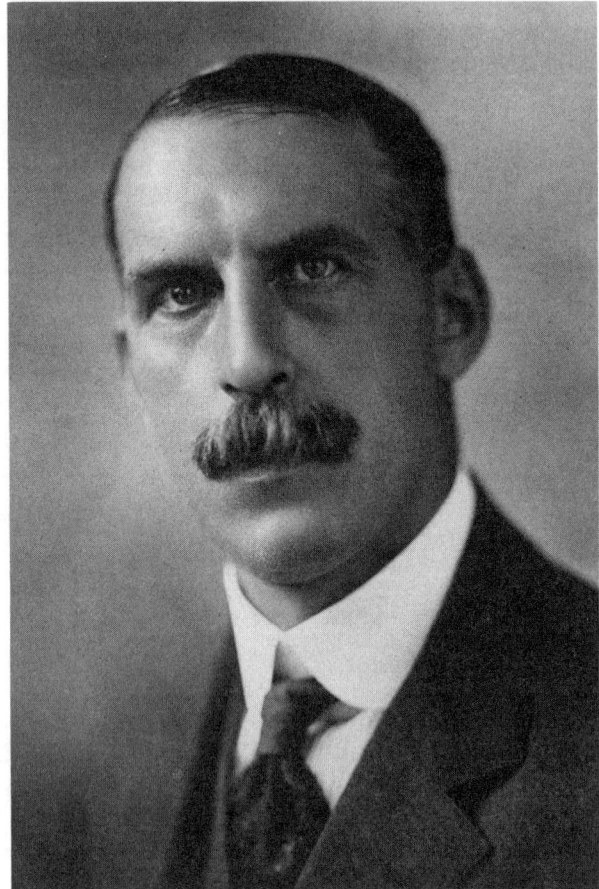

FIGURE 15:3   Frederick Hughes Scott, 1923. Courtesy Mn U Archives.

While at University College London, Scott also published pioneering investigations of the effects of hypercapnia and hypoxia on the respiratory drive.[31] In 1908, when Scott came to Minnesota as an assistant professor, he brought with him the spirit and the intellectual tools of modern physiological research. Unfortunately, at Minnesota his heavy teaching load in the medical school and severe lack of research funds limited the amount of research he could accomplish. At Minnesota, Frederick Scott published several papers on fluid balance in the blood, tissues, and organs, and on the effects of the contractibility of the spleen in hemorrhage, exercise, and asphyxia. He also supervised graduate student research on the chemistry of the blood, blood coagulation, and on chemical changes in the blood in various disease states.[32]

Both Scott and Lyon understood the importance of biochemistry to modern physiological research. Accordingly, Lyon incorporated in his department the staff of a subdepartment of physiological chemistry. Among his new appointees, Jesse

F. McClendon proved a brilliant choice. Born in 1880 at Lanette, Alabama, McClendon was educated at the University of Toronto, Canada, where he received an M.Sc. degree in 1904; in 1906 he received a Ph.D. degree in zoology at the University of Pennsylvania. McClendon came to Minnesota from Cornell in 1914 to teach physiological chemistry, appointed because of his demonstrated competence as a biochemist.[33]

Jesse McClendon directed research on the physiological changes effected by changes in the hydrogen ion concentration of extracellular fluids. He studied also the effect of alkali reserve and CO_2 tension on hydrogen ions. In the course of this work, McClendon and his colleagues developed more accurate and efficient methods for the determination of pH in body fluids and in sea water.

Between 1911 and 1926, some six vitamins were identified and vitamin deficiencies were proved to cause such serious diseases as beriberi, pellagra, rickets, and scurvy. Such diseases were, therefore, preventable, and the study of nutrition became a subject of urgent interest in medical research.[34] At Minnesota, Jesse McClendon and his colleagues became deeply immersed in nutritional studies. McClendon published numerous studies concerning the distribution of vitamins A, B, C, and D in foodstuffs and on the preservation of vitamin C in foods. He worked extensively on the pathology of the teeth and bones in deficiencies of vitamins C and D. McClendon studied also the relation of vitamin D deficiency to deficiencies of phosphorus and calcium, respectively, and demonstrated the distinct pathology resulting from each such deficiency.

At Minnesota between 1914 and 1939, McClendon published five books and more than 165 scientific papers.[35] McClendon's vitamin and nutrition research is summarized in his book *Advances in the science of nutrition*. Perhaps McClendon's most important contribution to nutrition research was embodied in his extensive studies of goiter, which included a survey of iodine in drinking water in the United States and part of Canada, presented in his book *Iodine and the incidence of goiter*. McClendon and his associates compared the iodine content of drinking water in various regions with the goiter records compiled by the Draft Board and the United States Public Health Service. They showed that regions with a high incidence of simple goiter were high also in the incidence of exophthalmic goiter, or Graves' disease, and that in such regions the drinking water tested low for concentrations of iodine, and thus the various forms of goiter resulted from a nutritional deficiency of iodine. McClendon's work led to the introduction of iodized salt, both for humans and domestic animals, an innovation that has virtually eliminated goiter from North America.

During the years before World War II, nutritional studies were but one of the important interests of physiological investigators. Since Claude Bernard's introduction in 1855 of the term *internal secretion,* numerous hormones had en isolated and described. The clinical importance of an accurate knowledge of hormones and their functions rapidly became apparent both in surgery and internal medicine. At Minnesota, both clinical and nonclinical departments became involved in endocrine research. In the Department of Physiology, McClendon led

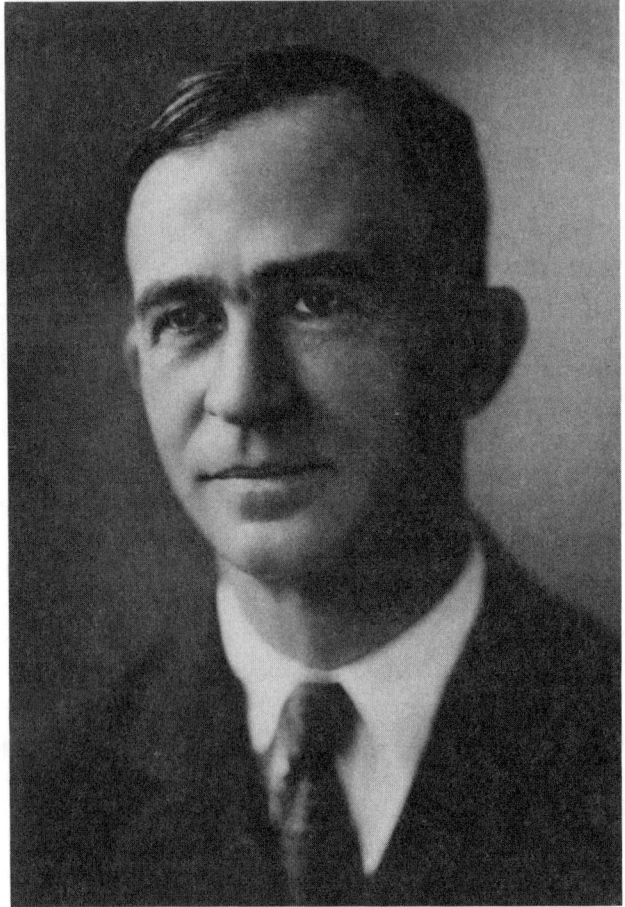

FIGURE 15:4 Jesse Francis McClendon, 1923. Courtesy Mn U Archives.

his colleagues in studies of the ovarian hormone. They worked to create methods and apparatus capable of yielding more precise data, spending six years developing the most perfect Wheatstone bridge for high-frequency electrical currents, and devising new equipment to measure basal metabolic rates and respiratory quotients.[36] In his hormone studies, McClendon demonstrated that the basal metabolic rate in women varies with both the menstrual cycle and with the blood level of ovarian hormone. Experimental injections of ovarian hormone were shown to raise low rates of basal metabolism.[37]

During the 1920s and 1930s several members of the physiology department also pursued research along other lines. From 1918 to 1936, Esther M. Gresheimer published several studies on respiratory irregularities including the effects of aluminum chloride, acidified Ringer's solution, and blood sugar on nerves.[38] She studied glycogen formation on various diets, to clear up questions relating to diabetes, and measured blood calcium levels in tuberculosis patients and in the aged.[39]

Bacteriology

In 1911 Winford P. Larson was appointed an instructor in the Department of Pathology, Bacteriology and Public Health. A native of Wisconsin, Dr. Larson was educated at Milton College at Milton, Wisconsin, and Union College at Lincoln, Nebraska, before entering the University of Illinois College of Medicine where he received the M.D. degree in 1904. After completing an internship, Larson spent three years in study in Europe, two years at the University of Berlin, one year at the Sorbonne in Paris, and a short period at Vienna.

When Larson arrived at Minnesota, he assumed primary responsibility for the teaching of bacteriology because Dr. Wesbrook, who had developed the courses in bacteriology, was occupied too heavily with his duties as department head and dean to spare much time for teaching. As a result of the reorganization of 1913 and the departure of Wesbrook, Harold E. Robertson was appointed professor of pathology and acting head of the department. At the same time a young man from Pennsylvania, Arthur T. Henrici, was appointed an instructor in the department. Dr. Henrici completed his medical degree in 1911 at the University of Pittsburgh, and then spent a year and a half as a pathologist for the St. Francis Hospital.

Soon after his arrival at Minnesota, Henrici began to collaborate with Dr. Thomas B. Hartzell, professor of oral surgery and clinical pathology in the dental college, in an investigation of the bacteria involved in pyorrhea and abscesses on the roots of teeth. Infections of the gums and teeth were then thought to possess a larger medical significance because of the theory of focal infection, and because statistical data gathered especially in England showed a connection between such infections and the occurrence of acute and chronic rheumatism. The patients whom Hartzell and Henrici studied usually suffered from either acute or chronic rheumatism: seventeen showed arthritic deformities, five were cases of acute rheumatic fever, and seven had endocarditis.

To distinguish the particular bacteria involved in infections from ordinary mouth bacteria, Hartzell developed a technique in which the tooth to be cultured was packed off and wiped dry with gauze. The surrounding area was painted with iodine, and if a local anesthetic were used, the gums around the neck of the tooth were seared with a cautery. After the tooth was pulled, the root tip, which usually had the abscess sac clinging to it, was nipped off with forceps and dropped into a tube of broth. In patients suffering from pyorrhea, as much pus as possible was squeezed out, the area was cleansed in the same manner, and cultures were made from material obtained by inserting a sterile curet into the pocket from which the pus came.

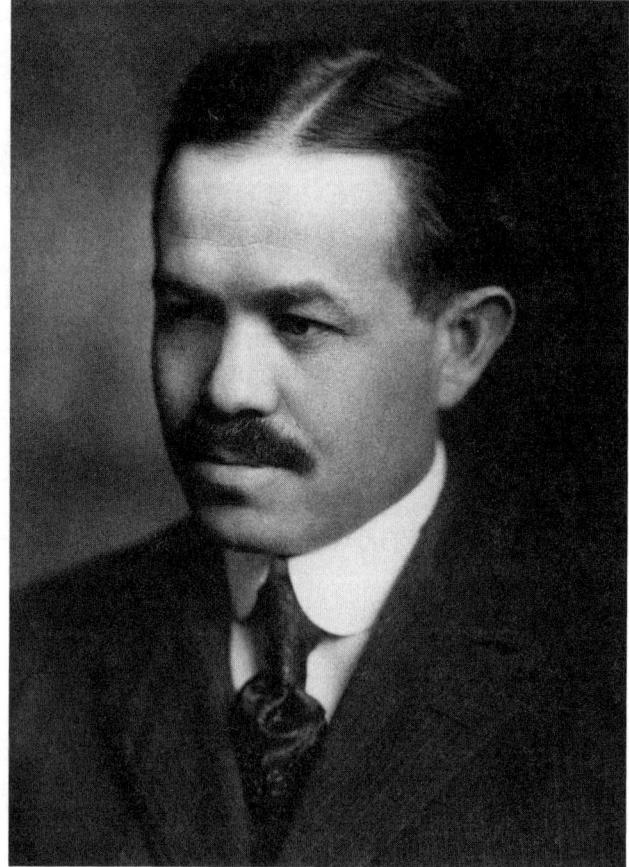

FIGURE 15:5   Winford P. Larson, 1914. Courtesy Mn U Archives.

In their bacteriological work, Hartzell and Henrici concentrated their attention on the streptococci because they found streptococci always present in tooth abscesses, and frequently the streptococcus was the only organism present. They thought, too, that since they were concerned primarily with the relationship of dental infections to rheumatism, the streptococci, which had already been suggested as the causal organism in rheumatic fever, would be most likely to yield results. Hartzell and Henrici took cultures from 162 patients and obtained streptococci from 150 of them. When healthy teeth were pulled they obtained sterile cultures. When Hartzell and Henrici grew the streptococci on plates of blood agar, there was no hemolysis, but the colonies, which appeared as small gray dots, were surrounded by a green halo. The organism, therefore, was Schotmüller's *Streptococcus viridans*. Almost every strain produced acid, and most also clotted milk.

To determine the pathogenic characteristics of the various strains of streptococci that they isolated, Hartzell and Henrici inoculated them into rabbits. After inoculation the rabbits continued to eat well, but grew progressively thinner and weaker. Some of the inoculated rabbits developed myocarditis and arthritis. The strains of streptococci isolated varied in their virulence, but three-quarters of the inoculated rabbits died and at autopsy were found to have heart lesions, kidney lesions, aortic lesions, or joint lesions. By contrast, among sixteen rabbits dead of rabies, there were no lesions comparable to those in rabbits inoculated with streptococci.

The heart lesions in rabbits inoculated with streptococci consisted of miliary nodules of small round cell infiltration in the heart muscle, which Hartzell and Henrici thought resembled the submiliary nodules described by Aschoff in the heart muscle of human patients dead from acute rheumatism. Nevertheless, while the Aschoff bodies were consistently present in cases of acute rheumatism and chorea, they were absent in bacterial endocarditis caused by *Streptococcus viridans*.

Hartzell and Henrici published their first work on mouth infections in 1915.[40] In 1916 they published a general discussion of the importance of the teeth as a portal for the entrance of infection to the body.[41] They noted that the tooth surface constantly possessed a rich bacterial flora, including streptococci, staphylococci, the pneumococcus, generally two spirochetes, macrodentium, and microdentium, and the fusiform bacillus. There were also two protozoa, Entamoeba buccalis and Trichomonas intestinalis. Furthermore, the flora and fauna of the mouth were always able to infect the soft tissue around the tooth. Although the surface of the gum was protected by a tough pavement epithelium, in the gingival crevice between tooth and gum there was almost no epithelial protection. When Henrici made sections through gum and tooth to illustrate the rich supply of blood vessels in the tissues surrounding a tooth, he discovered the absence of mucous membrane protection in the gingival crevice, an absence which meant that organisms growing on the surface of the tooth could easily enter the lymph spaces and renicles at the bottom of the gingival crevice and thence pass on into the deeper tissues in the lymph or circulating blood. The entrance of organisms would be aided by the formation of calculus or plaque along the margin of the tooth. The movement of the teeth in the gums during mastication might also exert a pumping action that would aid the invasion of microorganisms. The ease of infection through the gingival crevice suggested how the pulps of teeth could become infected even when the enamel remained perfectly sound.

During 1915 Hartzell and Henrici came to distinguish acute dental abscesses from chronic ones. In acute abscesses on teeth, the active organism was a staphylococcus whereas in chronic abscesses the most common organism was *Streptococcus viridans*. They recorded the cases of a number of patients who developed severe infections in the jaw or elsewhere in the body as a result of a primary infection of one or more teeth.

In 1917, in a study of the multitude of different organisms that occur in the mouth, Hartzell and Henrici concluded that the most important group in infectious diseases of the mouth were the streptococci. Streptococci were always abundant in the mouth and might live there without causing disease, but, when disease did occur, streptococci were usually involved. When Hartzell and Henrici took care to exclude surface organisms and made their cultures only from the deeper diseased tissues, they found, they said, "that the deeper you go into the tissues the more simple and uniform does the flora become, until ultimately streptococci alone remain."[42]

Hartzell and Henrici concluded that whatever other factors might be involved in tooth decay, the microorganisms active in the decay process were streptococci. Streptococci were also found uniformly in dental abscesses, although staphylococci might also be present in acute abscesses as a secondary infection. Similarly, when they made cultures from the deep tissues in pyorrhea, they usually obtained pure cultures of streptococci. Hartzell and Henrici believed that the streptococci must come from the mouth. Other investigators had suggested that dental abscesses might arise from the localization of streptococci in the circulating blood, but Hartzell and Henrici thought the hypothesis unlikely because most people with abscesses on their teeth gave no other evidence of streptococcal infection. They found, too, that cultures from the tissues surrounding the roots of healthy teeth two or even three teeth away from an abscess yielded growths of streptococci and they said that this could "only be explained as a spreading of the infection thru the regional lymphatics."[43] If the streptococci could invade through the lymphatics they could reach the roots of healthy teeth from the gingival crevice. They emphasized the inability of the nonhemolytic *Streptococcus viridans* to produce pus in the body and offered this fact as evidence that *Streptococcus viridans* was the cause of both pyorrhea and chronic alveolar abscess. Neither disease was primarily suppurative, but instead granulomatous in character.

In 1917 Henrici was promoted to assistant professor and the same year, with the entrance of the United States into the First World War, he joined the United States Army Medical Corps in which he served as a captain. He went to France with his unit, where he was posted to a hospital near Vichy and where he remained until after the armistice in November 1918.

When Henrici returned to the university in 1919, he resumed the work on tooth infections with Hartzell, this time on the organisms involved in infected pulps. They sought first to determine whether a vital pulp contained bacteria, and if so, how frequently and under what conditions. They cracked open freshly extracted vital teeth under sterile conditions, removed the pulp, and placed it in a liver peptone medium, which had proven useful in the study of the bacteria in war wounds because streptococci grew well on it.[44] They found that the pulps of healthy teeth were sterile, but that if pyorrhea or caries were present, about half the pulps were infected with microorganisms, usually streptococci, even though they appeared to be normal. They concluded that microorganisms were present long before actual necrosis of the tissues took place.[45] If microorganisms were present, they should produce inflammatory changes in the pulp tissue, and Henrici and Hartzell next made a histological study of the pulps of infected teeth to look for signs of inflammation. Although the pulps were of normal appearance, under the microscope they showed multitudes of minute granulomatous areas indicative

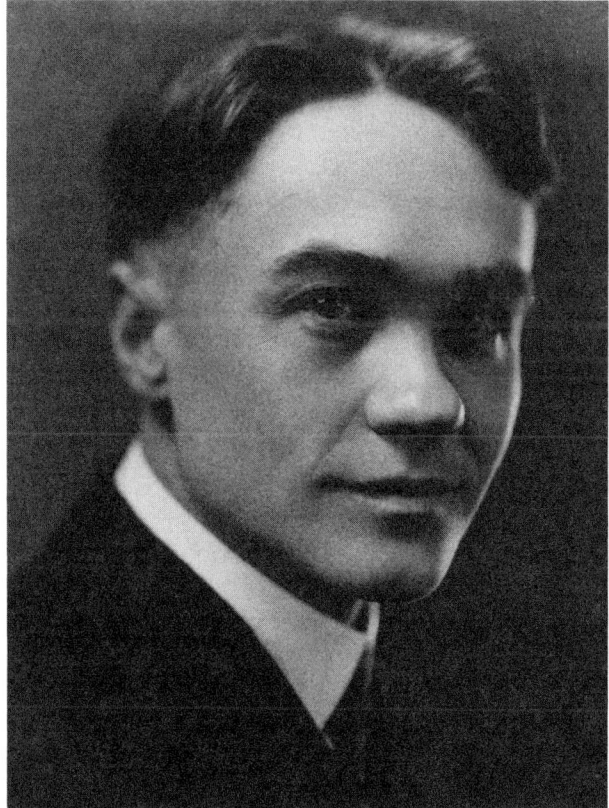

FIGURE 15:6 Arthur T. Henrici, 1922. Courtesy Mn U Archives.

of inflammation and also fibrotic changes, which were a normal sequel to inflammation.[46] Hartzell and Henrici thus confirmed that the pulp of a tooth might be invaded by microorganisms long before it was exposed by caries, and the pulp might be injured repeatedly before it underwent necrosis.[47]

In 1921 Henrici began a new line of investigation when he was called upon to identify the cause of a peculiar pneumonia. He found it to be caused by a fungus, a new species of *Actinomyces*.[48] With E. L. Gardner he made a study of the acid fast actinomycetes followed by a study with E. Nelson of their immunological characteristics.[49] Henrici's studies of actinomycetes culminated in 1930 in the publication of his classic book, *Molds, yeasts and actinomycetes*.

During the 1920s, Henrici's investigations took a new turn influenced by his reading of the book *On growth and form* published in 1917 by the Scottish zoologist D'Arcy Wentworth Thompson. Thompson analyzed the forms of animals and plants in terms of forces acting on them during their growth. Henrici studied the changes in the forms of various microorganisms as a colony or culture grew. His first such investigation was a statistical study of the "form and growth" of the colon bacillus.[50] During the active growth of a culture, the cells of the colon bacilli grew longer and relatively more slender, although their absolute diameters were greater. As the culture grew older and its rate of growth slowed down, the cells became shorter and smaller. Henrici compared the growing bacterial cells to the embryonic cells of a multicellular organism. D'Arcy Thompson had suggested that the forces of surface tension would act powerfully on bacterial cells and would tend to make them spherical. When bacterial cells become elongated instead of spherical, "there must be present," said Henrici, "some axially disposed force, some polar distribution of substances . . . to give them this oval or cylindrical or filamentous form."[51] When Henrici added a small quantity of a soap to the medium of a rapidly growing bacterial culture to lower the surface tension, the bacterial cells became even longer and more slender, assuming a filamentous form.

In another study of cultures of *Bacillus megatherium,* a microorganism selected for the relatively large size of its cells, Henrici showed an inverse mathematical relationship between the number of cells in a culture and the average length of the cells. He found, too, that the growth curve of a culture was influenced by the size of the seeding with which the culture was started. If cells from a rapidly growing culture were transplanted, they continued to grow at a maximum growth rate in the new medium. If they were transplanted from a mature culture in which growth had stopped, there was a lag period in the new medium before they again began to grow.

Henrici studied also the growth patterns and morphologic changes of a diphtheria-like bacillus and of the cholera vibrio. The characteristic form of the cholera vibrio was thought to be elongated and curved, resembling a comma, but Henrici showed that only mature cholera vibrios that had stopped growing adhered to the curved comma-like shape. Rapidly growing cholera vibrios were large, plump, and straight. When cholera cultures were old and dying, the forms of the cells became very variable, some retaining the slender curved form, others becoming spherical.

Since the pioneering bacteriological work of Ferdinand Cohn and Robert Koch fifty years earlier, species of bacteria had been recognized by their shape. If their cell were spherical, they were a coccus; if rod-shaped, a bacillus; and if rod-shaped with a spiral twist, a spirillum. By showing that bacterial cells were changing in form at all stages of their growth, Henrici shook the foundations of bacterial classification. In 1928, Henrici gathered his various studies of the morphological changes in bacteria during growth into a book, *Morphologic variation and the rate of growth of bacteria* . This small monograph of fewer than 200 pages established his international reputation as a bacteriologist.

In the late 1920s Henrici began to collaborate with Robert G. Green in a study of tularemia among wild animals in Minnesota. Tularemia had been discovered only in 1921 by Edward Francis as epizootic among jack rabbits in Utah. The disease was transmitted by deer flies from jack rabbits to man to cause what was known in Utah as *deer fly fever.*[52] In 1926 tularemia was discovered also among wild rats, and in 1928 among meadow mice in California.[53] At Minnesota in

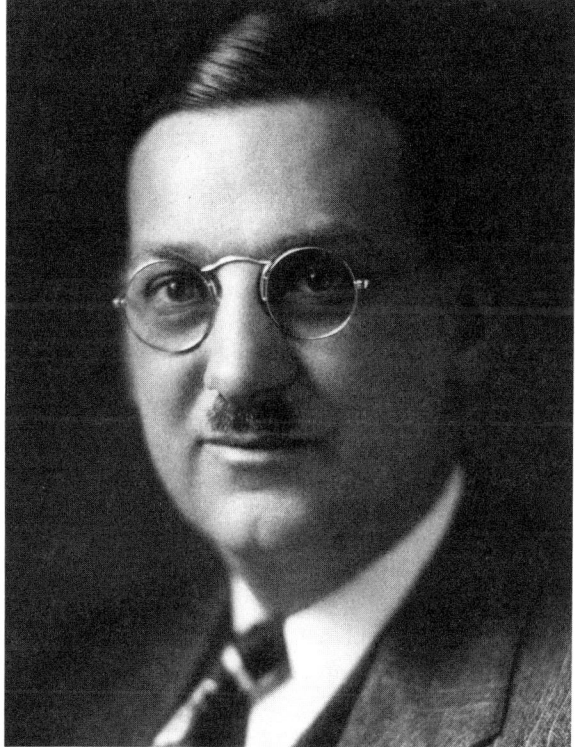

FIGURE 15:7   Robert G. Green, 1931. Courtesy Mn U Archives.

1928, Green and E. M. Wade showed that ruffed grouse could be infected experimentally with tularemia and in 1929 they found tularemia occurring naturally in quail.[54] The discovery of tularemia among game birds increased the possibilities for human infection as did also the discovery in 1924 that wood ticks could become infected with tularemia and could transmit the disease. Green, therefore, began a systematic study of the possibilities for the transmission of tularemia. On an island in Lake Alexander in north central Minnesota, he introduced tularemia-infected ticks into pens of grouse, pheasants, snowshoe hares, jack rabbits, cottontails and other species of wild animals to determine whether they would become infected.

Green invited Henrici to collaborate in the tularemia work and Henrici began to go to Lake Alexander during the summers, but instead of working on tularemia he became interested in the bacteria living in the water of the lake. Henrici was aware that the ordinary methods of growing pure cultures of bacteria on artificial media gave only a very incomplete representation of the varied populations of microorganisms that formed the microbic flora in natural environments. Most work on water bacteria had been carried out for purposes of sanitation and gave very little information about the bacteria living naturally in fresh water. In his laboratory at the university, Henrici had an aquarium which developed a growth of algae on its glass walls. Thinking that if he put some microscope slides in the aquarium, the algae would also grow on them and permit him to study the algae in situ, he placed some slides in the aquarium. When after a week he removed them and stained them, Henrici was astonished to find on the slide in addition to the algae a thin uniform coating of bacteria of various forms. He knew that the bacteria were growing on the glass because he could see microcolonies of steadily increasing size. Since the waters of an unpolluted lake or stream were ordinarily clear, Henrici decided that water bacteria were not ordinarily free floating organisms, but grew on submerged surfaces. Henrici repeated the aquarium experiment in a natural environment and was astonished by the great variety of morphologic types present in lake water. The bacteria were almost all Gram-negative. Some occurred in filaments or chains, others either singly or in irregular clusters of cells. There were minute spherical forms, larger round or oval cells, and rods of varying length and thickness. There were comma-shaped and spirillum forms of various sizes.[55] In 1935 with Delia Johnson, Henrici described a number of the forms, all new species, which he placed in a new order, the stalked bacteria.[56]

In 1936 in his third paper on fresh water bacteria, Henrici said: "A study of these slides presents a problem somewhat similar to the ideal ecological problem, the population of an island suddenly upthrust in the ocean. The immersion of the slide at once creates a new habitat, a surface upon which sessile organisms may grow; and it is not long before this habitat is found by such organisms."[57] In Henrici's thought there is an echo of Charles Darwin's *Voyage of the Beagle,* as if in those slides in Lake Alexander, Arthur Henrici saw a counterpart to the naked volcanic surface of the Galapagos Islands when they first emerged from the ocean. The particular organisms that colonized the slides would reflect the populations of the surrounding water. He observed bacteria as a naturalist, and often he described them in the language of a poet. But despite his naturalist's bent, or perhaps because of it, Henrici was also a physician. In 1939 he devoted his presidential address to the Society of American Biologists to the characteristics of fungal diseases, a group of diseases that have become of increasing importance.

Henrici distinguished the superficial fungal diseases of the skin such as Athlete's foot and ringworm from the deep-seated diseases such as actinomycosis or blastomycosis, which were progressive until they ended in death. He suggested that the organisms causing deep-seated fungal diseases were actually saprophytes that became established in such tissues as the lungs. The fungus was at first unable to multiply and spread through the tissues, but after a time a change occurred which permitted it to grow. "If one assumes," said Henrici, "that the fungus can multiply only in dead tissues or products of these, that it has very little toxicity itself, but that its continued presence in the host eventually gives rise to hypersensitivity to the products of the fungus, then one can explain the characteristic course of such infections."[58] His theory suggested why most fungal diseases were occupational diseases in which the disease developed because the patient was exposed to the fungus repeatedly over an extended period of time.

Pathology

Basic research in the Department of Pathology was established on a very high level at Minnesota by one of the medical school's most gifted faculty members, Elexious Thompson Bell. During the twenty-nine years Dr. Bell directed the department, he carried on an extraordinary research program, provided first-rate clinical and laboratory teaching for medical students, residents, and staff members, and maintained an extremely successful working relationship between the clinical and the basic science sections of the medical school.

E. T. Bell came to Minnesota in 1910 as an associate professor of anatomy, but in 1911 transferred to the Department of Pathology, Bacteriology and Public Health. Born in 1880 on a farm in Rolls County, Missouri to a rural physician-farmer and his wife, Bell completed both his undergraduate and medical school training at the University of Missouri. While a second-year medical student, he became a teaching assistant in anatomy under Clarence M. Jackson. Later during the term, Jackson went to Germany to study and left young Bell in charge of teaching both histology and gross anatomy and managing the research-in-progress. At the same time, Bell struggled to keep up with his own medical studies. Bell survived the experience, which he described as the most rigorous year of his life, emerging as a mature student of the discipline. He remained on the faculty of the anatomy department at Missouri for eight years, from 1902 to 1910, taking only a sabbatical year in 1905 to study embryology at the University of Bonn in Germany. In 1906, Bell was compelled to refuse an attractive offer to become a professor of anatomy at Johns Hopkins because the University of Missouri would not release him from a commitment to serve at least one year following a sabbatical leave.[59]

At Minnesota, Bell undertook immediately both a heavy teaching load and a demanding research program. In 1921, when he replaced Harold Robertson as department head, Bell had already published seventeen scientific papers based upon research done at Minnesota. In this early work, Bell collaborated extensively with investigators in the Department of Bacteriology and published jointly with others, including Winford Larson, Arthur Henrici, and Thomas Hartzell. With Larson, Bell explored the pathogenic properties of *Bacillus proteus,* an organism frequently implicated in kidney infections.[60] In cooperation with Arthur Henrici, Bell's interest in the pathology of the kidney deepened during their study of renal tumors in rabbits.[61] Later, E. T. Bell and Thomas Hartzell explored kidney disease from several perspectives. Their investigations on the effects of foreign protein on the kidney demonstrated the ability of proteins associated with invading bacteria to inflict damage to the ultrastructure of the kidney, particularly to the glomerulus.[62] Bell's research with Hartzell was concerned with nephritis and glomerulonephritis and with hypertension, especially in relation to disease of the heart and kidney.[63]

In a study of thirty-two cases of acute glomerulonephritis, Bell and Hartzell recognized degenerative, exudative, and proliferative types of inflammation in

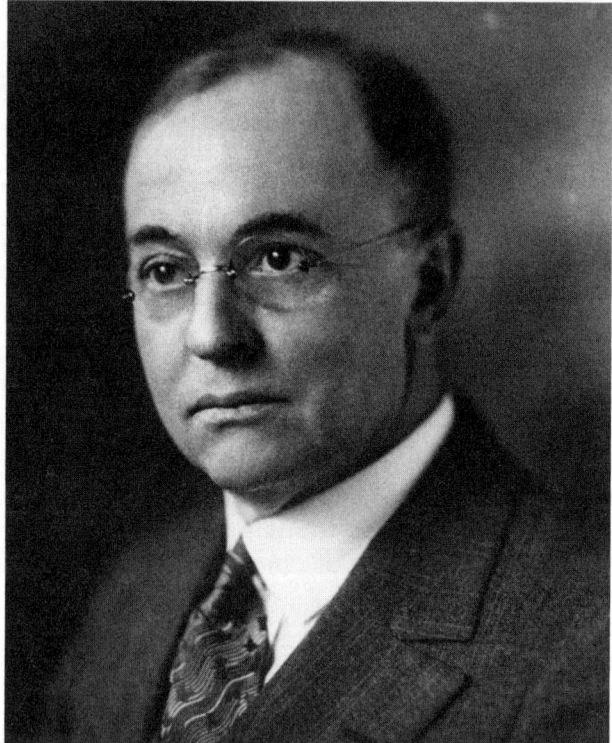

FIGURE 15:8   Elexious Thompson Bell, 1929. Courtesy Mn U Archives.

the glomeruli. Permanent glomerular damage occurred most frequently as a consequence of proliferative inflammation. Bell and Hartzell found that in acute glomerulonephritis, an infectious process, usually a streptococcal infection, was the immediate cause. Injury to the glomerular epithelium appeared to result from direct contact with circulating bacteria. Bell and Hartzell concluded that the clinical and pathological varieties of glomerulonephritis reflected the extent of permanent injury inflicted upon the glomerulus by the infection.[64]

As head of the Department of Pathology, Bell worked to strengthen its ranks, both by appointment and by encouraging promising medical and science students to prepare for careers in pathology. Among Bell's appointments, James S. McCartney, who came in 1920, and Benjamin J. Clawson, appointed the following year, became outstanding investigators and educators. McCartney, who had received training at Washington University, Jefferson Medical College, and the Johns Hopkins medical school, and as a surgical fellow at the Mayo Clinic, concentrated his research on cirrhoses of the liver. His studies of the cases of cirrhoses treated at Minnesota over several decades served to clarify the nature of that disease.[65] Pulmonary embolism, particularly post-traumatic pulmonary emboli, also interested McCartney.[66] He was, furthermore, a skilled forensic pathologist.[67]

A medical graduate of Rush Medical College with a Ph.D. degree from the University of Chicago, Benjamin J. Clawson joined forces with E. T. Bell and Thomas Hartzell in their studies of valvular heart disease.[68] Together they examined the effects of acute rheumatic fever and of subacute bacterial endocarditis upon the cardiac valves.[69] In his continued investigations of rheumatic fever and rheumatic heart disease, Clawson observed that various structural changes occur in the valves during the progress of rheumatic heart disease and demonstrated that rheumatic fever was caused by streptococcal infection. Clawson also showed that hypersensitivity to streptococci was an important factor in recurrences of rheumatic heart disease.[70] By 1930 Clawson had laid an experimental foundation for the possible development of vaccine therapy in acute rheumatic fever.[71] He anticipated that vaccines might be especially valuable in preventing recurrences of rheumatic fever. Despite encouraging laboratory results, Clawson's vaccine against rheumatic fever was never tested on human subjects. Following this disappointment, Clawson expanded his research to include studies of the immune response to BCG vaccine in tuberculosis and to other aspects of allergic and immune reactions.

Through the 1930s and 1940s, E.T. Bell intensified his research on renal pathology. His detailed correlations of the clinical and histopathological features of glomerulonephritis and nephroses and of diabetic and hypertensive renal pathology received international recognition. In 1946, he summarized the work of decades in a lengthy monograph on kidney diseases.[72] In 1960, he published a monograph containing the results of his numerous studies on diabetes mellitus, which dealt with the vascular and renal complications of that disease and with the histopathology of the diabetic pancreas.[73]

Students and colleagues alike regarded E. T. Bell as an extraordinarily gifted teacher. His method was Socratic, his standards uncompromising, his manner firm but unfailingly kind. In the 1920s, Bell began his highly successful weekly clinical-pathological conferences. At these Wednesday noon meetings, the more interesting surgical specimens collected during the week were discussed. On Thursday mornings Bell and McCartney held a second series of clinical-pathological conferences at the Minneapolis General Hospital for the benefit of the students and residents there.

The contributions of Minnesota's pathology department were presented to countless students through the eight editions of Bell's *Textbook of pathology*, for which McCartney and Clawson served as coauthors.

Pharmacology

In 1907 the medical school invited Edgar D. Brown of Western Reserve University to head a new Division of Pharmacology within the Department of Physiology. Although Brown was encouraged to begin a research program at Minnesota, he was given little time or space, and even less money for such research.

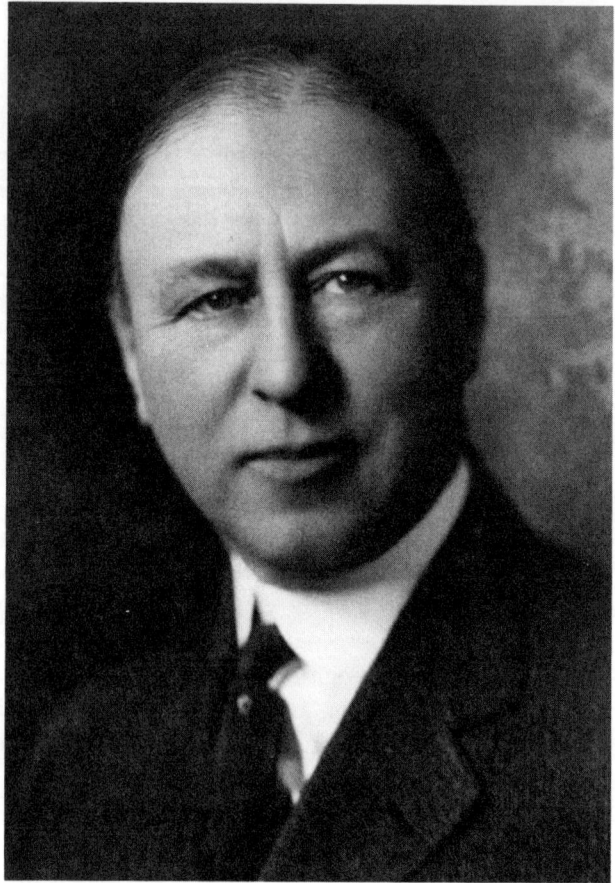

FIGURE 15:9   Arthur Hirschfelder, 1923. Courtesy Mn U Archives.

Even so, drawing upon his own considerable skills as a glassblower, wood, and metal craftsman, Brown managed to assemble a respectable, if rudimentary, laboratory for pharmacological research. In 1913, the administrative board formed a Department of Pharmacology separate from physiology, and appointed Arthur D. Hirschfelder to head it.[74] At John Hopkins Hirschfelder had accomplished classical work on problems related to the circulation and wrote the first comprehensive monograph on cardiology published in America.[75]

Arthur Hirschfelder was born in San Francisco in 1879, son of Dr. Joseph O. Hirschfelder. The elder Hirschfelder, who had studied in Germany under Carl Ludwig and Franz Hoffman, was a professor of medicine at Cooper Medical College (later Stanford Medical School), where he was known as a distinguished clinical teacher and investigator. In 1897, at the age of eighteen, Arthur Hirschfelder became the University of California's youngest recipient of the bachelor of science degree, and then he went to Europe to study chemistry and biological sciences at

Heidelberg before returning to the United States to study medicine at Johns Hopkins. Early in his career, Hirschfelder was attracted to medical investigation. In 1905, Lewellys Barker placed him in charge of the physiological laboratory of the medical clinic at the Hopkins, one of three clinical research laboratories that Barker had established. Under Hirschfelder, the physiological laboratory produced important new information about cardiovascular diseases based upon measurements of function.

At Minnesota, Hirschfelder worked to apply chemistry to pharmacology and to chemotherapy. He had planned to continue to practice medicine at Minnesota, but he could not obtain a medical license in Minnesota because he had not had the required course in physical diagnosis. Therefore, he was obliged to devote his full time to pharmacology.[76] Hirschfelder and his associates studied the mode of action, penetration, and effectiveness of various antiseptics. Hirschfelder admired Paul Ehrlich, the German biochemist who had discovered in Salvarsan an effective chemotherapeutic treatment for syphilis. Like Ehrlich, Hirschfelder believed that specific chemotherapeutic agents might be either discovered or synthesized to treat diseases caused by specific microorganisms. Following Ehrlich's example, Hirschfelder and his colleagues tested a large number of drugs in search of antibiotic agents. In the course of this work, Hirschfelder and his associate, M.C. Hart, synthesized a drug which they called Saligenin. Although Saligenin lacked antibacterial properties, it proved extremely useful as a local anesthetic, rapidly becoming the anesthetic of choice for use in cystoscopic procedures. Subsequently, a chemical derivative of Saligenin was compounded with mercury and used in the treatment of clinical gonorrhoea.

Cardiac Physiology

In 1936 Maurice B. Visscher returned to Minnesota to succeed Dean Lyon as head of the Department of Physiology. A native of Holland, Michigan, where he was educated at Hope College, Maurice Visscher first came to Minnesota in 1922 to pursue graduate study in physiology under Frederick Scott. After receiving the Ph.D. degree in 1925, Visscher went to England, probably at Scott's urging, to spend a year at University College London in postdoctoral work with the physiologist Ernest Starling, then very near the end of his career. In 1927 Starling and Visscher published a classic paper in which, using the heart-lung preparation introduced by Starling in 1910, they showed that the oxygen consumption of the heart was related directly to its volume in diastole, without regard to the amount of work it was doing in pumping blood. Thus if the heart were enlarged so that its diastolic volume was increased, it would consume more oxygen without accomplishing more work, so that its efficiency would be reduced.[77]

During 1926–27, Maurice Visscher pursued research in physiology with A. J. Carlson at the University of Chicago. He taught physiology at the University of

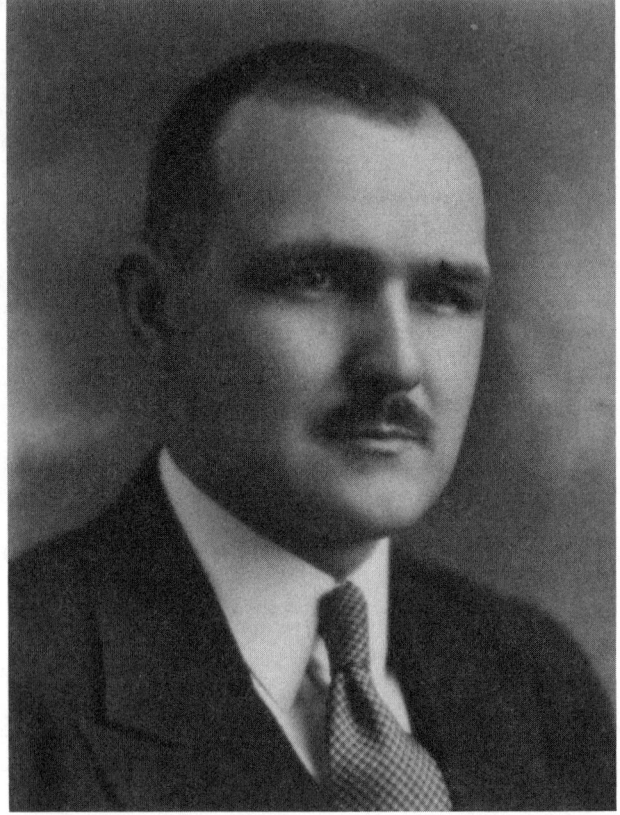

FIGURE 15:10   Maurice B. Visscher, 1936. Courtesy Mn U Archives.

Tennessee for two years and then at the University of Southern California. During the summers Visscher took undergraduate work in the medical school at Minnesota, and in 1931 completed the requirements for the M.D. degree. The same year he went to the University of Illinois as professor and head of the department of physiology.

At the University of Illinois, Visscher continued his research on the heart, particularly on conditions of heart failure. In 1936, with Howard Peters, Visscher showed that in failure the heart was no longer working efficiently; that is, it was continuing to consume oxygen and release energy, but it was able to convert less of that energy to useful work in pumping blood. Cardiac glucosides, of the digitalis group, had the effect of increasing the efficiency of the heart, as did also calcium. By contrast, other drugs, including certain reputed heart tonics, reduced the efficiency of the heart.[78]

At Minnesota, Visscher continued to study the physiological changes that occurred in heart failure. An understanding of the mechanism of heart failure was, he insisted, essential to the rational treatment of patients suffering from heart failure.[79] In 1939, with Gordon K. Moe, Visscher confirmed that the fundamental change that occurred in the failure of the mammalian heart was a loss of efficiency.[80] He also traced the cause of heart failure to a reduction in the flow of blood through the coronary arteries, a reduction that reduced the supply of oxygen to the heart muscle. Injection of very small amounts of the pituitary hormone *pitressin* into a heart-lung preparation reduced the coronary blood flow as much as 80 percent. The ventricles of the heart, deprived thereby of much of their oxygen supply, became enlarged in diastole because of the weakness of the heart muscle. Only by such enlargement could the heart continue to perform its work, but the enlarged heart worked less efficiently. Visscher and his colleagues thus demonstrated that heart failure occurred as a consequence of reduced coronary circulation, whether the blood flow in the coronary arteries drops suddenly or gradually.[81] His work threw valuable light on the mechanism of heart disease resulting from sclerosis or blockage of the coronary arteries. Aware of the many aspects of cardiac physiology that might be of importance to surgery, Visscher also collaborated with Owen Wangensteen in conducting a regular physiology-surgery conference that proved invaluable in acquainting surgical residents with the techniques of experimental physiology.

NOTES

1. J.A. Myers, "Clarence Martin Jackson — a great physician (a personal appreciation)," *J.-Lancet*, 1942, *62*, 142–145, p. 143. During the Jackson years, the anatomy department produced physical evidence of its enormous productivity by bringing out a sixteen volume set of papers published by members of the faculty from 1909 to 1939. University of Minnesota, Department of Anatomy, *Contributions* [reprinted from various periodicals].

2. J. A. Myers, "Andrew T. Rasmussen," *J.-Lancet*, 1953, *73*, 417–422. Born in Spring City, Utah, in 1883, Rasmussen earned his B.A. degree at Brigham Young University and then taught biology there for four years while pursuing summer studies in bacteriology, physiology, neuroanatomy, and psychology at the University of Chicago.

3. Andrew T. Rasmussen, "A method for the volumetric study of the human hypophysis cerebri with illustrative results," *Proc. Soc. exp. Biol. Med.*, 1922, *19*, 416–423; idem, "The proportions of the various subdivisions of the normal human adult hypophysis cerebri and the relative number of the different types of cells in *pars distalis*, with biometric evaluation of age and sex differences and special consideration of basophilic invasion into the infundibular process," *Proc. Ass. Res. nerv. ment. Dis.*, 1938, *17*, 118–150.

4. Andrew T. Rasmussen, "The hypophysis cerebri of the woodchuck (Marmota monax) with special reference to hibernation in inanition," *Endocrinology*, 1921, *5*, 33–66.

5. Andrew T. Rasmussen, "Experimental demonstration of the entire course of four descending tracts (fasciculus Rubrospinalis, Radix Mesencephalica Trigemini, fasciculus Longitudinalis Medialis, fasciculus Tectospinalis) by a single alcoholic injection in the mid-brain of the cat," *Proc. Soc. exp. Biol. Med.*, 1922, *20*, 104–107.

6. A. T. Rasmussen, "Secondary vestibular tracts in the cat," *J. comp. Neurol.*, 1932, *54*, 143–177.

7. A. T. Rasmussen and W. T. Peyton, "Origin of the ventral external arcuate fibers and their continuity with the striae medullares of the fourth ventricle of man," *J. comp. Neurol.*, 1946, *84*, 325–338; idem, "The course and termination of the medial lemniscus

in man," *J. comp. Neurol.*, 1948, *88*, 411–424; Andrew T. Rasmussen, *Atlas of cross section anatomy of the brain. Guide to the study of the morphology and fiber tracts of the human brain*.

8. Edith Boyd, "Richard E. Scammon. An obituary and a biographical sketch," *Anat. Rec.*, 1953, *116*, 257–262.

9. Richard E. Scammon and L. A. Calkins, *The development and growth of external dimensions of the human body in the fetal period;* J. A. Harris et al., *The measurement of man*.

10. Hal Downey and C. A. McKinlay, "Acute lymphadenosis compared with acute lymphatic leukemia," *Archs intern. Med.*, 1923, *32*, 82–112.

11. Hal Downey, ed., *Handbook of haematology*.

12. Lemen J. Wells and C. A. McKinlay, "Hal Downey, Ph.D. 1877–1959," *J.-Lancet*, 1960, *80*, 445–448. The most complete and authoritative study of Downey's work is Jane M. Tang, "Hal Downey and the development of hematology in America."

13. Edward A. Boyden, "The gall-bladder in the cat, — its development, its functional periodicity, and its anatomical variation as recorded in twenty-five hundred specimens," *Anat. Rec.*, 1923, *24*, 388–389.

14. Evarts A. Graham and Warren H. Cole, "Roentgenologic examination of the gallbladder: Preliminary report of a new method utilizing the intravenous injection of tetrabromphenolphthalein," *J. Am. med. Ass.*, 1924, *82*, 613–614.

15. Edward A. Boyden, "The effect of natural foods on the distention of the gall bladder, with a note on the change in pattern of the mucosa as it passes from distention to collapse," *Anat. Rec.*, 1925, *30*, 333–364.

16. Edward A. Boyden, "A study of the behaviour of the human gall bladder in response to the ingestion of food; together with some observations on the mechanism of the expulsion of bile in experimental animals," *Anat. Rec.*, 1926, *33*, 201–256; A. C. Ivy and Eric Oldberg, "A hormone mechanism for gall-bladder contraction and evacuation," *Am. J. Physiol.*, 1928, *86*, 599–613.

17. Edward A. Boyden and Leo G. Rigler, "A cholecystographic and fluoroscopic study of the reaction of the human gall bladder to faradic stimulation of the stomach and duodenum," *Anat. Rec.*, 1934, *59*, 427–447.

18. Edward A. Boyden, "The 'Phrygian cap' in cholecystography: a congenital anomaly of the gallbladder," *Am. J. Physiol.*, 1928, *86*, 599–613.

19. Edward A. Boyden, "The pars intestinalis of the common bile duct, as viewed by the older anatomists (Vesalius, Glisson, Bianchi, Vater, Haller, Santorini, etc.)," *Anat. Rec.*, 1936, *66*, 217–232; idem, "The sphincter of Oddi in man and certain representative mammals," *Surgery*, 1937, *1*, 25–36.

20. Rudolph Kramer and Amiel Glass, "Bronchoscopic localization of lung abscess," *Ann. Otol. Rhin. Lar.*, 1932, *41*, 1210–1220.

21. William Ewart, *The bronchi and pulmonary blood vessels—their anatomy and nomenclature* .

22. Edward D. Churchill and Ronald Belsey, "Segmental pneumonectomy in bronchiectasis," *Ann. Surg.*, 1939, *109*, 2, 481–499.

23. R. C. Brock, "Observations on the anatomy of the bronchial tree, with special reference to the surgery of lung abscess," *Guy's Hosp. Rep.*, 1942, *91*, *111*–130; 1943, *92*, 26–37, 82–88, 123–144; 1944, *93*, 90–107.

24. Edward A. Boyden, "The intrahilar and related segmental anatomy of the lung," *Surgery*, 1945, *18*, 706–731.

25. Edward A. Boyden, *Segmental anatomy of the lung*.

26. F. H. Scott, "On the metabolism and action of nerve cells," *Brain*, 1905, *28*, 506–526, p. 521.

27. Ibid., p. 522.

28. F. H. Scott, "On the relation of nerve cells to fatigue of their nerve fibres," *J. Physiol., Lond.*, 1906, *34*, 145–162.

29. Ibid., p. 162.

30. Dr. H. Blaschko of Oxford University has drawn attention to the historical importance of Scott's early work. See H. Blaschko, "Frederick Hughes Scott and his contribution to the early history of the transmitter concept," *Notes Rec. R. Soc. Lond.*, 1982, *37*, 235–247.

31. J. A. Myers, *Masters of medicine: an historical sketch of the College of Medical Sciences, University of Minnesota*, pp. 321–383.

32. "Ten years activity in the fields of scientific research at the University of Minnesota: summary of research in the Medical School," University of Minnesota, *President's report for . . . 1928–30*, 513–522, p. 520.

33. *American men of science: Physical and biological sciences*, 10th ed., s.v. "McClendon, Jesse F."

34. "Ten years activity" (n. 32), pp. 521–522.

35. Jesse F. McClendon, *Physical chemistry of vital phenomena;* Jesse F. McClendon and Grace Medes, *Physical chemistry in biology and medicine;* Jesse F. McClendon, *A manual of biochemistry;* idem, *Advances in the science of nutrition* ; idem, *Iodine and the incidence of goiter*.

36. Jesse McClendon and C. V. Van Slyke, "An indirect calorimeter for the determination of O_2 and CO_2," *Proc. Soc. exp. Biol. Med.*, 1927, *24*, 925; Jesse McClendon et al., "A simple respiration apparatus for determination of O_2 and CO_2 in indirect calorimetry," *J. biol. Chem.*, 1928, *77*, 413–420; Jesse McClendon, "Polarization capacity as measured with a Wheatstone bridge with sine-wave alternating currents of high and low frequency," *Am. J. Physiol.*, 1929, *91*, 83–93.

37. Jesse McClendon and G. Burr, "Basal metabolism of a woman not secreting ovarian hormone, after its injection," *Proc. Soc. exp. Biol. Med.*, 1928, *26*, 782–783; Jesse McClendon, G. Burr, and C. Conklin, "Basal metabolism (oxygen) of normal women in relation to injection of Follicular hormone," *Proc. Soc. exp. Biol. Med.*, 1928, *26*, 265–266; C. V. Conklin and J. F. McClendon, "The basal metabolic rate in relation to the menstrual cycle," *Archs intern. Med.*, 1930, *45*, 125–135.

38. Myers, *Masters of medicine* (n. 31), p. 385. Dr. Esther M. Gresheimer earned a Ph.D. degree in physiology at the University of Chicago and the M.D. degree at Minnesota in 1923. She first came to Minnesota in 1918 as an instructor in physiology, and left the institution in 1936 to accept a position as professor of physiology at the Women's Medical College in Philadelphia.

39. University of Minnesota, *President's report* (n. 32), p. 520.

40. Thomas B. Hartzell and Arthur T. Henrici, "A study of streptococci from Pyorrhea alveolaris and from apical abscesses," *J. Am. med. Ass.*, 1914, *64*, 1055–1060.

41. Thomas B. Hartzell and Arthur B. Henrici, "The dental path: its importance as an avenue to infection," *Surg. Gynec. Obstet.*, 1916, *22*, 18–27.

42. Thomas B. Hartzell and Arthur T. Henrici, "The pathogenicity of mouth streptococci and their role in the etiology of dental diseases," *J. natn dental Ass.*, 1917, *4*, 477–498.

43. Ibid., p. 492.

44. Arthur T. Henrici and Thomas B. Hartzell, "The bacteriology of vital pulps," *J. dent. Res.*, 1919, *1*, 419–422, p. 420.

45. Ibid., p. 422.

46. Arthur T. Henrici and Thomas B. Hartzell, "A microscopic study of pulps from infected teeth," *J. dent. Res.*, 1920, *2*, 537–550.

47. Ibid., p. 549.

48. Arthur T. Henrici and E. L. Gardner, "A case of pulmonary infection with a new species of acid fast *Actinomyces,*" *Minn. Med.*, 1921, *4,* 443-445.

49. Arthur T. Henrici and E. Nelson, "Immunologic studies of actinomycetes, with special reference to the acid-fast species," *Proc. Soc. exp. Biol. Med.*, 1921-22, *19,* 251.

50. Arthur T. Henrici, "A statistical study of the form and growth of *Bacterium coli,*" *Proc. Soc. exp. Biol. Med.*, 1923, *21,* 215-217.

51. Arthur T. Henrici, *Morphologic variation and the rate of growth of bacteria,* p. 94.

52. Edward Francis, "Tularemia, Francis 1921: A new disease of man," *J. Am. med. Ass.,* 1922, *78,* 1015-1018.

53. L. V. Dieter and B. Rhods, "Tularemia in wild rats," *J. infect. Dis.,* 1926, *38,* 541-546; J. C. Perry, "Tularemia among meadow mice (Microtes californicus aestuerinus) in California," *Pub. Hlth Rep.,* 1928, *43,* 260-263.

54. R. G. Green and E. M. Wade, "Ruffed grouse are susceptible to tularemia," *Proc. Soc. exp. Biol. Med.,* 1928, *28,* 515-517; R. G. Green and E. M. Wade, "A natural infeciton of quail by B. tularense," *Proc. soc. exp. Biol. Med.,* 1929, *26,* 626-627.

55. Arthur T. Henrici, "Studies of freshwater bacteria. I. A direct microscopic technique," *J. Bacteriol.,* 1933, *25,* 277-286.

56. Arthur T. Henrici and Delia E. Johnson, "Studies of freshwater bacteria, II. Stalked bacteria, a new order of Schizomycetes," *J. Bacteriol.,* 1935, *30,* 61-92.

57. Arthur T. Henrici, "Studies of freshwater bacteria. III. Quantitative aspects of the direct microscopic method," *J. Bacteriol.,* 1936, *32,* 265-280, p. 265.

58. Arthur T. Henrici, "Characteristics of fungous diseases," *J. Bacteriol.,* 1940, *39,* 113-138.

59. Among numerous biographical and obituary articles on E. T. Bell, see Lemen J. Wells, "In honor of Elexious Thompson Bell," *J.-Lancet,* 1960, *80,* 41-44; J. Arthur Myers, "Tommy Bell," *J.-Lancet,* 1964, *84,* 237-238; Reuben Berman, "Our senior educators, Elexious Thompson Bell," *Minn. Med.,* 1962, *45,* 1263-1265.

60. E. T. Bell and W. P. Larson, "A study of lesions produced by Bacillus proteus," *J. infect. Dis.,* 1913, *13,* 510-516; idem, "A study of pathogenic properties of Bacillus proteus," *J. exp. Med.,* 1915, *21,* 629-644.

61. E. T. Bell and A. T. Henrici, "Renal tumor of the rabbit," *J. Cancer Res.,* 1916, *1,* 108-112, 157-167.

62. E. T. Bell and T. H. Hartzell, "Effects of foreign protein on the kidney," *J. infect. Dis.,* 1919, *24,* 618-627.

63. E. T. Bell and Thomas Hartzell, "Spontaneous nephritis in rabbits and its relation to chronic nephritis in man," *J. infect. Dis.,* 1919, *24,* 628-635; idem, "Etiology and development of glomerular nephritis," *Archs intern. Med.,* 1922, *29,* 768-820; idem, "Studies on hypertension: relation of age to size of heart," *J. med. Res.,* 1924, *44,* 478-487.

64. E. T. Bell and T. H. Hartzell, "Etiology and development of glomerularnephritis," *Archs intern. Med.,* 1922, *29,* 768-820.

65. James S.McCartney, "Latent portal cirrhosis of the liver," *Archs Path.,* 1933, *16,* 817-838; idem, "Diseases of the liver and gallbladder," in E. T. Bell, ed., *Textbook of pathology,* pp. 579-599.

66. James S. McCartney, "Pulmonary embolism following trauma," *Surg. Gynec. Obstet.,* 1935, *61,* 369-379.

67. J. Arthur Myers, *Masters of medicine* (n. 28), p. 335.

68. Ibid., pp. 335-336.

69. E. T. Bell and B. J. Clawson, "Comparison of acute rheumatic and subacute bacterial endocarditis," *Archs intern. Med.,* 1926, *37,* 66-81; idem, "Valvular diseases of the

heart with special reference to pathogenesis of old valvular defects," *Am. J. Path.*, 1926, *2*, 193–234.

70. Benjamin J. Clawson, "Experimental streptococcal inflammation in normal, immune, and hypersensitive animals," *Archs Path.*, 1930, *9*, 1141–1153.

71. B. J. Clawson and G. E. Fahr, "Experiments leading to a possible basis for vaccine therapy in acute rheumatic fever," *Proc. Soc. exp. Biol. Med.*, 1930, *27*, 964–965; B. J. Clawson and P. K. Allen, "Intravenous vaccine treatment for staphylococcic infections," *Archs Derm.*, 1931, *23*, 894–900; B. J. Clawson, "Experiments relative to a possible basis for vaccine treatment of acute rheumatic fever," *J. infect. Dis.*, 1931, *49*, 90–97.

72. E. T. Bell, *Renal diseases*.

73. E. T. Bell, *Diabetes mellitus, a clinical and pathological study of 2,529 cases*.

74. A. McGhee Harvey, "Arthur D. Hirschfelder: Johns Hopkins's first full-time cardiologist", *Johns Hopkins med. J.*, 1978, *143*, 129–139, pp. 136–137.

75. Arthur D. Hirschfelder, *Diseases of the heart and aorta*.

76. Because the Minnesota Medical Practice Act required completion of a formal course in physical diagnosis, the State Board of Medical Examiners refused to allow Hirschfelder a license to practice either by reciprocity or by examination on the grounds that Hirschfelder's training at the Hopkins had not included such a course. Such rigidity on the part of the State Board of Medical Examiners may have reflected the bitterness engendered by the reorganization of the medical school in 1913. Hirschfelder could have taken the required course in physical diagnosis at Minnesota, but did not.

77. E. H. Starling and M. B. Visscher, "The regulation of the energy output of the heart," *J. Physiol., Lond.*, 1926–27, *62*, 243–261. In 1927, the year that their paper appeared, Ernest Starling died. Maurice Visscher was one of his last students.

78. Howard C. Peters and Maurice B. Visscher, "The energy metabolism of the heart in failure and the influence of drugs upon it," *Am. Heart J.*, 1936, *11*, 273–291.

79. Maurice B. Visscher, "Physiological principles of importance in heart failure and its treatment," *J.-Lancet*, 1937, *57*, 309–311.

80. Gordon K. Moe and Maurice B. Visscher, "The mechanism of failure in the completely isolated mammalian heart," *Am. J. Physiol.*, 1939, *125*, 461–473.

81. M.B. Visscher, "The restriction of the coronary flow as a general factor in heart failure," *J. Am. med. Ass.*, 1939, *113*, 987–990.

CHAPTER 16

Developments in Biochemistry, the Laboratory of Physiological Hygiene, and the Identification of Risk Factors in Coronary Heart Disease

On his return to Minnesota in 1936, Maurice Visscher was dissatisfied with the state of physiological chemistry under the brilliant, but eccentric, Jesse McClendon.[1] In 1938 Visscher arranged for McClendon to be offered a research professorship at Hahnemann Medical College. When McClendon hesitated to accept the Hahnemann offer, President Guy Stanton Ford put on his straw hat and went down the street to see him. Ford told McClendon, "Prepare yourself for ten years of dry rot at the University of Minnesota if you decide not to take the Hahnemann offer."[2] Neither Visscher nor Ford evidently attached much value to McClendon's outstanding work on the role of iodine deficiency in the incidence of goiter, and in 1939 McClendon left for Hahnemann.

In 1940 George O. Burr was appointed director of a newly established Division of Physiological Chemistry within the Department of Physiology. Although Burr was a biochemist, he had previously held an appointment as professor of plant physiology in the Department of Botany at Minnesota. A native of Arkansas, George Burr came to Minnesota in 1920 to do graduate study in biochemistry under Ross Gortner, chief of the Division of Biochemistry in the College of Agriculture. After receiving his Ph.D. degree in 1924, he went to the University of California at Berkeley as a research associate in the department of anatomy. At Berkeley, Burr worked with Herbert M. Evans in investigations of the chemical nature of vitamin E, which Evans and Katherine J. Bishop had discovered in 1922.[3] In 1926 Evans and Burr attempted to concentrate vitamin E, but Evans and his coworkers did not succeed in isolating it as α-tocopherol until 1935.[4] Meanwhile, in 1927 George Burr and his wife and coworker, Mildred Burr, left Berkeley to return to Minnesota. They made the journey across the mountains and the plains in their Model-T Ford car, taking with them in cages a colony of the Long-Evans strain of laboratory rats, the strain which Joseph Long and Herbert Evans had used to carry out their classic study of the oestrous cycle of the rat at Berkeley.[5] At overnight stops at hotels, the Burrs smuggled the rat cages into their room to protect the rats from the nighttime chill.[6]

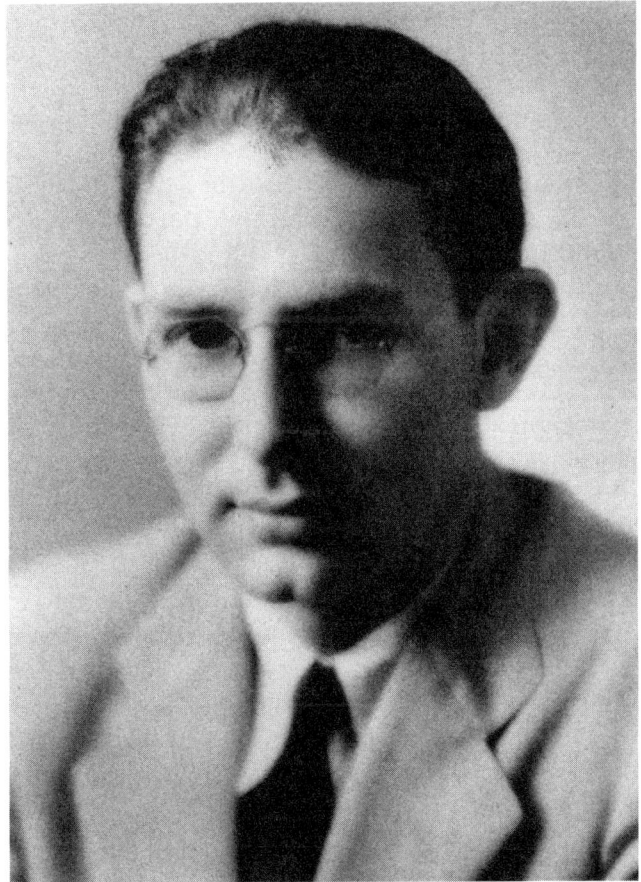

FIGURE 16:1   George O. Burr, 1930. Courtesy Mn U Archives.

After George and Mildred Burr settled into their laboratory in the Botany Building, directly across the street from the university hospital, George Burr received a grant from the Medical Research Fund of the University of Minnesota to continue their nutritional studies on rats. While working at Berkeley with Evans, Burr had suspected that fat might play a more significant role in the diet than the mere provision of calories. When Evans and Burr added small amounts of fat to the diet of rats fed upon a highly purified diet lacking in fat, the growth and ovulation of the rats improved significantly. Furthermore they found that the improvement was brought about by the fatty acid portion of the fat, not by the glycerol nor by the unsaponifiable fraction in which vitamins A, D, and E were carried.[7] At Minnesota, George and Mildred Burr attempted to raise rats on a completely fat-free diet that was otherwise nutritionally complete. After about three months on the fat-free diet, the rats developed a characteristic disease, marked first by a scaly condition of the skin. Later the tips of the rats' tails became inflamed and swollen, and the whole tail was soon heavily scaled and ridged. Gradually the tip of the tail became necrotic, eczema developed over the whole body, the hair fell out in patches, and sores often appeared on the skin. After another three or four months the animals died. Nevertheless, if a small amount of lard were added to their diet, the rats would recover quickly. The Burrs determined that the essential part of the fat resided in the fatty acids, and that the fatty acids in lard were adequate to cure the disease.[8] In 1930, George and Mildred Burr showed further that the fatty acids capable of curing the deficiency disease in the rats were unsaturated fatty acids, and that linoleic acid, occurring in lard, and in olive oil, corn oil, and other vegetable oils, was far more effective than the oleic acid of butter.[9]

George and Mildred Burr's demonstration that certain unsaturated fatty acids were essential for nutrition was a major discovery in biochemistry. Across the street at the university hospital, Dr. Arild Hansen of the Department of Pediatrics saw immediately that certain childhood skin diseases, such as infantile eczema, were suspiciously similar to the fatty-acid deficiency disease described by the Burrs in rats. When he tested the blood of ten children suffering from infantile eczema, Dr. Hansen found that their blood serum did contain lower levels of unsaturated fatty acids than the blood sera of normal children.[10] Hansen and Burr together found that rats on fat-free diets also had lower serum levels of fatty acids and cholesterol than rats on the normal control diet.[11] In 1933 very little was known of the fatty acids present in human blood serum. Four years later, in 1937, William R. Brown and Arild E. Hansen found that the levels of two fatty acids, arachidonic acid and linoleic acid, were much lower than normal in patients suffering from eczema.[12] They also tested the effect of a very low fat diet on an adult human subject for a period of six months. Although no change occurred in serum level of cholesterol or total fatty acids, the serum fatty acids became progressively more saturated. The body weight decreased gradually during the first three months on the diet, and the average blood pressure fell about 10 mm. of mercury. The subject no longer felt tired, and after about six weeks on the diet, ceased to have migraine attacks which previously had occurred every seven to ten days. The decline in unsaturated fatty acids over the six-month period suggested that humans could not synthesize unsaturated fatty acids, which therefore needed to be provided in the diet. During the six months of the experiment, the subject was living upon his body's stores of unsaturated fatty acids and probably could not have continued to subsist indefinitely on the low fat diet.[13]

In the course of his work on dietary fats, George Burr discovered a process for converting various oils, such as cotton, corn, soybean, peanut, or linseed oils, into oils with quick-drying properties similar to those of tung oil. The war in China had made tung oil, used in the manufacture of varnishes, shellacs, and lacquers, difficult to obtain in the United States. Burr's discovery of a means to convert nondrying oils into drying oils provided cheap and abundant substitutes for tung oil and was therefore of far-reaching economic and strategic significance during World War II.

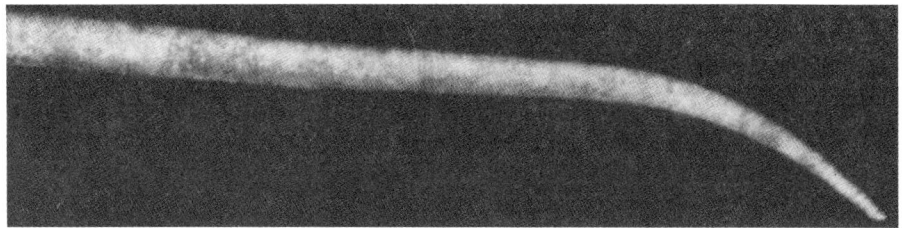
a.

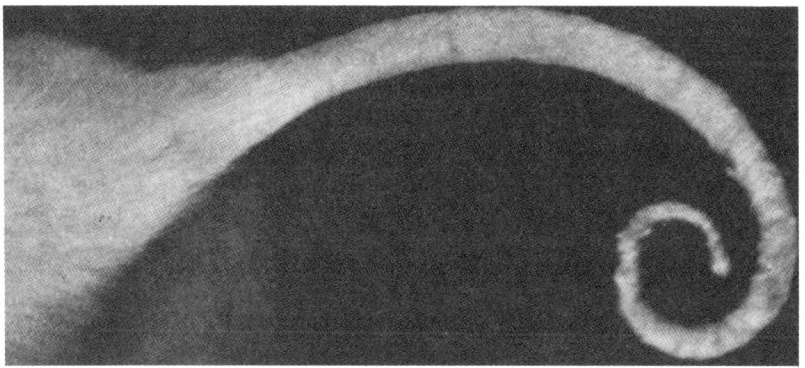
b.

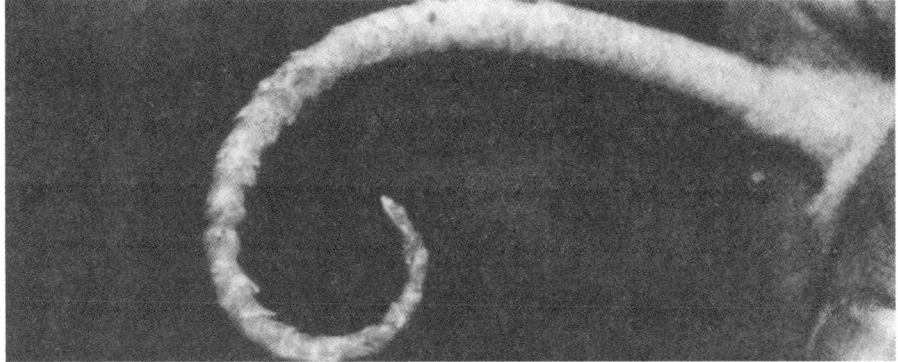
c.

FIGURE 16:2 Fatty acid deficiency disease in rats (Burr and Burr, 1930). Courtesy *Journal of Biological Chemistry*. a. Tail of rat fed on fat-free diet + 10 drops of lard daily. Entirely normal in appearance. b. Tail of rat fed on fat-free diet + 5 drops of glycerol daily. Glycerol gives no protection. c. Tail of rat fed on fat-free diet + the non-saponifiable matter from 10 drops of lard daily. There is no protection from the disease.

By 1940 when George Burr was appointed director of the new Division of Physiological Chemistry, he was one of the outstanding biochemists in the United States. In view of his greater responsibilities, Dr. Visscher and Dean Diehl both recommended—indeed assumed as a foregone conclusion—that Burr's salary would be increased from the $4,750 that he had been receiving as a professor of botany to the level of $5,500 that his predecessor, Dr. McClendon, had been paid. Such was not to be the case. Over the strenuous objections of Maurice Visscher and Harold Diehl, Burr received only a $250 increase to $5,000. In 1942 Burr received a further increase of $200, but not until 1944 did his salary rise above that which McClendon had been paid in 1939. Meanwhile, Burr had reorganized the teaching in physiological chemistry and made Minnesota a world center for research in lipids and mineral metabolism.

George Burr's salary at Minnesota was much lower than the salaries for comparable positions at other universities. At the same time his salary was necessarily the highest paid to any faculty member in physiological chemistry. In the circumstances, the inevitable happened. In succession three very able young biochemists resigned, two to go to important research positions in industry, and one to become head of the department of biochemistry at another university, all three at salaries substantially above what Burr was receiving at Minnesota. In 1946 George Burr himself left to become director of biochemical research for the Hawaiian Sugar Planters Association at Honolulu. In his final year at Minnesota, Burr's salary was $5,900. Two years earlier Dr. Visscher and Dean Diehl pleaded urgently that it be increased to $6,000, a figure which, although still inadequate, Dr. Burr would accept as evidence that the university administration approved of his work. Instead the university set his salary at that time at $5,700.

In 1946, following the departure of George Burr, the Board of Regents elevated physiological chemistry to the status of a department of the medical school and appointed Professor Wallace D. Armstrong as its head. Then at the age of forty-two, Wallace Armstrong was already famous for his discovery of the role of fluoride in the prevention of tooth decay and for his pioneering work in the use of radioactive isotopes in metabolic studies. A native of Texas, Dr. Armstrong came to Minnesota in 1928 to begin graduate study in physiological chemistry under Jesse McClendon. When he was ready to begin research, McClendon suggested that Armstrong study the biological relationships of fluorine because it was the one halogen that had not yet been studied, and Armstrong's first published paper dealt with a method for the colorimetric determination of fluorine.[14] In 1936 Armstrong introduced a much more accurate method for the determination of the very small amounts of fluorine that occur in teeth and other tissues.[15] In certain areas of the United States such as western Texas, Colorado, and Montana, the drinking water contained levels of fluoride high enough to produce mottling of the teeth, and dentists had noted that such mottled teeth rarely contained caries. In 1938 Dr. Armstrong and Dr. P. J. Brekhus of the School of Dentistry showed that the enamel of carious teeth contained little more than half as much fluorine as the enamel of sound teeth.[16] They concluded that optimal amounts of fluorine in tooth enamel might confer an increased resistance to tooth decay, without producing the unsightly mottling associated with excessive amounts of fluorine.

Following the observation by Armstrong and Brekhus that sound teeth contain much more fluorine than decayed teeth, various field studies showed a lower incidence of tooth decay in geographic areas of endemic mottled enamel. Other studies carried out from 1938 to 1942 showed that in areas where the fluoride content of drinking water was as high as one part per million, the incidence of tooth decay was low, even though there might not be sufficient fluoride to produce mottling of the teeth.[17] In 1941 Mabel Perry and Wallace Armstrong showed that when laboratory rats were given drinking water containing higher than normal levels of fluoride, the fluorine content of the tooth enamel was increased while that of the dentin remained unchanged. Their observation indicated that the enamel of the teeth had taken up fluoride directly from the drinking water, rather than from the circulating blood, and suggested that it might be possible to increase the fluorine content of the enamel of human teeth by the direct application of fluoride solutions to the surface of the teeth.[18]

In April 1942 John W. Knutson, a dental surgeon with the United States Public Health Service, came to Minnesota to collaborate with Wallace Armstrong on a controlled study of the effect of topical treatments of the teeth of three groups of Minnesota school children with sodium fluoride solutions. The results were striking. Among teeth that received topical treatment with sodium fluoride, 40 percent fewer carious teeth developed than among untreated teeth.[19] Their findings reinforced those of H. Trendley Dean and his colleagues at the United States Public Health Service who showed, as a result of the examination of more than 7,000 children in twenty-one cities, that in cities where the water supply contained little or no fluoride, the incidence of dental caries was two to three times greater than in cities where the water supply contained one part per million or more of fluoride.[20]

By 1943 it was clear that the incidence of dental caries could be reduced by fluoride treatment, which might be given either by the addition of one part per million of fluoride to municipal water supplies or by the direct application of fluoride solution to the surface of the teeth. The addition of fluoride to water supplies provided more effective prevention of dental caries than topical applications. It was also a far cheaper and more easily administered method to prevent dental caries in whole populations using a common water supply. Nevertheless, the complete fluoridation of municipal water supplies would still leave about a third of the population of the United States unprotected because they depended on separate, private sources of water. Therefore, both methods would have to be used in a general program to reduce the incidence of dental caries.[21]

Over the next thirty years Wallace Armstrong played an active role in the campaign to achieve the fluoridation of municipal water supplies. Many states, including Minnesota, passed laws requiring the fluoridation of public water supplies, a requirement that frequently evoked strong opposition from individuals and groups who assumed mistakenly that fluoridation might be harmful. Dr.

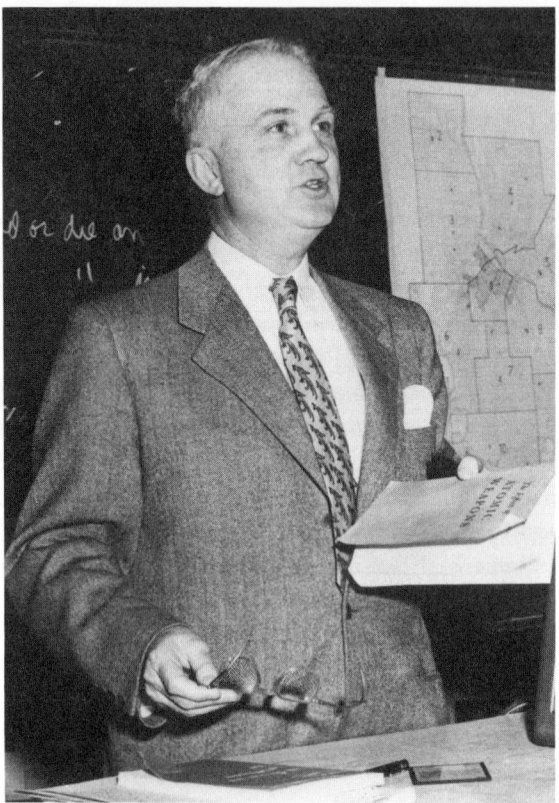

FIGURE 16:3 Wallace D. Armstrong, circa 1946. Courtesy Mrs. Armstrong.

Armstrong worked to inform the public that fluoridation of water supplies at the appropriate levels was not only harmless but immensely beneficial in reducing the incidence of tooth decay. In April 1963, Armstrong went to Ireland to testify before the Irish High Court at Dublin on the medical and physiological effects of fluoridation in a lawsuit challenging an act passed by the Irish Parliament to permit the fluoridation of water supplies in Ireland. In Minnesota, the result of Wallace Armstrong's efforts may be seen today in the very low incidence of dental caries among Minnesota school children, many of whom have perfect teeth with no cavities whatever—a state of affairs very different from that of fifty years ago.

The Laboratory of Physiological Hygiene

In 1937 Ancel Keys came from the Mayo Clinic to join the Department of Physiology. Then thirty-three years old, Dr. Keys had pursued research in respiratory physiology and the study of human fatigue at Cambridge University in England and at Harvard University before coming the year before to the Mayo Foundation in Rochester. In his studies on respiration, fatigue, and high altitude physiology, Dr. Keys had come to realize the need for greater knowledge of human physiology for the maintenance of human health. He wished to investigate the physiological responses of the human body to such variables as exercise, food, and changes in the air breathed, designating such studies as physiological hygiene. In Millard Hall he set up a laboratory with special equipment either donated by local firms or made in the medical school's workshop in the basement, a laboratory that quickly became known as the Laboratory of Physiological Hygiene.

In his initial work at the medical school, Keys' primary interest was in the effects of environmental factors such as temperature and altitude (air pressure) on the functions of the heart, lungs, and circulation. In 1938 Keys and Friedell used x-ray photographs to compare the size of the heart in college students trained for strenuous sports with its size in moderately athletic and nonathletic students. Previously, physiologists had believed that the heart was enlarged in athletes and that such enlargement might be harmful. Keys and Friedell found to the contrary, that in all three groups of students the heart in its contracted state (systole) was the same size, but in its dilated state (diastole), the heart was much larger in the athletes so that at each beat it pumped a larger quantity of blood.[22] Keys and his colleagues went on to develop the use of the slit x-ray cardiogram combined with techniques to measure both the output of the heart and its efficiency, especially in patients suffering from defective heart valves or congenital heart defects such as patent ductus arteriosus.[23] They were able thereby to measure the severity of valve leakages or congenital heart defects.

Since these studies possessed obvious significance for the ability of soldiers to perform under various conditions of stress, the United States Army asked Keys to carry out investigations for them. In 1940 at Fort Snelling, Keys and Henschel tested the effect of vitamin supplements when added to ordinary army rations and found that they had no influence on the output or efficiency of the hearts of soldiers performing strenuous exercise. Changes in the lactic acid content of the blood and the blood sugar level were exactly the same with or without supplementary vitamins in the diet.[24] Their findings contradicted the popular belief, then widespread, that additional vitamins would confer unusual stamina or greater resistance to stress.

In the spring of 1941 Ancel Keys and his colleagues developed for the army light, compact rations for the use of the parachute troops in training. After field tests the army adopted the rations, named K rations for Keys, for general use as emergency combat rations for American troops in World War II.

In 1942, pressed by the need for more space in which to house the human subjects used in their research, Keys and his colleagues moved their laboratory out of Millard Hall to improvised quarters beneath the university football stadium. The space was provided by the Department of Physical Education, which was interested in the laboratory's studies of physical exercise and athletic performance,

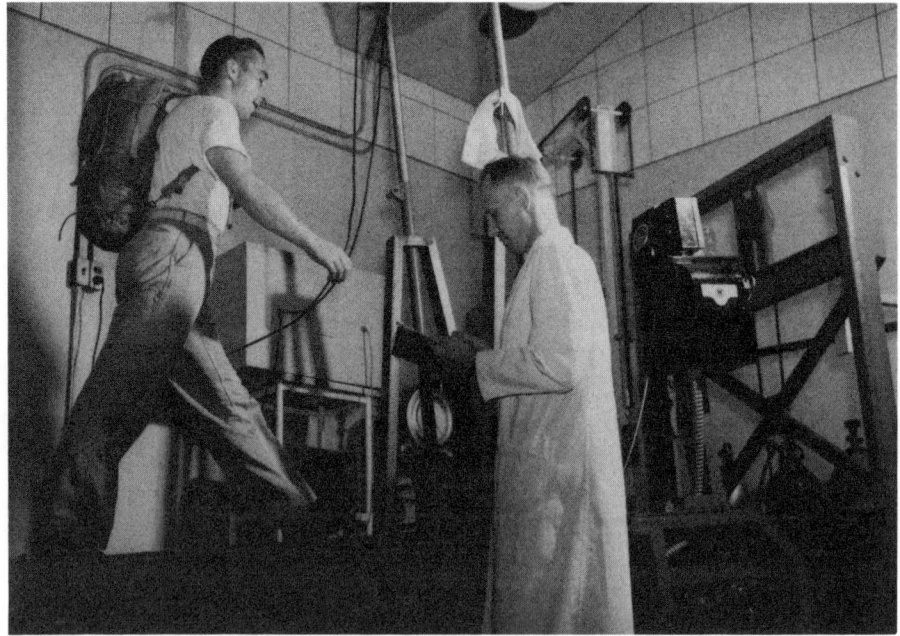

FIGURE 16:4 Studying the effect of exercise on the heart, Laboratory of Physiological Hygiene. Courtesy Mn U Archives.

and much of the work of the laboratory was supported by the receipts from football games and other athletic events.

During World War II with the financial help of the Society of Friends, the Church of the Brethren, and the Mennonites, the laboratory obtained the permission of the Selective Service System to use volunteers from among conscientious objectors as subjects for physiological experiments. At the beginning of 1944, Keys and his staff, realizing that as a result of the war there would be widespread starvation in Europe, were astonished to discover that very little was known about the effects of prolonged hunger on people. Nevertheless, they knew that the undernourished person was different both physiologically and psychologically from one who was well fed. They decided, therefore, to seek volunteers from among conscientious objectors to carry out a controlled study of the effects of prolonged starvation and refeeding. From more than a hundred volunteers, they selected thirty-six young men who in November 1944 entered upon what was to be known as the Minnesota Experiment. After an initial twelve-week control period, the young men were placed on a semistarvation diet for twenty-four weeks, followed by twelve weeks of controlled refeeding. Their capacity for physical performance, their physiology, and their psychology were monitored regularly until the conclusion of the experiment in October 1945.

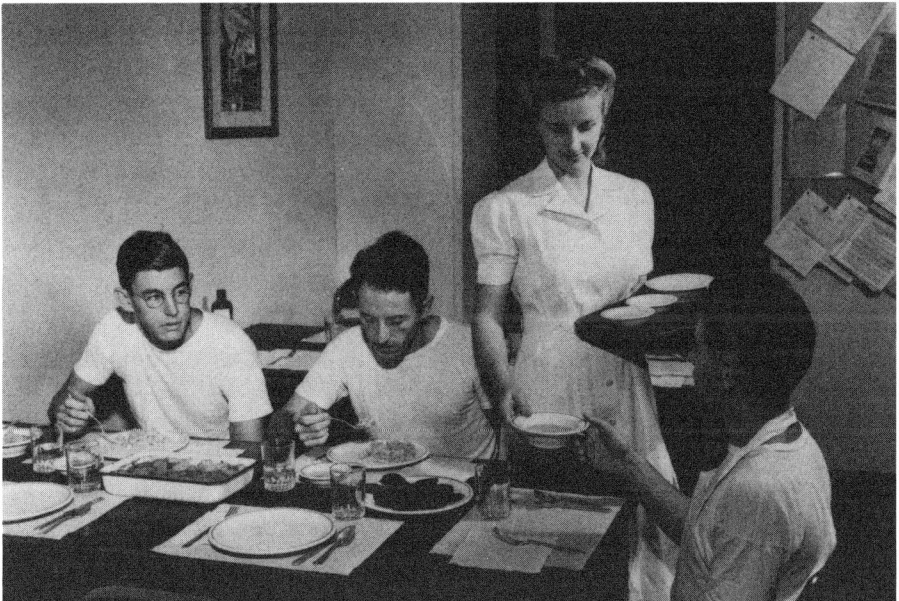

FIGURE 16:5 The Minnesota Experiment, 1945—eating dinner. Courtesy Mn U Archives.

The Minnesota Experiment was designed to duplicate the conditions of severe famine, the diet consisting mainly of potatoes, turnips, and cereals in amounts calculated to bring about in six months a loss of one-fourth of the body weight. Most of the weight loss was from the muscles, and the heart became shrunken, with resultant loss of strength and endurance. The starved subjects were always cold and slept under several blankets, even through the heat of July. Even more than from the cold, they suffered from unceasing hunger, weakness, mental depression, and a sense of being old, although their intelligence, memory, and reasoning power were unimpaired. Most of the men developed a distinctive blotchy skin pigmentation that looked much like dirt. They developed starvation edema, despite the fact that their plasma proteins remained normal, and they showed no signs of heart failure. One of the subjects recalled the experience later: "We lost our semblance of humanity . . . . I remember seeing a guy on a corner in Minneapolis and I got mad at him because he could go and have something to eat. A couple of days later I saw a kid on a bicycle. My first thought was 'how could anybody get that much energy.' Then I thought, 'he is probably going home to supper. I hate him.' "[25] The Minnesota Experiment showed that in relieving victims of starvation, the greatest need was simply for a sufficient supply of ordinary foods. No special foods or vitamin supplements were needed. Nevertheless, recovery occurred slowly and might require as long as a year.[26]

In 1946, with the war over, the Laboratory of Physiological Hygiene turned its attention to the effects of aging and particularly to the problem of coronary heart disease, which was then increasingly epidemic among American men. They began a long-term study of two groups of healthy men, one group of young men, seventeen to twenty-four years of age, the other group of middle-aged business and professional men. They found that the physiological differences between the younger and older men were generally less than anticipated except for the serum cholesterol level which was markedly higher among the older men. On further investigation of men over a range of ages, they found that the serum cholesterol level began to rise after age thirty, reaching a plateau in the forties and fifties, and declined slightly in later years.[27] In 1950 Ancel Keys and his colleagues showed from the study of two male patients with inborn hypercholesteremia that the serum cholesterol level could be lowered by the elimination of fat from the diet, but it was not influenced by cholesterol in the diet.[28] At the same time Dr. Carleton Chapman, who worked both in the Laboratory of Physiological Hygiene and the Department of Medicine, showed that the fat-free rice-fruit diet used to control hypertension also lowered the level of serum cholesterol.[29]

To determine what characteristic of the rice-fruit diet caused the serum cholesterol level to fall, Joseph T. Anderson and Ancel Keys began in 1949 a series of controlled dietary experiments on male schizophrenic patients at Hastings State Hospital. Twenty-six patients were divided into two comparable groups. For four weeks one group was fed a high fat diet while the other received a diet moderate in fat. Then the first group changed from a high fat to a moderate fat diet and after a further four weeks their serum cholesterol levels had fallen sharply. Meanwhile, the second group switched from a moderate fat to a high fat diet, and their serum cholesterol levels rose somewhat more than those of the first group had fallen.[30] Anderson and Keys concluded that neither the rice, the fruit, the low salt, nor the absence of cholesterol caused the level of serum cholesterol to drop on the rice-fruit diet; instead the critical factor was simply the absence of fat.[31] Nevertheless, the primary role of fat in the diet, as opposed to cholesterol itself, in determining the level of serum cholesterol, and therefore susceptibility to atherosclerosis, was denied by other investigators who produced atherosclerosis experimentally by feeding cholesterol in large doses to chickens.[32]

In 1951 Ancel Keys went to England to spend a year as a Fulbright Fellow at Oxford University where he continued his research on nutrition and heart disease. In Great Britain as in the United States, the incidence of coronary heart disease had risen sharply during the preceding decades. In February 1952 Ancel Keys left England to spend several weeks at Naples in Italy where with the help of his wife, Margaret Keys, and Italian colleagues at the University of Naples, he determined the serum cholesterol levels among some eighty-four Neapolitan firemen and other municipal employees varying in age from eighteen to fifty-four years. Among the young Italians up to the age of thirty-five, serum cholesterol levels corresponded closely to those of the young Minnesotans whom Keys had studied at Minneapolis, but whereas in Minnesota the serum cholesterol continued to rise from age thirty-five to age fifty-five, among the Naples working men it remained level, being essentially the same at age fifty as at age thirty-five. The Naples working

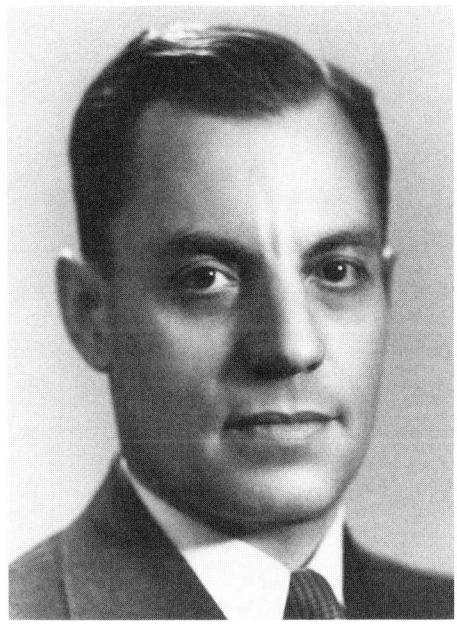

FIGURE 16:6 Ancel Keys, 1945. Courtesy Mn U Archives.

men were poorly paid and lived mainly on bread, spaghetti, and vegetables, with meat or fish only once or twice a week.[33] Coronary heart disease was almost unknown among them, but the Italian physicians told Keys that it did occur at Naples among the rich, whose diet was more like that of Americans.

After his return to England in March 1952, Keys was able to take the serum cholesterol levels of a group of forty-eight Englishmen at the Industrial Health Clinic at Slough near London, but he did not calculate the results immediately because in May he and his wife went to Spain. The Institute of Medical Research at Madrid arranged for him to determine the serum cholesterol levels of a group of Spanish working men. The institute also collected information on the diet of the men, which consisted largely of bread and potatoes with small amounts of fish, meat, vegetables, and fruits.[34] As at Naples, the serum cholesterol levels of the Spanish working men did not rise after age thirty-five as they did among Minnesota men, nor as they did among Spanish doctors, whose diet, although different, contained as much fat as the average American diet. Although he did not have data on the occurrence of coronary heart disease at Madrid, the Spanish physicians thought that it occurred much more commonly among the rich than the poor people there. In June 1952 Keys wrote from Madrid: "In any case here is a solid set of facts showing a marked change in the age trend of something we can measure and it is unquestionably associated with differences in diet which we also can measure. I think this is something new in the embryonic science of the quantitative study of later ontogeny of man."[35] It was. Keys' preliminary studies in England, Italy, and Spain in 1952 provided a model for later studies of the epidemiology of coronary heart disease that the Laboratory of Physiological Hygiene helped to organize in Finland, Greece, Hawaii, Japan, South Africa, and Yugoslavia. In 1957 Keys and his colleagues developed protocols and methods for an international collaborative study of the epidemiology of coronary heart disease by full-scale field trials in villages in southern Italy and the Greek island of Crete. From 1957 to 1964 the international collaborative study was carried out, using sixteen cohorts, including more than 12,000 middle-aged men (ages 40–59) in seven countries: the United States, Japan, Yugoslavia, Finland, Italy, the Netherlands, and Greece.[36] The seven countries' study revealed that the principal risk factors for coronary heart disease were age, arterial blood pressure, and serum cholesterol level. Other anticipated relationships proved inconclusive, showing that the problems were more complex than had been expected. Nevertheless, the epidemiological method has proved a powerful tool in the search for preventive measures against coronary heart disease.

During the years that the seven countries' study was in progress, Ancel Keys and his colleagues, Joseph Anderson and Francisco Grande, also carried out a series of controlled dietary experiments using male patients at the Hastings State Hospital and mentally retarded inmates at the Faribault State School and Hospital. They were assisted in performing the experiments by volunteers from the Church of the Brethren, who lived with the subjects in the institutions throughout the course of the experiments. In 1957 Keys and his colleagues determined the effect on the level of serum cholesterol of changing the proportion of saturated to unsaturated fat in the diet, and developed equations to predict serum cholesterol levels from given changes in the fat component of the diet.[37] In 1965 they determined that the degree of unsaturation of fatty acids did not affect the level of serum cholesterol. They showed also that reduction of the quantity of cholesterol in the diet reduced the level of serum cholesterol, but the effect was small, varying as the square root of the reduction in dietary cholesterol.[38] Anything short of a cholesterol-free diet, which must necessarily be a completely vegetarian diet, appeared to make only a small difference to the level of serum cholesterol. Nevertheless, in 1984 in a review of the whole question of the relation of the level of serum cholesterol to cholesterol in the diet, based both on work done at the Laboratory of Physiological Hygiene and at other laboratories, Ancel Keys concluded that if the amount of saturated fat in the diet were reduced from 18 percent of total calories to half that amount, serum cholesterol would fall on average by 23 mg. per 100 ml. If, at the same time, the amount of dietary cholesterol were cut in half, the level of serum cholesterol would fall an additional 7 mg. per 100 ml, a change which Keys said was "certainly not negligible."[39] Four decades of research, both intense and wide ranging, at the Laboratory of Physiological Hygiene give his words the weight of authority.

NOTES

1. David A. Zarkin, "Visiting Dr. Maurice B. Visscher," *Minn. Med. Fndn Med. Bull.*, Spring 1982, pp. 2–4.
2. Quoted in Owen H. Wangensteen, *Owen H. Wangensteen*, pp. 35–36.
3. H. M. Evans and Katherine S. Bishop, "On the existence of a hitherto unrecognized dietary factor essential for reproduction," *Science*, 1922, 56, 650–651.
4. Herbert M. Evans and George O. Burr, "The antisterility vitamin fat soluble E," *Mem. Univ. Calif.*, 1927, 8, 1–176; Herbert M. Evans, O. H. Emerson and Gladys A. Emerson, "The isolation from wheat germ oil of an alcohol, α-tocopherol, having the properties of vitamin E," *J. biol. Chem.*, 1936, 113, 319–332.
5. Joseph A. Long and Herbert McLean Evans, *The oestrous cycle in the rat and its associated phenomena*.
6. Ralph Holman, "George Burr: the discovery of essential fatty acids" [lecture delivered in the Department of History of Medicine, University of Minnesota, 2 November 1987].
7. Herbert M. Evans and George O. Burr, "A new dietary deficiency with highly purified diets. III. The beneficial effect of fat in the diet," *Proc. Soc. exp. Biol. Med.*, 1927–28, 25, 390–397.
8. George O. Burr and Mildred M. Burr, "A new deficiency disease produced by the rigid exclusion of fat from the diet," *J. biol. Chem.*, 1929, 82, 345–367.
9. George O. Burr and Mildred M. Burr, "On the nature and role of the fatty acids essential in nutrition," *J. biol. Chem.*, 1930, 86, 587–621.
10. Arild E. Hansen, "Study of iodine number of fatty acids in infantile eczema," *Proc. Soc. exp. Biol. Med.*, 1933, 30, 1198–1199.
11. Arild E. Hansen and George O. Burr, "Studies on iodine absorption of serum in rats fed on fat-free diets," *Proc. Soc. exp. Biol. Med.*, 1933, 30, 1200–1201; Arild E. Hansen and George O. Burr, "Iodine numbers of serum lipids in rats fed on fat-free diets," *Proc. Soc. exp. Biol. Med.*, 1933, 30, 1201-1203.
12. William R. Brown and Arild E. Hansen, "Arachidonic and linoleic acid of the serum in normal and eczematous human subjects," *Proc. Soc. exp. Biol. Med.*, 1937, 36, 113–117.
13. W. R. Brown et al., "Observations on human subject subsisting six months on a diet extremely low in fat," *Proc. Soc. exp. Biol. Med.*, 1937, 36, 281–283; William Redman Brown et al., "Effects of prolonged use of extremely low fat diet on an adult human subject," *J. Nutr.*, 1938, 16, 511–524.
14. Wallace D. Armstrong, "Colorimetric determination of fluorine," *Ind. Engng Chem. analyt. Edn*, 1933, 5, 300–302.
15. Wallace D. Armstrong, "Microdetermination of fluorine. Elimination of effect of chloride," *Ind. Engng. Chem. analyt. Edn.*, 1936, 8, 384–387.
16. Wallace D. Armstrong and P. J. Brekhus, "Possible relationship between the fluorine content of enamel and resistance to dental caries," *J. dent. Res.*, 1938, 17, 393–399.
17. H. Trendley Dean, "Endemic fluorosis and its relation to dental caries," *Pub. Hlth Rep.*, 1938, 53, 1443–1452; H. T. Dean et al., "Domestic water and dental caries including certain epidemiological aspects of oral L. acidophilus," *Pub. Hlth Rep.*, 1939, 54, 862–888.
18. Mabel W. Perry and W. D. Armstrong, "On the manner of acquisition of fluorine by mature teeth," *J. Nutr.*, 1941, 21, 35–44.
19. John W. Knutson and Wallace D. Armstrong, "The effect of topically applied sodium fluoride on dental caries experience," *Pub. Hlth Rep.*, 1943, 58, 1701–1715; idem, " . . . II. Report of the findings for second study year," *Pub. Hlth Rep.*, 1945, 60,

1085–1090; idem, ". . . Report of findings for the third study year," *Pub. Hlth Rep.*, 1946, *61*, 1683–1689.

20. H. Trendley Dean et al., "Domestic water and dental caries," *Pub. Hlth Rep.*, 1942, *57*, 1155–1179.

21. John W. Knutson and Wallace D. Armstrong, "Post-war implications of fluorine and dental health. The use of topically applied fluorine," *Am. J. pub. Hlth*, 1943, *34*, 239–343.

22. Ancel Keys and H. L. Friedell, "Size and stroke of the heart in young men in relation to athletic activity," *Science*, 1938, *88*, 456–458.

23. Ancel Keys and H.L. Friedell, "Quantitative measurement of cardiac stroke and valvular leakage in man," *J. clin. Invest.*, 1939, *18*, 476; Ancel Keys et al., "The Roentgen kymographic evaluation of the size and function of the heart," *Am. J. Roentg.*, 1940, *44*, 805–833; Ancel Keys et al, "The valvular efficiency in mitral and aortic insufficiency," *Am. J. Physiol.*, 1940, *52*, 101–102.

24. Ancel Keys and Austin F. Henschel, "High vitamin supplementation (B_1, nicotinic acid and C) and the response to intensive exercise in U.S. Army infantrymen," *Am. J. Physiol.*, 1941, *133*, 350–351; Ancel Keys and Austin F. Henschel, "Vitamin supplementation of U.S. Army rations in relation to fatigue and the ability to do muscular work," *J. Nutr.*, 1942, *23*, 259–269. In 1943 Keys and his colleagues confirmed their initial studies. See Ancel Keys et al., "Absence of rapid deterioration in men doing hard physical work on a restricted intake of vitamins of the B complex," *J. Nutr.*, 1944, *27*, 485–496.

25. Samuel Legg, "Excerpts from a talk," *J. Am. diet. Ass.*, 1946, *22*, 587.

26. Ancel Keys, "Human Starvation and its consequences," *J. Am. diet. Ass.*, 1946, *22*, 582–587. Cf. Ancel Keys et al., *The biology of human starvation*.

27. Ancel Keys, "Some preliminary findings from the research program on cardiovascular degeneration at the Laboratory of Physiological Hygiene," *Bull. Univ. Minn. Hosp. & Minn. med. Fndn*, 1948–49, *20*, 403–410; Ancel Keys et al., "The concentration of cholesterol in the blood serum of normal man and its relation to age," *J. clin. Invest.*, 1950, *29*, 1347–1353.

28. Ancel Keys et al., "The relation in man between cholesterol levels in the diet and the blood," *Science*, 1950, *112*, 79–81.

29. Carleton Chapman et al., "The effect of the rice-fruit diet on the composition of the body," *New Engl. J. Med.*, 1950, *243*, 899–905.

30. Joseph T. Anderson and Ancel Keys, "Dietary fat and serum cholesterol," *Fed. Proc.*, 1953, *12*, 169.

31. Ancel Keys, "Diet and the incidence of heart disease," *Bull. Univ. Minn. Hosp. & Minn. med. Fndn*, 1952–53, *24*, 376–388. See especially pp. 382–383.

32. E.g. Louis N. Katz, "Experimental atherosclerosis," *Circulation*, 1952, *5*, 101–114. Cf. Edgar V. Allen, ed., "Atherosclerosis: a symposium," *Circulation*, 1952, *5*, 98–100.

33. Ancel Keys, "Notes from a medical journey," *J.-Lancet*, 1952, *72*, 205–207; Ancel Keys et al., "The trend of serum cholesterol levels with age," *Lancet, Lond.*, 1952, *263*, 209–210; Ancel Keys et al., "Studies on serum cholesterol and other characteristics of clinically healthy men in Naples," *Archs intern. Med.*, 1954, *93*, 328–336.

34. Ancel Keys, "Notes from a medical journey," *J.-Lancet*, 1952, *72*, 340–342.

35. Ancel Keys, "Notes from a medical journey," *J.-Lancet*, 1952, *72*, 380–382, p. 381. Cf. Ancel Keys et al., "Studies on the diet, body fatness and serum cholesterol in Madrid, Spain," *Metabolism*, 1954, *3*, 195–212.

36. Ancel Keys et al., "Epidemiological studies related to coronary heart disease: characteristics of men aged 40–59 in seven countries," *Acta med. Scand.*, 1966, *Suppl. 460*; Ancel Keys, *Seven countries: a multivariate analysis of death and coronary heart disease*.

37. Ancel Keys et al., "Prediction of serum-cholesterol responses of man to changes in fats in the diet," *Lancet, Lond.*, 1957, *ii*, 957–966.

38. Ancel Keys et al., "Serum cholesterol response to changes in the diet," *Metabolism*, 1965, *14*, 759–787.

39. Ancel Keys, "Serum cholesterol response to dietary cholesterol," *Am. J. clin. Nutr.*, 1984, *40*, 351–359.

CHAPTER 17

The Medical School in the Second World War, 1941–1945

Early in March 1940 when in Europe the Great Powers were already at war, Dean Diehl received a letter from the United States surgeon general, who outlined a plan for the organization of general hospitals along the lines of the base hospitals that had proven so effective in the First World War. Each such hospital would be affiliated with a medical school and would be staffed with doctors and nurses from the affiliated school, so that from the beginning the staff of a general hospital would know each other and be accustomed to work together. The War Department invited the University of Minnesota to organize such a general hospital to be ready in case of a national emergency and suggested that it should be called the 26th General Hospital to perpetuate the tradition begun by Base Hospital No. 26 in World War I.

On 9 April 1940 the administrative committee approved the surgeon general's proposal in principle.[1] After a visit to Washington in May 1940, during which he conferred with Colonel Fitz at the War Department, Dean Diehl reported to the medical school that until a national emergency should require the mobilization of the general hospital, the members of the professional staff would not be required to attend summer camp, ordinarily required of members of reserve units. The general hospital should be staffed with people who could be spared from teaching in the medical school, because in the event of war, the War Department wanted the medical schools to continue to train physicians. If war broke out, medical students in the United States Army Reserve would be assigned to continue in medical school, and all medical students except freshman, whether in the reserve or not, would be required to continue in medical school. Dean Diehl suggested to the War Department that freshman medical students and the best of the premedical students should remain in school as well. The War Department said that at the request of the medical school members of the medical faculty who already held commissions in the reserve might be transferred to the 26th General Hospital.

The administrative committee decided to write to the faculty to ask for volunteers for the 26th General Hospital and Chauncey McKinley, Leo Rigler, and Owen Wangensteen were appointed a committee to work with Dean Diehl in organizing the unit.[2]

In September 1940 Dean Diehl announced that the recently passed Selective Service Act postponed military service for all college and university students through the academic year 1940–41, but so far no special provision had been made to defer medical students until their courses were completed. The War Department estimated that during the coming year 8,000 physicians would be needed in the armed forces, whereas there were then only 1,000 physicians available in the regular Army and the National Guard. The War Department estimated, therefore, that during the coming year they would have to call up 7,000 of the 15,000 members of the Medical Reserve Corps. Dean Diehl said also that during a recent visit to Washington he had learned that the surgeon general planned to increase the staff of the 26th General Hospital from forty-five to seventy-three physicians, and that he had transferred fifteen members of the faculty holding reserve commissions to the 26th General Hospital.[3]

On 1 October 1940 Dean Diehl notified those members of the faculty who had been selected to form the staff of the 26th General Hospital. Such faculty members who were not already reserve officers then applied for commissions in the Medical Reserve Corps and they underwent physical examinations. During February and March 1941 they received official letters of appointment from the adjutant general's office. Lieutenant Colonel L. Haynes Fowler, chief of the surgical service, was appointed acting director of the hospital until a commanding officer was appointed.

Shortly after the organization of the 26th General Hospital was announced, nurses also began to apply for appointment to the staff. Nurses who were already enrolled in the Red Cross Nursing Service could request transfer to the hospital, and those who were enrolling in the service for the first time could also request assignment directly to the hospital. On 2 January 1941 the School of Nursing recommended Miss Cecilia Hauge to be chief nurse for the 26th General Hospital, and their recommendation was approved by Dean Diehl and by the surgeon general. Cecilia Hauge then became responsible for all appointments to the nursing staff. Early in 1941 appointments to the professional staff of the 26th General Hospital were completed, but the staff remained at their posts in the university hospital to await events.

A few days after the attack on Pearl Harbor on 7 December 1941, all of the officers of the 26th General Hospital were ordered to report to Fort Snelling for their final physical examinations. At the station hospital many of the examining physicians were graduates of the medical school who subjected their former teachers to a little gentle ragging, but most of the officers were found to be physically fit for duty. In mid-January, Dean Diehl and Lieutenant Colonel Fowler were notified that probably within a few weeks the 26th General Hospital would be ordered to active duty at Fort Sill, Oklahoma. The orders to report to Fort Sill came on 1 February, and the officers were notified that they would be ordered to active duty on 15 February. On 10 February the medical faculty held a farewell banquet attended by a thousand persons at the University of Minnesota Union for the officers and nurses of the 26th General Hospital. Mrs. Arthur A. Law, widow of the director of Base Hospital No. 26 in World War I, and her daughter presented the 26th General Hospital with a large United States flag, and Dr. S. Marx White presented the hospital with checks for almost $3,000 (equivalent to ten times that sum today), which had been contributed by former members of Base Hospital No. 26 and other friends. Major General Ellard A. Walsh, representing the state of Minnesota, spoke prophetically when he told the hospital staff: "There will be lots of mud that will turn to dust; there will be cold which will turn to heat; and you will never be satisfied. You have had poor meals, but there will be worse ones."[4]

On 15 February 1942 the officers of the 26th General Hospital boarded the train at Minneapolis to go to Fort Sill, and the nurses followed them on 26 February. At Fort Sill the officers and nurses lived in barracks, received immunizations, and worked to organize the various services for the hospital. A regular army officer, Colonel Floyd V. Kilgore of the Station Hospital at Fort Sill, was appointed commanding officer of the 26th General Hospital. The men of their medical detachment came largely from Fort Niagara, New York, so that the 26th General Hospital became a Minnesota-New York group. On 6 March thirty-eight Minnesota men, who had enlisted specifically for service with the 26th General Hospital, arrived from Fort Snelling. They were men with special skills as clerks, stenographers, cooks, bakers, barbers, pharmacists, and even embalmers.[5]

After more than seven months of training at Fort Sill, the 26th General Hospital departed by train on 12 October, and a week later they boarded ship at Staten Island to cross the Atlantic. During the first day at sea, their ship, the liner S. S. *Mariposa,* was part of a large convoy, but when they came on deck the second day they found themselves alone in the vastness of the ocean. After landing at Liverpool on 29 October, they went by train to Great Barr, near Birmingham, where they were quartered in an unoccupied housing development, called Pheasey Estates, and assigned to the Second Army Corps. When the Allies landed in North Africa on 8 November 1942, the United States Second Army Corps Headquarters in London planned to have the 26th General Hospital land at Oran on 24 November. The hospital's equipment and supplies, which had been assembled at Fort Sill and transported to Liverpool on the same ocean liner that had brought the officers and men, had been unloaded and stored at Liverpool. Early in November the equipment and supplies were sent by train to Glasgow where they were transferred to a ship sailing for North Africa. On 20 November Colonel Kilgore was notified that the 26th General Hospital's orders for movement were cancelled. Meanwhile, its equipment and supplies were on board ship at Glasgow, guarded by Sergeant Gasparich. Faithful to his orders to stay with the equipment, Sergeant Gasparich sailed to North Africa while the rest of the hospital personnel remained in England.

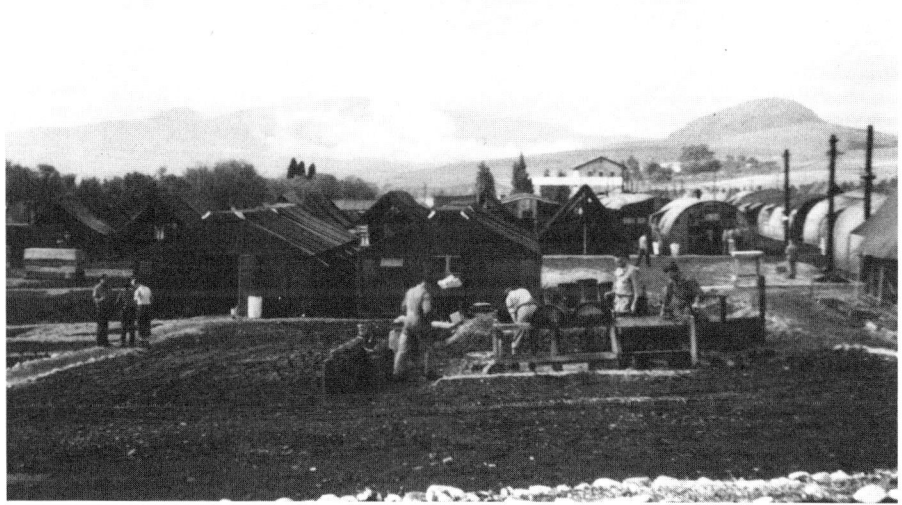

FIGURE 17:1   26th General Hospital, Assi Ameur, North Africa, 1943—under construction. Courtesy Mn U Archives.

The 26th General Hospital remained in England over the Christmas season, and on 24 December they helped to arrange a Christmas party for Birmingham children. Finally, on 20 January 1943 they left Pheasey Estates by train for Gourock, Scotland, where the next day they boarded ship, and on 1 February landed at Oran in Algeria. After a further delay the officers and men of the 26th General Hospital arrived on 27 March 1943 at Bizot, near Constantine, where they were to set up their hospital on an open, windswept hillside called Assi Ameur.

When the hospital personnel arrived at Assi Ameur, United States Army Engineers were already at work building roads and walkways, and pouring the concrete slabs that were to serve as floors for the ward tents and Nissen huts to house the hospital. Men of the medical detachment of the 26th General Hospital were assigned immediately to help the engineers, and during the next several weeks medics and engineers worked together with pick and shovel, digging and leveling, pushing wheelbarrows, and mixing concrete. They laid water pipes and sewage drains, and finally erected the Nissen huts and pitched the ward tents. When the Nissen huts and tents were in place, they were fitted with plumbing and electric wiring. The operating theaters, laboratories, x-ray equipment, clinics, and administrative offices were set up in the Nissen huts, barrel-shaped prefabricated structures of corrugated iron, while beds and cots were set up in the ward tents. Because most of the 26th General Hospital's equipment, which had arrived in North Africa in November 1942, had been requisitioned for use by other hospitals, the 26th General Hospital faced difficulties not unlike those that had confronted the old Base Hospital No. 26 in the summer of 1918. They had to build

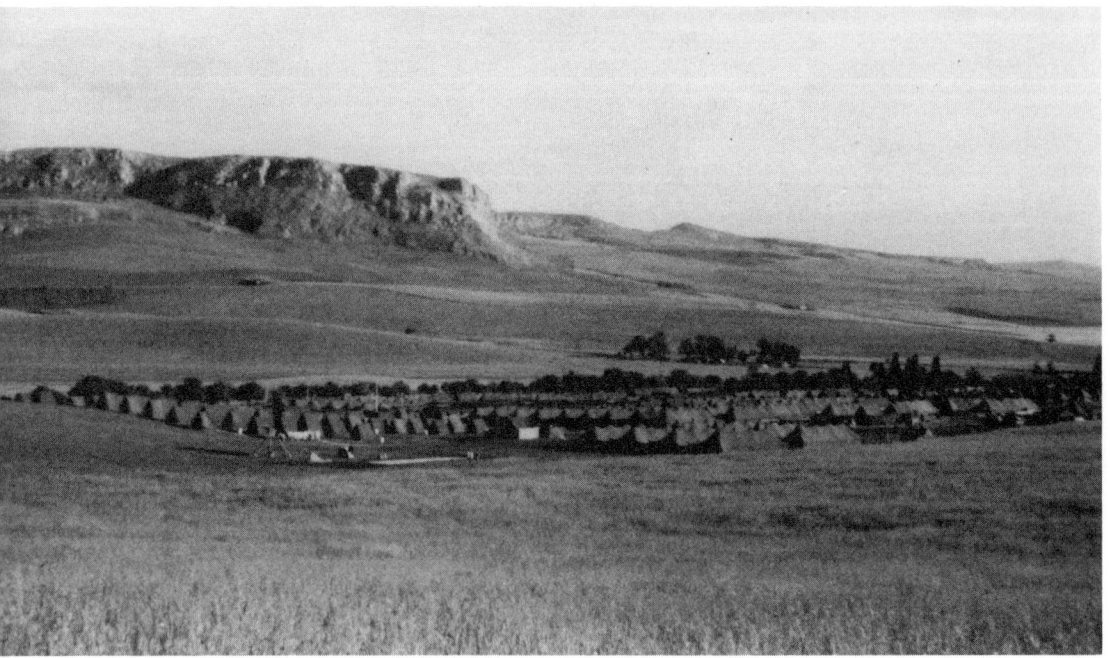

FIGURE 17:2   26th General Hospital, Assi Ameur—looking southeast. Courtesy Mn U Archives.

or improvise much of what they needed. The utilities section built partitions, cabinets, desks, laboratory benches, tables, and other furniture. They made sinks and tubs out of empty oil drums, and containers for surgical dressings from tin cans. They created a gasoline heating unit to provide hot water for the messes, and made other improvisations.

While they were building the hospital in April 1943, successive rains turned the camp site into a sea of mud. Because the surrounding country was intensely malarious—Bizot lay in the region where Alphonse Laveran had first observed malaria parasites in 1882—the 26th General Hospital launched a mosquito control program. The men systematically oiled all surface water in ditches, pools, and ponds within two to three kilometers of the hospital to prevent the breeding of mosquitoes. Toward the same end they also cut and burned swamp brush. As a result of these control measures, during the time that the hospital was at Bizot, it had only two cases of malaria among its personnel.

In less than one month, on 23 April, the 26th General Hospital was ready for patients, and three days later the first contingent of 110 patients arrived by ambulance convoy. Within another week the hospital had admitted 1,300 patients. They were men of the American Second Corps, which together with the British Eighth Army was engaged in battle with the German Army under General Rommel. The patients were pale, tired, and dirty. All were bandaged and many wore

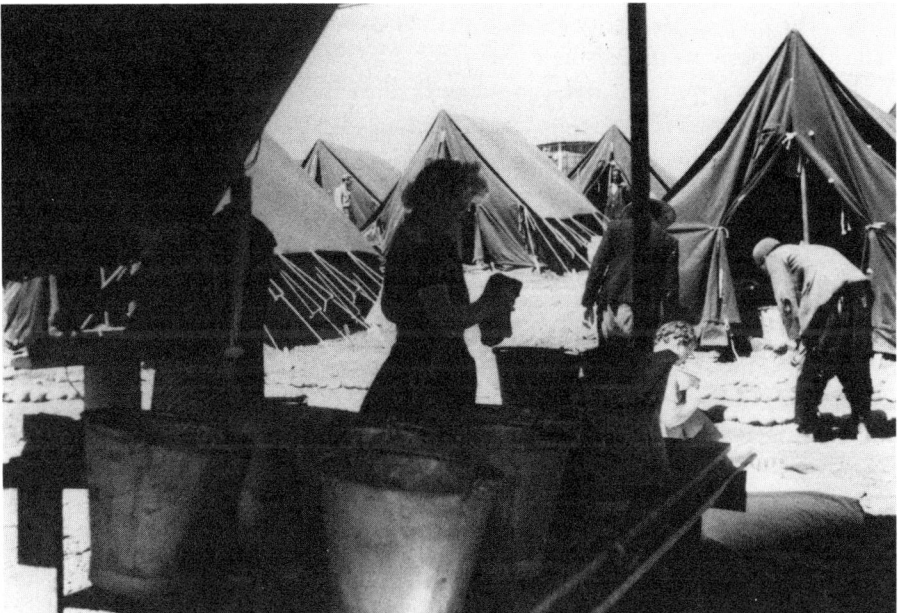

FIGURE 17:3 Nurses' laundry, 26th General Hospital, Assi Ameur.
Courtesy Mn U Archives.

splints or casts. They were mostly infantrymen who told of savage fighting in the mountains against a determined and resourceful enemy, who fought from prepared positions. As the wounded were brought into the receiving hut on litters, the expression of relief in their faces told of their many hours of suffering in the mud and cold.

Although most of the patients were surgical, the 26th General Hospital was desperately short of surgical equipment. The staff improvised Wangensteen suction sets out of bottles, tubing, and rubber stoppers. They made drapes and wrappers out of bed sheets. Always they fought against the ever present flies. They screened the Nissen huts to keep out flies and used fly spray and fly swatters constantly, but it was difficult to keep wounds free of maggots unless they kept the patient under a bar of mosquito netting.

On 18 May the hospital began to admit large numbers of wounded Italian and German prisoners of war. After the invasion of Sicily on 9 July 1943, many soldiers began to arrive at the 26th General Hospital with malaria, so that in addition to surgical patients there were now many medical patients. A few days after the United States Fifth Army landed in Italy on 9 September, patients began to arrive also from Italy. The morale of the hospital, strong from the beginning, remained high as the staff realized that they were overcoming all obstacles to provide a very high level of medical and surgical care to sick and wounded soldiers from the various fronts. The hospital mortality was only 0.132 percent, a very low rate for the treatment of seriously wounded men.

During the summer of 1943, in the peak of the fly season, many soldiers were brought into hospital suffering from diarrheal diseases, including the various forms of bacillary dysentery. Beginning in August men suffering from malaria began to arrive. Most were recurrent infections with Plasmodium vivax (benign tertian malaria) originating in North Africa or Sicily. Infectious hepatitis also became a severe problem in the late summer of 1943.

With the beginning of autumn, the 26th General Hospital gradually emptied as patients returned to duty, were evacuated to other hospitals, or were sent home. By October there was no longer need for a general hospital in the Constantine area. Bizot was too far from the Italian front to serve the troops there effectively, and since the fighting was over in North Africa, the 26th General Hospital needed to move to Italy. On 29 October 1943 Colonel Kilgore went to Italy to look for a new site for the hospital. At Bari on the Adriatic coast he was delighted to find a relatively new Italian military hospital, the Ospedale Militare Lorenzo Bonomo, built in 1936, which he was able to requisition for the 26th General Hospital. The harbor of Bari was a hive of activity with ships arriving daily with supplies for the British Eighth Army and the American Fifteenth Air Force. On 5 November, because it was anticipated that in Italy the 26th General Hospital would be caring mainly for airmen of the Fifteenth Air Force, it was transferred from the Second Army Corps to the Twelfth Air Force Service Command.

On 10 November 1943 most of the officers and men of the hospital left Bizot by train for Bizerte. The next day the remaining officers and the nurses set out for Bizerte by motor convoy. On 25 November, Thanksgiving Day, the officers and men landed at Taranto in Italy, especially thankful to be there after a rough voyage across the Mediterranean in British landing craft. The nurses arrived several days later by hospital ship. On 26 November the officers went on by train to Bari to begin the task of establishing the 26th General Hospital in Italy. Although the Ospedale Militare Lorenzo Bonomo was new, it had been neglected by the Italians and damaged before their departure. The building was extremely dirty and had to be thoroughly cleaned. Bedbugs and cockroaches had to be eliminated by treatment with a mixture of kerosene and cresol. The plumbing, which had been sabotaged, needed to be repaired. The most serious deficiency was a lack of hospital equipment.

On 2 December an enemy bombing attack on the harbor of Bari — one of the most destructive attacks of the war — sank the ship carrying equipment and supplies intended for the 26th General Hospital. There were many casualties, both among sailors on ships sunk or damaged in the harbor and among the people of the city. The explosion of a United States ship carrying mustard gas caused many mustard gas injuries. Two days after the attack, the 26th General Hospital, still lacking equipment and supplies, admitted its first patients at Bari, most of whom were mustard gas casualties. Because, without equipment, the hospital could care for only a limited number of patients, a number of anesthetists, technicians, and

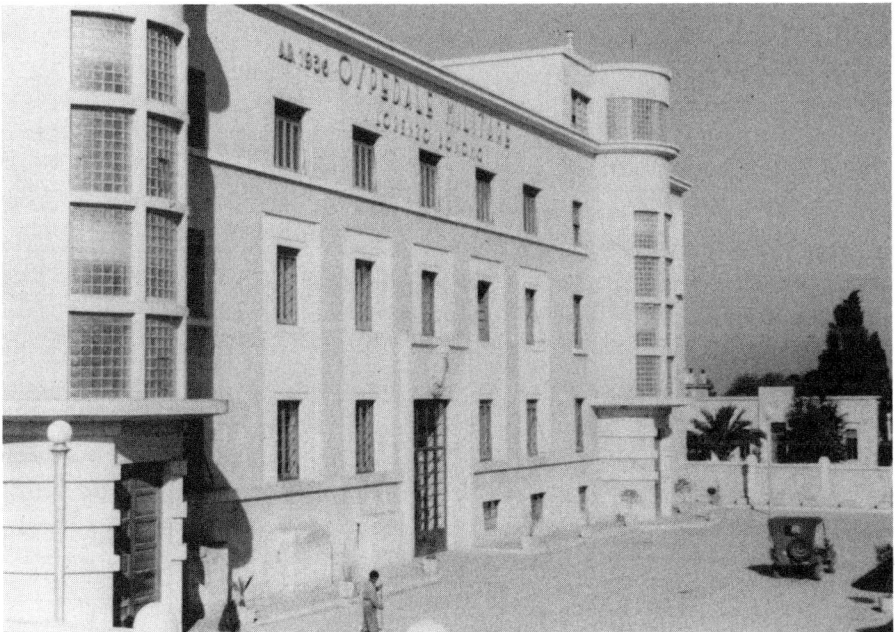

FIGURE 17:4 Home of the 26th General Hospital, Bari, Italy. Courtesy Mn U Archives.

nurses were detached to assist during the emergency at the 98th British General Hospital. Finally on 29 December a second ship carrying supplies for the 26th General Hospital was unloaded at Bari, and by 15 January 1944 the hospital was in full operation with a capacity of 1,000 beds.

At Bari the 26th General Hospital supplied hospital facilities for all American armed forces in the Adriatic region of Italy, but primarily it served the men of the Fifteenth Air Force. The hospital staff established close liaison with the flight surgeons of squadrons, groups, and wings of American air units in southern Italy so as to give the most prompt and effective treatment to airmen injured by antiaircraft fire during bombing raids or by fire from enemy aircraft. At the request of the United States Fifth Army, the hospital sent surgical teams to the front to help with the emergency care of the wounded at field hospitals. Sometimes, when the need for their assistance was over, the surgeons had difficulty finding transportation back to Bari. But in such cases they could usually get help from their friends in the air force.

As had been true in North Africa, so also in Italy, the 26th General Hospital provided a high level of medical and surgical care. During 1944 the hospital admitted 16,832 patients, with among them only 45 deaths for a mortality rate of 0.267 percent, and the staff performed more than 4,000 surgical operations. In April 1944, when cases of malaria began to appear among the hospital personnel, the men searched the area within a radius of one and a half miles of the hospital for breeding places of mosquitoes. In each of 180 villas, they found at least one mosquito breeding place and other breeding places in open water. A hospital team treated all open water with oil to kill mosquito larvae. They covered garbage dumps with earth and treated enclosed breeding places such as gutters and cisterns with kerosene once a week. As a result of their efforts, malaria practically disappeared from among the hospital personnel. In May 1944 they also began to use DDT to eliminate flies from the hospital.

In August 1944 when the United States Air Force began to evacuate Allied prisoners of war, most of them United States airmen from Roumania, the liberated prisoners were given physical examinations at the 26th General Hospital, and those needing medical attention were admitted to hospital. On 1 September the hospital staff examined more than a thousand liberated prisoners from Roumania, and on 17 September examined another 367 United States airmen rescued from Bulgaria. Altogether in 1944 they examined 4,262 liberated prisoners, and during the first six months of 1945, another 1,140.

In December 1944 the 26th General Hospital spent its third Christmas overseas. To help overcome the homesickness that both staff and patients felt, the hospital obtained from the 801st Engineers, who were operating a sawmill in the Italian mountains, enough Christmas trees to place one in every ward. The patients decorated the trees, making tinsel from metal chaff and ornaments from a great variety of objects. They cut stars and bells from tin cans and scraps of plexiglass, and painted empty penicillin bottles and broken Ping-Pong balls. From the staff of the University of Minnesota came many gifts, including a maroon and gold banner for the hospital.

On 1 June 1945 the 26th General Hospital, by then the oldest general hospital in the Mediterranean Theater in length of overseas service, received a Meritorious Unit Service Plaque. After summarizing the hospital's care of approximately 8,000 patients, and mentioning especially its service to liberated American prisoners of war "who were in dire need of proper medical attention," the plaque stated, "The outstanding services rendered to the sick and wounded members of the Armed Forces of the United States reflect the highest credit upon the personnel of the 26th General Hospital and the Medical Department of the Army of the United States."[6]

On 13 June many of the enlisted men and officers and nearly all of the nurses of the 26th General Hospital were transferred to the 45th General Hospital, and on 21 June the remaining staff of the 26th General Hospital left Bari to go home. The remaining patients, equipment, and supplies were transferred to the 45th General Hospital. Thus as an organizational unit, the 26th General Hospital was going home, but most of its personnel remained in Italy through the summer of 1945 and maintained the policies and practices of the 26th General Hospital. Late in October 1945 the last of the personnel of the 26th General Hospital returned to the United States.

NOTES

1. School of Medicine, Administrative Committee, Minutes, 9 April 1940.
2. School of Medicine, Administrative Committee, Minutes, 21 May 1940.
3. School of Medicine, Administrative Committee, Minutes, 23 September 1940.
4. Ellard A. Walsh in *Bull. Minn. med. Fdn,* 1942, *2* (no. 12), 8.
5. George S. Bergh and Reuben F. Erickson, eds., *A history of the Twenty-Sixth General Hospital,* p. 21. The account of the 26th General Hospital in this chapter is drawn largely from Bergh's and Erickson's *History*.
6. Ibid., p. 272.

CHAPTER 18

The Mayo Memorial Campaign and Campaigners

In 1939 the Doctors Mayo died, Charles H. Mayo on 26 May and William J. Mayo on 28 July. The deaths so close together of the two famous brothers, who had made the Mayo Clinic known throughout the world, evoked a feeling, widespread and deep, that some memorial, proportioned to the greatness of their contributions to Minnesota, ought to be created within the state. In September 1940, Governor Harold E. Stassen appointed a Mayo Memorial Commission of Minnesota citizens, with Senator Richardson of Rochester, Minnesota, as chairman, to consider the form that such a memorial to the Mayo brothers should take. Shortly thereafter, Dean Diehl wrote to the secretary of the commission, Dr. George Earl of St. Paul, that an appropriate memorial ought to " . . . occupy a central place and play an important role in medical education and medical research" in Minnesota for generations to come. Such a commemoration would be superfluous in Rochester, said Dean Diehl, where the Mayo Clinic, the Mayo Foundation, and the various hospitals together constituted so massive and permanent a memorial that any additional tribute there would be insignificant and meaningless.

> Clearly [wrote Dean Diehl] the most appropriate place for a memorial to these two great physicians of Minnesota is on the campus of the Medical School of the University to which they gave not only several millions of dollars but also years of unselfish service, "Doctor Will" as a member of the Board of Regents and "Doctor Charlie" as Professor of Surgery.[1]

As Dean Diehl wrote the above words he knew—no one could have known better—that the large endowment which the Mayo brothers had entrusted to the university for the Mayo Foundation did not benefit the university directly, and certainly not the medical school. The income of the Mayo Foundation could be used to support medical education and research only at Rochester, in effect at the Mayo Clinic. The millions of dollars which the Mayos had given were, therefore, in fact an endowment of the Mayo Clinic. Nevertheless, during their lifetimes the Mayos had consistently professed their devotion to the university, while managing to contribute almost nothing to its support or development. In fact, the twofold aim of the Mayos, at least since 1913, and probably from the time of William Mayo's election to the Board of Regents in 1907, was to restrict the development of the university hospital as a medical center, while at the same time attaching the prestige of the University of Minnesota to the Mayo Clinic. Now with unspoken and perhaps unconscious irony, Dean Diehl was to use the image of unselfish devotion to the university, which the Mayos had projected during their lifetimes, to accomplish a purpose that in life they did their utmost to prevent—namely, the large scale development of the medical school as a clinical and research center. As a memorial " . . . that would keep the name of these two great men, their accomplishments and their ideals, constantly before the future generations of students . . . ," Dean Diehl suggested that there might be built a Mayo memorial building for medical research, to be located within the quadrangle formed by the university hospitals. The building might house laboratories for the various clinical departments of the medical school and for the Departments of Pathology and Bacteriology. Such a building would be appropriate because the great genius of the Doctors Mayo, said Dean Diehl, lay in the successful application of advances in the medical sciences to the practical art of medicine. As alternatives to a Mayo memorial building, Dean Diehl suggested that the commission might also consider a Mayo endowment fund for medical research, a Mayo memorial medical library at the university, a loan fund for medical students, or endowed professorships, but his deepest desire was for a large building for medical research.[2]

There had been no expansion of the university hospitals since 1929, and the medical school was housed in the Institute of Anatomy and Millard Hall, both completed in 1912, twenty-eight years before. By 1940 the basic science departments of the medical school were extremely crowded, and the space for clinical research laboratories severely limited.

Dean Diehl discussed the proposal both with President Guy Stanton Ford and with Dr. Donald C. Balfour, director of the Mayo Foundation, who, as Dr. Will Mayo's son-in-law, could speak for the Mayo family. Ford immediately threw his support behind the idea.[3] Both he and Balfour agreed that a Mayo memorial building on the medical campus of the university would be a fitting memorial to the Doctors Mayo. In January 1941 Dean Diehl wrote again to Dr. Earl to urge a Mayo memorial building at the university. "I can think of nothing more appropriate," wrote Dean Diehl, "to keep alive the memory of two men who devoted their own lives unselfishly, as did Doctor 'Will' and Doctor 'Charlie,' to the improvement of medical service through better medical education and medical research."[4]

The first meeting of the Mayo Memorial Commission, attended by Mrs. Charles H. Mayo and members of the Mayo Clinic, was held at Rochester on 1 February 1941. Representatives of the clinic, including Dr. Balfour, said that since the Doctors Mayo always looked to the future of medicine, the most fitting memorial would be one that would contribute to the advancement of medicine.

Dean Diehl urged his suggestion for a building for medical research at the university.[5] Donald J. Cowling, president of Carleton College at Northfield, Minnesota, was appointed chairman of a planning committee to study proposals for a suitable memorial.

Dr. Cowling suggested that the memorial might take the form of an institute for medical research and medical education in one of the South American countries, preferably Argentina, to be administered jointly by a university in the country concerned and the University of Minnesota. Dean Diehl, who knew that the state of Minnesota was unable or unwilling to support adequately its own medical school, must have been startled at the thought of the state's undertaking to create an entirely new medical research institution in a foreign country. Cowling's suggestion showed also how little acquainted he was in 1941 with the problems confronting the medical school. Dean Diehl pointed out that the cost of a medical research institute would be prohibitive. For a fraction of the amount the state could create at the University of Minnesota a memorial to the Mayos, "which," said Dean Diehl, "for all time would assure Minnesota of a place of leadership in scientific medicine and medical education." After pointing out further difficulties in Cowling's South American scheme, Diehl added: "No memorial could be so appropriate nor so permanent as to have on the University Campus a Mayo Memorial Institute of such distinction that students, scholars and scientists, not only from South America, but from all over the world would come here to study."[6] Cowling was persuaded, reluctantly but completely. He asked Diehl to send more details about the proposed building, how it would be used, and how much it might cost.[7] A few days later he invited Diehl to present his ideas to a meeting of the planning committee of the Mayo Memorial Commission.[8]

Dean Diehl's initial proposal for a Mayo memorial building was a distinctly monumental building to be placed in the center of the university hospital quadrangle, rising one or two stories above the hospital buildings and possibly surmounted by a carillon tower. The building would contain the research laboratories for the various clinical departments and laboratories for bacteriology and pathology. It would contain a pathological museum, an auditorium large enough to assemble the whole medical student body, and possibly new surgical operating rooms. He estimated its cost at $500,000 to $600,000. Dean Diehl suggested also that the medical faculty could make excellent use of an endowment that would provide $50,000 to $100,000 annually to support medical research.[9]

At the meeting on 15 April, Dean Diehl evidently succeeded in winning over the planning committee, because three days later the Board of Regents decided to have the university architect prepare sketches for the proposed Mayo building to be presented to a meeting of the full Mayo Memorial Commission on 15 May.[10] At that meeting the commission voted unanimously and enthusiastically to raise a fund of not less than $1 million to erect a Mayo memorial building at the university and to provide an endowment for medical research.[11]

In the enthusiasm of that spring day in 1941, who could imagine that nearly fourteen years, two wars, and a galloping inflation would have to be endured before the Mayo Memorial tower would appear on the campus skyline. By foresight and tenacity, Dean Diehl had succeeded in gaining the proposed Mayo memorial for the medical school, but it would remain an empty victory until the funds to create the memorial were actually raised. In the autumn the University of Minnesota Press published *The Doctors Mayo* by Helen Clapesattle, a book that proved an immediate and sensational success; 20,000 copies were printed before publication and a second printing of 20,000 copies was soon required. Clapesattle portrayed the Mayo brothers as selfless physicians and described the rise of the Mayo Clinic to world fame. The Mayo brothers were the most famous Minnesotans of their time, and Clapesattle presented a fascinating account of their character and achievements. Her book increased the enthusiasm for a suitable memorial to the Mayo brothers. Nevertheless, Senator Richardson called no further meetings of the Memorial Commission, and on 16 October Harold Diehl wrote to Donald Balfour to ask how they might stir the commission to action.[12]

Part of the reason for delay may have been that members of the Mayo Memorial Commission and university officials thought that the Mayo Clinic or Mayo Properties Association would themselves wish to contribute a large part, if not the whole, of the proposed memorial. Guy Stanton Ford thought so, but his expectations were disappointed.[13] Ford, who had resigned as president of the University of Minnesota to go to the American Historical Association at Washington, D. C., wrote Diehl that although the time might not be right for a fund-raising campaign, they should go ahead anyway.

After the entry of the United States into World War II in December 1941, plans for the Mayo memorial were suspended. Diehl and Cowling, who were friends and, during the summer, neighbors at their cottages on Starr Island in Cass Lake, continued to discuss the project at intervals. In 1943 after Senator Richardson had failed for more than two years to call a meeting of the Mayo Memorial Commission, they decided it was dead so far as the original commission was concerned.[14] At Dean Diehl's request, Dr. Cowling presented the problem to Governor Stassen. The governor agreed that the only way to revive the enterprise would be to discharge the existing commission, which he was willing to do provided Dr. Cowling would serve as chairman of the new committee.[15] Cowling agreed, with the stipulations that he be allowed to nominate other members of the committee, and that the new committee should be established by action of the Minnesota legislature. He undertook the task because he hoped that, by helping the university, he would strengthen relations between the university and the state's private colleges. In April 1943, at the request of Governor Stassen, the Minnesota legislature passed a resolution creating a Committee of Founders of the Mayo Memorial, and immediately Governor Stassen appointed Donald J. Cowling chairman.[16] From long experience as a college president, Cowling was thoroughly familiar with the social, cultural, political, and financial forces active in the life of the United States, and especially in the state of Minnesota. The committee had eighteen members, three from the House of Representatives, three from the Senate, and additional members to be appointed by Governor Stassen. The last group

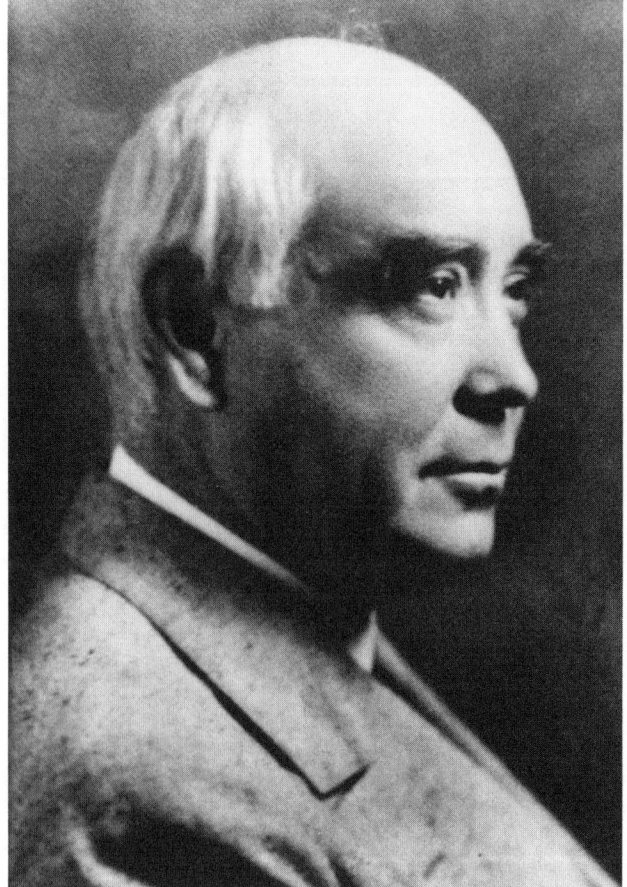

FIGURE 18:1   Donald J. Cowling, circa 1945. Courtesy Mn U Archives.

would include such prominent Minnesotans as Mrs. George Chase Christian, Jay C. Hormel of the Hormel meat packing company at Austin, James Ford Bell of General Mills, Archbishop John G. Murray, and Ignatius A. O'Shaughnessy, oil magnate of St. Paul.

Dr. Cowling immediately began to lay plans to seek gifts for the Mayo memorial. Since the memorial was to be a building on the university campus, the Board of Regents expressed formally to Dr. Cowling their appreciation that he had undertaken to bring the Mayo memorial into being.[17] Mrs. W. J. Mayo gave her personal support, and the staff of the Mayo Clinic and the faculty of the Mayo Foundation also expressed their approval and offered their support.[18]

In the spring of 1943, when the legislature was about to create the Mayo memorial committee, the trustees of the Mayo Properties Association told Dean Diehl informally that they were interested in supporting work in public health at the medical school. They suggested that they might endow a Mayo professorship of public health and provide funds to create a school of public health.[19] Dr. Gaylord Anderson, professor of medicine and public health, was then in Washington for the duration of the war as director of medical intelligence in the surgeon general's office, but Dean Diehl was looking ahead to the development of public health teaching at Minnesota after the war. Such a school would provide a much needed regional training center in public health for a vast area in the north central United States. Once established, it might also attract financial support from the Rockefeller Foundation, which focused much of its work on public health.[20] In December 1943 the Mayo Properties Association made a gift to the university of $500,000 to endow a school of public health, and the Board of Regents changed the status of the Department of Preventive Medicine and Public Health to that of the School of Public Health.[21]

In April 1944 the university submitted a request to the Rockefeller Foundation for a grant of $500,000 to erect a building for the School of Public Health, but the request was turned down.[22] Regent James Ford Bell, who accompanied Dean Diehl to New York City, said that Dr. Diehl made "a marvellous presentation." Bell commented bitterly: "I don't think these people have an appreciation of the needs of our prairie country and the isolated conditions compared with those in places where they have seen fit to center their efforts and which already enjoy unusual facilities."[23] While the request to the Rockefeller Foundation was pending, Dean Diehl wished to keep the School of Public Health separate from the Mayo memorial, but after the Rockefeller request was turned down, public health necessarily became part of the Mayo memorial.

Meanwhile, on 20 December 1943 Dr. Cowling came to the university to spend most of the day looking around the medical school and the university hospital, so that he might become familiar with the needs that the proposed Mayo memorial building might be expected to meet. He had lunch at the Campus Club with President Coffey, Dean Diehl, and other university officials. Their goal was to raise $1 million, but Dr. Cowling thought that they should secure at least $400,000 in pledges privately from large donors before they launched a public campaign. Dr. Cowling said that the campaign would require a full-time executive secretary in addition to the volunteer efforts of himself and other members of the committee.[24] Early in 1944 Dr. Cowling obtained the help of Byron W. Shimp, director of the Minnesota War Service Fund (the U.S.O. fund-raising organization), who had an office in the Northwestern Bank Building in Minneapolis. Dr. Cowling had known Byron Shimp since 1922, when Shimp had helped to direct a fund drive for Carleton College. Mr. Shimp said that he would need two assistants and funds for office expenses and travel in connection with the campaign, and Dean Diehl undertook to obtain funds to pay such expenses from the Minnesota Medical Foundation.[25] The foundation granted $1,000 to get the campaign started. By April Dr. Cowling had settled on eleven persons to be added to the Committee of Founders, who were then appointed by Governor Stassen's successor, Governor Edward J. Thye, bringing the total membership of the committee to eighteen. While Dr. Cowling was getting a fund-raising campaign organized, Dean Diehl was working with the heads of departments in the medical school on their detailed needs, and it was already clear that the building as first conceived was too small. The architects estimated that a building of sufficient size would cost $1,250,000, with at least $250,000 needed for equipment.[26] This was the earliest realization that both the scale of planning and estimates of the cost of the Mayo memorial might be too small.

On 16 June the Committee of Founders of the Mayo Memorial met formally at the Minneapolis Club for permanent organization. The committee decided to seek $1.5 million for a building for medical education and research to be located on the medical school campus. When the committee met next on 2 October, estimates of the cost of the proposed Mayo memorial building had risen from $1.5 to $2.1 million.[27] Dr. Cowling apparently doubted that the committee could raise such a large sum entirely from gifts, so on 9 November the Committee of Founders decided to ask the legislature to appropriate $1 million for the Mayo memorial on condition that the committee raise another $1 million from voluntary contributions, which they hoped to do by July 1945.[28] A member of the committee, Jay C. Hormel of Austin, Minnesota, undertook to approach businessmen in outstate areas to ask them to form local committees to solicit gifts for the memorial from business interests.

At the beginning of 1945, Byron Shimp obtained a six-month leave of absence from the Minnesota War Service Fund to work full time as director of fund raising for the Mayo memorial. He prepared a booklet to describe the facilities for medical research and medical education to be included in the building. As the primary intent of the Mayo memorial, namely, to serve the needs of medical research and medical education, emerged more clearly, the leading members of the Mayo Foundation were won over to its support.[29] Dr. Cowling arranged to have bills introduced into the Minnesota House and Senate during the 1945 session to appropriate $1 million for the Mayo memorial, on condition that an equal amount be raised by private contributions.[30] He also set up fund-raising committees in each of the larger cities of Minnesota. By March 1945 the Minneapolis committee, which had a goal of $500,000, had already raised $200,000. The St. Paul committee undertook to raise $200,000 and Duluth $100,000. The State Medical Association undertook to organize committees in the various counties of the state with a total goal of $100,000. Other committees were organized in large cities throughout the United States to seek special gifts, without attempting any general solicitation.[31]

The campaign for the Mayo memorial was sailing along smoothly when suddenly and unexpectedly it struck a rock. On Friday, 23 March, the Finance Committee of the Minnesota Senate tabled the bill to provide a $1 million appropriation for the Mayo memorial, even though the Minnesota House had passed the appropriation for the Mayo memorial unanimously. Dr. Cowling was appalled at the Senate Finance Committee's action, because he realized that the failure of the Minnesota legislature to provide the matching appropriation would effectively kill the campaign for gifts to the Mayo memorial. The next morning, Saturday, much discouraged, he went to see Governor Edward J. Thye at his office in the state Capitol and told the governor that the Mayo memorial had failed. Without a state appropriation there was no hope of obtaining private contributions, and Dr. Cowling thought that he should resign as chairman of the Committee of Founders. Governor Thye, saying that he did not believe all was yet lost, called Senator Oscar Swenson, a senior member of the Senate, and asked him to come to his office.[32] Senator Swenson came, and the three men talked the matter over. Senator Swenson had forgotten that the legislature had itself created the Committee of Founders of the Mayo Memorial two years before. He thought that the committee was merely a private group coming with a request to the legislature. Dr. Cowling suggested that the mass resignation of the Committee of Founders would evoke a violent public reaction, and would be seen as an attempt by the senators to reverse the policies of former Governor Stassen. The Mayo memorial campaign had received an unusual amount of publicity outside Minnesota, including an article in *Collier's* magazine, a type of publicity given ordinarily only to such national groups as the War Service Fund or the Red Cross. If the legislature were to repudiate its commitment to the Mayo memorial of only two years before, it would make Minnesota the laughing stock of the whole country.

The last point struck home. Donald Cowling had not led Carleton College through thirty-seven years for nothing. He knew the people of the state. He knew, too, the men with whom he was duelling, quietly but tensely, in the governor's office that morning. Uneasily aware that their actions might frequently border on the absurd, the senators did not wish to expose themselves, or the state, to ridicule. Senator Swenson agreed that the Finance Committee would be called back into session, and that he would try to have the committee reconsider its action.

Dr. Cowling did not rest. On Monday morning he wrote to another member of the Senate Finance Committee, A. J. Rockne, senator from Goodhue County, who over many years had time and time again reduced or obstructed appropriations for the university. In a handwritten letter Senator Rockne replied: ". . . our tax levy will be thirteen mills, which will be the greatest levy ever made in the State of Minnesota . . . . From the demand that is being made by the University and other committees like yours, it appears to me as tho we will soon throw the state and nation into bankruptcy, and all we will have left is a lot of buildings . . . ." Nevertheless, Senator Rockne concluded by expressing his great admiration for the Mayo brothers whom, he said, he knew very well—especially Will Mayo.[33] Dr. Cowling replied in a long, polite, but very firm letter. He noted that the concurrent resolution establishing the memorial committee two years before had passed both the House and the Senate unanimously, which meant that both Senator Rockne and Senator Swenson must have voted for it. The committee included three members of the House and three from the Senate, as well as the governor, and the members from the legislature had participated actively in establishing the goal of $2 million for the Mayo memorial. Dr. Cowling wrote:

> We started our part of the campaign on January 1, believing that the members of the Senate and House would be pleased if we could show a substantial amount of private contributions before the Legislature made its appropriation. The response so far on the part of the citizens of Minnesota has been wonderful. I have never had anything to do with any project which has made such a universal appeal. We have secured gifts amounting to about $325,000, most of it already paid in cash.[34]

Nevertheless, wrote Cowling, a decision by the Senate Finance Committee to postpone any action on an appropriation for the Mayo memorial would kill the campaign for private contributions. He described the acute need for enlarged facilities for medical research at the university and concluded by pointing out that the Senate Finance Committee ought to be glad to obtain such facilities at half their cost. Without the Mayo memorial campaign, the state would have to pay the whole.

After unrelenting pressure from Dr. Cowling, Governor Thye, and others, the Senate Finance Committee in late April 1945 approved an appropriation of $750,000 for the Mayo memorial on condition that an equal sum was to be raised by voluntary contributions. At the same time, legislators friendly to the Mayo memorial assured Dr. Cowling that an additional appropriation of $250,000 could probably be obtained at a later session of the legislature. The Committee of Founders pressed ahead with their campaign for $1 million in contributions. Much of the enthusiasm which had sustained the campaign during the winter had been lost as a result of the wrangle with the Senate Finance Committee, but Dr. Cowling sought to revive morale by a large public dinner at Coffman Memorial Union on 28 May at which the surgeon general of the navy, Admiral Ross T. McIntire, spoke. By the end of June 1945, $704,000 had been contributed to the Mayo memorial fund.[35] Early in July Dr. Cowling sent out a message to his campaign workers: "We have passed $800,000!!! Less than $200,000 to go."[36]

In September 1945 Dr. Cowling retired as president of Carleton College and moved from Northfield to St. Paul. He began to devote his full time to the Mayo memorial campaign, taking the place of Byron Shimp who moved to New York City to work in fund-raising for the National Association of Manufacturers. The campaign was carried on from the same small, two-room office in the Northwestern Bank Building in Minneapolis.[37] That summer James Lewis Morrill came from the University of Wyoming to become eighth president of the University of Minnesota. A thoughtful, liberal-minded, and kindly man, Morrill was confronted almost immediately with the immense problems created by the thousands of students returning to the university from the armed services after the war.

By September 1945 contributions to the Mayo memorial fund exceeded $932,000, and after expenses had been deducted, there was together with the legislative appropriation approximately $1,650,000 available toward the building.[38] Dr. Cowling thought that it was time to prepare detailed plans and specifications for the building, and on 22 September the Board of Regents authorized the architects to prepare plans.[39] Even that fall, Dr. Cowling thought that the earlier architect's estimates of $2.1 million would be too small.[40] Accordingly, the

Committee of Founders decided to increase their goal from $1 million to $1,250,000. By late December gifts to the fund had risen to $1,040,000 so that the original goal had already been exceeded.[41]

When the memorial committee began late in 1945 to consider detailed plans for the Mayo building, they were faced with the medical school's acute need for increased space for all its activities. The teaching and research activities of the medical school had grown greatly. Although there were more faculty and more students in the medical school, the school continued to carry on most of its teaching and research, including clinical research, in the Institute of Anatomy and Millard Hall. Splendid as those buildings had been when erected in 1912, by 1945 they were severely crowded and inadequate. The medical school was also planning new buildings for the School of Public Health and for the medical library, which was then housed in the university library building, two blocks away from the medical school and university hospital. The Minnesota division of the American Cancer Society also wished to put up a building for a cancer research institute in connection with the medical school. In the circumstances the Board of Regents asked the Chicago architectural firm of Schmidt, Garden & Erickson, who were experienced in hospital design, to review the plans for the Mayo memorial and other buildings contemplated. After thorough study this firm recommended that for economy and greater convenience the buildings proposed for the School of Public Health, the medical library, and the cancer research institute should all be incorporated into the Mayo memorial building. They developed a plan for a main nineteen-story building that would be connected by six-story wings to the existing units of the university hospitals. The auditorium would be in a separate but attached building, and a large underground garage was planned beneath the forecourt of the main Mayo memorial building. The total estimated cost was $5 million—$3 million for the Mayo memorial and auditorium, and $2 million for the other connected buildings.

In May 1946, before the new plans for the Mayo memorial were complete but when it was already clear that the cost would be more than double previous estimates, Dr. Cowling made a trip east in search of additional contributions. At New York City, Byron Shimp arranged various interviews for him. Mr. Shimp had already obtained a gift of $10,000 from a New York physician, Emanuel Libman, with whom Dr. Cowling had a pleasant visit. He also had satisfactory interviews with Mr. Arch Davis of the International Business Machines Corporation, who promised a further contribution to the Mayo memorial, and with Whitelaw Reid, publisher of the *New York Herald Tribune*. This last interview resulted in an editorial in the *Herald Tribune* on 9 May in support of the Mayo memorial campaign.[42]

After the revised estimates for the Mayo memorial had been obtained and studied, Dr. Cowling called a meeting of the Committee of Founders of the Mayo Memorial for 20 December 1946, at which time he recommended that the committee ask the legislature for a further appropriation of $750,000, raising the total state appropriation to $1.5 million. The committee should then undertake to raise an equal sum from private contributions. Since gifts for the Mayo memorial had already reached $1,164,000, the committee would have to raise an additional $336,000.[43] The critical decision that the Committee of Founders had to make was whether to request another $750,000 from the Minnesota legislature. The committee decided to do so, and Dr. Cowling wrote immediately both to Governor Thye and to Governor-elect Luther W. Youngdahl asking them to support the additional appropriation.[44] Dr. Cowling also went to see Governor-elect Youngdahl, who assured him of his support.

On 22 April 1947 the legislature passed the further appropriation of $750,000 for the Mayo memorial. In anticipation, Dr. Cowling had already arranged to have Byron Shimp come out to Minneapolis to direct the campaign for the approximately $350,000 needed in voluntary contributions, and by 25 April Mr. Shimp was at work. He and Dr. Cowling did not think that it would be easy to raise the additional funds because in the 1945 campaign they had canvassed all possible sources of gifts. In July, Dr. Cowling obtained one gift of $50,000, but otherwise the campaign went slowly. A year later, in August 1948, they were still $92,600 short of the $1.5 million goal, and during the first nine months of 1948 the Mayo memorial fund received only $27,000.[45] In May 1947 the university requested $1,250,000 from the federal government in Hill-Burton Construction Act funds to make up the total of $5 million required for the building, and in October 1947 Dean Diehl and Dr. Cowling attended a meeting of the Governor's Advisory Council on Hospital Construction in Minnesota in support of the request. During the fall of 1947, however, the architects advised university officials that construction costs had risen another 15 percent since the new plans were developed the year before, and the cost of the Mayo memorial and related buildings would now be about $6 million.[46]

When the Committee of Founders met in December 1947 they realized that they would either have to secure much more money, or else cut drastically the whole plan for the Mayo memorial. The latter option had become for Dean Diehl and Dr. Cowling unthinkable, because it would inflict a devastating blow to the morale of the medical faculty. In 1947 the medical school was led by an extraordinary group of first-rate men, several of them internationally famous, and all occupying leading positions in their respective fields. Yet as Dean Diehl had pointed out repeatedly to the university administration, even the most eminent professors in the medical school were paid salaries far below those at other American medical schools. Most of the department heads had received more than one offer to move elsewhere to positions at much higher salaries, sometimes more than double what they were receiving at Minnesota. They had declined such offers out of loyalty to the medical school, and in the hope that both their salaries and the old and inadequate buildings in which they worked would soon improve. If plans for the Mayo memorial had to be cut drastically, hopes for improved facilities would be dashed for many departments, and the most able and brilliant members of the medical faculty might leave.

With building costs rising steadily from month to month during the postwar years, it became a desperate race to raise money before building costs got entirely beyond them. The architects had not yet prepared detailed plans for the proposed buildings so that the estimates of costs were very approximate. In November 1947, the Board of Regents decided that they must move ahead, and they authorized the architects to prepare plans and specifications for a Mayo memorial building not to cost more than the $5,126,000 available.[47] Unfortunately, buildings cannot be designed that way. Architects have to decide upon the size and layout of a building, then prepare detailed plans and specifications, and only when the plan and specifications are complete can they make accurate estimates of costs. During 1948 the architects, C. H. Johnston and Company of St. Paul, worked to prepare plans for the Mayo memorial, and the university anticipated that they would be ready by 1 December. With the intention of remaining within the cost limitations imposed by the Board of Regents, the architects planned for a seventeen-story building, but extended some of the lower floors to keep the total cubic footage space the same. In August 1948, the Committee of Founders were still $92,600 short of their $1.5 million goal, but Dr. Cowling hoped to complete the fund raising by the end of the year. At that time he anticipated that the committee would have to go back to the legislature at its next session to request an additional appropriation of at least $1.5 million.[48] In mid-1948, the architects provided a revised estimate of $6.9 million for the Mayo memorial building, which with other costs brought the total to just over $7 million. Dean Diehl and Dr. Cowling decided to apply for federal funds available under the Hill-Burton Act and late in the fall of 1948 the university received a promise of a federal grant of $1,250,000 for the Mayo memorial, bringing the available funds to more than $6 million.

In January 1949 when the university finally received from the architects completed estimates for the construction of the Mayo memorial, they were for almost $11 million.[49] Dean Diehl and Dr. Cowling were faced with a major crisis. The second campaign of 1947 had demonstrated that sources of private gifts for the Mayo memorial were almost exhausted. Similarly, while some additional funds might be obtained from the federal government, any such grants would fall far short of the amounts needed. The only possible source of help on the scale required was the Minnesota legislature. When the Committee of Founders met in January 1949, their only options were either to reduce the size of the Mayo memorial building drastically or to ask the legislature for an additional appropriation of $5.5 million, a sum more than three and a half times the combined appropriations of 1945 and 1947 previously obtained. Dr. Cowling said that at first the size of the request seemed almost breathtaking.[50] Fortunately, the legislative representatives on the Committee of Founders were willing to support the request, and in 1949 the mood of both House and Senate was different from what it had been in 1945, partly because of the effect of the Mayo memorial campaign in making the public aware of the needs of the medical school. Governor Youngdahl supported the request strongly, and legislators recognized that the request simply reflected the increase in building costs caused by inflation. Dr. Cowling

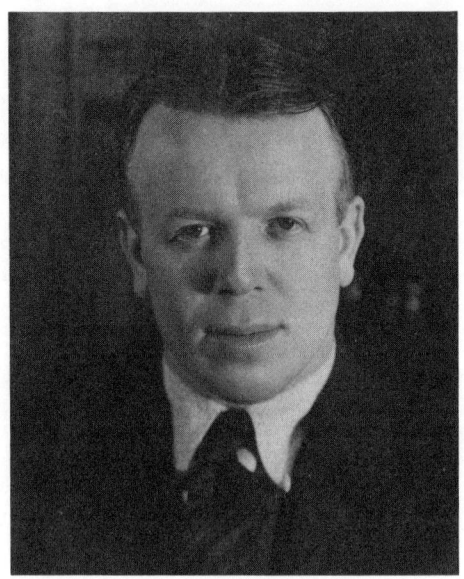

FIGURE 18:2 Raymond M. Amberg, 1930. Courtesy Mn U Archives.

did not fail to remind the governor and the legislators that for several years the university had been receiving over $1 million a year to support medical research and training projects, almost all of which came from outside the state. If the Mayo memorial building could be completed as planned, the members of the medical faculty who attracted such a steady flow of research funds would most likely remain in Minnesota.[51]

On 19 April 1949 the Minnesota Senate approved a $5.5 million appropriation for the Mayo memorial, the House having already passed the bill. Two days later President Morrill wrote to Dr. Cowling to thank him " . . . for a magnificent rescue from a situation which can only be regarded as desperate in the ongoing of the University's medical and scientific enterprise."[52] At the end of 1949 when Dr. Cowling was winding up the affairs of the Committee of Founders, President Morrill wrote to him again to express more fully his appreciation of all that Dr. Cowling had done, saying: "Not only good management of the gifts-campaign but also the strength of your prestige and influence in the State Legislature have made possible the realization of the Mayo Memorial."[53] The influence of the director of the university hospitals, Ray Amberg, who possessed the confidence of key legislators, played a critical role. Cigar in mouth, Amberg spent endless sessions at the state Capitol. He alone knew how to talk on a fraternal basis to the state legislators. The high respect accorded Dean Diehl was likewise important in obtaining a building appropriation of unprecedented size.[54] Perhaps, too, the leadership of President Morrill was an essential factor in the ultimate victory. Since his arrival at Minnesota in 1945, Morrill had won an ever-increasing measure of trust from both the faculty and the legislature. Morrill claimed nothing, giving

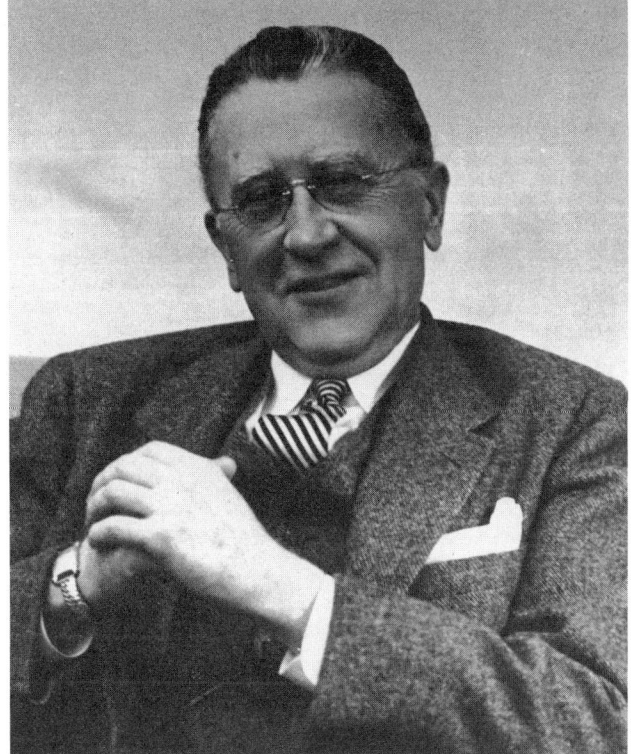

FIGURE 18:3 James L. Morrill, circa 1955. Courtesy Mn U Archives.

all credit for the success of the Mayo memorial to others, a fact which may itself be significant.[55] The mutual respect and trust which linked together all who worked for the Mayo memorial was essential in gaining the wholehearted support of the legislature.

During 1949 Dean Diehl obtained further grants of federal funds in the amount of $1,192,000 for the Mayo memorial to bring the total sum available to more than $12.2 million.[56] At the end of 1949, the work of the Committee of Founders finished, Dr. Cowling closed its office.

After the legislature made the $5.5 million appropriation in April 1949, the university authorized the preparation of plans for the full twenty-two stories of the Mayo memorial building, the original plans having included specifications for foundations and structure to carry twenty-two stories, even though they were drawn for only nineteen. Dean Diehl hoped that construction could begin in January 1950, but the architects, C. H. Johnston and Associates of St. Paul, were not ready. The university revised the schedule with construction planned to begin by 1 July 1950, but after several months the architects still did not have the plans for the whole building ready to be submitted for bids. The university revised the

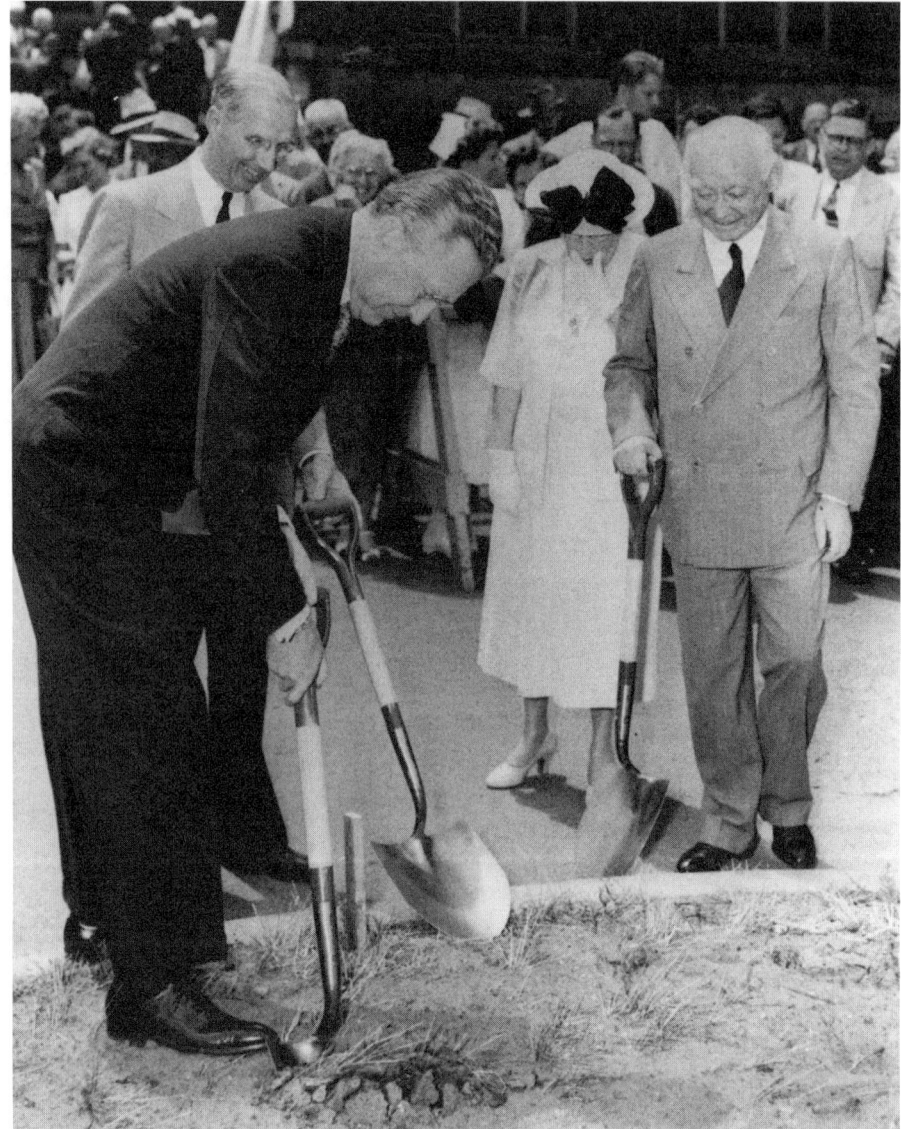

FIGURE 18:4 Ground-breaking for the Mayo Memorial, 5 July 1950. From left to right: President Morrill, Dean Diehl, Mrs. George Chase Christian, Dr. Cowling. Courtesy Mn U Archives.

schedule so that work on excavations and footings could begin in July 1950, while contracts for the superstructure were postponed. The delay by the architects proved disastrous. After the outbreak of the Korean conflict in June 1950, contractors' bids for construction jumped from 10 to 30 percent.[57] President Truman canceled construction of all Veterans' Administration hospitals that were not already under contract, shortages of structural steel and other building materials developed, and the prospect of realizing the Mayo memorial building, which the year before had seemed assured, was again imperiled. Nevertheless, on 5 July 1950 the university held a ground-breaking ceremony to begin excavation for the Mayo memorial, and on that occasion Dr. Cowling reviewed the ten-year history of efforts to achieve the memorial.[58]

While the foundations of the Mayo memorial were being laid that fall, the architects still had not completed the plans and specifications for the building itself. They had promised to have final drawings and specifications completed by 1 October, but, despite urgings from university officials, failed to meet successive deadlines for completion of portions of the work.[59] In December the university finally received the complete plans and specifications so that they could send them out for bids. When the bids came in on 2 March 1951, the lowest bid was approximately $3 million more than the funds available. After studying the project to see what might be omitted or postponed, Dean Diehl decided that they might omit funds allocated for equipment and for remodeling the existing university hospital. Yet after deducting those items, there was still a shortage of about $2.5 million. Again, the only possible source for such an amount was the legislature. Dr. Cowling immediately called a meeting of the Committee of Founders who decided to request a supplementary appropriation of $2.5 million from the legislature. Unfortunately, in 1951 the legislature proved recalcitrant. The House passed an appropriation bill, but in the Senate the session ended without any action on the request. In 1949 Dr. Cowling and other members of the Committee of Founders had assured the legislators that the $5.5 million that they were requesting at that time would be sufficient to complete the building, and that they would not be back for more money. In 1951 the legislators had difficulty in understanding why the Mayo memorial building had not been started two years before, when the money for it became available.[60]

When the legislature adjourned without acting on the requested appropriation, the university was confronted with a dilemma. Should they wait two years until the 1953 session of the legislature to repeat their request for a supplementary appropriation, or should they reduce their plans to bring the cost of the building within the funds available. Since the Mayo memorial project had been in contemplation for more than ten years, and the first fund-raising campaign had begun six years before, further delays would be heartbreaking, especially to the medical faculty. Dean Diehl acted promptly. After careful study, the university decided to reduce the size of the Mayo memorial building from twenty-two to fourteen stories. The loss of eight stories eliminated space for the medical library, cancer research, biophysics, histological and cytological chemistry, pathology, and a pathological museum. To reduce costs the architects also eliminated one elevator, and wherever possible substituted less expensive materials. The fourteenth floor would be left unfinished until funds became available to complete it. The revised plans were submitted for new bids which came within the funds available. The

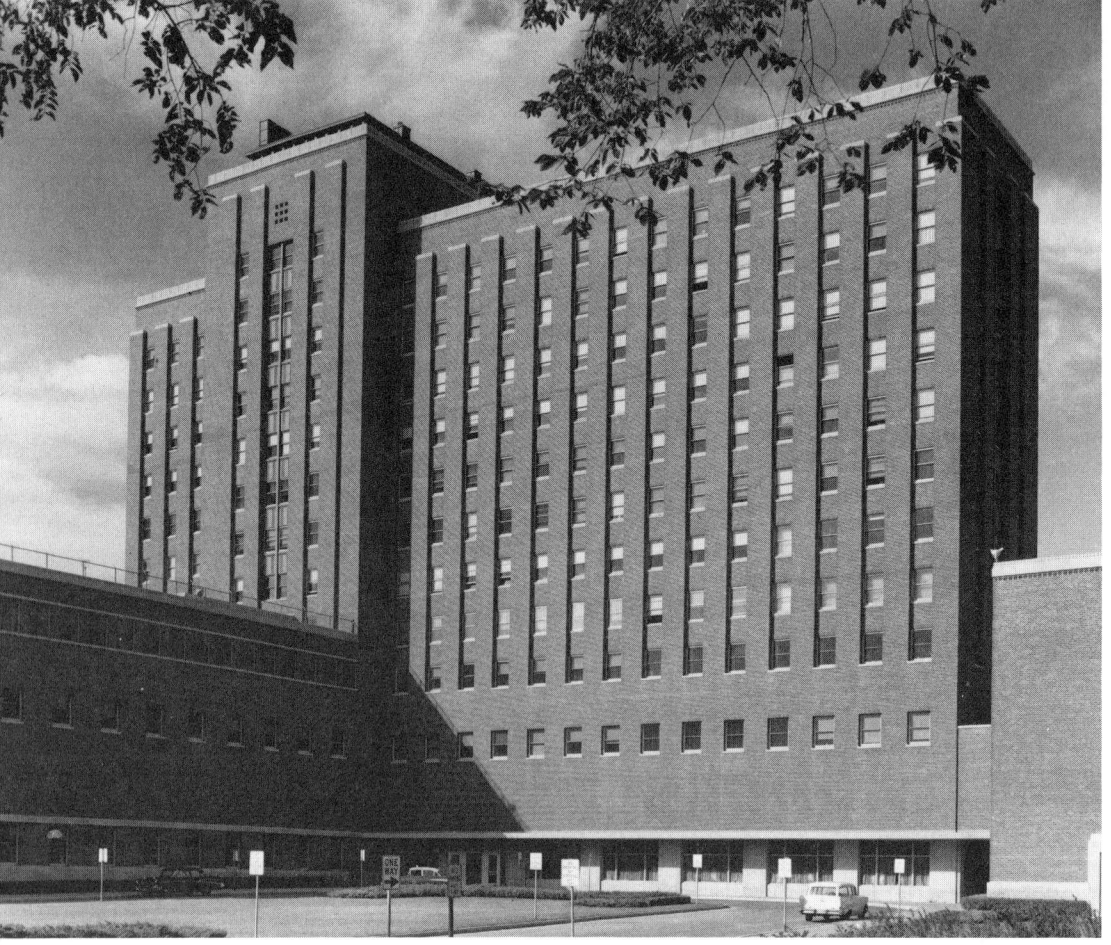

FIGURE 18:5 Mayo Memorial Building, 1955. Courtesy Mn U Archives.

contract was let and in September 1951 construction of the Mayo memorial resumed.

The Mayo Memorial Building was completed during the summer of 1954, and on 21 October the university dedicated the building in a day-long program during which a series of speakers discussed the promise of medical education and medical research in the years ahead. In the fourteen-story tower section of the Mayo Memorial and its three six-story wings there were facilities for 104 additional patients, 14 operating rooms, 2 floors for patient rehabilitation, medical research laboratories, the School of Public Health, and the Department of Bacteriology. In addition to operating rooms and clinical research laboratories, the Mayo Memorial Building contained the other central service units of the university hospital such as the diagnostic laboratories, blood bank, x-ray department, administrative offices, pharmacy, record rooms, central supply rooms, visitor's entrance, and main lobby of the hospital. Underground there were animal quarters and surgical research laboratories. In a distinct but connected building was the Mayo Memorial Auditorium with seating for 550 persons and two classrooms, each capable of holding 180 students. Beneath the auditorium was a two-level underground garage capable of holding 240 cars. Toward the cost of the Mayo Memorial Medical Center, the legislature had appropriated $7 million; $3,122,000 had come from federal funds; and private individuals and foundations had contributed $2,225,000.[61]

Apart from the Variety Club Heart Hospital, which was a separate and special unit of the university hospital, the Mayo Memorial Building was the first addition to the general facilities of the university hospitals since 1929, and the first addition to the facilities of the medical school since 1912. This great building complex was a memorial to the Mayo brothers, embodying their vision of the future promise of medicine, and that was sufficient. As President Morrill said at the dedication:

> Step by step, in more than a decade, the resources have been mobilized to make possible the Memorial, the building and its equipment. Steadily new sources of support have been recruited or have sprung up almost spontaneously in response to the appeal, and the potential, of this facility for the struggle against human suffering and the needless loss of life.[62]

Although in retrospect the Mayo Memorial Building might have seemed to have proceeded inevitably to its completion, Dean Diehl knew how often the project was on the brink of total failure. Until the end he did not take for granted that the Mayo Memorial would finally be realized. After the building was completed and his own office was established in the tower, he found it difficult to believe that the project was finally finished. "Even though we have been occupying and using it for sometime," said Dean Diehl in the fall of 1954, "I still feel like touching the walls to see whether they are real or whether they are a continuation of the dreams which we have had about this building for the past fifteen years."[63] The walls were real, and from the moment that the Mayo Memorial Building came into use, the operating rooms became scenes of extraordinary drama in the pioneering development of open heart surgery in Minnesota.

The Minnesota Medical Foundation[64]

In 1939 when the medical school celebrated its first half century, members of the Medical Alumni Association conceived the idea of establishing a medical foundation to advance the educational and research work of the medical school. At that time the Medical Alumni Association was a relatively small organization, containing only a fraction of the alumni. Many of the alumni were for various reasons unhappy with the medical school, or indifferent to it. In August 1939 the

Medical Alumni Association appointed a special committee under the chairmanship of Erling S. Platou, a Minneapolis pediatrician, to plan the creation of a medical foundation.[65] In a series of meetings through the fall of 1939, Dr. Platou's committee worked out the details of the proposed foundation. Although it would be devoted entirely to the interests of the medical school, the foundation would be incorporated separately from the university as a nonprofit tax-exempt foundation. Its management would be independent of the school. On 24 November 1939 the Medical Alumni Association called a meeting to organize the foundation, and seventy-three persons came. The assembled founders approved the articles of incorporation and bylaws submitted by the committee and elected officers. Erling S. Platou became the first president of the foundation.[66] Five days later when the articles of incorporation were filed with the Minnesota Secretary of State, the Minnesota Medical Foundation became a legal entity.

Early gifts to the foundation were mostly small, but Dr. Leo J. Madsen gave the then considerable sum of $1,000. With the threat of war then looming over the country, all gifts were invested in United States Defense Bonds. During 1940 the foundation enrolled 415 members and was entrusted with the administration of various funds given to the medical school for particular purposes. The entry of the United States into World War II in December 1941 slowed the growth of the foundation, and the urgent demands of wartime reduced gifts to a trickle. One part-time secretary in Dean Diehl's office was easily able to attend to all of the foundation's affairs. Nevertheless, by 1944 the foundation's finances had grown sufficiently that it was able to contribute $1,000 to launch the campaign for the Mayo memorial.

Erling Platou remained president of the foundation until 1949 when he was succeeded by Owen Wangensteen, who, like Dr. Platou, worked valiantly to increase the foundation's membership and to obtain gifts and bequests. That fall the foundation awarded its first scholarships to five medical students. In 1950 Dr. Wangensteen persuaded two laymen, Donald J. Cowling and Senator Gerald T. Mullin, both of whom had played leading parts in the Mayo memorial campaign, to accept election to the board of trustees of the foundation. Dr. Cowling remained an active trustee until 1963 and was instrumental in raising a substantial endowment to provide scholarships for medical students. In recognition of Dr. Cowling's long-time presidency of Carleton College, Cowling scholarships were awarded to medical students who were graduates of Minnesota's private liberal arts colleges.

In 1959 the foundation appointed its first full-time executive secretary, Eivind O. Hoff, Jr. Mr. Hoff began an active and successful campaign to increase the endowment base. In 1961, the receipt of a $200,000 bequest made a substantial increase to the endowment for medical research; in 1967 a bequest of $4 million was received from the estate of Royal A. and Olive W. Stone of St. Paul for an endowment to support research in heart disease and cancer. The Stone bequest increased dramatically the scale of the foundation's resources, and the endowments have continued to grow. They provide scholarships for medical students and funds to support medical research.

The Elias P. Lyon Memorial Laboratory

When the space for cancer research was eliminated from the Mayo Memorial Building, the university could not use the $300,000 given by the Minnesota Cancer Society for its construction. Dean Diehl, therefore, planned another, smaller building for cancer research and heart research to be located in the open space along Washington Avenue between the Institute of Anatomy and Millard Hall. He used the $300,000 gift from the Minnesota Cancer Society together with a grant from the National Heart Institute to pay for it.[67] The building was named in memory of Dean Lyon, who had also served as professor of physiology. The Lyon Laboratory was sadly the last nail in the coffin of the noble plan that Cass Gilbert had conceived for the medical campus, but that plan had been abandoned in 1931 when Owre Hall was built, blocking the open vista between buildings from Washington Avenue to the Elliot Hospital. Gilbert had envisioned open spaces between buildings, arranged to create extended vistas, for the campus as a whole. But President Vincent strangled the Gilbert plan almost at its birth, and on the medical campus the desperate improvisations of later years destroyed it utterly. With a seemingly active contempt for the work of his predecessors, the architect did not try to make the Lyon Laboratory compatible with the handsome older buildings on either side of it. Instead, it protrudes like a wart between them.

The Masonic Memorial Hospital

In December 1954, Dr. C. W. Delplaine of Minneapolis was late for a meeting of the Grand Council of the Minnesota Masons. When he arrived he explained that he had stopped at homes of two patients, each dying of cancer. Both patients needed more care than they could receive at home, and in addition to the suffering caused by their illness, both were worried that they were a burden to their families. Such patients were all too common, and the Masons decided to try to help them. Judge Leroy E. Matson wrote to Masonic lodges throughout Minnesota to invite them to attend a meeting to be held in Minneapolis on 14 January 1955 for the purpose of discussing the urgent need for hospital care for indigent people with cancer and other incurable diseases, a sadly neglected group of patients, and asking, "What can members of the craft do to supply leadership in filling this great need?"[68] Judge Matson appointed Donald J. Cowling chairman of a committee to plan the January meeting. When Dr. Cowling informed Dean Diehl that the Masons might be willing to build a new unit of the university hospital

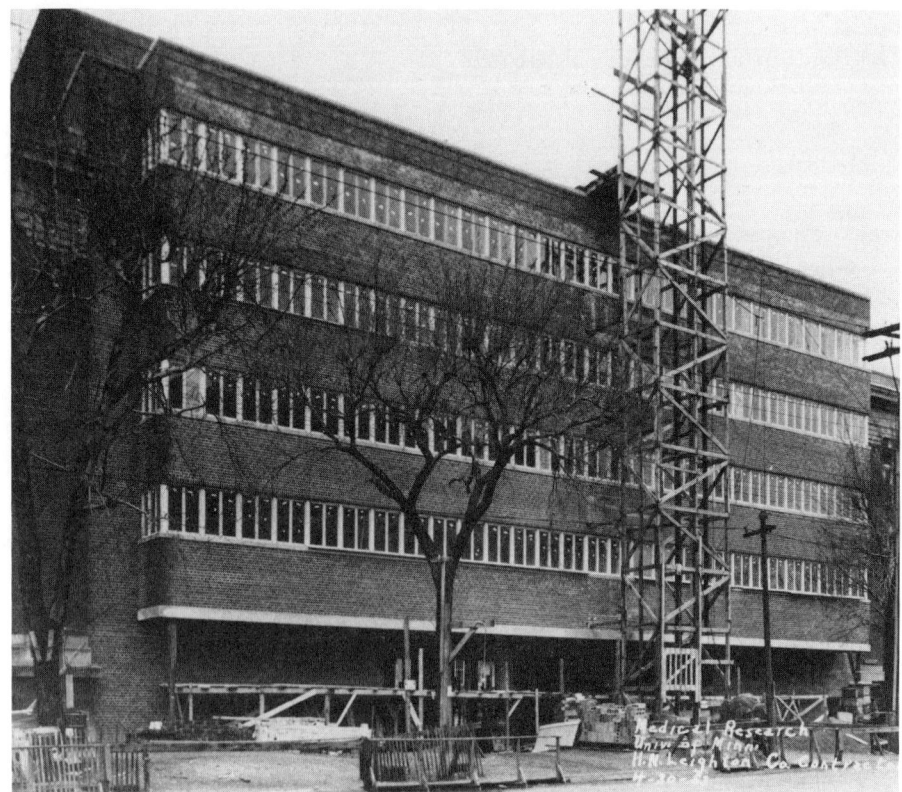

FIGURE 18:6 Elias P. Lyon Memorial Laboratory under construction, 1953. Courtesy Mn U Archives.

especially for the care of patients with advanced cancer, Diehl invited him to present the idea to a meeting of the administrative committee of the medical school. The response was enthusiastic.[69] Not only was there an urgent need for a special hospital for cancer patients, but such a unit would permit medical students to gain experience in the care of patients with terminal cancer. Much could be done to make the final weeks, months, or years of such patients less painful and less disruptive for their families. The hospital should have a capacity of about fifty beds and include facilities for research on cancer.[70]

The Masons decided to pursue the question of a cancer hospital and appointed an executive committee chaired by Dr. Cowling. Since the medical faculty were eager to have the proposed cancer hospital as part of the university hospital, Cowling and Diehl decided that it should be built on a site close to the university hospital and be connected to the latter by a tunnel or overpass. Dean Diehl suggested that they proceed as with the Variety Club Heart Hospital; that is, if the Masons would raise the necessary funds and turn them over to the Board of Regents, the university would build and operate the proposed cancer hospital.[71] The estimated cost of such a fifty-bed hospital with associated research laboratories was $1 million, but Dean Diehl thought that the university might obtain federal matching funds for half the amount.[72]

On 29 April 1955 a group of nearly one hundred Masons from various places in Minnesota met at Minneapolis to organize as the Masonic Cancer Relief Committee of Minnesota, with Judge Matson as chairman. Donald Cowling was elected chairman of an executive committee for the purpose of raising at least $500,000 for a cancer hospital in connection with the university hospitals.[73] The Board of Regents promptly accepted the Mason's offer.[74]

The campaign did not begin until the fall of 1955, but once started it developed vigorously. On 14 January 1956 some 500 members of Masonic cancer committees in communities throughout Minnesota came to the university for a Masonic Cancer Day. The medical faculty presented a program on the existing knowledge and treatment of cancer and the directions of cancer research.[75] Although originally the university had hoped to obtain federal matching funds to pay perhaps as much as half the cost of the proposed cancer hospital, in May 1956 the university learned that if any federal funds could be obtained, they would be much less than the $500,000 that the Masons were seeking to raise.[76] In June when the Masons had nearly reached their goal of $500,000, they decided to go on to raise a much larger sum. The excess over $500,000 was to be kept by the university in a special trust fund until the Masonic Cancer Relief Committee decided how it should be used.[77] By August the Masons had raised about $650,000, and the university architects were preparing preliminary plans for a cancer hospital expected to cost $1.2 million to be located at the corner of Harvard and Essex Streets.[78] By December 1956 the Masons had raised more than $800,000, largely from their own members.[79] The Masons thereupon raised their goal to $1 million and continued their campaign.[80]

The university began construction of the Masonic cancer hospital in May 1957 and the building was completed and dedicated on 4 October 1958. On 15 October the first patients were admitted. By May of the following year, the Masons had turned over almost $991,000 to the university and were confident that by the end of June they could raise the remaining $9,000 needed to meet their goal.[81]

The Masonic Memorial Hospital was designed to create a cheerful and comfortable atmosphere for patients and their families in a hospital that nevertheless contained all of the most modern equipment for the diagnosis and treatment of cancer. The hospital contained eighty beds, most in two-bed rooms each with its own bath, clothes closets, and telephones. On the first floor there was a lounge and dining room with a common fireplace between them.[82] The hospital proved so successful that in May 1963 the Masons undertook a second campaign to raise another $1 million to build two additional floors to contain forty more beds.[83] On 19 April 1966 they presented the university with a solid gold check for $1.1 million to pay for the addition. In 1970 the Masons also established a Masonic professorship of oncology and provided funds to support research and teaching on the cure of cancer patients.

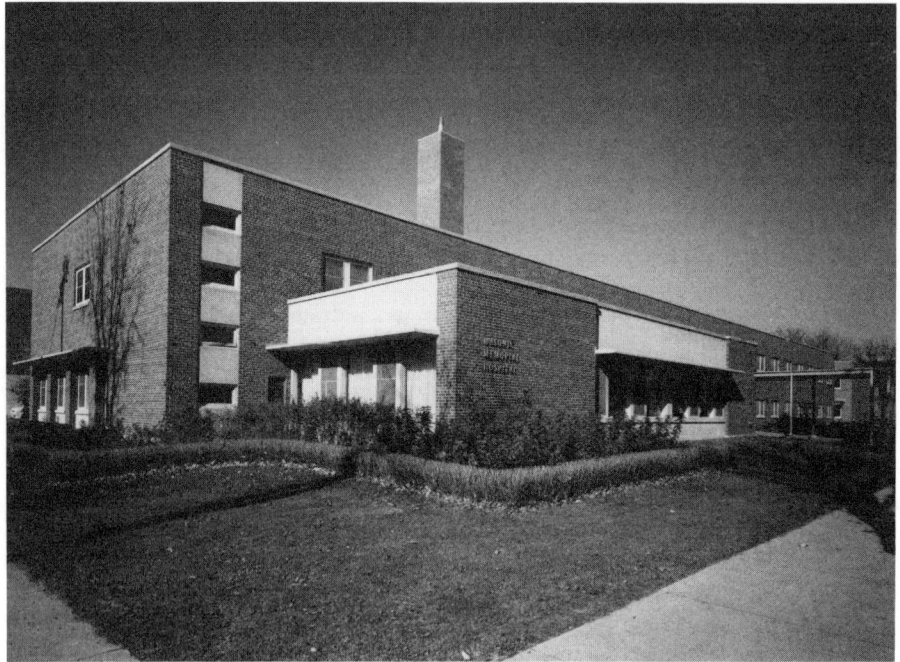

FIGURE 18:7 Masonic Memorial Hospital, circa 1959. Courtesy Mn U Archives.

During its first years the Masonic Memorial Hospital provided for cancer patients a level of care intermediate between that of a hospital and that of a nursing home. The advent of successful chemical therapy for cancer in the mid-1960s required more intense patient care, usually over a shorter period of time. More medical and nursing staff were required to perform the special diagnostic procedures and to care for patients following treatment with toxic chemotherapeutic agents. Thus the Masonic Hospital evolved from being a parahospital, designed for the prolonged nursing care of terminal cancer patients, to a hospital for the intensive treatment of cancer patients for relatively brief periods of time, the average length of stay declining from thirty-two days to eight days. A majority of patients treated recover to go home.[84]

The Masonic Memorial Hospital has given the medical students an opportunity to learn about cancer as a disease, and the various treatments used to combat it. The student may learn at first hand the art of controlling pain and other effects of cancer, including the anxiety, depression, anger, and grief of both the patient and the patient's family and friends. The student learns the need for the special skills of the social worker, and the minister, priest, or rabbi in dealing with the economic and emotional consequences of prolonged illness.[85] When the American Board of Internal Medicine created a subspecialty in medical oncology in 1972, the Masonic Memorial Hospital became a training center for cancer specialists.

While the Masons were raising money for the cancer hospital, the Veterans of Foreign Wars also were raising funds for a building to be devoted to cancer research. By September 1956 they had raised $200,000 and the medical school decided to seek federal matching funds for the proposed building, which was expected to cost about $610,000.[86] The Veterans of Foreign Wars Cancer Research Institute was built at the corner of Harvard and Delaware Streets, attached to the north end of the Masonic Hospital where it provided additional space for laboratories devoted to cancer research.

The Medical-Biological Library

Dean Diehl's greatest disappointment when the Mayo Memorial Building had to be reduced to fourteen stories in 1951 was the necessity to eliminate the space for the medical-biological library. When Harold Diehl and Owen Wangensteen were medical students thirty-five years earlier, the medical library had been in Millard Hall, and both faculty and students used it extensively. It was a good library assembled from the gifts and bequests of former faculty members, nurtured devotedly for years by Professor Thomas G. Lee, and after 1911 by the staff of the university library, and growing steadily from the inflow of books and journals. After 1924 when the medical library was moved out of Millard Hall to the university library about two blocks away from the medical school, it was used much less regularly by either faculty or students. As a young faculty member in the 1920s, Dr. Wangensteen spent every Saturday afternoon in the library reading current medical journals, but the distance of the library from the medical school, and somewhat greater distance from the university hospital, made more frequent visits to the library difficult. If weary, harassed, and overworked interns and residents were to use the library, it must be close at hand, especially during the bitterly cold weather of a Minnesota winter. Dean Diehl knew that medical students, interns, residents, and faculty all must read—all must be familiar with the medical and scientific literature—if they were to be competent and creative physicians. Furthermore, by the 1950s the main university library was becoming so overcrowded that an addition would have to be made to it unless the medical- biological library could be moved elsewhere.

In 1943 the university planned to erect a building for a medical-biological library in a vacant space on the corner of Church Street and Delaware Street between the Institute of Anatomy and Owre Hall. In that location the library would be connected directly to the medical and dental schools and would be just across the street from both the university hospital and the botany and zoology buildings. But the medical school shelved the plan when it decided to include the library in the Mayo Memorial Building. After the library had to be omitted from the Mayo Memorial, Dean Diehl sought to revive the former plan. He wished to have the university request the necessary appropriation for a library at the 1953 session of the legislature.[87] However, when Dean Diehl informed the dean of the dental school, William H. Crawford, of his proposal, Dean Crawford objected. If a building were to be placed in the vacant corner between the Institute of Anatomy and Owre Hall, said Dean Crawford, it should be used to provide additional space for the dental school, which was severely overcrowded.[88] Dean Crawford suggested that the medical-biological library might be placed across Union Street on land already owned by the university and then being used as a parking lot.[89] At a conference held by President Morrill on 7 October 1952, there was a general consensus that a new site should be sought for a medical-biological library and after the conference President Morrill, at the urging of Dean Diehl, included $800,000 for a medical-biological library among requests to the Minnesota legislature at the 1953 session, but the legislature denied the request.[90]

The following year with the library question still unresolved, Deans Crawford and Diehl decided that a better solution for the medical-biological library would be to build a new building for the dental school across Union Street from Millard Hall and to place the library in Owre Hall where the large room used for the dental clinic would make an ideal library reading room. The medical-biological library would also occupy the ground floor of Owre Hall and the ground floor of a new building to be placed in the vacant corner between Owre Hall and Jackson Hall (before 1954 the Institute of Anatomy) with book stacks in a deep excavation beneath the new building.[91]

In 1955 the university submitted to the legislature a request for $900,000 for a medical-biological library. At the same time the transfer of bacteriology, the School of Public Health, and the animal research laboratories out of Millard Hall into the Mayo Memorial required a request for $330,000 to remodel Millard Hall so that the vacated space could be used for physiology, biochemistry, and pharmacology laboratories. Similarly, a request for $1 million was needed to remodel parts of the university hospital when the various activities housed in them were moved to the Mayo Memorial Building. Dean Diehl also needed to ask for additional salary funds to staff the enlarged facilities created by the Mayo Memorial Building. Among so many requests in 1955, the legislature did not provide appropriations for a new dental building, and only $400,000 of the $900,000 requested for a medical-biological library.

The failure of the legislature to provide an appropriation for a new dental building meant that the plan to locate the library on the corner between Jackson Hall and Owre Hall and within Owre Hall itself had to be abandoned, yet $400,000 was not nearly sufficient to build a separate library building. Dean Diehl was also carefully husbanding about $100,000 from royalties on Copavin, a cold medicine which he had patented and given to the university in the 1930s, so that he had about $500,000 of the estimated $1 million needed to build the library.

In August 1956, Dean Diehl asked President Morrill to include a request for $500,000 for the medical library among requests to the legislature in 1957. It was first among proposed legislative requests for the medical school and university hospital amounting to almost $2.3 million. In 1956 the federal government was providing no funds for the construction of medical libraries. Apart from any private gifts that might be obtained, the state would have to pay the full cost of building a library. During the fall of 1956 there was some disagreement between the pathology department and dental school over the dental school's proposal to place a new building on the corner between Jackson Hall and Owre Hall.[92] Both the dental school and the pathology department were working under extremely crowded conditions, their faculties were frustrated, and they faced increasing demands for teaching. The failure to act earlier on their needs had created an acute situation.

In November 1956 a ray of hope appeared. From Florida, Mr. I. A. O'Shaughnessy of St. Paul wrote to Dr. Wangensteen that if Dean Diehl could raise $150,000, he would give another $150,000 for medical research facilities.[93] Then at the age of seventy-one, Ignatius Aloysius O'Shaughnessy was a successful businessman, who in 1917 organized the Globe Oil & Refining Company and later other companies in the oil and gas industry. A native of Stillwater, Minnesota, Mr. O'Shaughnessy was educated at the College of St. Thomas in St. Paul. He was a generous donor to his alma mater as well as other worthy purposes, but this was his first substantial gift to the medical school. Within a month Dean Diehl had firm commitments for his share, and with the matching funds from Mr. O'Shaughnessy, the first $300,000 was available for the research laboratories needed to take the place of those that had to be omitted from the Mayo Memorial Building. The laboratories were planned to extend out underground from the east wing of the university hospital beneath Union Street. Although the total construction cost of the laboratories would exceed $1.5 million, Dean Diehl intended to seek half the amount from the federal government in matching funds.[94] At Washington in December 1956, Dean Diehl talked with congressmen and senators concerned with health appropriations, including Senator Edward J. Thye of Minnesota, to urge the inclusion of construction funds in forthcoming appropriations.[95] Meanwhile, Dr. Wangensteen was writing in all directions to potential donors in search of the additional private funds needed for the research laboratories.[96] By the following summer, Dean Diehl requested that the university commission architects to prepare plans for the new underground research laboratories to cost no more than $1,575,000. By October 1957, Dean Diehl and Dr. Wangensteen had accumulated gifts for the new laboratories totaling $589,721 so that they were within sight of their goal of $835,000 to match the contingent federal grant for the amount needed to build and equip the laboratories.

In the spring of 1957, the Minnesota legislature approved a second appropriation of $400,000 for a bio-medical library building to make a total of $800,000 available for its construction. Although the director of libraries, Edward B. Stanford, was anxious to move ahead quickly with the planning and construction of the library before rising costs made the appropriations insufficient, by 1957 the funds were already insufficient.[97] The architects estimated that an adequate building for the library would cost $1.6 million, twice the amount available. Furthermore, federal matching funds could not be used for the construction of libraries.

In April 1958 Dr. Wangensteen approached I. A. O'Shaughnessy, who had provided a library for the College of St. Thomas, to try to interest him in providing a library for the medical school.[98] Mr. O'Shaughnessy did not reply or show any interest in Dr. Wangensteen's suggestion, but the following December he told Dr. Wangensteen that he would be interested in watching one of the open heart operations for which the university was then famous. Dr. Wangensteen arranged for Mr. O'Shaughnessy to come to the university hospital on 20 January to observe from the operating room observation dome while Drs. C. Walton Lillehei and Herbert Warden operated on the heart of an eleven-month-old baby boy. The older man watched with wonder and admiration while the young surgeons worked together to save the child's life. He was impressed deeply by the coordinated organization in the operating room that made such surgery possible. At lunch afterwards in Dr. Wangensteen's office, Mr. O'Shaughnessy remarked that in the operation he had just seen, clinical accomplishment had at last caught up with research. From the window where they were eating lunch, they could look out at the large hole in the ground where the new research laboratories, which Mr. O'Shaughnessy's gift two years before helped to make possible, were being built. The next day Dr. Wangensteen wrote to Mr. O'Shaughnessy to tell him of the medical school's urgent need of funds for the medical library.[99] Two weeks later Dr. Wangensteen wrote also to Dr. Cowling to plead for his help in finding funds to build an adequate library.[100]

Meanwhile, the medical school decided to build as much library building as could be built with the funds available. The architects designed a very plain, square building, with two floors below ground level and one above, to be located at the corner of Essex and Union Streets adjoining the new underground research laboratories. The bottom floor was to be used for medical research and would connect directly with the existing laboratories. The funds used for its construction were exclusive of the library appropriations, but they would provide the foundation for the library building to be built above. The economic recession of 1958 kept building costs down so that the university was able to plan for three floors for the library (two above ground), although the additional floor would have to remain an unfinished shell. The plans were completed and bids obtained by June 1958, and excavation for the building began that summer.

In June 1957, Dean Diehl told the administrative committee of the medical school that he was resigning as dean effective 30 June 1958 to become senior vice president for research and medical affairs at the American Cancer Society in New York City. He was sixty-six years old, three years short of the age of compulsory retirement at the University of Minnesota, but so many years of raising of funds that seemed never sufficient to meet the rising costs of buildings, of pressures from the legislature to increase the size of classes in the medical school before the classrooms and laboratories had been enlarged to accommodate them, and the resultant acrimonious exchanges with President Morrill and the vice presidents—the strain of all such things had taken their toll. Dean Diehl was accustomed to say that time and patience would deal with many of the problems that harass people.

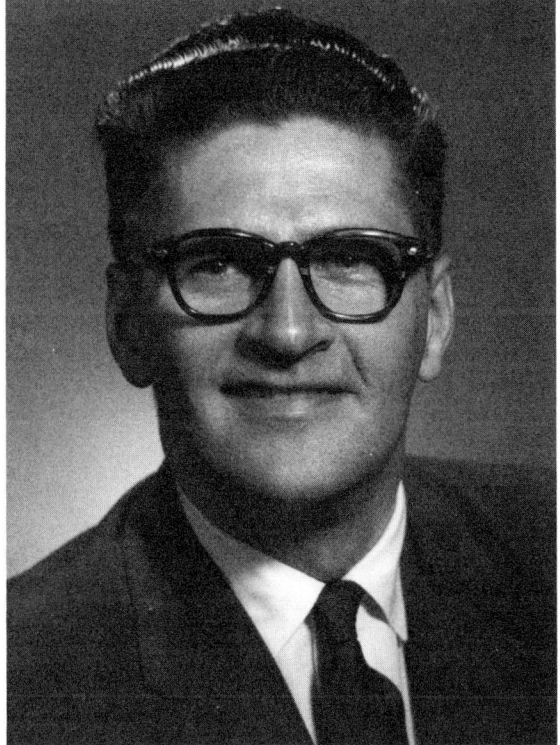

FIGURE 18:8 Robert B. Howard, 1958. Courtesy Mn U Archives.

Nevertheless, the passage of years and the exercise of infinite patience still left the medical school with a seemingly endless array of acute problems.

Dean Diehl's announcement stunned the administrative committee, and as the news spread throughout the school, the faculty were dismayed. On 14 June the administrative committee reconvened itself without the dean and elected a committee, consisting of Maurice Visscher, Owen Wangensteen, and Cecil Watson, to urge Dean Diehl to reconsider. Noting that the years of Dr. Diehl's deanship had seen the medical school emerge as one of the strong schools of the country, they said that his "wise, courageous, and patient leadership" had stimulated and sustained the development of the school. They pleaded that his work was not yet finished and that the school would "lose immeasurably" if he left prematurely. The committee wrote: "We want and need your vision and guiding hand. Above all we want you to know the warmth of the affection and the great esteem which every member of the Administrative Committee holds for you." They pledged their support and begged him to remain.[101]

It was to no avail. Dean Diehl's mind was made up. Intuitively he knew that he was reaching the limits of his strength. In December 1957 while driving his car, he suffered a dizzy spell and went off the road. As a result of the accident

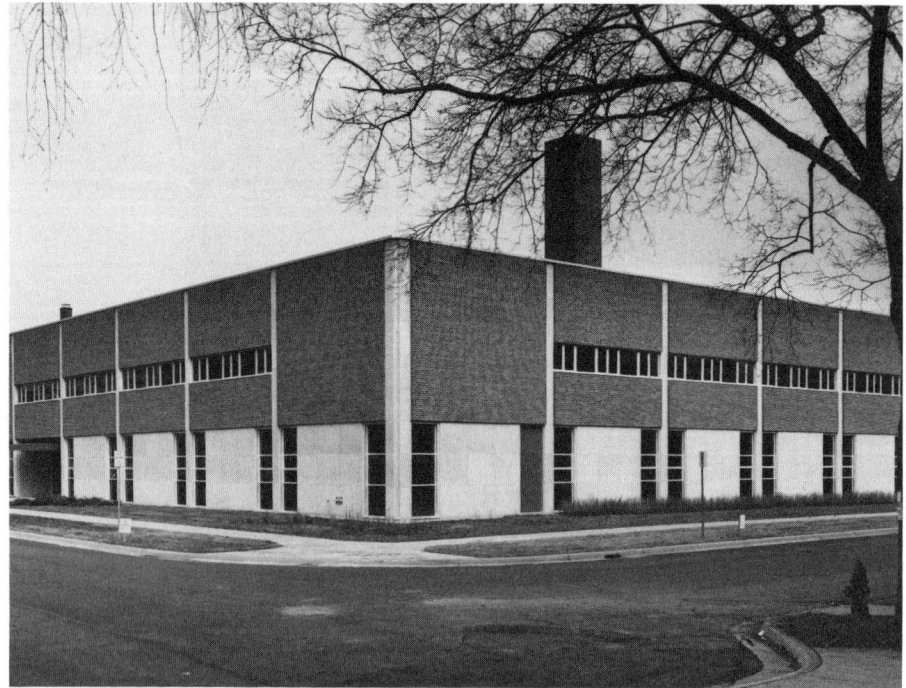

FIGURE 18:9   Diehl Hall, 1961. Courtesy Mn U Archives.

he was for a time in hospital. In January 1958 Mrs. Diehl wrote to Dr. Cowling, "Harold is a very tired man . . . ."[102]

When Dean Diehl's departure was announced publicly in July, the *Minneapolis Star* published an editorial entitled "A Great Dean." Of Dean Diehl's success in obtaining funds for buildings, equipment, research, and scholarships, the *Star* commented: "The story is told that a prominent eastern doctor once asked Dean Diehl at a medical convention how the money was obtained. The reply was 'Oh, it just comes.' " Nevertheless, those who knew how Dean Diehl had worked "night and day, in season and out" to obtain funds for the medical school, knew how casual the remark was. The *Star* said also: "It is well known that the University medical school has less friction, less rivalry and less jealousy than any other similar organization in the country," because of the atmosphere that Dean Diehl had maintained. Finally, with pardonable pride the *Star* said that Dean Diehl's leadership and ideas went far to explain why "Minnesota's medical school is now one of the greatest — if not the greatest — in the world."[103]

Although Dean Diehl continued as dean through 1957–58, during much of that year Associate Dean Robert B. Howard administered the medical school. In July 1958 Dr. Howard was appointed dean. The following September the university decided that the new building to contain research laboratories and the medical-biological library should be named Diehl Hall.

Early in 1959 Dr. Wangensteen renewed his plea to Mr. O'Shaughnessy for funds to complete Diehl Hall. The top floor (level 4) of Diehl Hall would remain an unfinished shell when the construction then underway was complete. He also sought Dr. Cowling's help in raising funds for the project.[104] Early in 1960 the medical school hoped to obtain federal matching funds for the completion of Diehl Hall, a possibility that spurred on Dr. Cowling's and Dr. Wangensteen's efforts to obtain gifts. In June 1960 Mr. and Mrs. John Sargent Pillsbury gave $100,000 to buy rare medical books for the library, and a week or two later Mr. O'Shaughnessy gave $225,000 for construction of the library, stipulating that his gift should remain anonymous.[105] In August 1960, a few weeks after Mr. O'Shaughnessy made his gift, the National Institutes of Health once again announced that federal construction funds could not be used for the construction of libraries.[106] When Mr. O'Shaughnessy learned of their decision, he decided to remove the anonymity from his gift in the hope that it might then serve to attract other gifts.[107] A few weeks later, through the sympathetic magic of Dr. Cowling, Dr. Wangensteen received from one of his former patients an anonymous gift of $300,000 toward the building of the library.[108] The arrival of the second gift, which brought funds for the further construction of Diehl Hall to a total of $525,000, coincided with the completion of the first phase of the building. In December 1960 two floors of Diehl Hall became ready for occupancy by the library, and during the Christmas vacation 145,000 volumes of books and journals were moved into them from the university library. In January 1961 the Bio-medical Library opened in Diehl Hall.

Although the architects' estimate of $610,000 to finish level 4 and construct level 5 of Diehl Hall was not very much greater than the $525,000 available from gifts, Dean Howard did not wish to begin construction until they had also obtained the funds to build level 6, which would complete the building to the height the foundations were designed to carry. Because level 6 would be used for research laboratories, federal matching funds could be used for its construction, but the medical school still had to find its part of any such matching funds. The Minnesota Medical Foundation was willing to contribute $25,000 from its funds. In January 1961 Dean Howard thought that he might be able to assemble from certain gifts and various research funds as much as $235,000 to match $235,000 presumed to be available in federal funds for the construction of research facilities.[109] Nevertheless, the combined $470,000 was still too far short of the $776,000 needed to build level 6. Besides, the medical school was once again climbing the slippery slope of rising costs. By March 1961 estimates for the cost of finishing level 4 and building level 5 had risen to $764,000 and the cost of level 6 to $822,000.[110] An additional $153,000 would be needed to finish level 5.[111] In August 1961 Dr. Wangensteen obtained another $40,000 in gifts.[112] In September, when Dr. Wangensteen thought that it would be necessary finally to appeal to small donors, he himself pledged $1,500 for the library.[113] In December Dr. Wangensteen was shocked to learn that in addition to the sums required to construct and finish level 5, a further $125,000 would be required to furnish it with library equipment.[114] There were no university funds for the purpose.[115] For their fortieth reunion the medical class of 1922–23 decided to raise funds for the medical library project.[116] Other gifts trickled in, some of them as large as $15,000, but the sum remaining to be raised was still formidably large.

Meanwhile, in April 1962 the university announced that in addition to the large Pillsbury gift, it had received several other gifts for the purchase of historical medical books. Dr. George D. Eitel had given funds for surgical books and a fund had been created in memory of Edgar T. Hermann for historical books in cardiology.

The same spring Dr. Wangensteen became severely ill with a peripheral neuritis that confined him to bed for several months. The immediate cause of his illness was a hypersensitive reaction to an immunization for foreign travel, but the months and years of anxious fund raising may have contributed to its severity. His illness tended to slow down the campaign for funds for Diehl Hall through 1962, although not in every case. In August, Alice O'Brien of St. Paul sent him a note of sympathy in his baffling and painful illness, and enclosed a check for $10,000. Miss O'Brien added: "I wish all of the checks I signed would give me as much pleasure as this one does. Due to your ability and kindness, research in the surgery field has become one of the most vital interests in my life."[117] Dr. Wangensteen added Miss O'Brien's gift to the library fund.

By September 1962 the estimates for the finishing of level 4 and construction of level 5 had risen to $965,000. Dr. Wangensteen had managed to raise $635,000, but the alarming amount of $355,000 remained to be found.[118]

Through the winter of 1963 the library fund grew slowly. In the spring, the medical school was faced with a crisis because, when construction bids were obtained, the medical school found that, even excluding the cost of equipment, they still lacked $108,000 of the amount needed to complete levels 4 and 5 of Diehl Hall.[119] In June 1963 Dr. Wangensteen received a pledge of $25,000 from a former student, Dr. Richard W. Giere, a gift made in memory of his father who had graduated from the medical school in 1892.[120] In July, Jay Phillips of Minneapolis, who had already given $30,000 for the library building, offered to match further gifts for the library up to an amount of $125,000. The only condition that Mr. Phillips attached to his commitment was that the library, when completed, should be named for Dr. Wangensteen. " . . . I feel strongly," wrote Mr. Phillips, "that a person who has devoted his life to the service of mankind, who has worked so hard and diligently as you have in the service, and who has been so closely identified with the University, deserves appropriate recognition in permanent form."[121]

Meanwhile Drs. A. B. Baker and Donald Hastings were struggling to raise the funds needed for the construction of level 6, which was to provide research laboratories for neurology, psychiatry, and pediatrics. In July 1963 they still had to obtain an additional $45,000 for the basic structure and were finding it difficult to do so.[122]

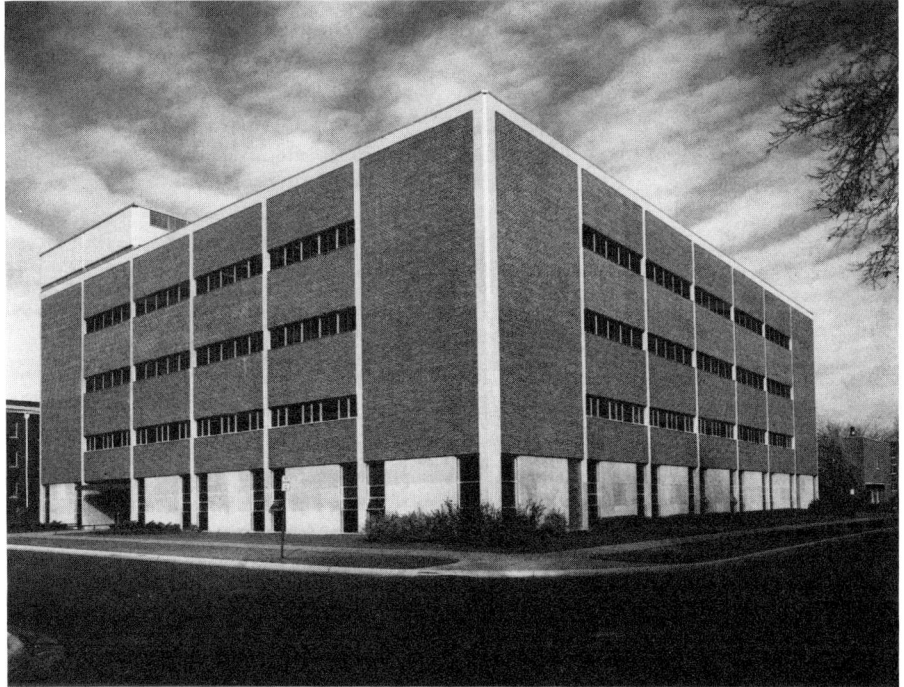

FIGURE 18:10 Diehl Hall, 1965. Courtesy Mn U Archives.

Despite such difficulties by the end of July 1963 Dean Howard decided that they were close enough to their goal to justify the letting of contracts for the completion of level 5 of Diehl Hall.[123] Nevertheless, while the new floors of Diehl Hall were under construction during the fall of 1963, the medical school was still about $110,000 short of the funds needed to complete and furnish them.

When the contractor turned over the 4th and 5th floors of Diehl Hall to the university in June 1964, the east side of the 5th floor remained unfinished and there were no funds available to furnish the finished portion.[124] However, by August Dean Howard used some funds remaining in a Diehl Hall contingency fund together with a special allotment from the Regents' Reserve Fund to complete and furnish the fourth and fifth levels of Diehl Hall.[125] During the following year the two new floors of the library were furnished and began to be used.

On Saturday evening, 27 November 1965, Dr. Cowling died quietly, his great work of fund raising for the university finally complete. For more than twenty years he had worked quietly, steadily, and effectively with donors and legislators. He liked people and possessed an unusual gift for winning their friendship. The Mayo Memorial, the Masonic Hospital, and Diehl Hall were each his monuments, as they would also be those of Dean Diehl and Dr. Wangensteen.

NOTES

1. Diehl to Earl, 24 September 1940 [copy], President's Office, Papers.
2. Ibid.
3. Ford to Diehl, 26 September 1940 [copy], President's Office, Papers. In 1921 the medical school lost a building when the Departments of Bacteriology and Pathology were required to move out of the former Institute of Public Health and Pathology. Pathology moved into the Institute of Anatomy and bacteriology into Millard Hall, but in order to provide sufficient space for bacteriology in Millard Hall, the medical library was transferred in 1924 to Walter Library, the new university library building, two blocks away from the medical school.
4. Diehl to Earl, 22 January 1941 [copy], President's Office, Papers.
5. "Mayo memorial pondered. University site proposed," *St. Paul Pioneer Press*, 2 February 1941.
6. Diehl to Cowling, 27 March 1941 [copy], President's Office, Papers. The Rockefeller Foundation had spent more than $40 million on the Peking Union Medical College in China, a sum far greater than the foundation had anticipated.
7. Cowling to Diehl, 5 April 1941 [copy], President's Office, Papers.
8. Cowling to Diehl, 10 April 1941 [copy], President's Office, Papers.
9. Diehl to Cowling, 12 April 1941 [copy], President's Office, Papers.
10. Middlebrook to Johnston, 19 April 1941 [copy], President's Office, Papers.
11. Diehl to Balfour, 16 October 1941 [copy], President's Office, Papers.
12. Ibid.
13. Ford wrote to Diehl: " . . . I really feel that the Clinic or Mayo Properties Association should do this thing out of hand themselves and avoid all possible misunderstanding." Ford to Diehl, 20 October 1941 [copy], President's Office, Papers.
14. Dean Diehl feared that the project would never be revived, but in the summer of 1942, Dr. Cowling thought it could still become a reality. Diehl to Cowling, 2 July 1942; Cowling to Diehl, 6 July 1942 [copies], President's Office, Papers. Cf. Merril E. Jarchow, *Donald J. Cowling,* pp. 390–396.
15. Diehl to Cowling, 12 March 1943 [copy], President's Office, Papers.
16. Stassen to Cowling, 27 April 1943, President's Office, Papers. During thirty-five years as president of Carleton, Donald Cowling had made it one of the outstanding liberal arts colleges in the United States.
17. Coffey to Cowling, 10 July 1943, President's Office, Papers.
18. Mayo to Coffey, 25 July 1943, President's Office, Papers ; Balfour to Coffey, 26 July 1943, President's Office, Papers.
19. Diehl to Coffey, 22 April 1943, President's Office, Papers.
20. Diehl to Cowling, 4 September 1943, President's Office, Papers.
21. Coffey to Lobb and Harwick, 15 December 1943 [copy], President's Office, Papers. Cf. Board of Regents, Supplement to the Minutes, 10 December 1943. The change was to take effect 1 July 1944.
22. Coffey to Fosdick, 15 April 1944 [copy], President's Office, Papers.
23. Bell to Coffey, 12 May 1944, President's Office, Papers.
24. Harold S. Diehl, "Memorandum of conference on the Mayo memorial," President's Office, Papers.
25. W. T. Middlebrook, "Memorandum . . . Mayo Memorial Committee," 1 February 1944, President's Office, Papers. Shimp to Middlebrook, 13 March 1944 [copy], President's Office, Papers. Mr. Shimp suggested that the new School of Public Health be included in the Mayo memorial campaign to add a human interest appeal to the campaign. Otherwise, Shimp thought the appeal became primarily intellectual, except for the emotional element in the life and work of the Doctors Mayo.

26. Shimp to Cowling, 6 April 1944, President's Office, Papers.
27. Harold S. Diehl, "Remarks . . . at the October 2, 1944 meeting of the Committee of Founders of the Mayo Memorial," President's Office, Papers.
28. Cowling to Thye, 10 November 1944 [copy], President's Office, Papers.
29. Balfour et al. to Cowling, 23 February 1945, President's Office, Papers. Balfour wrote: "As the purpose of this memorial becomes increasingly evident, the Graduate Committee [of the Mayo Foundation] wishes to assure you . . . of its deep appreciation of this recognition of the lives and work of the Doctors Mayo. . . . Such a center of medical research on the University campus, by providing important educational facilities for contributing to the advancement of medicine, will surely bring to the University further prestige and renown as a great educational institution."
30. Cowling to Lunden, 17 February 1945, President's Office, Papers. Dr. Cowling suggested that as the university received gifts for the Mayo memorial the funds should be invested in interest-bearing securities until they were actually needed to pay for construction. The interest thus earned, Dr. Cowling hoped, might be sufficient to pay the expenses of the campaign so that the full amount of all gifts could be used for the Mayo memorial.
31. Diehl to Stassen, 7 March 1945 [copy], President's Office, Papers.
32. This account is based on Senator Thye's recollections at the time of the Mayo Memorial Building dedication. Thye to Morrill, 4 October 1954, President's Office, Papers.
33. Rockne to Cowling, 29 March 1945, Cowling papers.
34. Cowling to Rockne, 31 March 1945 [copy], President's Office, Papers.
35. Cowling to Chairman and Committee Members, 29 June 1945. President's Office, Papers; Shimp to Morrill, 3 July 1945, President's Office, Papers. Byron Shimp thought that in July they were just where they would have been in April if it had not been for the difficulty with the Senate Finance Committee.
36. Cowling to all chairmen and committee members, 13 July 1945, President's Office, Papers.
37. Byron Shimp wrote later: "We certainly accomplished a great deal in those two small rooms with the very small staff which we employed. As a matter of fact, I don't see sometimes how we got the work done. Mrs. Robinson and her small staff certainly accomplished a tremendous volume of work." Shimp to Cowling, 27 December 1945, President's Office, Papers.
38. Harold S. Diehl, "Memorandum of conference on Mayo Memorial," 19 September 1945, President's Office, Papers.
39. Morrill to Cowling, 24 September 1945, President's Office, Papers.
40. Diehl (n. 38).
41. Cowling to Shimp, 22 December 1945 [copy], President's Office, Papers.
42. Cowling to Shimp, 6 June 1946 [copy], President's Office, Papers.
43. The $2 million required for connected buildings could be obtained from other university funds, including the Mayo Properties Association gift for the School of Public Health, gifts from the American Cancer Society for a cancer research institute, and funds that Dean Diehl had been accumulating for years in the Copavin fund for a medical library.
44. Cowling to Thye, 30 December 1946 [copy]; Cowling to Youngdahl, 23 December 1946 [copy], President's Office, Papers.
45. Cowling to Shimp, 30 August 1948, President's Office, Papers.
46. Harold S. Diehl, "Memorandum for Hospital Survey and Planning Committee," 13 November 1947, President's Office, Papers.
47. Middlebrook to Jones, 28 November 1947, President's Office, Papers.
48. Cowling to Shimp, 30 August 1948 [copy], President's Office, Papers.

49. Middlebrook to Diehl, 10 January 1949 [copy]; Jones et al. to Middlebrook, 6 January 1949, President's Office, Papers.
50. Donald J. Cowling, "The Mayo Memorial," *J.-Lancet,* 1950, *70,* 383–385, 407, p. 384.
51. Cowling to Youngdahl, 1 March 1949 [copy], President's Office, Papers.
52. Morrill to Cowling, 21 April 1949, President's Office, Papers.
53. Morrill to Cowling, 29 November 1949, President's Office, Papers.
54. Morrill to Amberg, 21 April 1949 [copy]; Morrill to Diehl, 21 April 1949 [copy], President's Office, Papers.
55. From Duluth, Dr. Edward L. Tuohy, a medical alumnus and member of the Committee of Founders, wrote to President Morrill: "From the standpoint of the general university development, permit me again to congratulate you. We have a masterly hand at the helm." Tuohy to Morrill, 14 May 1949, President's Office, Papers.
56. A commitment for $200,000 came from the National Cancer Institute, $243,000 from the National Heart Institute, and $750,000 from the United States Public Health Service. Cowling to the Committee of Founders, 2 November 1949, President's Office, Papers.
57. Diehl to Johnston, 1 August 1950 [copy], President's Office, Papers.
58. Cowling (n. 50).
59. Ibid.; Cf. Holmes to Middlebrook, 23 August 1950, President's Office, Papers.
60. Madden to Cowling, 26 March 1951, Cowling papers.
61. Jarchow, *Cowling* (n. 14), p. 426.
62. J. L. Morrill, "Mayo Memorial Dedication [address]," 21 October 1954, President's Office, Papers.
63. Harold S. Diehl, "The Mayo Memorial dedicated," *Minn. Med.,* 1954, *37,* 780–783.
64. This account of the Minnesota Medical Foundation is based upon that by Eivind O. Hoff, "The Minnesota Medical Foundation, 1939–1966," in Jay Arthur Myers, *Masters of medicine,* pp. 661–674.
65. The other members of the committee were Theodore Anderson, Gordon Kamman, Jennings C. Litzenberg, Maurice B. Visscher, and Owen H. Wangensteen.
66. The other officers were Maurice B. Visscher, vice president; Jennings C. Litzenberg, treasurer; and Robert L. Wilder, secretary.
67. Diehl to Middlebrook, 31 August 1951 [copy], President's Office, Papers.
68. Cowling to Diehl, 16 February 1955, Cowling papers. Dr. Cowling's role in raising funds for the Masonic Hospital is described in Jarchow, *Cowling* (n. 14), pp. 430–432.
69. Amberg to Cowling, 12 January 1955, Cowling papers.
70. Diehl to Cowling, 4 February 1955, Cowling papers.
71. Diehl to Cowling, 25 February 1955 [copy], Cowling papers.
72. Diehl to Cowling, 3 March 1955, Cowling papers.
73. Cowling to Diehl, 4 May 1955 [copy], Cowling papers.
74. Middlebrook to H. S. Diehl, 25 May 1955 [copy], Cowling papers.
75. Hegman to Nunn, 18 January 1956, President's Office, Papers.
76. Lunden to Middlebrook, 9 May 1956, President's Office, Papers.
77. Matson and Cowling to Diehl, 20 June 1956; Diehl to Cowling, 25 June 1956 [copy], President's Office, Papers.
78. Diehl to Morrill, 29 August 1956, President's Office, Papers.
79. Cowling to Amberg, 4 December 1956 [copy], Cowling papers.
80. Middlebrook to Humphrey, 19 February 1957 [copy], President's Office, Papers. In February 1957 the United States Public Health Service approved a grant to the university of $202,279 to help with the construction of the proposed Masonic cancer hospital.

Nunn to Cowling, 17 January and 23 January 1958 [copies], President's Office, Papers. When the United States Public Health Service grant was announced publicly in November 1957, Dr. Cowling became concerned that such a grant would diminish the identity of the cancer hospital with the Minnesota Masons. The director of university relations, William L. Nunn, wrote to reassure him that the $1 million goal set by the Masons would provide the funds needed to construct the cancer hospital. The federal grant would pay for the tunnels to connect the cancer hospital to the university hospital and for equipment and furnishings.

81. Cowling to Howard, 11 June 1959 [copy], Cowling papers.

82. B. J. Kennedy and John Westerman, "Parahospital," *J. Am. Hosp.*, 1962, *36*, pp. 39–43, 56–64.

83. Construction of the additional floors began in March 1965 and was completed in September 1966.

84. B.J. Kennedy, "Masonic Memorial Hospital: A special cancer center for the study of advanced malignant diseases," *Minn. Med.*, 1974, *57*, 527–531.

85. Anastasias Theologides, [Editorial] "Oncology service in a teaching hospital," *J. chron. Dis.*, 1971, *23*, 601–603.

86. Wipperman to Morrill, 8 August 1957, President's Office, Papers . In 1957 the university sought a federal grant of $172,000 to assist with its construction.

87. Diehl to Morrill, 7 March 1952, President's Office, Papers.

88. Crawford to Morrill, 11 March 1952, President's Office, Papers.

89. Crawford to Morrill, 20 March 1952, President's Office, Papers.

90. Diehl to Cowling, 3 November 1952; Wangensteen to Cowling, 27 February 1953, Cowling papers. Wangensteen to Mullin, 13 March 1953 [copy], President's Office, Papers. In February 1953 Dr. Owen H. Wangensteen asked Dr. Cowling to help support the library request before the legislature and wrote to legislators to urge their support.

91. Harold S. Diehl, "Memorandum for file," 19 June 1954; Harold S. Diehl, "Self-survey of building needs, College of Medical Sciences," [1954]; Diehl to Morrill, 29 July 1954; Stanford to Diehl, 16 July 1954 [copy]; Diehl to Morrill, 1 October, and 27 October 1954, President's Office, Papers.

92. Crawford to Morrill, 19 October 1956; Dawson to Diehl, 24 October 1956; Crawford to Morrill, 24 October 1956, President's Office, Papers.

93. O'Shaughnessy to Wangensteen, 19 November 1956 [copy]; Diehl to O'Shaughnessy, 21 November 1956 [copy], President's Office, Papers.

94. Diehl to Morrill, 13 December 1956; Diehl to O'Shaughnessy, 11 January 1957 [copy], President's Office, Papers.

95. Diehl to Youmans, 14 December 1955 [copy], President's Office, Papers.

96. Wangensteen to Cowling, 18 July 1957, Cowling papers.

97. Stanford to Middlebrook, 8 May 1957, President's Office, Papers.

98. Wangensteen to O'Shaughnessy, 12 April 1958 [copy], President's Office, Papers.

99. Wangensteen to O'Shaughnessy, 21 January 1959 [copy], Cowling papers.

100. Wangensteen to Cowling, 6 February 1959, Cowling papers.

101. Visscher, Wangensteen, and Watson to Diehl, 15 June 1957, Harold S. Diehl file, Personnel records, University of Minnesota.

102. Diehl to Cowling, 4 January 1958, Cowling papers.

103. [Editorial] "A Great Dean," *Minneapolis Star,* 27 July 1957.

104. Wangensteen to O'Shaughnessy, 21 January 1959 [copy]; Wangensteen to Cowling, 6 February 1959, Cowling papers.

105. Wangensteen to Cowling, 8 July 1960, Cowling papers.

106. Howard to Cowling and Wangensteen, 17 August 1960, Cowling papers.

107. Wangensteen to Howard, 8 November 1960 [copy], Cowling papers.

108. Wangensteen to Cowling, 30 November 1960; Howard to Cowling, 2 December 1960, Cowling papers.

109. Howard to Cowling, 18 January 1961, Cowling papers.

110. Fleeson to Cowling, Wangensteen, and Howard, 22 March 1961, Cowling papers.

111. Robert B. Howard, "Diehl Hall. Summary of construction, funds available and funds needed, July 15, 1961," Wangensteen papers.

112. Wangensteen to Howard, 31 August 1961 [copy], Cowling papers.

113. Wangensteen to Howard, 19 September 1961, Wangensteen papers.

114. Stanford to Wangensteen, 5 December 1961; Wangensteen to Stanford, 12 December 1961, Wangensteen papers.

115. Stanford to Wangensteen, 29 December 1961, Wangensteen papers.

116. Oppegard to Members of the Class in Medicine 1922–1923, 1 February 1962, Wangensteen papers.

117. O'Brien to Wangensteen, 20 August 1962, Wangensteen papers.

118. Stanford to Wangensteen, 10 September 1962, Wangensteen papers.

119. Howard to Wangensteen, 7 May 1963, Wangensteen papers.

120. Giere to Wangensteen, 11 June 1963; Wangensteen to Giere, 13 June 1963 [copy], Wangensteen papers.

121. Phillips to Wangensteen, 1 July 1963, Wangensteen papers. Although the Board of Regents had a strict rule against the naming of any building for an active member of the faculty, in 1972, five years after Dr. Wangensteen's retirement, the library which he worked so hard to create was named the *Owen H. Wangensteen Historical Library of Biology and Medicine.*

122. Hastings to Wangensteen, 16 July 1963, Wangensteen papers.

123. Howard to Lund, 30 July 1963 [copy], Wangensteen papers. Part of the additional cost was for an enclosed overpass to connect the new level 5 of Diehl Hall with the fifth floor of the university hospital, which could be omitted with a resultant saving.

124. Gault, Jr. to Wangensteen, 27 May 1964, Wangensteen papers.

125. Howard to Wangensteen, 6 August 1964, Wangensteen papers.

CHAPTER 19

The Fusion of Basic and Clinical Research at Minnesota 1942–1960

Cancer

During the 1930s Dr. Wangensteen became increasingly concerned with surgery for cancer, especially cancers of the alimentary canal. Such cancers were all too common and were estimated to cause more than half of the 150,000 cancer deaths that occurred annually in the United States. They fell into two principal groups: cancers of the stomach and cancers of the colon and rectum. When Clarence Dennis came to the Department of Surgery in 1935 to begin a residency, he brought with him familiarity with the slow, exact, and careful operative techniques originated at the Hopkins by William Stewart Halsted and taught to Dennis by the associate professor of surgery, Warfield M. Firor. At Minnesota, Dr. Dennis used the Hopkins principles to perform a closed intestinal anastomosis after removing a gangrenous intussusception from an infant, who made a smooth recovery. Fascinated by Dennis's technique, Dr. Wangensteen suggested to him that they work together to develop the same type of closed anastomosis to join together the stomach and jejunum following gastric resection. Dennis declined, thinking that the technique would be difficult to apply to the stomach and jejunum. Dr. Wangensteen then asked whether Dr. Dennis minded if he went ahead to work on it and Dennis said, "No, indeed." Recalling this incident, Dr. Dennis admitted, "I felt very foolish because he did it beautifully and it was a very productive contribution."[1] The new technique of aseptic anastomosis for the reconnection of portions of stomach or intestine after the removal of a cancer or an ulcer, introduced by Dr. Wangensteen in 1940, reduced the incidence of peritonitis, particularly after gastric surgery, and with it the rate of postoperative mortality.[2] For patients suffering from advanced gastric cancer, removal of part or the whole of the stomach was merely a palliative procedure that permitted the patient to live in reasonable comfort for an interval of usually no more than two years. Nevertheless, if cancer were detected early enough, it could be removed completely and the patient cured. From 1936 through 1945, Dr. Wangensteen

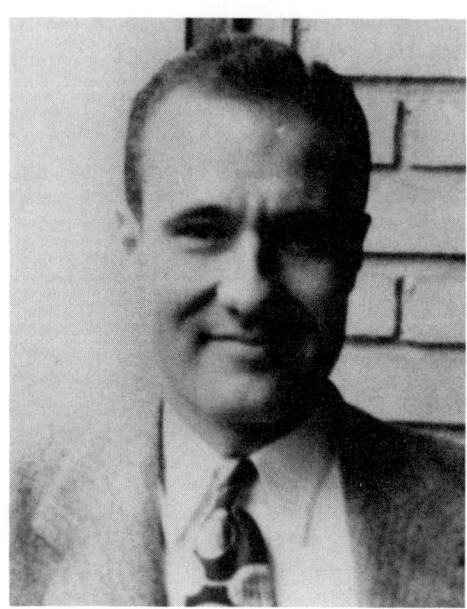

FIGURE 19:1   Stanley Friesen, circa 1950. Courtesy Mn U Archives.

and his colleagues found that they were able to operate upon an increasing proportion of cancers, and remove more of them, while during the same period the operative mortality rate dropped to less than a fifth of what it had been in 1936. The reduced mortality reflected not only improved surgical procedures but also better nutritional preparation to overcome the effects of semistarvation caused by stomach cancer, better control of the patient's fluid balance, and by 1945 the availability of antibiotics, especially penicillin. More than 20 percent of patients who had undergone gastrectomy for stomach cancer survived the operation more than five years, indicating that they had been cured permanently. The survival rate might have been higher except that many of the operations were performed on patients whose cancers were too far advanced to be curable, the purpose of the surgery being to make their final months more comfortable. Only about a quarter of the patients with stomach cancer were suitable candidates for a curative type of operation. If stomach cancer could be detected earlier, more patients might be curable. The difficulty was that a stomach cancer might become inoperable before the patient was aware of any symptoms.

Frequently after a radical operation for cancer of the stomach, Dr. Wangensteen learned from the pathologist that cancer cells were still present in the tissues of the stomach wall along the line of resection. In such patients, he observed that there was an interval of eighteen months to two years before symptoms of stomach cancer recurred. A Minnesota surgeon, Dr. Stanley R. Friesen, designated the period before symptoms of stomach cancer reappeared as *the silent interval,* a period he found to be about twenty months, followed by about two months of illness before death. Because a similar silent interval might also follow surgery for cancer of the colon and rectum, Dr. Wangensteen suggested in 1949 that when at operation patients were found to have lymph node metastases of their cancer, they should undergo a second operation after a period of three to four months to remove any cancerous growths that might have developed in the interval. Such second operations were known as *the second look,* for which the Minnesota surgical clinic became famous.[3]

By 1940 an increasing number of cancer patients were being referred to the university hospital for diagnosis and treatment. In 1937, the National Cancer Institute designated the University of Minnesota one among several regional centers for special training in cancer. In addition to surgery, an increasing number of patients were being treated for cancer at the university hospital with radiation. In June 1938, the Citizens Aid Society provided the radiology department with an additional 220 kilovolt x-ray machine for deep radiation treatments. Radiation treatments were supervised by Karl Wilhelm Stenstrom who was trained as a physicist rather than in medicine, but who had become an acknowledged authority on radiation therapy for cancer. Stenstrom found that an extended series of daily treatments with a large total dose of radiation was better tolerated and more effective than fewer but more severe radiation treatments. Stenstrom began to give such a series of radiation treatments for carcinoma of the cervix before surgery or radium therapy.[4] In 1937, Dr. Harold O. Peterson joined the Department of Radiology where he studied especially tumors of bone and of the central nervous system. Grants from the Citizens Aid Society also provided fellowships for the study of radiological diagnosis of cancer and the pathology of cancer. The fellow in pathology spent most of his time performing post-mortem examinations, which were especially valuable because during life the patients autopsied had received such thorough clinical study in the university hospital.

The Citizens Aid Society supported the mimeographed bulletin of the university hospital staff meeting. Since 1929 the university hospital staff had met for luncheon every Friday from October to June. During the 1930s and 1940s they met in the recreation room in Powell Hall, the nurses residence. After luncheon they held a scientific meeting at which one of the clinical departments presented a program. Papers delivered at the meeting were then published in the mimeographed *University of Minnesota Hospitals Staff Meeting Bulletin.* During the thirties more than two-thirds of the programs related to some aspect of cancer.

In April 1940 the annual George Chase Christian lecture, provided from the Citizens Aid Society grant, was delivered by John J. Bittner, associate director of the Roscoe B. Jackson Memorial Laboratory at Bar Harbor, Maine. Although only thirty-six years of age, Dr. Bittner was already well known for his discovery in mice of a cancer-producing factor that was transmitted through the mother's milk while nursing. In 1928 as a graduate student in zoology and genetics at the University of Michigan, Bittner had started breeding cancerous mice in an effort to identify the cause of cancer in them. After he obtained his Ph.D. at Michigan in 1930, Bittner went to the Jackson Laboratory where he developed inbred lines of mice,

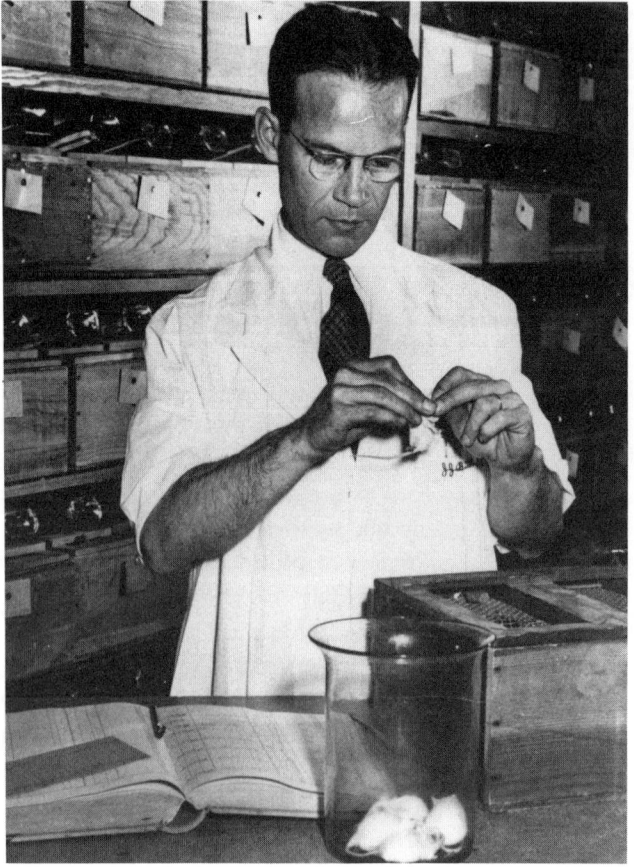

FIGURE 19:2 John J. Bittner, circa 1945. Courtesy Mn U Archives.

some of which showed a high incidence of breast cancer, others a low incidence. When he crossed female mice of a high-cancer line with males of a low-cancer line, the resulting female hybrid mice showed the same high frequency of breast cancer as their mothers. By contrast, when he crossed high-cancer males with low-cancer females, the female offspring showed a low incidence of breast cancer. Bittner concluded that some nongenetic factor must influence the development of breast cancer in mice, and in 1936 he traced it to a factor transmitted through the mother's milk while nursing.[5] In his Christian lecture in 1940, Bittner showed that susceptibility to breast cancer in mice was inherited through a single dominant gene, but the actual development of breast cancer was influenced strongly by the factor transmitted through the milk of female mice of high-cancer lines and by the influence of ovarian hormones on the mammary gland.[6]

Dr. Bittner's results offered a promising lead into the baffling problem of cancer, which was the central concern of the George Chase Christian Cancer Hospital

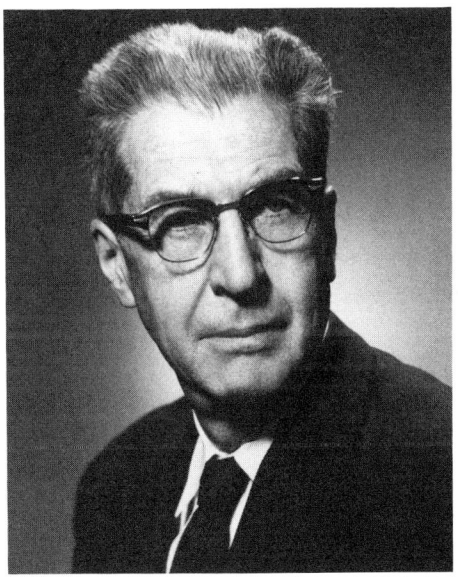

FIGURE 19:3 William Peyton, 1958. Courtesy Mn U Archives.

at Minnesota and of members of the faculty in various departments of the medical school, including Robert Green in bacteriology and Maurice Visscher in physiology. For several years the Citizens Aid Society of Minneapolis had made an annual grant of $10,000 to the Christian Cancer Hospital that was used to provide stipends for instructors and fellows, to support cancer research, and for social work related to the needs of cancer patients.[7] In 1942 the Citizens Aid Society made an additional grant to the university to support a George Chase Christian professorship in cancer research. John Bittner was appointed to the new chair and became director of a Division of Cancer Biology within the Department of Physiology.

Bittner's invitation to Minnesota came about because a group of faculty in the medical school were seriously interested in cancer. In addition to members of the surgery department who faced the practical problem of cancer in their day to day work, Dr. Robert Green in the Department of Bacteriology had studied cancer in wild animals. In 1936 Green helped to show that rabbit papilloma disease, known to be caused by a virus, was transmitted by the bites of ticks.[8] He also argued that viruses, as obligate parasites which could live and multiply only within the living cells of a host, may have developed by retrograde evolution of unicellular organisms. The virus could grow only by complementing its own limited vital processes with the functions of the surrounding host protoplasm.[9] Viruses might stimulate the metabolism and proliferation of the host cells, thereby producing the uncontrolled growth of host cells found in cancer. In 1940, with William Peyton and others, Green described the transmission of a virus-caused human papilloma to monkeys.

Even before John Bittner came to Minnesota in 1943, he had begun to collaborate with Green and Visscher in an effort to identify the cancer-producing factor in mouse's milk, which they isolated and found to have the characteristics and molecular size of a virus.[10] Visscher and Green established colonies of Bittner's mouse lines at Minnesota, but in the fall of 1942 the grants supporting their research ran out and they were forced to maintain their mouse colonies with small month-to-month grants from the graduate school research fund.[11] In 1943, with the energetic help of Regent James Ford Bell and Governor Stassen, the university obtained grants from foundations and from the Minnesota legislature to carry on the cancer research program on a more stable basis. The difficulty that the medical school experienced in obtaining research funds for such established investigators as Bittner, Green, and Visscher suggests how few and inadequate were the sources of research funds in the early 1940s.

In 1946 Green demonstrated that when the mouse cancer milk factor was injected into rabbits or rats, it stimulated the production of antibodies that would prevent the growth of cancer cells in mice. The observation provided further evidence that the mouse cancer milk factor was a virus and suggested a possible line of investigation toward the treatment of cancer.[12] This promising research was not to be. On 8 September 1947, Dr. Robert Green died suddenly of a heart attack, only a few months after he had been appointed to succeed Winford Larson as head of the Department of Bacteriology, Larson having died suddenly earlier in 1947. Within four years bacteriology at Minnesota lost by death three of its leading investigators, Arthur Henrici in 1943, and Winford Larson and Robert Green in 1947. In 1948 Jerome T. Syverton was appointed to succeed Dr. Green and the name of the department was changed to microbiology to reflect the broadening scope of its researches in virology and fungal diseases in addition to bacteriology.

In 1946 the study of cancer in the Department of Surgery took a new turn when Dr. George Moore, then a surgical resident, began to inject sodium fluorescein into patients who were to be operated upon for stomach cancer, in the hope that under ultraviolet light there might be revealed a difference in the amount of fluorescence between normal and malignant tissues. At first Dr. Moore found no variations in fluorescence, but when he injected the sodium fluorescein several hours before operation, patches of cancerous tissue on the surface of the peritoneum fluoresced with a vivid yellow color that distinguished them sharply from the surrounding normal tissue.[13] Nevertheless, if the tumor tissue lay even a few millimeters below the surface, it did not fluoresce, probably because the ultraviolet light could not penetrate much below the surface of the tissue. Colon, stomach, and breast cancers were less likely to fluoresce, but when biopsies were taken from brain tumors and placed under ultraviolet light they fluoresced consistently. During the following year Moore pursued the application of fluorescein dye to the localization of brain tumors. Using radioactive iodine, he prepared diiodofluorescein. Two to four hours after radioactive diiodofluorescein was injected into a patient, a Geiger counter detected an increase in radiation over the suspected tumor. In one patient in whom the Geiger counter outlined a definite area on the surface

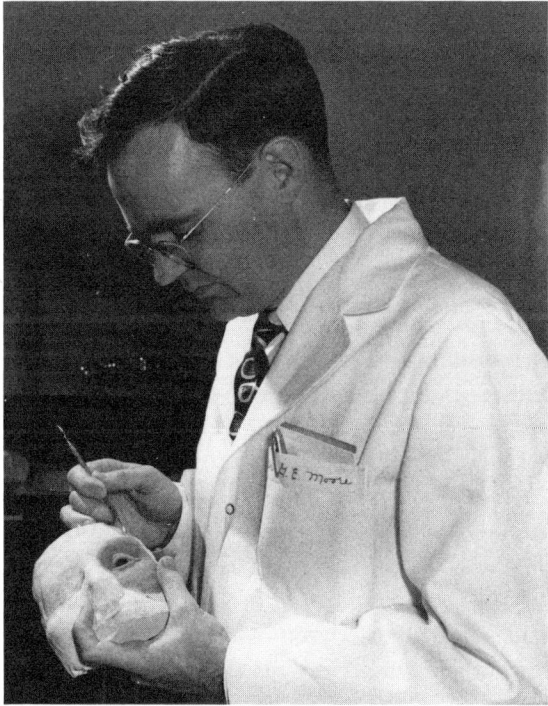

FIGURE 19:4   George E. Moore, 1952. Courtesy Mn U Archives.

of the skull, the outlined area coincided closely with a meningeoma found at operation.[14] However, radioactive diiodofluorescein proved less useful than injection of sodium fluorescein.[15] Brain tumors were so often accompanied by cerebral edema that neurosurgeons frequently could not determine the size and location of a tumor before operation, and consequently did not know where best to open the dura mater. They had been accustomed to make a needle biopsy and to section the biopsied tissue in order to locate a tumor before opening the dura mater. Nevertheless, such procedures were time consuming and difficult. In a patient who had been injected with fluorescein, they could simply place the biopsied tissue under ultraviolet light. If it were tumor rather than normal brain tissue, it showed a brilliant yellow green fluorescence. By March 1948 Moore had used the fluorescein technique on forty-six patients on Dr. William Peyton's neurosurgical service and had determined the presence or absence of tumor tissue correctly in forty-four of them, thereby demonstrating clearly the clinical value of the method. When ultraviolet light was shone into the cavity after surgical removal of a brain tumor, it sometimes revealed small pieces of tumor tissue that had previously been overlooked, so that the fluorescein method provided a check on the completeness of the surgery.[16]

Immune deficiency diseases

In 1952 Colonel Ogden C. Bruton, a pediatrician at the Walter Reed Army Hospital in Washington, D.C., published an account of an unusual patient, an eight-year-old boy, whom he had been observing for more than three years. At the age of four and a half the child had been admitted to the hospital suffering from a high fever and other signs of severe infection. Two days after he was started on a course of penicillin, the child's temperature dropped to normal, and he appeared well. Nonetheless, because his fever was thought to be caused by osteomyelitis, the penicillin was continued for twenty-eight days. He was then discharged from the hospital. Two weeks later he was back with pneumonia, and thereafter was in and out of hospital with successive infections, each of which was treated successfully with antibiotics. When the child twice suffered from pneumonia caused by the same pneumococcus, Bruton decided that he was not forming antibodies against it. He was then given a pneumococcal vaccine, but he still failed to form antibodies against the pneumococcus. He proved similarly incapable of forming antibodies against other pathogenic organisms. Something appeared to be wrong with his gamma globulins, from which antibodies are formed, and when his blood serum was analyzed by electrophoresis the gamma globulins were found to be completely absent. Thereafter, monthly injections of human gamma globulin prevented the child's recurrent bouts of infection. Ogden concluded that the child was suffering from a congenital failure to form gamma globulin or *agammaglobulinemia*.[17]

A year later Dr. Charles A. Janeway and his colleagues at the Harvard Medical School reported that they had collected nine cases of agammaglobulinemia, six from their own clinic and three from other parts of the country. All the patients were children and all were male, suggesting that the disease was inherited as a recessive sex-linked gene. They noted that the disease had been "unmasked by the antibiotic age," because before the availability of penicillin and other antibiotics such children would have died of overwhelming infections before their condition could be studied.[18]

Once agammaglobulinemia was described, many cases began to be recognized. At the University of Minnesota during the first nine months of 1954, Dr. Robert A. Good discovered and studied seven patients with agammaglobulinemia, including five children and two adults. All the children were boys; of the adults one was a woman. Although they were unable to resist bacterial infections, they seemed to possess normal defenses against viral infection. In both of the adults, the agammaglobulinemia appeared to be acquired rather than inborn. The male patient, a fifty-eight-year-old man, also suffered from a large tumor of the thymus gland and lacked eosinophils almost completely in both his blood and bone marrow. In fact, all of the patients with agammaglobulinemia lacked plasma cells in their blood. The absence of plasma cells was especially significant to Dr. Good because four years earlier he had collaborated with Fred Kolouch in showing that plasma cells originated from the reticuloendothelial tissue of the bone mar-

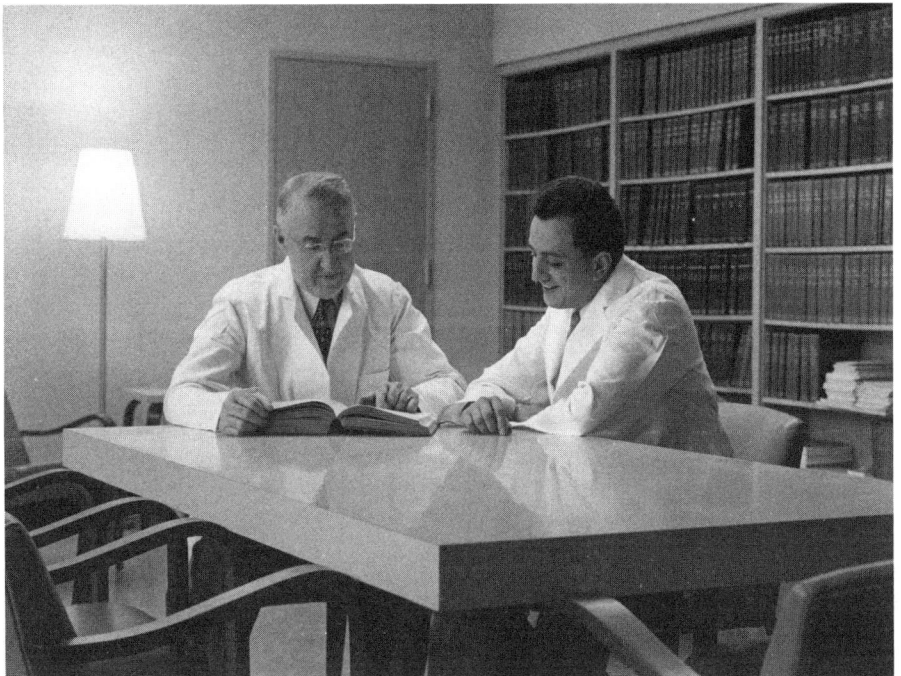

FIGURE 19:5 Robert A. Good (right) with Irvine McQuarrie in the Pediatrics conference room, 1955. Courtesy Mn U Archives.

row.[19] Nevertheless, patients with agammaglobulinemia showed the same acute reaction as normal persons—chills, fever, and malaise—to the injection of endotoxins, showing that the acute reactions to infection were distinct from the production of antibodies. Dr. Good regarded agammaglobulinemic patients as invaluable experiments of nature from which physicians might gain understanding of immunological systems. Of special interest was the observation that a skin graft from an adult to a seven-year-old boy with agammaglobulinemia took, grew, and continued to survive seven months after application.[20] The successful skin graft provided further evidence that the reason why transplanted organs normally failed to survive was because they were rejected by the host's immunological system.

In 1955, as a result of further studies on agammaglobulinemia patients, Robert Good confirmed the absence of plasma cells in them. He suggested that plasma cells must be involved in the formation of antibodies and gamma globulin, and noted Hal Downey's early observation that plasma cells possessed many of the characteristics of secretory cells.[21] Meanwhile in April 1954 a fifty-eight-year-old man, from whom a large thymic tumor had been removed in November 1951, was readmitted to the university hospital because of recurrent severe bacterial infections, including bouts of pneumonia and several attacks of septicemia.

Electrophoretic analysis of his blood serum showed an absence of gamma globulin. While in hospital the patient developed intense jaundice and died on Christmas Day 1954. The association of acquired agammaglobulinemia with a tumor of the thymus in this patient suggested that the thymus gland might play a role in antibody production. Lloyd D. Maclean, a surgical resident, and three colleagues, including Robert Good, tested the relationship by removing the thymus gland from rabbits but observed no effect on the immune system.[22]

During the later 1950s, Robert Good and his colleagues continued to study patients with agammaglobulinemia, testing their receptivity to transplants of skin and of lymph nodes.[23] By 1960 Good and his group had studied nineteen boys with the inherited sex-linked recessive form of agammaglobulinemia and nine adults with acquired agammaglobulinemia, and they had helped to establish the diagnostic and pathological features of the disease. Ten of the twenty-eight patients had died of various infectious diseases. Victims of agammaglobulinemia suffered from gross immunological deficiencies, unable to form antibodies against bacterial infections or such viral diseases as mumps, herpes simplex, and poliomyelitis.[24] Despite the lack of antibodies against viral diseases, the agammaglobulinemic patients possessed normal resistance and developed normal immunity to viral diseases. Patients with agammaglobulinemia lacked plasma cells and failed to produce plasma cells in response to antigens. The lymphatic tissues in their lymph nodes, bowel, spleen, and bone marrow were generally undeveloped. Good and his colleagues concluded that agammaglobulinemia resulted from a basic defect in the blood-forming cells of the reticuloendothelial tissue of the bone marrow and lymph nodes.

In 1960 August Mueller and his colleagues at the University of Wisconsin published their work on the bursa of Fabricius in chickens, an organ that develops as an outgrowth of the wall of the cloaca. They found that when they either prevented the development of the bursa of Fabricius by injection of an androgenic hormone (19-nortestosterone) into the incubating egg, or removed the bursa of Fabricius surgically from chicks at the age of one week, the birds' ability to form antibodies was markedly reduced. But if the bursa were not removed until the chickens were ten weeks old, its removal had no effect on antibody production.[25] Since the function of the bursa of Fabricius was thought to be the same as that of the thymus, Robert Good and his colleagues at Minnesota realized that the reason for the failure of their 1958 experiments in removing the thymus from rabbits might have been that the rabbits were already mature at the time of thymectomy. Working in Good's laboratory at Minnesota, Olga Archer and J.C. Pierce proceeded to remove the thymus from young rabbits when they were only five to seven days old, and they found that the thymectomized rabbits were unable to form antibodies. They concluded that the thymus was essential for the normal development of the immune response in the rabbit.[26] In 1962 Good and his colleagues confirmed that surgical removal of the thymus from newborn rabbits and mice prevented the development of any capacity to form antibodies. The mouse proved more suitable than the rabbit for the demonstration of the role of thymus, because at birth the mouse had almost all of its lymphoid tissue restricted to the thymus. Good and his colleagues suggested that in the course of development lymphoid cells were distributed from the thymus to reticuloendothelial tissues in the spleen, lymph nodes, bowel, and other sites.[27] Ben Papermaster and Robert Good compared the embryological development of the bursa of Fabricius in chickens with that of the thymus in mammals and found a rich development of lymphocytes in both glands.[28]

The discovery that the thymus gland played a critical role in the establishment of the immune system in early life led to the identification in the late 1960s of two important classes of lymphocytes, the T-lymphocytes derived from the thymus and the B-lymphocytes which originate independently of the thymus. During the 1960s investigators demonstrated that the lymphocytes originate in the thymus from precursor cells that have migrated to that organ from the bone marrow.[29] The discovery of the essential role of the thymus in immunity thus was a key that opened a door to a broad array of questions in immunology.

Rheumatic Fever and Streptococcal Infections

In 1952 Lewis W. Wannamaker came to the medical school as an instructor in pediatrics. Dr. Wannamaker was a native of South Carolina, who had been educated at Emory University and had studied medicine at Duke University. As a medical student and later as a house officer on the pediatric wards of Duke Hospital, Wannamaker became interested in the frequency of skin infections in children suffering from acute nephritis, and in the laboratory he attempted to isolate hemolytic streptococci from such skin infections. After completing a residency in pediatrics at Duke in 1948, Dr. Wannamaker entered the United States Army, and immediately he was assigned to a new Streptococcal Diseases Laboratory at the Francis A. Warren Air Force Base at Cheyenne, Wyoming. The Warren Air Force Base had an average strength of 8,000 men, who were there to take short training courses; there was a turnover of about a thousand men per month. Epidemics of streptococcal throat infections and rheumatic fever among the men were a continual problem. In the 1940s 200,000 to 250,000 new cases of rheumatic fever occurred annually in the United States, and each person who developed rheumatic fever not only suffered prolonged illness, but might also be left with a permanently damaged heart. In the armed services rheumatic fever was an especially serious problem because when thousands of young men were brought together in the crowded conditions of large training camps, they became exposed to a multitude of respiratory infections, including streptococcal infections, and in a certain proportion of patients streptococcal infections resulted in rheumatic fever. At Fort Warren, Lewis Wannamaker worked with Drs. William R. Brink and Floyd Denny under Charles H. Rammelkamp, director of the Streptococcal Diseases Laboratory, who, however, was absent much of the time because of his responsibilities at Western Reserve University. Rheumatic fever occurred frequently among the airmen in training at Fort Warren and had been a great problem in the armed services during World War II. The group, therefore, began to investigate whether rheumatic fever might be prevented by vigorous treatment of streptococcal sore throat infections. In patients who had already suffered an attack of rheumatic fever, prophylactic treatment with sulphonamides appeared to prevent a repetition of rheumatic fever, but sulphonamides were unable to prevent the initial attack of rheumatic fever in a patient who was already suffering from an acute streptococcal throat infection. The Fort Warren group decided to try treatment of streptococcal throat infections with penicillin, and in order to avoid delay in treatment they began to give penicillin immediately to soldiers who came to sick call with a sore throat. They assigned soldiers randomly to treatment or control groups and among those treated, they tested three different level of penicillin dosage.[30] By late in 1949, the Fort Warren group established, in contrast to the observations of earlier workers, that prompt treatment of acute streptococcal infections with large doses of penicillin would prevent the development of rheumatic fever almost completely.[31] Later Lewis Wannamaker and his colleagues confirmed their initial findings in a study of more than 2,000 patients. They found also that penicillin prevented the formation of antibodies against streptococci, a finding which suggested that the penicillin had eliminated the streptococcal infection from the patient's body.[32]

The success of the Fort Warren group in the prevention of rheumatic fever with penicillin was the reason why, at the conclusion of their period of army service, both Lewis Wannamaker and Floyd Denny came to Minnesota in 1952. One of the principal purposes of the Variety Club Heart Hospital, which had just opened, was the study of rheumatic fever, and the director of the laboratories, Lewis Thomas, was eager to develop a team of investigators to pursue research in rheumatic fever.

In the late summer of 1953, a little over a year after Wannamaker's arrival at Minnesota, six members of one family, including both parents and four of five children, were admitted to the Minneapolis General Hospital suffering from acute nephritis associated with streptococcal infections. The family epidemic was so striking that the chief of pediatrics, Irvine McQuarrie, encouraged Lewis Wannamaker to investigate it as an expanded "experiment of nature," and provided funds from the limited resources of the pediatrics department to support the research. Wannamaker found that in each member of the family attacked, acute nephritis appeared about six days after the streptococcal infection. The source of the epidemic appeared to be exposure to scarlet fever in the family of an aunt, a sister of the father, who lived in a crowded tenement in Minneapolis where some of the other residents were Indians who had recently come from the Red Lake Indian Reservation in northern Minnesota. The State Health Department had learned that on the Red Lake Indian Reservation there was also an epidemic of scarlet fever

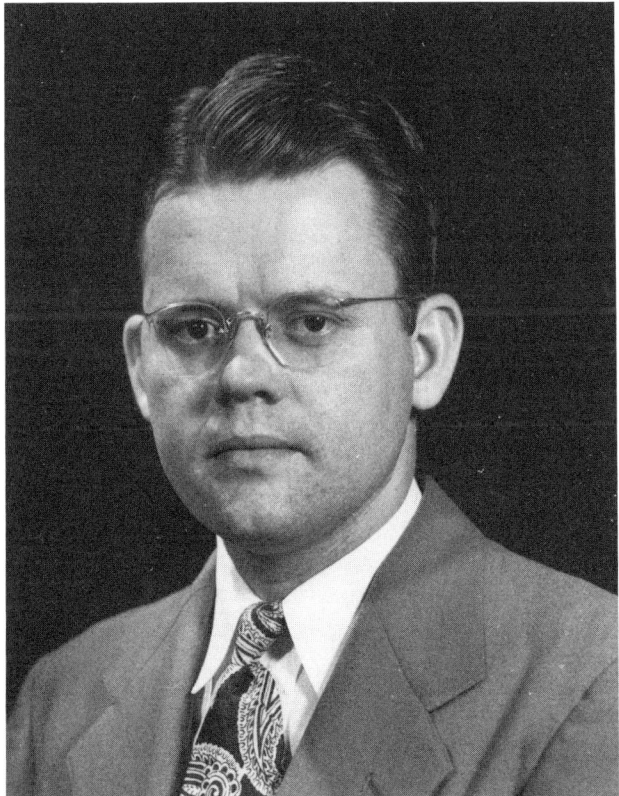

FIGURE 19:6 Lewis Wannamaker, circa 1952. Courtesy Doreen Bower.

and acute glomerulonephritis, the latter frequently accompanied by pyodermic skin infections, that is, impetigo. Since the family epidemic at Minneapolis appeared to be connected with the epidemic at Red Lake, Dr. Wannamaker arranged for two patients with skin infections to be sent from Red Lake to the university hospital for study. The streptococcal infections associated with acute nephritis in the family at Minneapolis and the streptococci associated with skin infection and acute nephritis among the Indians at Red Lake were both of a new and unknown serological type that Lewis Wannamaker and Howard Pierce designated *type 49*.[33]

From his initial study of the familial epidemic of acute glomerulonephritis at Minneapolis and its connection with the Red Lake epidemic, Lewis Wannamaker continued for more than thirty years to study streptococcal infections and their complications, especially rheumatic heart disease and glomerulonephritis. Wannamaker and his colleagues confirmed that rheumatic fever occurred as a sequel to streptococcal throat infections, but did not follow upon streptococcal infections of the skin. They showed that the streptococci causing skin infections were different from those causing throat infections, and indeed belonged to types that had not previously been identified.[34] In 1958 Dr. Wannamaker was appointed a career investigator of the American Heart Association, an appointment that permitted him to work at any institution he cared to select. He chose to continue at Minnesota, where, apart from sabbaticals, he remained until his untimely death in the spring of 1983. His work on streptococcal disease is continued by an active group of colleagues whom he helped to develop.

Staphylococcic Infections

In 1942 Dr. Wesley Spink received from the committee on medical research of the Office of Scientific Research and Development in Washington, D.C., a small supply of penicillin to be tested for its effectiveness against staphylococcic infections. On 10 July 1942 Dr. Spink and his colleague Dr. Wendell Hall used penicillin to treat a seven-year-old girl who was gravely ill with acute osteomyelitis, staphylococcal pneumonia, and septicemia, and expected to die. Instead of dying, the child recovered rapidly with penicillin treatment. Over the next two years, Spink and Hall treated some 200 patients with penicillin and were able to reduce the death rate from staphylococcic septicemia from 80 percent to 35 percent. They generally reserved penicillin for staphylococcic infections because the sulphonamides had already proven effective against streptococci. They found that penicillin could reduce the death rate from pneumococcic and staphylococcic meningitis and lung abscesses, and even offered hope for victims of that dread disease bacterial endocarditis. It was the drug of choice for the treatment of gonorrhea.[35] Nevertheless, quite early in the use of penicillin, resistant strains of staphylococci began to appear, and hospitals began to experience epidemics of staphylococcal sepsis. In 1947 Wesley Spink and Viola Ferris showed that penicillin-resistant strains of staphylococci were particularly common in hospitals, such as the university hospital, where penicillin had been used extensively.[36] By 1951 the problem of resistant organisms was even greater. Sulphonamide-resistant strains of gonococcus and hemolytic streptococcus made the sulphonamides no longer reliable for the treatment of gonorrhea or streptococcal infections. At the university hospital, Dr. Spink found that penicillin-resistant strains of staphylococcus were increasing at an alarming rate and that such resistant strains could overcome the effects of even high concentrations of penicillin because they produced an enzyme, penicillinase, that destroyed the penicillin.[37] Dr. Spink and his colleagues found again and again that when penicillin failed clinically to control a staphylococcal infection, the staphylococcus responsible for the infection produced penicillinase. So frequently was penicillin resistance encountered by 1951 that Dr. Spink could no longer use it confidently for the treatment of staphylococcal infections. Fortunately Dr. Spink and his colleagues found that penicillin-resistant staphylococci could usually be treated effectively with other antibiotics, especially with aureomycin. Resistance to aureomycin developed more slowly and gradually than resistance to other antibiotics.

Through the 1950s the problem of antibiotic-resistant strains of staphylococci grew ever more serious. Strains of staphylococci resistant to a particular antibiotic appeared about in proportion to the frequency with which the antibiotic was used. Dr. Spink found that in the university hospital patients and staff tended to become colonized with antibiotic-resistant staphylococci in their noses and throats. In 1959 Paul Quie reported the appearance of staphylococci resistant to neomycin, an antibiotic that had been available for about ten years, but the use of which had been limited because of its toxic side effects.[38]

Since antibiotics were no longer reliable for the treatment of staphylococcal infection, Dr. Spink decided to return to an older method of strict isolation of the patient with staphylococcal sepsis in order to avoid transmission of the infections in the hospital. In February 1961 the university hospital established station 52 as a seventeen-bed isolation unit for patients from all hospital services with staphylococcal infections. At the entrance to the isolation unit all staff on duty changed to surgical gowns and caps and changed their shoes. When treating patients they also wore masks and gloves, which were discarded immediately afterward. Floors were mopped several times daily with antiseptic detergents that were used also to wash the shoes of everyone and the wheels of all carts leaving the isolation unit. The isolation unit proved a remarkable success. The number of staphylococcal infections declined throughout the hospital, and the whole hospital staff, including janitors and elevator operators, became alert to the importance of isolation technique. The morale of patients in the isolation unit was also good because they received the benefit of intensive nursing. The combination of epidemiologic study of the staphylococci causing the infections with strict antisepsis brought the problem of hospital-induced staphylococcal disease under control.[39]

Because of the limited value of antibiotics against staphylococcal infections, during the 1960s Paul Quie began to study the natural defenses against staphylococci. A native of Minnesota, Dr. Quie was educated at St. Olaf College in Northfield and studied medicine at Yale. In 1954 he began a residency in pediatrics at the university hospital and in 1958 joined the faculty of the Department of Pediatrics. In 1961, with Lewis Wannamaker, Dr. Quie described an assay for antistaphylokinase, an antibody against staphylococci.[40] In 1967, in the McQuarrie tradition of studying "experiments of nature," Quie showed that in children suffering from granulomatous disease, an immune deficiency disease described at the university hospital in 1957, the polymorphonuclear leukocytes possessed a reduced capacity to kill bacteria that they had ingested in phagocytosis.[41] His observations suggested that the cellular process of phagocytosis was separate from the process of digestion of the bacteria within the leukocyte, and thus he threw light on the fundamental nature of the body's defenses against disease.

In 1971, with Cynthia Curry, Dr. Quie showed that patients who were subject to prolonged intravenous catheterization for parenteral feeding frequently developed fungal septicemia.[42] Their results led to the greater use of disposable, hermetically sealed, sterile reservoirs for intravenous fluids, sterile disposable catheters, and regular changes of the intravenous site. In 1974 Harry Hill and Paul Quie found that three children suffering from chronic eczema and a succession of severe abscesses caused by staphylococcal infection each had a defective neutrophil granulocyte chemotaxis, a condition now known as the Hill-Quie Syndrome.[43] In 1978 Dr. Quie and his colleagues identified peptidoglycan as a component of the cell walls of staphylococci that was active in the opsonization of the organisms, and therefore in the action of the immune system of the host.[44] This research first identified the key role of the staphylococcal cell wall in the development of staphylococcal infections.

NOTES

1. Clarence Dennis to Leonard G. Wilson, 20 October 1987, personal communication, deposited in Mn U Archives.

2. David State, George Moore, and Owen H. Wangensteen, "Carcinoma of the stomach: A ten year survey (1936 to 1945 inclusive) of early and late results of surgical treatment at the University of Minnesota Hospitals," *J. Am. med. Ass.*, 1947, *135*, 262–267.

3. O.H. Wangensteen, "Cancer of the colon and rectum with special reference to: 1) earlier recognition of alimentary tract malignancy; 2) secondary delayed re-entry of the abdomen in patients exhibiting lymph node involvement; 3) subtotal primary excision of the colon; 4) operation in obstruction," *Wisc. med. J.*, 1949, *48*, 591–597.

4. K.W. Stenstrom, "Roentgen therapy," *Univ. Minn. Hosp. staff Meet.*, 1939, *10*, 383–386.

5. John J. Bittner, "Some possible effects of nursing on the mammary gland tumor incidence in mice," *Science*, 1936, *84*, 162.

6. John J. Bittner, "Breast cancer in mice as influenced by nursing," *J. natn Cancer Inst.*, 1940, *1*, 155–168. This paper was the published text of the George Chase Christian Lecture.

7. Diehl to Mrs. George Chase Christian, 8 April 1942 [copy], President's Office, Papers.

8. C.L. Larson, J.E. Shillinger, and R.G. Green, "Transmission of rabbit papillomatosis by the rabbit tick, Haemaphysalis leporis palustris," *Proc. Soc. exp. Biol. Med.*, 1935–36, *33*, 536–538.

9. Robert G. Green, "On the nature of filterable viruses," *Science*, 1935, *82*, 443–445.

10. Maurice B. Visscher, Robert G. Green, and John J. Bittner, "Characterization of milk influence in spontaneous mammary carcinoma," *Proc. Soc. exp. Biol. Med.*, 1942, *49*, 94–96.

11. Green and Visscher to Blegen, 5 December 1942 [copy]; Blegen to Coffey, 5 December 1942, President's Office, Papers.

12. Robert G. Green, Marye M. Moosey, and John J. Bittner, "Antigenic character of the cancer milk agent in mice," *Proc. Soc. exp. Biol. Med.*, 1946, *61*, 115–117; Robert G. Green, "Virus aspects of carcinoma," *Minn. Med.*, 1946, *29*, 277–279.

13. George E. Moore, "Fluorescein as an agent in the differentiation of normal and malignant tissues," *Science*, 1947, *106*, 130–131.

14. George E. Moore, "Use of radioactive diiodofluorescein in the diagnosis and localization of brain tumors," *Science*, 1948, *107*, 569–571.

15. G.E. Moore, S.W. Hunter, and T.B. Hubbard, "Clinical and experimental studies of fluorescein dyes with special reference to their use for the diagnosis of central nervous system tumors," *Ann. Surg.*, 1949, *130*, 637–642.

16. George E. Moore et al., "The clinical use of fluorescein in neurosurgery," *J. Neurosurg.*, 1948, *5*, 392–398.

17. Ogden C. Bruton, "Agammaglobulinemia," *Pediatrics*, 1952, *9*, 722–728.

18. Charles A. Janeway et al., "Agammaglobulinemia," *Trans. Ass. Am. Physns*, 1953, *66*, 200–202.

19. Fred Kolouch, Robert A. Good, and Berry Campbell, "The reticuloendothelial origin of bone marrow plasma cells in hypersensitive states," *J. lab. clin. Med.*, 1948, *32*, 749–755.

20. Robert A. Good, "Agammaglobulinemia - a provocative experiment of Nature," *Bull. Univ. Minn. Hosp. & Minn. Med. Fndn*, 1954, *26*, 1–19. Cf. Robert A. Good and Richard L. Varco, "Successful homograft of skin in a child with agammaglobulinemia," *J. Am. med. Ass.*, 1955, *157*, 713–716.

21. Robert A. Good, "Studies on agammaglobulinemia," *J. lab. clin. Med.*, 1955, *46*, 167–181. Cf. Hal Downey, "The origin and structure of the plasma cells of normal vertebrates, especially of the cold-blooded vertebrates and the eosinophils of the lung of Amblystoma," *Folia haemat.*, 1911, *11*, 275–314.

22. Lloyd D. Maclean et al., "Thymic tumor and acquired agammaglobulinemia: A clinical and experimental study of the immune response," *Surgery*, 1956, *40*, 1010–1017; L.D. Maclean et al., "The role of the thymus in antibody production: an experimental study of the immune response in Thymectomized rabbits," *Transpl. Bull.*, 1957, *4*, 21–22.

23. Robert A. Good et al., "Transplantation studies in patients with agammaglobulinemia," *Ann. N. Y. Acad. Sci.*, 1957, *64*, 882–928.

24. Robert A. Good et al., "Clinical investigation of patients with agammaglobulinemia and hypogammaglobulinemia," *Pediat. Clin. N. Am.*, 1960, *7*, 397–433.

25. August P. Mueller et al., "Precipitin production in chickens. XXI. Antibody production in bursectomized chickens and in chickens injected with 19-nortestosterone on the fifth day of incubation," *J. Immunol.*, 1960, *85*, 172–179.

26. Olga Archer and J.C. Pierce, "Role of thymus in development of the immune response," *Fed. Proc.*, 1961, *20*, 26.

27. Robert A. Good et al., "The role of the thymus in development of immunologic capacity in rabbits and mice," *J. exp. Med.*, 1962, *116*, 773–796. Cf. B.W. Papermaster et al., "Suppression of antibody forming capacity with thymectomy in the mouse," *Proc. Soc. exp. Biol. Med.*, 1962, *111*, 41–43.

28. Ben W. Papermaster and Robert A. Good, "Relative contributions of the thymus and bursa of Fabricius to the maturation of the lymphoreticular system and immunological potential in the chicken," *Nature*, 1962, *196*, 838–840.

29. William L. Ford, "The lymphocyte — its transformation from a frustrating enigma to a model of cellular function," in Maxwell M. Wintrobe, ed., *Blood, pure and eloquent*, pp. 457–508.

30. Maclyn McCarty, "Lewis Wannamaker in the campaign against rheumatic fever," *Zentbl. Bakt. Mikrobiol. Hyg.*, 1985, ser. A, *260*, 151–164.

31. Floyd W. Denny et al., "Prevention of rheumatic fever: Treatment of the preceding streptococcic infection," *Am. J. med. Ass.*, 1950, *143*, 151–153.

32. Lewis W. Wannamaker et al., "Prophylaxis of acute rheumatic fever by treatment of the preceding streptococcal infection with various amounts of depot penicillin," *Am. J. Med.*, 1951, *10*, 673–695.

33. Lewis W. Wannamaker and Howard C. Pierce, "Family outbreak of acute nephritis associated with type 49 streptococcal infection," *J.-Lancet*, 1961, *81*, 561-571. Cf. Herman Kleinman, "Epidemic acute glomerulonephritis at Red Lake," *Minn. Med.*, 1954, *37*, 479-483, 489.

34. Lewis W. Wannamaker, "The chain that links the heart to the throat (T . Duckett Jones Memorial Lecture)," *Circulation*, 1973, *48*, 9-18.

35. Wesley W. Spink and Wendell H. Hall, "Penicillin therapy at the University of Minnesota Hospitals: 1942-1944," *Ann. intern. Med.*, 1945, *22*, 510-525.

36. Wesley W. Spink and Viola Ferris, "Penicillin-resistant staphylococci: mechanisms involved in the development of resistance," *Ann. intern. Med.*, 1947, *26*, 379-393.

37. Wesley W. Spink, "Clinical and biological significance of penicillin-resistant staphylococci, including observations with streptomycin, aureomycin, chloramphenicol, and terramycin," *J. lab. clin. Med.*, 1951, *37*, 278-293.

38. Paul Quie et al., "Neomycin-resistant staphylococci," *Lancet, Lond.*, 1960, *279, ii*, 124-126.

39. Ward E. Bullock et al., "A staphylococcal isolation service: Epidemiologic and clinical studies over one year," *Ann. intern. Med.*, 1964, *60*, 777-789. Cf. Wesley W. Spink, *Infectious diseases: Prevention and treatment in the nineteenth and twentieth centuries*, pp. 282-287.

40. Paul G. Quie and Lewis W. Wannamaker, "Serum antibodies in staphylococcal disease," *Pediatrics*, 1964, *33*, 63-70.

41. P.G. Quie et al., "In vitro bactericidal capacity of human polymorphonuclear leukocytes: Diminished activity in chronic granulomatous disease of childhood," *J. clin. Invest.*, 1967, *46*, 668-679. Cf. H. Berendes et al., "A fatal granulomatosus of childhood: the clinical study of a new syndrome," *Minn. Med.*, 1957, *40*, 309-312.

42. Cynthia Rapp Curry and Paul G. Quie, "Fungal septicemia in patients receiving parenteral alimentation," *N. Engl. J. Med.*, 1971, *285*, 1221-1225.

43. Harry R. Hill and Paul G. Quie, "Raised serum-Ig E levels and defective neutrophil chemotaxis in three children with eczema and recurrent bacterial infections," *Lancet*, 1974, *i*, 183-187.

44. Philip K. Peterson et al., "The key role of peptidoglycan in the opsonization of *Staphylococcus aureus*," *J. clin. Invest.*, 1978, *61*, 597-609.

CHAPTER 20

The Development of Cardiac Surgery at Minnesota 1940–1960

The bold approach to open heart surgery introduced in the mid-1950s by young surgeons at the University of Minnesota opened the way for the successful treatment of many fatal or crippling cardiac defects and focused international attention on the medical school. Within a few months, Minnesota was a mecca for inquiring surgeons and patients needing cardiac repair. *Hypothermia, cross circulation,* and *bubble oxygenator* became bywords at surgical gatherings throughout the world. Time and place were ripe for such a burst of originality. The development of open heart surgery can be understood only in relation to the historical forces that converged to produce it.

On 1 September 1939, Dr. Owen Wangensteen, using a technique introduced the year before by Dr. Robert E. Gross at the Children's Hospital in Boston, successfully ligated a patent ductus arteriosus in a child at the university hospital.[1] During fetal life, the ductus arteriosus transfers a large part of the blood pumped by the right ventricle of the heart directly into the aorta, thereby by-passing the circulation through the lungs. Normally at birth, the ductus arteriosus closes off so that all blood pumped by the right ventricle must pass through the lungs in order to reach the left side of the heart. If the ductus remains open, retaining a direct connection between the pulmonary artery and the aorta, the pressure in the pulmonary artery must be essentially the same as in the aorta, and blood circulates through the lungs under much higher pressure than normal. Although patent ductus arteriosus is not itself a defect of the heart, it has consequences identical in several respects to those caused by defects in the interior of the heart. It makes the heart work inefficiently as a pump; it forces the right side of the heart to work against the same pressure as the left; and it raises pressure in the pulmonary arteries far above normal.

Although Robert Gross's introduction in 1938 of a method for tying off the ductus made the operation possible, physicians initially were hesitant to recommend such surgery. In 1940 the risks of surgical operation were far higher than today. The control of anesthesia was imperfect, surgical shock was an ever-present threat, and the understanding of fluid and electrolyte balance rudimentary. Despite such risks, the promise of heart surgery was too great to ignore.

Cardiac operations were of particular interest to the Minneapolis physician Morse J. Shapiro who, on his graduation from the Minnesota medical school in 1917, had served in the United States Army as a medical officer in World War I. In the examination of soldiers at Camp Dodge, Iowa, Dr. Shapiro had become impressed with the large number of men with heart defects who gave a history of rheumatic fever during childhood. After his return to Minneapolis, Dr. Shapiro continued his work on heart disease at the Lymanhurst Health Center for tuberculous children where he established a forty-bed hospital for children with rheumatic fever or rheumatic heart disease.

In examining children for rheumatic heart disease, Dr. Shapiro also came across children with congenital heart defects. In 1941 with Dr. Ancel Keys, he published a valuable study of twenty-three patients with patent ductus arteriosus, whom he had studied at the Lymanhurst clinic between 1922 and 1940.[2] Shapiro and Keys concluded that since most patients with patent ductus arteriosus were free of symptoms and led normal, unrestricted lives, they should not be subjected to the considerable risk of ligation of the ductus as recently announced by Dr. Robert Gross. Two years later in 1943, Shapiro and Keys had changed their minds. Further study of a larger series of patients revealed that although most of them suffered no serious disability throughout most of their lives, few survived beyond the age of thirty-five. About 40 percent developed subacute bacterial endocarditis—an invariably fatal disease before the introduction of antibiotics—while the remainder died of congestive heart failure.[3] Even though patients with patent ductus arteriosus might appear to be in good health, they carried a lethal defect. Their life expectancy could be increased greatly by closure of the ductus, and the operation should be performed before the abnormally high blood pressure in the pulmonary arteries had damaged the lungs. By 1943 surgical operations to ligate or sever the ductus were demonstrably successful. At the university hospital, Owen H. Wangensteen had operated on ten patients for patent ductus arteriosus, the last eight cases with complete success.[4] But if all patients with patent ductus arteriosus were to have surgical operations, the need for such surgery would exceed the existing capacity of the university hospital.

Meanwhile, the university hospital was receiving increasing numbers of children with rheumatic fever and rheumatic heart disease, but their facilities could not provide the prolonged periods of bed rest with medical treatment that such cases required. Instead, many children from small towns and rural areas in Minnesota had to stay in boardinghouses in the neighborhood of the hospital in order to visit the clinic as outpatients.[5] Frequently they were forced by poverty to return to their homes in isolated parts of the state where they might remain bedridden for months with little or no medical attention. At this time even the Twin Cities had only two rheumatic fever clinics, one at the university and the other at Children's Hospital in St. Paul.

The scope of cardiac surgery was dramatically enlarged by Dr. Alfred Blalock's operation in 1944 at the Johns Hopkins Hospital to help the congenital condition known as tetralogy of Fallot (stenosis of the pulmonary artery, ventricular septal defect, enlargement of the right ventricle, and right location of the aorta). Following a suggestion of his colleague, the pathologist Helen B. Taussig, Blalock connected the left subclavian artery to the left pulmonary artery to provide additional blood supply to the lungs. Although the first patient, a fifteen-month-old girl, died six months after the operation, the next two children were transformed from a breathless, cyanotic state, in which they could hardly walk, to normal health and activity.[6] The Blalock-Taussig procedure was carried on thereafter on so-called bluebabies, not only at Johns Hopkins but at medical centers throughout the world.

The Variety Club Heart Hospital

In 1944 Mr. Al W. Steffes, owner of motion picture theaters in Minneapolis and Chief Barker of Tent 12 of the Minneapolis unit of the Variety Club, a service organization of people in the entertainment business, paid a visit to the Glen Lake Tuberculosis Sanatorium. His particular interest was in the children's rheumatic fever clinic conducted by his friend Dr. Morse J. Shapiro. The incidence of tuberculosis had declined so much that the sanatorium was partially empty, and Dr. Shapiro's rheumatic fever clinic and hospital had been moved to Glen Lake from the Lymanhurst Health Center in Minneapolis to make room for Elizabeth Kenny's treatment of victims of poliomyelitis. Glen Lake was west of the city of Minneapolis and about twelve miles from the university, making it difficult for school children to get there for examination and for Dr. Shapiro to combine his work at Glen Lake with his duties as associate professor of medicine at the university hospital.[7]

When Al Steffes recognized the lack of facilities in Minneapolis for the treatment of children with rheumatic heart disease and the difficulty of using the clinic at Glen Lake for the teaching of medical students, he invited Shapiro to present his ideas to the Variety Club. In the fall of 1944 Morse Shapiro, accompanied by his colleague and friend, Jay Arthur Myers, spoke to a meeting of Tent 12 of the Variety Club. Dr. Myers was known throughout Minnesota for his work on tuberculosis. Shapiro and Myers described the acute need for a special heart hospital in connection with the university hospital to serve the needs of children throughout the Northwest. The club members responded enthusiastically, and on 25 January 1945 made a formal offer to the Board of Regents to raise at least $150,000 for the construction of a Variety Club Heart Hospital on the campus in connection with the university hospital and to pledge a minimum of $25,000 annually for its support. The Board of Regents accepted the offer and Tent 12 began a fundraising campaign.

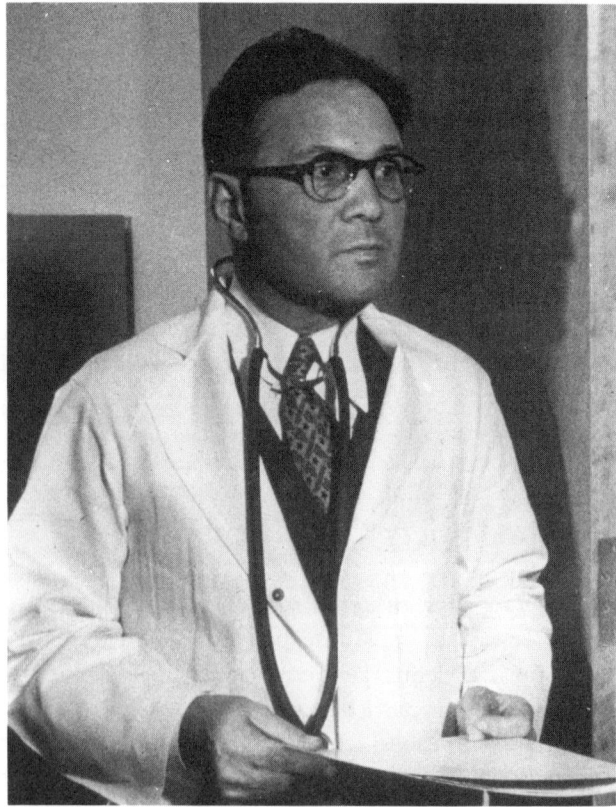

FIGURE 20:1   Morse J. Shapiro. Courtesy Mn U Archives.

In the 1940s, the motion picture industry was at its height in America. Television had not yet appeared, and every night of the week the movie theaters were filled. On weekend evenings, even in the depths of winter, long lines formed in the street to buy tickets to popular films. Since many of the Variety Club members were connected with the motion picture industry, they decided to use the movies to appeal to the public. Warner Brothers Studio in Hollywood made without charge a short movie on the urgent need for a heart hospital. In the film, actor Ronald Reagan appealed to movie audiences to join in the battle against heart disease by contributing to the proposed hospital. The film was shown as a trailer to the main feature in hundreds of theaters throughout the Northwest.

In May 1945 the campaign for the heart hospital received a significant boost from the announcement by Blalock and Taussig of their successful blue-baby operations. As the possibilities for the surgical treatment of congenital heart defects became more apparent, the need for a special heart hospital became ever more urgent and the Variety Club rose to the challenge.[8] In the end the Variety Club raised more than $500,000 for the heart hospital, while the federal govern-

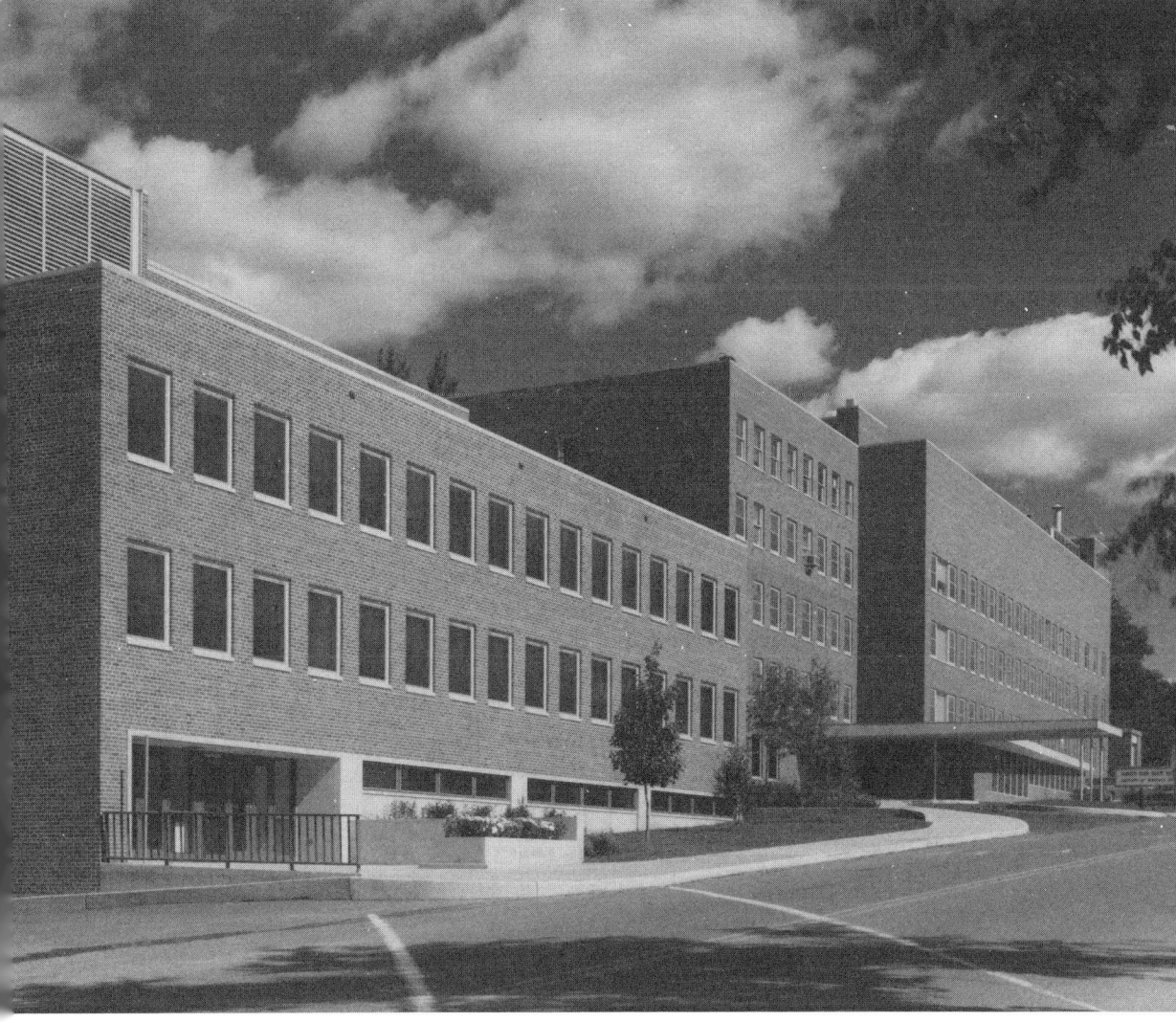

FIGURE 20:2 Variety Club Heart Hospital. Courtesy Mn U Archives.

ment provided $600,000, and the university contributed $400,000 from other gifts and special funds. When completed in March 1951 at a cost of more than $1.5 million, the Variety Club Heart Hospital was a four-story building, standing on the slope overlooking the Mississippi River and connected to the original Elliot block of the university hospital by a bridge on the top floor.[9] It was the first hospital in the United States to be devoted entirely to heart patients, and the first addition to the university hospital to be opened since 1929.

Late in 1945, when the drive for the heart hospital was in full swing, Maurice B. Visscher, head of physiology, and Owen H. Wangensteen, chief of surgery, suggested to Clarence Dennis, associate professor of surgery, that he undertake to develop a mechanical heart-lung apparatus that would permit the complete bypass of the heart and lungs during surgical operations on the heart. Dr. Dennis was the son of Warren Dennis, a St. Paul surgeon and a former member of the medical faculty. Clarence Dennis graduated M.D. in 1935 from Johns Hopkins and then came to Minnesota for his residency in surgery under Dr. Wangensteen. In accordance with Dr. Wangensteen's custom of requiring residents to study physiology, he spent the year 1938–39 working with Dr. Visscher in the Department of Physiology. After he completed his Ph.D. in surgery in 1940, Dr. Dennis was appointed to the faculty in the Department of Surgery. When World War II broke out in 1941, Dennis found himself physically disqualified from entering military service, so he was obliged to remain at the medical school. During the war years, when the department was short staffed, Clarence Dennis was occupied more than fully with surgical teaching and the care of patients.

With the end of the war in 1945, the whole situation changed. Faculty who had been with the 26th General Hospital, or who had served elsewhere with the services, returned to the medical school. At the same time, large numbers of young doctors who had gone directly into the services from medical school returned to begin residencies. Thus the faculty, restored to its prewar strength, had crowds of young physicians to train. In 1945 the medical school was unusually well prepared to meet the situation. Most of its departments were led by men still in their forties and at the peak of their energies, who had established international reputations in their respective fields. In radiology, Leo Rigler was a leading figure in x-ray diagnosis and Karl Wilhelm Stenstrom in radiation therapy; in medicine, Cecil Watson was a world authority on liver diseases and Wesley Spink, renowned for his work on brucellosis, was doing important research on the clinical use of sulfa drugs and penicillin; in physiology, Maurice Visscher was an acknowledged authority on the heart and circulation; and in physiological chemistry, Wallace Armstrong was known for his discovery of the role of fluoride in the prevention of tooth decay. Finally, in surgery, Owen Wangensteen was famous for his work on intestinal obstruction and the discovery of gastric suction. In American military hospitals in every theater of the war, the wards containing soldiers with abdominal wounds had become known as "Wangensteen alleys" because of the rows of Wangensteen suction tubes, one attached to each wounded man.

In addition to the brilliance of his own work, Dr. Wangensteen had created in the Department of Surgery conditions for the training of surgical residents that were unusual, if not unique. Each member of the surgical faculty was expected to pursue some line of research, on which residents might work with him. Dr. Wangensteen thought that surgical residents should spend only a limited part of their time in the care of patients and attendance at operations. They needed to learn to operate, certainly. They must also learn to perform such routine duties as the insertion of intravenous tubes, but once mastered little more was to be learned by the endless repetition of such tasks. Surgical residents, Dr. Wangensteen thought, needed time to read and to think, and to try out their ideas in the laboratory. He would not have them mere intellectual parasites, using ideas and methods developed by others. They must contribute, he said, to the patrimony of their subject.

Dr. Wangensteen believed these things, believed them passionately, and worked furiously to bring them about. From a multitude of sources he obtained funds to enable him to appoint large numbers of residents so that there would be plenty of residents to do the necessary hospital work while the rest were learning experimental physiology, doing research in the laboratory, or reading in the library. If the training that a resident needed was not available in the medical school, Dr. Wangensteen would send him to another university. In the early 1930s he sent Charles Rea to the University of Chicago, and other residents to the University of Illinois to study physiology with Maurice Visscher. After Visscher returned to Minnesota in 1936, he and Wangensteen developed a joint physiology-surgery seminar, and Dr. Wangensteen sent many residents, as he had Clarence Dennis, to spend a full year working in physiology with Maurice Visscher.

Shortly after he became chief of surgery, Dr. Wangensteen introduced into the routine of the department a weekly review of complications that had occurred during surgical operations, including a merciless analysis of how and why mistakes were made, and how in future they might be avoided. In such sessions the surgical staff were unsparing of one another, not with intent to be cruel, but in order to avoid the perpetuation of false ideas or slipshod practices. The atmosphere thus created was not comfortable, but it was stimulating. The Canadian surgeon Dr. Morley Cohen, who visited from Winnipeg several times in the early 1950s before coming to Minnesota to take a residency, commented: " . . . I was impressed with the broad yet fundamental approach to a multitude of surgical problems during these sessions, which were carried on in an atmosphere of competitive informality. The staff said what they thought to be right (and no doubt many were wrong but they were certainly sure nonetheless). Few pussyfooted around the accomplishments or deficiencies of the clinical and research problems . . . brought forward at these sessions." Dr. Cohen added that he could not help but be impressed by the frequently imaginative suggestions made by Dr. Wangensteen during the discussions. After Dr. Cohen came to Minnesota as a surgical resident, he found the training program often seemingly chaotic, residents disappearing to the research labs for extended periods of time, then returning, and sometimes leaving again for another interval. Nevertheless, such constant change and unpredictability stimulated residents to do their utmost to accomplish some research that would establish their identity.[10] A further feature of the surgical program at Minnesota, unusual at the time, was that it was open to anyone of ability, regardless of race, creed, or color. People of diverse races and from many countries came to Minnesota for surgical training. In this active and inquiring atmosphere, Clarence Dennis took up the search for an effective heart-lung machine.

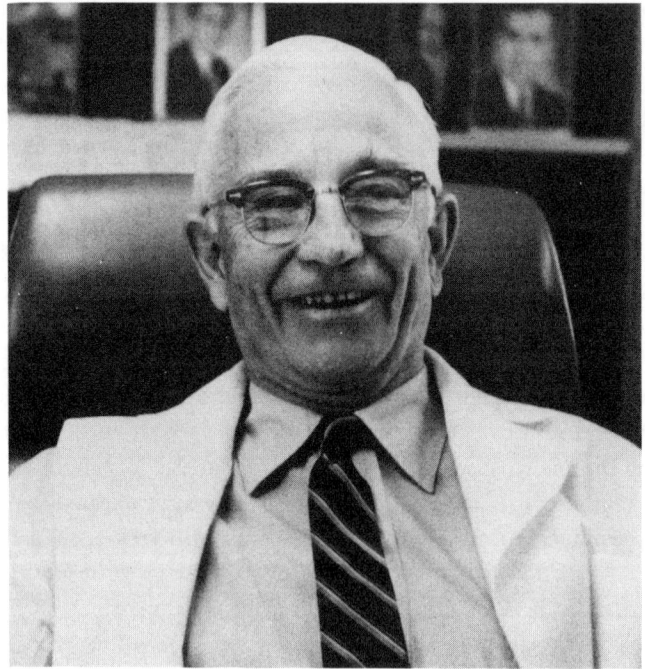

FIGURE 20:3   Owen H. Wangensteen, "the Chief," 1954. Courtesy Mn U Archives.

The concept of a heart-lung machine was not new. In 1931 when Dr. John Gibbon was a surgical fellow under Dr. Edward D. Churchill at the Massachusetts General Hospital, he conceived the idea of a machine to assist the heart and lungs after watching a patient dying from a massive pulmonary embolism. Although Dr. Churchill had operated rapidly to remove the embolus, the patient died on the operating table.[11] Gibbon realized that, if they could have oxygenated the blood and maintained the circulation even during the brief period of the operation, the patient might have been saved. In 1934, during his second surgical fellowship at the Massachusetts General Hospital, Gibbon began research on a heart-lung machine and by 1937 had developed a machine that would maintain respiration and circulation in experimental animals for thirty to forty minutes during complete heart-lung by-pass.[12] Nevertheless, at the conclusion of by-pass the normal function of the heart and lungs was restored in only three of his animals, and they survived only a few hours.

At Jefferson Medical College at Philadelphia in 1937, Gibbon built a new heart-lung machine, using two of the roller pumps introduced by Michael De Bakey in 1934. The new machine had sufficient capacity to perform the work of the heart and lungs in experimental cats, but it was too small to serve for dogs or man.[13] The outbreak of World War II brought Gibbon's research to a halt. When he returned from war service to become professor of surgery at Jefferson, he resumed work on a larger and more effective heart-lung machine. Thus in late 1945, when Clarence Dennis began work on a heart-lung machine at the University of Minnesota, John Gibbon was taking up the project on which he had worked for seven years before the war.

In 1946 John Gibbon sought the help of skilled engineers.[14] Ultimately an IBM engineer built a new heart-lung machine for him, designed to minimize hemolysis and to prevent air bubbles from entering the circulation.[15] The blood circuit was enclosed within a cabinet kept at body temperature, and the blood flow was carefully controlled to maintain a constant blood volume. With it John Gibbon was able by 1947 to create a complete heart-lung by-pass in small dogs in order to perform surgery inside their hearts. Although at first 80 percent of the dogs died, Gibbon and his colleagues gradually learned how to avoid air embolism as a result of opening the heart, and within three years they were able to reduce the mortality rate to 10 percent.[16]

When Clarence Dennis attempted to construct a blood oxygenator at Minnesota, he studied the kinds of apparatus that had been devised by other investigators. The requirements of an oxygenator were that it would use as little blood and do as little damage to the blood cells as possible, and that it would achieve a high level of oxygenation with a minimum of foaming. Dennis first tried passing the blood through tubes of cellulose sausage casing in an oxygen atmosphere. The sausage casing was intended to serve as a dialysing membrane, which, by separating the blood from direct contact with the oxygen, would prevent both foaming and bacterial contamination of the blood. Nevertheless, the rate of oxygenation through the cellulose membrane was too low to make the method practical. Therefore, the blood must be brought into direct contact with the oxygen. Dennis and his colleagues next injected oxygen directly into the blood flowing through the membranous tubes, but they immediately began to lose an excessive amount of blood by foaming. A system of slowly revolving horizontal cylinders likewise produced excessive foaming. When they distributed the blood on the inner surface of a vertical rotating plexiglass cylinder containing oxygen, they found, as had Gibbon, that the blood did not foam and that it was oxygenated sufficiently for experiments on animals, although the machine was still limited in its oxygenating capacity. A vertical revolving funnel showed characteristics similar to the revolving cylinder, but did reduce the damage to the red blood cells.[17]

Dennis and his colleagues next built a modified Gibbon pump consisting of a nest of vertical revolving stainless steel cylinders mounted over a revolving funnel in which the blood, oxygenated on the walls of the cylinders, was collected. They checked every detail of design and construction to minimize injury to the red blood cells. In place of De Bakey roller pumps they used modified Dale-Schuster pumps because the latter resulted in less hemolysis. The resultant apparatus was cumbersome, difficult to sterilize, and difficult to clean. More serious still, most of the dogs on which it was used died, either during perfusion with the machine or shortly afterward. Among sixty-four dogs on which they operated, they had only nine survivors, and while some of the deaths occurred during the developmental testing of the machine, many others occurred after it was complete.

Dennis and his colleagues found that although they had succeeded in reducing the hemolysis of red cells, other drastic changes occurred in the blood of the experimental dogs. Half of the plasma protein was lost during thirty minutes of perfusion, the platelets fell to one third, and the white blood cell count was cut in half. Frequently a marked acidosis developed that was followed by a fatal gastrointestinal hemorrhage a few hours later.[18] Dennis and his colleagues did not know why such changes occurred, nor how to prevent them. During the next year Dr. Russell M. Nelson found that the destructive changes in the blood were identical with those produced by infection of the blood with a paracolon bacillus. With this clue, the oxygenating apparatus was found to be contaminated. Once contamination was identified as the source of trouble, they changed the method of sterilization to eliminate it. They also changed the design of the oxygenator, abandoning the nest of revolving vertical cylinders in favor of the application of a film of blood by jets on to multiple screen discs, rotating slowly on a shaft, a method introduced by a Swedish investigator, Viking Bjork. The multiple screens provided an oxygenator with capacity sufficient for an adult human.

During the designing and testing of the new multiple screen oxygenator, Dennis and his colleagues learned much about how to avoid the factors causing hemolysis. They redesigned the blood pumps to reduce turbulence, crushing of cells, and sudden changes in pressure. When they began experiments on dogs, they first kept the dogs under observation for two weeks during which time they were well fed, checked for distemper, and de-wormed. The night before the operation they were given penicillin and streptomycin. Despite such precautions, the death rate among dogs subjected to heart operations while perfused with the machine remained formidably high. On 5 April 1951, Dennis and his colleagues used the new blood oxygenator for an open heart operation on a six-year-old girl, breathless and cyanotic because of a large defect in her interatrial septum. At the time of operation, the child was suffering from pulmonary edema. Her heart was enlarged and was failing rapidly. During the operation Dennis was astonished at the amount of blood returning into the right ventricle of the heart from the Thebesian veins, about 250 cc. per minute, or fifteen times the quantity they had observed coming from the Thebesian veins in the hearts of dogs. So much blood from the Thebesian veins was aspirated from the heart that they were forced, without having planned for it, to return the aspirated blood to the oxygenator.

Although the patient died shortly afterward, Clarence Dennis was encouraged by the performance of the blood oxygenator during the operation. He and his colleagues had learned much about the planning and organization required to perform heart surgery with an oxygenator. The team included two physician-anesthetists, four surgeons, four men to run the oxygenator and pumps, one man to run the intra-arterial transfusion apparatus, one man to take blood samples, two technicians, and two nurses — or a total of sixteen persons in the operating room. Dennis thought that the blood oxygenator as it then existed offered a prac-

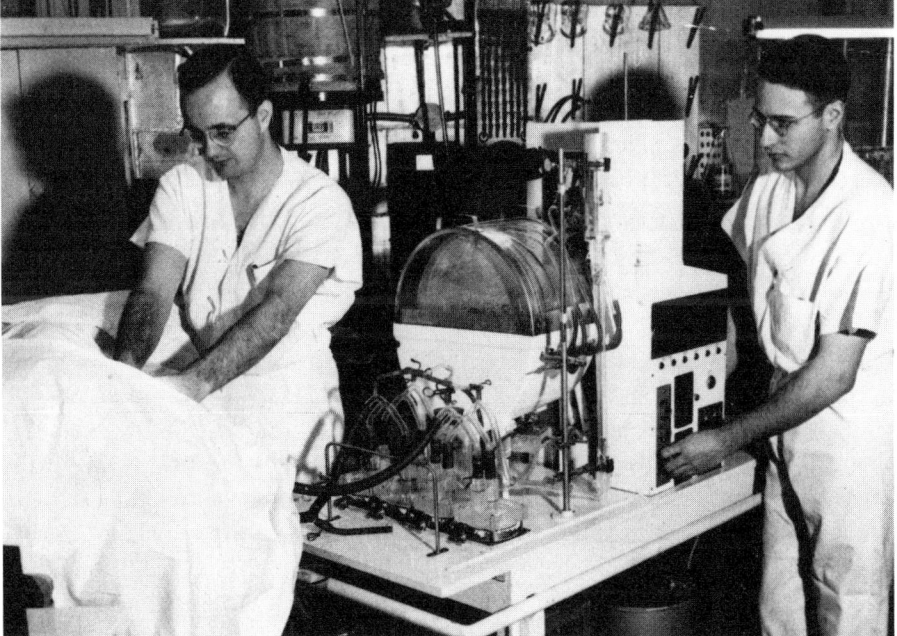

FIGURE 20:4 Clarence Dennis and W. Harris preparing for heart surgery, using the multiple screen blood oxygenator, 1951. Courtesy Mn U Archives.

ticable means to provide a chance of survival to cardiac patients who otherwise would surely die. He attributed the loss of his patient to the unexpectedly large flow of Thebesian blood, and consequent loss of blood. They did learn that to permit the heart to fill with blood from the Thebesian and coronary veins at the end of the operation was sufficient to avoid air embolism.

Clarence Dennis and his colleagues were not alone in the difficulties that they encountered in the use of a mechanical blood oxygenator. At Philadelphia, John Gibbon's team, using the oxygenator designed for him by IBM engineers, consisting of a battery of fixed screens over which films of blood were allowed to flow within an oxygen chamber, continued to experience similarly high mortalities among their experimental dogs. Among twenty-one dogs that had been maintained on the heart-lung apparatus for periods of from twenty minutes to more than an hour and a half, fourteen died. Although half of the deaths were from obvious causes that might be avoided in future, the reasons for the other deaths remained obscure.[19] Some of the dogs that did survive suffered fairly severe hemolysis during the operation.

In 1951 when the Minnesota and Philadelphia groups each presented their results with blood oxygenators to the American Surgical Association, they had overcome one defect of earlier blood oxygenators—insufficient oxygenating capacity—only to find that far too many of the dogs on which they operated were dying from unknown causes. The year before at Toronto, Canada, W. G. Bigelow and his colleagues showed that if experimental dogs were cooled down to 20° C., their oxygen consumption fell to about 15 percent of normal, and their hearts could be isolated from the circulation for as long as fifteen minutes and operated on with survival. Because many of the dogs died from fibrillation of the heart, either in the cold state or on rewarming, Bigelow and his colleagues used electric shocks to defibrillate such hearts, and even used an artificial pacemaker to deliver repeated electric impulses at the desired heart rate for fifteen minutes. Nevertheless, as with the blood oxygenator, many of the dogs died for reasons that could not be identified.[20]

In July 1951, Clarence Dennis became professor of surgery at the State University of New York Downstate Medical Center at Brooklyn, New York, and took his blood oxygenators with him. The Downstate Medical Center paid the University of Minnesota some $16,000 for the equipment, thereby creating a fund with which to continue research on heart surgery at Minnesota. Fortunately, Dr. C. Walton Lillehei, appointed associate professor of surgery in 1951, wished to pursue research in heart surgery. Then at the age of thirty-three, Dr. Lillehei was one of those young physicians who in 1946 returned from war service to begin a surgical residency. He had completed his surgical residency the year before, but the day after he completed his residency, he underwent radical surgery on his head, neck, and chest for a lymphosarcoma that had appeared on his right ear.

While a surgical resident, Dr. Lillehei spent the year 1948-49 working with Dr. Maurice Visscher in physiology. In his research of that year, Lillehei found that when he created large arteriovenous fistulas in dogs so as to require their hearts to work much harder to pump a larger volume of blood, the dogs invariably developed bacterial endocarditis and kidney disease (glomerulonephritis). Lillehei saw immediately that the endocarditis and glomerulonephritis produced by overloading the heart might explain why bacterial endocarditis developed so frequently among patients with congenital heart defects.[21] Frequently persons with such congenital heart defects as interatrial and interventricular septal defects or patent ductus arteriosus also developed lesions of the heart valves, which reduced the pumping efficiency of the heart even further. Lillehei suggested that the valvular lesions might be the result of one or more attacks of bacterial endocarditis brought about by stress on the heart created by the congenital defect.[22] If congenital heart defects led regularly and inevitably to the development of bacterial endocarditis, then the correction of heart defects became urgent, even when such defects might appear superficially benign. Thus in 1951 on experimental grounds, Dr. Lillehei arrived at the same conclusion for congenital heart defects of all kinds that Morse Shapiro and Ancel Keys had reached in 1943 on purely clinical evidence for patent ductus arteriosus alone.[23] Since the only hope of curing congenital heart defects lay in the development of open heart surgery, which would permit the surgeon to operate under direct vision, Dr. Lillehei decided to pursue research on open heart surgery. A number of times at autopsies on patients who had died with tetralogy of Fallot, the pathology resident permitted Lillehei to perform mock operations to correct the defects. He found that through an incision in the outflow tract of the right ventricle he could, operating under direct vision, correct the anatomical defects with two or three well-placed stitches.[24] Lillehei knew, therefore, that if they could once gain access to the interior of the heart to operate under direct vision, the surgery itself would be relatively simple. By 1951 physicians were also coming to realize that congenital heart defects occurred far more commonly than previously thought. Statistics from two large series of autopsies, one in Massachusetts and the other in Minnesota, showed that congenital heart defects were responsible for about one percent of all deaths.[25] Moreover, because heart defects caused death at an early age, they occurred even more commonly than the autopsy figures suggested. In 1952 a survey of preschool age children in Colorado found over 15 cases of congenital heart defects per 1,000.[26] The Blalock-Taussig procedure, introduced in 1944, certainly helped victims of tetralogy of Fallot, but the procedure did not correct the fundamental defect. Such children still had an inefficient, overworked heart, and could not be expected to live out a full life. The adequate correction of congenital heart defects depended on the development of open heart surgery, which would permit the surgeon to operate inside the heart under direct vision. Thus when Dr. Wangensteen asked him what his research interest would be, Dr. Lillehei replied "open heart surgery" and Dr. Wangensteen accepted it without question.

From what Lillehei knew in 1951 of the various kinds of mechanical heart-lung apparatus that had been developed by Gibbon, Dennis, and others, he thought them complex, difficult to sterilize, and therefore difficult to use repeatedly. The mechanical heart-lung, which was the product of intensive scientific and engineering development over the preceding five years, still required experienced and highly skilled teams to make it work, and a majority of the dogs operated upon died mysteriously, often after having recovered initially from the effects of the operation. Lillehei concluded that if open heart surgery were to be accomplished, heart-lung by-pass must be achieved by some simpler, more easily controlled means.

In 1952 the British surgeon Anthony Andreasen and his assistant, Frank Watson, working at the laboratories of the Royal College of Surgeons at the Buckston Browne Farm (on the former estate of Charles Darwin) at Downe, Kent, were investigating the conditions under which dogs might survive after occlusion of the vena cava for the purpose of surgery on the interior of the heart. Andreasen noted that the various investigators who had attempted to isolate the heart from the circulation by clamping off the superior and inferior vena cava all failed to state clearly whether they had, or had not, shut off the flow from the azygos vein. Yet, if the return of venous blood to the heart were to be prevented completely, the azygos vein would have to be shut off. In preliminary experiments, Andreasen and Watson found that if they shut off the two venae cavae, while leaving the azygos vein open, dogs would survive for longer than ten minutes. If the azygos vein were closed, the dogs showed signs of brain damage after five minutes, and none survived after ten minutes' closure. By contrast, if they left the azygos vein open, dogs could survive without signs of brain damage for up to forty minutes with both venae cavae shut off. In other words, the flow of blood through the azygos vein supplied sufficient blood to the brain to prevent brain damage for periods as long as forty minutes. When Andreasen and Watson measured the azygos flow, they found that it rose sharply when the venae cavae were shut off and then declined slowly throughout the period of the experiment. The initial azygos flow was sufficient to enable the dogs to survive without brain damage, and although declining steadily, the flow did not drop below the minimum needs of the brain until after forty minutes.[27]

In 1948 at Guy's Hospital, London, Russell Brock operated successfully to relieve stenosis of the valves in the pulmonary artery.[28] The operation required a small opening into the right ventricle of the heart through which a curved valvulotome was passed and inserted into the pulmonary artery, cutting apart the fused valves. At Johns Hopkins, Alfred Blalock adopted Brock's procedure, and during 1949–50 Russell Brock served as an exchange professor of surgery at the Johns Hopkins Medical School. By March 1950 operations for pulmonary stenosis using Brock's technique had been performed on nineteen patients at the Johns Hopkins Hospital.[29] Until operation the patients were in a dangerous condition. Some of them had previously undergone a Blalock-Taussig procedure to increase the blood supply to the lungs. After the opening of their stenosed pulmonary valves, such patients required a second operation to close the artificial ductus created by the Blalock-Taussig procedure.

When Dr. John Paine returned to the Minnesota surgery department from the 26th General Hospital in 1946, he took over from Dr. Wangensteen responsiblity for patent ductus operations and for the early Blalock-Taussig procedures on children suffering from tetralogy of Fallot, and when Dr. Paine left a year later to go to the University of Buffalo, Dr. Richard Varco, assistant professor of surgery, became primarily responsible for such procedures.

At the University of Minnesota, Dr. Varco, using the Blalock-Taussig procedure, was accustomed to open the pericardium widely enough to check for the presence of the valvular type of stenosis in the pulmonary artery. He found that about 30 percent of tetralogy of Fallot patients suffered also from pulmonary stenosis, whereas Dr. Blalock thought that patients with tetralogy of Fallot rarely suffered from the valvular type of pulmonary stenosis. Since it seemed worthwhile to correct stenosis of the pulmonary valve in patients with tetralogy of Fallot in order to reduce the number of defects, Dr. Varco and his colleagues explored the ability of the heart to withstand the cutting off of the inflow of blood through the superior and inferior venae cavae and the azygos vein. With their work on dogs, they found that they could isolate the heart for as long as four minutes with eventual recovery of the animal; this finding they applied to patients and began to use a very brief interruption of cardiac inflow in order to correct the pulmonary valvular stenosis under direct vision.[30] Nevertheless, because the Minnesota surgeons realized that they knew very little about the ability of the normal heart to tolerate a complete stoppage of venous inflow, in 1951 Morley Cohen, who came to Minnesota after three years of postgraduate training in surgery at the University of Manitoba, began experiments on the interruption of the inflow of blood to the hearts of dogs. Dr. Cohen and his colleagues found that the dogs recovered well from up to five minutes of complete venous occlusion (including ligation of the azygos vein). After six minutes occlusion, the dogs showed some paralysis, mostly in the hind legs, and after seven minutes they suffered severe and irreversible brain damage. By repetition of periods of venal occlusion alternated with periods of recovery, Cohen and his colleagues were able to gain up to fifteen minutes of complete venous occlusion during which they first created and then closed defects in the interatrial septum.[31]

When Andreasen's and Watson's work on azygos flow was published in 1952, Lillehei realized its possible significance for cardiac surgery. He and Cohen carried out quantitative experiments to determine the amount of blood returning to the heart through the azygos vein, with the two venae cavae ligated, and the ability of the azygos flow to sustain the life of an animal without damage to the brain or other organs. They confirmed Andreasen's and Watson's finding that the amount of blood flowing through the azygos vein, after the two venae cavae were ligated, was sufficient to maintain the vital organs undamaged for extended periods of time. "This conclusion was surprising to us," wrote Cohen and Lillehei, "but nonetheless inescapable."[32] They then undertook to measure directly the amount of the azygos flow in a series of animals subjected to thirty minutes of vena caval occlusion, recording at the same time systemic blood pressure and pulse rate. In contrast to Andreasen and Watson, Cohen and Lillehei found that the azygos flow did not decline over the thirty-minute period of vena caval occlusion, but remained steady and sometimes even increased. The quantity of flow was related to body weight, but increased more rapidly with increasing body weight than did body weight itself.

The significance of the observations of azygos flow was that they showed that the level of blood flow required to maintain life in the animal without damage to the brain or other organs was only about 8 to 9 percent of the normal basal output of the heart of an anesthetized dog. If the body could be maintained without damage by a flow of blood less than one-tenth of the resting output of the heart, the requirements for maintaining the body during the time that the heart must be isolated from the circulation for open heart surgery were radically less than had been presupposed. Cohen and Lillehei suggested that under conditions of reduced blood circulation, the blood vessels, including the capillary beds of such organs as the brain and the heart, became dilated so as to receive a larger proportion of the limited blood supply, and the tissues removed from the circulating blood a much larger proportion of the oxygen than under conditions of normal circulation. In fact, they demonstrated experimentally that in dogs maintained on azygos flow, the oxygen level of venous blood was only about one-tenth its normal level.[33]

Dr. Lillehei and his colleagues believed strongly that they might avoid many of the difficulties of mechanical blood oxygenators by using normal lung tissue,

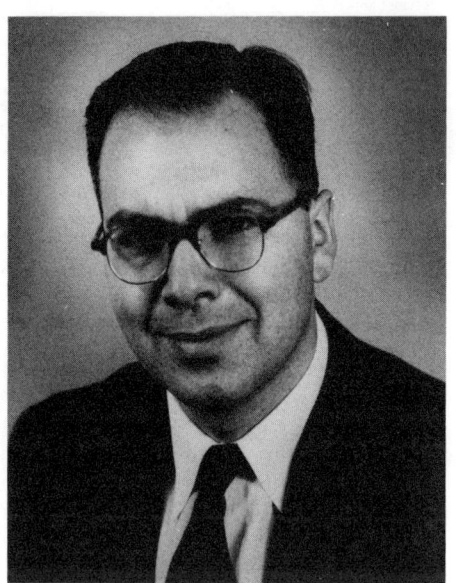

FIGURE 20:5   Morley Cohen, circa 1954. Courtesy Mn U Archives.

whether in patient or donor, for blood oxygenation. A mechanical blood oxygenator inevitably removed platelets and fibrinogen from the blood so that it might create postoperative-clotting problems. Then, too, passage of the blood through the lungs served to filter harmful particles from it, including bacteria.

On the assumption that a flow of oxygenated blood equal to the azygos flow would be sufficient to maintain the body unharmed during complete heart by-pass, Cohen and Lillehei performed cardiac by-pass operations on a series of dogs, using just one lobe of the lung, the cardiac lobe, as a blood oxygenator. In each dog they first inserted cannulae into the right external jugular vein and the right common carotid artery. Next they opened the chest, ligated the azygos vein and placed loops of tape around the two venae cavae. They inserted a cannula into the branch of the pulmonary artery supplying the cardiac lobe of the lung and another cannula into the pulmonary vein from the same lobe. The cannulae were then attached to the pump circuits so that they would withdraw venous blood from the jugular vein, circulate it through the cardiac lobe of the lung where it would become oxygenated, and supply it to the arterial system through the right common carotid artery. The pumps maintained the circulation at a level corresponding to the azygos flow, and the two venae cavae were tied off by tightening the loops around them.

Among the first eighteen dogs operated on while the techniques were still being perfected, thirteen survived and five died. In a second group of thirty-two dogs, each subjected to thirty minutes of perfusion during complete cardiac by-pass, there were no deaths. Cohen and Lillehei then performed cardiac surgery on the auricles of a series of five dogs during complete cardiac by-pass, again with

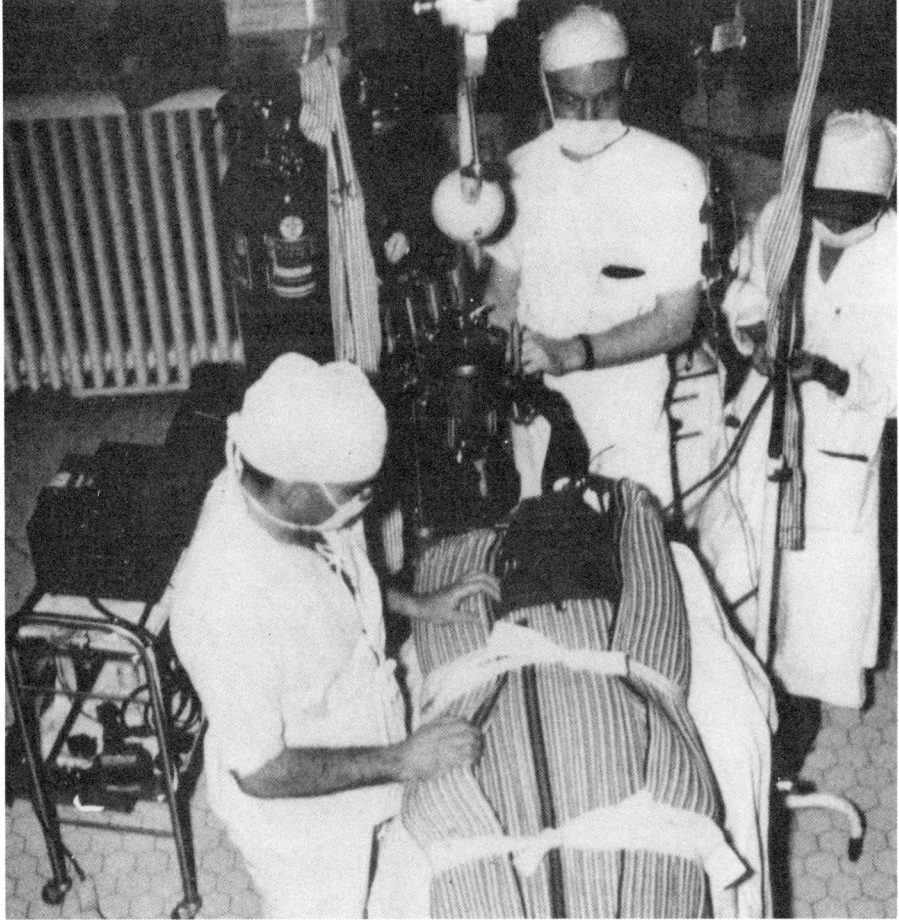

FIGURE 20:6 Anesthetized patient shown wrapped in the refrigerating blankets for heart surgery, 1953. (Lewis, Varco, and Taufic, 1954.) Courtesy *Surgery*.

no deaths. Such results were strikingly different from those experienced by Gibbon, Dennis, and others with mechanical heart-lung machines and suggested that the unexplained deaths in previous attempts at cardiac by-pass may have been connected with the much higher rates of perfusion that they used. Cohen's and Lillehei's technique was much simpler than any previous method used to by-pass the heart. They used a single pump to drive both the pulmonary and systemic circuits; their oxygenator was simply one lobe of the subject's lungs used in place; the simple external blood circuit required only a small volume of blood and could be disposed of after each operation so that it did not have to be cleaned or sterilized; and the amount of blood perfused was very small, in accordance with the azygos flow concept. A further advantage of perfusion at the level of azygos flow

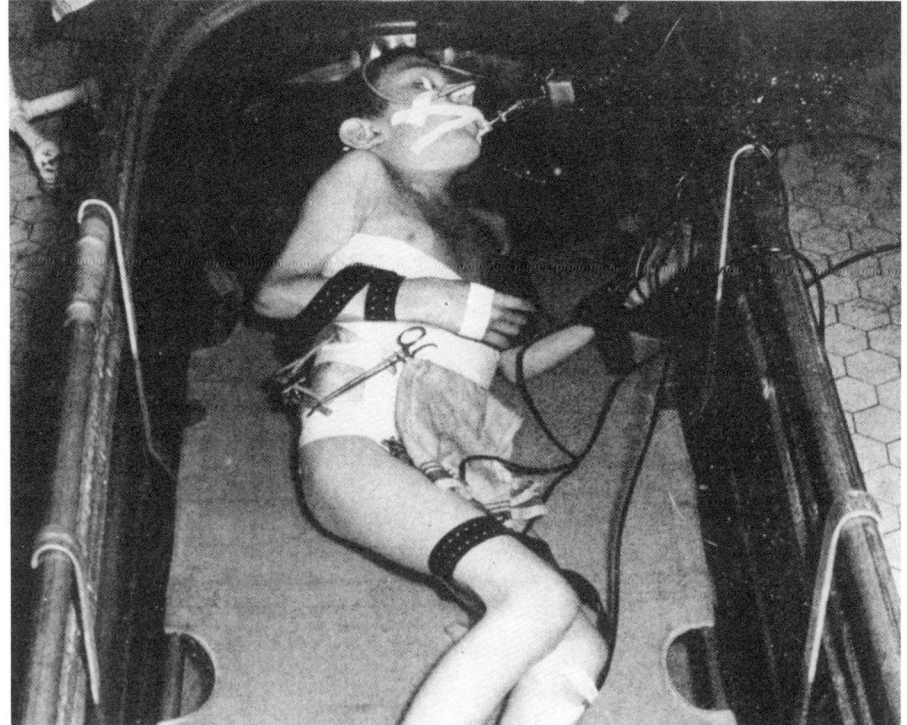

FIGURE 20:7 Patient being warmed in the hot water bath which was kept at 45° C. (Lewis, Varco, and Taufic, 1954.) Courtesy *Surgery*.

was that the return of blood through the coronary veins was reduced; hence the amount of blood lost during surgery on the heart was reduced correspondingly.

In physiologic studies before and after the period of heart by-pass, Cohen and another resident, Herbert Warden, together with Lillehei measured changes in blood pressure, red cell count, plasma hemoglobin levels, kidney and liver function, and respiratory exchange. They found that oxygen uptake and elimination of carbon dioxide were quite efficient. A slight acidosis developed from accumulation of acid metabolites.[34]

Cohen's and Lillehei's goal was to achieve a safe, simple method of total cardiac by-pass for the limited periods of time required to perform surgery within the heart. Because lowering the body temperature would reduce the oxygen requirements of the tissues, they suggested that hypothermia might be used to prolong the by-pass period if operations on the heart should require more time.[35] At Minnesota, F. John Lewis and Mansur Taufic began experimenting with the use of hypothermia to lower the oxygen requirements of dogs while they first created and later corrected defects in the atrial septum. Using hypothermia, Lewis and Taufic first produced atrial septal defects in thirty-nine dogs, of which only twenty-seven survived the operation. As Bigelow had found at Toronto, the chief cause of death was ventricular fibrillation. They then operated on twenty-six of the surviving dogs to close the defect under direct vision, again using hypothermia to reduce the oxygen requirements of the body during cardiac by-pass. Four dogs died during anesthesia or cooling, before the heart was opened, and in one the defect was found to have healed spontaneously. Among the twenty-one dogs on which Lewis and Taufic operated to correct their atrial defects, seventeen survived the surgery. Although the mortality for intracardiac operations under hypothermia was still high, Lewis and Taufic were able to identify the cause of all but one of the operative deaths. Most of them occurred early in the series before they had perfected their technique. One of the chief causes of death was ventricular fibrillation resulting from coronary air embolism. Among the last ten operations for closure of the atrial defect, there was only one death, and in every survivor the septal defects healed soundly.

By the late summer of 1952, Lewis, Varco, and Taufic felt sufficiently confident of their hypothermic technique to attempt an operation on a patient, and on 2 September 1952 they operated for atrial septal defect on an underdeveloped, sickly five-year-old girl. When her body temperature was lowered to 28° C. (82° F.), they opened the chest and stopped the venous inflow to the heart for five and a half minutes while they closed an opening two centimeters in diameter in her atrial septum. The child recovered uneventfully, and on the eleventh day after the operation went home. Her cardiac murmur was gone.[36] The operation was the first in history to be performed on the open heart under direct vision.

By February 1954 Lewis and his coworkers, using hypothermia, had performed open heart surgery to correct atrial septal defects on eleven patients. Two patients died during the operation, while in a third patient the heart went into ventricular fibrillation during the cooling process so that surgery was not attempted; the patient recovered. Ventricular fibrillation occurred also in three other patients following surgery but was overcome by electric shocks, administered by an apparatus built at Minnesota especially for surgical use, accompanied by massage of the heart. One of the operative deaths was due to hemorrhage because the defect was more complicated than Lewis had anticipated. The second death occurred from heart block three days after the operation. Among the patients whose defects were closed successfully, most showed clinical improvement within a few weeks after operation. Their hearts decreased in size, and cardiac catheterization showed that the interatrial shunt had been eliminated.[37]

Most of the patients upon whom Lewis and his colleagues operated for atrial septal defect were adults, and their success demonstrated that adults could safely be subjected to hypothermia. Frequently atrial septal defect was not detected until the patient reached adulthood because only in adulthood did it reveal itself by symptoms, usually breathlessness on exertion. Nevertheless, atrial septal defect was a serious lesion that led ultimately to heart failure, and patients with it did not live very long.[38] Adults with such defects were, therefore, suitable candidates for surgery under hypothermia. Children, on the other hand, were not. If a child

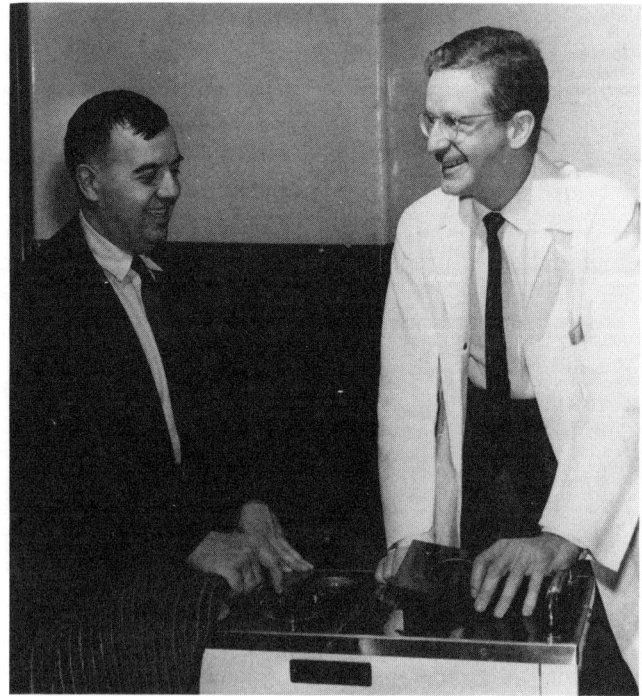

FIGURE 20:8 Richard Varco, left, with cooling blanket for hypothermia in his hands; F. John Lewis, right, leaning on cooling machine, October 1953. Courtesy Mn U Archives.

showed symptoms of atrial septal defect, it probably also had some additional defect in the interventricular septum which could not be corrected under hypothermia.

Through 1953 while John Lewis and Mansur Taufic were doing open heart surgery under hypothermia, C. Walton Lillehei and his coworkers continued their search for a means to oxygenate the blood during complete heart by-pass for the purpose of open heart surgery. Although one lobe of a dog's own lung served very well as an oxygenator during heart by-pass, the procedure required both a number of delicate cannulations of the pulmonary vessels and the inflation of the lungs while surgery proceeded on the open heart. The inflated lungs tended to get in the surgeon's way as he operated on the heart, and too frequently pulmonary edema developed in the lobe used as an oxygenator. The work did show that they could perform open heart surgery for limited periods of time if they could provide the body with a relatively small, but continuous and dependable, supply of oxygenated blood. In one of the discussions between Drs. Morley Cohen and Herbert Warden, it occurred to them that all pregnant mothers provided just such a supply of oxygenated blood for their offspring in the uterus. When they considered how to create an artificial placenta, they thought it might be done by connecting the circulation of the patient to the circulation of a donor, so that the donor's heart

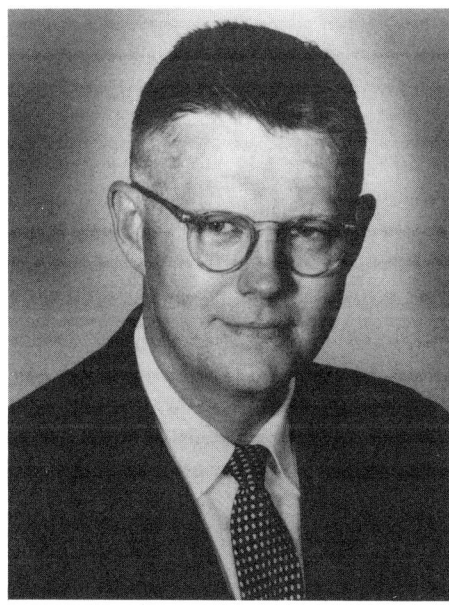

FIGURE 20:9   Herbert Warden, circa 1954. Courtesy Mn U Archives.

and lungs would pump and oxygenate the blood just as the maternal circulation oxygenates the blood of the fetus through the placenta.

In 1953 Andreasen and Watson in England published their experiments on controlled cross circulation in dogs in which they were able to support a recipient dog in heart by-pass for thirty minutes.[39] They found that the cross circulation must be controlled, or else the donor animal would bleed excessively into the recipient. Warden and Cohen proposed to connect the circulation of a donor directly to that of the heart by-pass recipient as Andreasen and Watson had done. Dr. Warden carried out experiments on a series of dogs in which he used as donors somewhat larger dogs than those used as recipients. Using plastic cannulae that passed through a control pump, he connected the femoral artery of the donor to the right common carotid artery of the recipient, and the external jugular vein of the recipient to the femoral vein of the donor. The cannula inserted into the recipient's jugular vein was passed down the jugular as far as the inferior vena cava and had holes in its sides so that it could receive venous blood from both the superior and inferior venae cavae. When the connections were completed and the cannulae filled with blood, the pump was turned on and set to circulate through the recipient at a rate of flow determined on the basis of the recipient's weight and the azygos flow factor.

In an initial group of thirty-one dogs (seventeen as recipients and fourteen as donors, three serving twice as donors), Warden and his colleagues established a complete heart by-pass, continued it for thirty minutes, and then restored the dogs' own circulation. They did not open the heart, but after the operation they

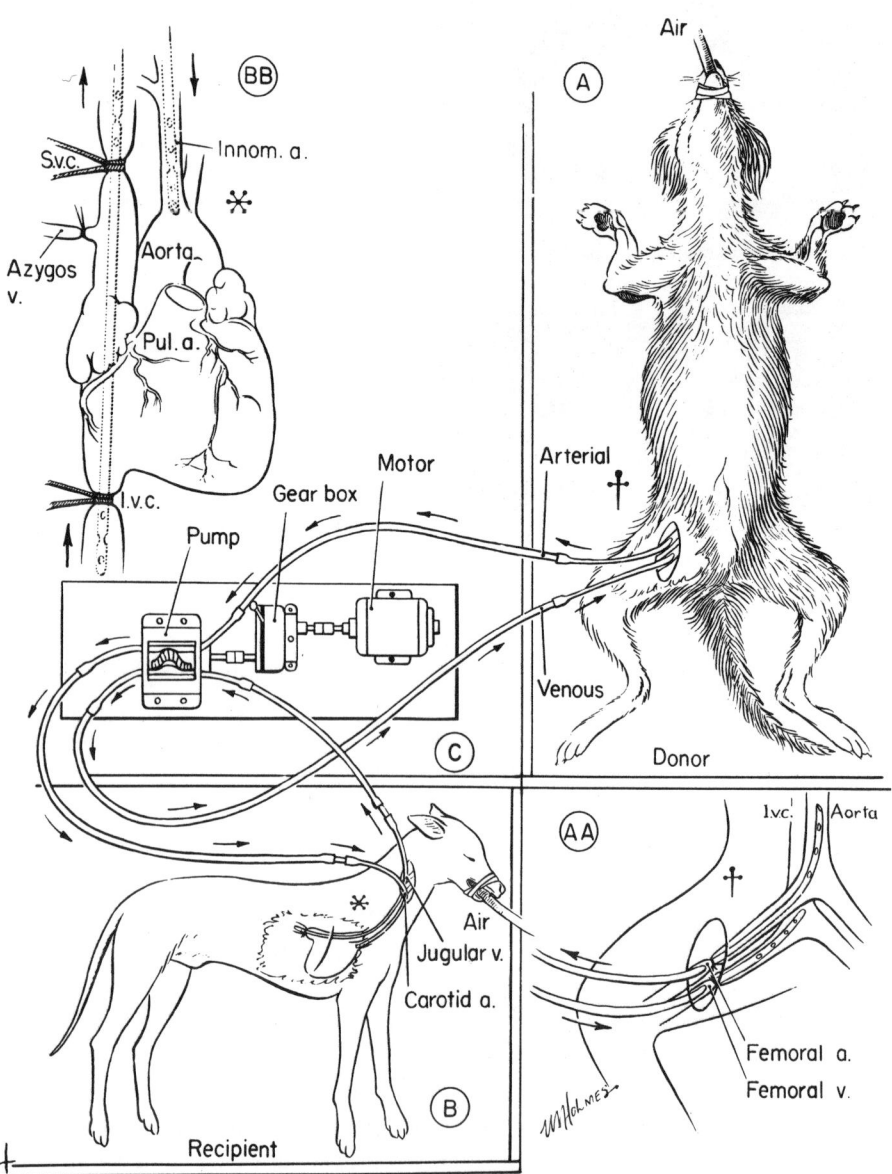

FIGURE 20:10 Experimental controlled cross circulation in dogs (Warden et al., 1954). Courtesy *Journal of Thoracic Surgery*.

carried out physiological and metabolic studies to determine the effectiveness of the cross-circulation method in the maintenance of the animal during thirty minutes of complete heart by-pass. They divided the dogs into three groups, which were perfused at the level of azygos flow, twice azygos flow, and three times azygos flow, respectively, and found that the blood pressure in the recipient corresponded roughly to the level of flow. At three times azygos flow, the blood pressure was about four-fifths normal systemic pressure. During by-pass there was some hemolysis, and the amount of hemolysis was roughly proportionate to the level of flow. The oxygen level of the recipient's blood declined sharply, but the decline was proportionately less at the higher levels of flow. In the study group there were no deaths among the donors. Three of the seventeen recipient animals died following the operation, but in each case the deaths were due to identifiable, and therefore preventable, causes.

In a second group of thirty-seven dogs subjected to thirty minutes of heart by-pass by cross circulation, Warden and his colleagues operated on the heart of each recipient dog to create a hole in the interventricular septum. Among twenty-three dogs who received less than three times the azygos flow, there were fifteen deaths, and two of the eight survivors suffered central nervous system damage. Among fourteen dogs who received from three to five and a half times the azygos flow, there were ten survivors (none showing signs of brain damage) and four deaths. Almost all the deaths among the dogs subjected to operations on the heart were from ventricular fibrillation. From their operative results, Warden and his colleagues concluded that the optimum level of perfusion during heart by-pass was somewhere between 30 and 50 percent of the resting heart output. A higher level of flow not only was not needed, but was actually harmful; when the heart was opened, the increased amount of blood flowing through the coronary system interfered with the surgeon's vision.[40]

In March 1954, Dr. Lillehei and his group judged that the technique of cross circulation was developed sufficiently that they might use it for open heart surgery on human patients. Because the method was new, and its risks to human patients and donors still unknown, they resolved to select at first only children with severe symptoms, accompanied by pulmonary hypertension, who were likely to live only a short time unless their heart defects were corrected.

On 26 March 1954, the Lillehei team operated on a one-year-old boy who had spent most of his short life in hospitals because of repeated attacks of pneumonia and heart failure. He was abnormally small, weighing only 6.9 kg., and during his episodes of pneumonia he turned decidedly blue. He had a pronounced systolic heart murmur with thrill, and cardiac catheterization showed that he had a hole in his interventricular septum. For the heart by-pass the boy's father served as the cross-circulation donor. Perfusion was carried on for thirteen minutes during which time Dr. Lillehei closed a large opening in the interventricular septum by direct suture. The operation went smoothly and the little boy appeared to be recovering well until he developed pneumonia with bronchitis and died eleven

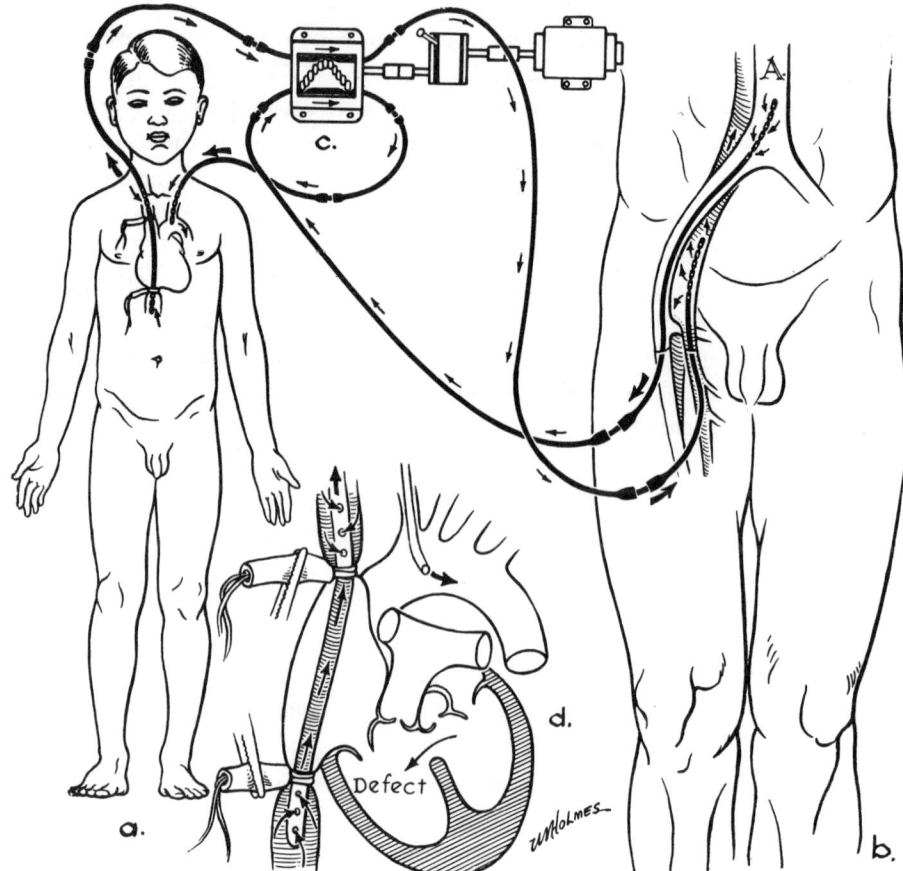

FIGURE 20:11 Open heart surgery, using cross circulation: a. Patient, showing cannulations in the superior and inferior venae cavae, and in the common carotid artery. b. Donor, showing cannulations in the femoral artery and great saphenous vein. c. Pump that controlled the rate of flow of blood between patient and donor. d. Diagram of patient's heart showing the position of the catheter so as to draw blood from both the superior and inferior venae cavae. (Lillehei et al., 1955.) Courtesy *Surgery, Gynecology and Obstetrics*.

days after surgery.[41] At autopsy the arterioles in his lungs were found to have their walls thickened so as to restrict the pulmonary circulation severely.[42]

Undaunted, Lillehei and his colleagues operated on a second patient, a four-year-old boy, on 20 April 1954, again using the child's father as donor. The second child also developed pneumonia following the operation, but this patient recovered and went home.[43] By the end of August 1954, Dr. Lillehei and his colleagues had performed eight open heart operations to close ventricular septal defects, with two deaths. In view of the drastic nature of the defects and the deteriorating condition of the patients at the time of operation, the record of the first eight cases was remarkably successful.

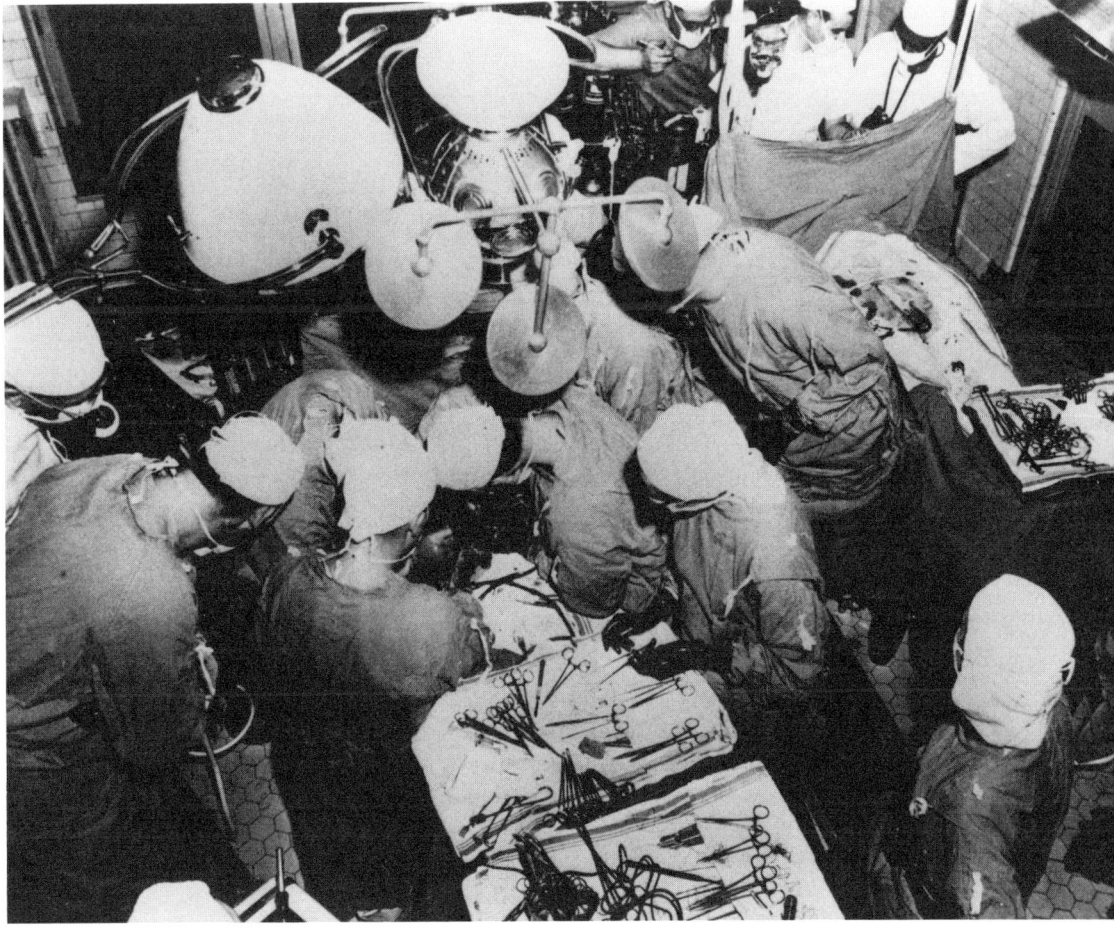

FIGURE 20:12 First successful open heart surgery, using cross circulation, 20 April 1954. Donor patient is on far right. Courtesy Mn U Archives.

In anticipation of the hoped-for development of open heart surgery in the near future, the Department of Surgery at Minnesota had since 1950 refrained from doing the Blalock-Taussig operation on children suffering from tetralogy of Fallot unless their condition were deteriorating significantly. The Minnesota surgeons thought that except in cases of emergency, it was better to refrain from a palliative procedure when there might be an opportunity presently to correct the defects completely. Dr. Lillehei was accustomed to attend the autopsy of every patient dying from a known or suspected heart defect. The autopsies were almost always performed by a pathology resident, who willingly allowed him to spend hours performing surgical operations on the cadaver to correct the heart defects found. Although Lillehei could only perform a relatively small number of such operations, the experience thus gained proved invaluable because the fresh, soft

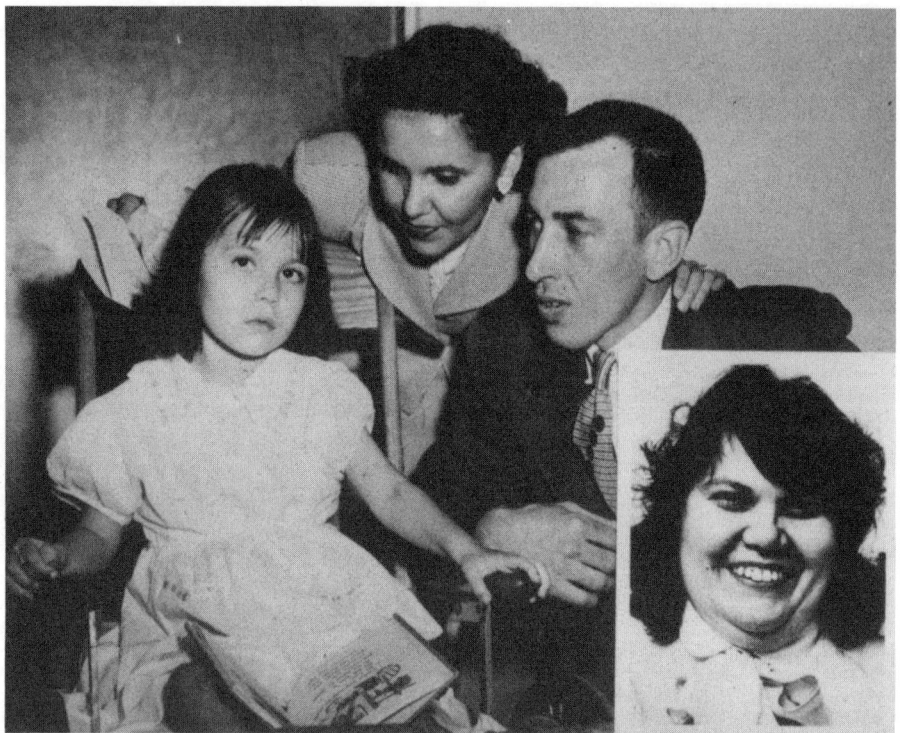

FIGURE 20:13 The second patient to have closure of a ventricular septal defect using cross circulation, seen seven days after operation on 23 April 1954, and (inset) thirty years later. Courtesy Dr. C. Walton Lillehei.

tissues were so different from the hard substance of the hearts preserved in pathological collections. From his autopsy experience, Lillehei learned that the rightward shift of the aorta in tetralogy of Fallot was usually more apparent than real and did not pose an obstacle to surgical correction. On 31 August 1954, the experience gained from autopsies was put to the test when Dr. Lillehei and his group operated on an eleven-year-old boy suffering from tetralogy of Fallot. Thin and small for his age, the child was noticeably blue in color. He could walk less than a block, with frequent stops for squatting, and he could no longer attend school. At the beginning of the operation, when the cannulae were in place, the child's heart stopped, but as soon as the cross circulation began, it resumed its regular beat. Dr. Lillehei and his colleagues closed an opening high in the interventricular septum and opened the stenosis of the pulmonary artery. The child recovered uneventfully and two weeks later went home. He was soon playing baseball and riding a bicycle. Even so, cardiac catheterization seven months after the operation showed that there remained a small opening in the interventricular septum and some stenosis of the pulmonary artery. The repair was, therefore, effective, without being perfectly complete.[44]

OPEN HEART SURGERY

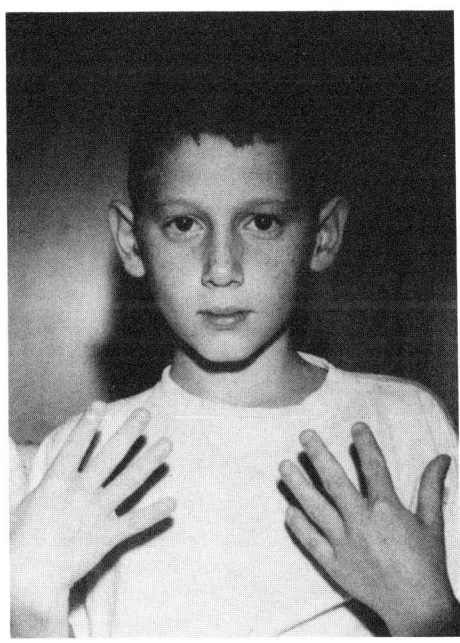

FIGURE 20:14 The first patient (M.S.) to have surgical correction of tetralogy of Fallot, 31 August 1954. Courtesy Dr. C. Walton Lillehei.

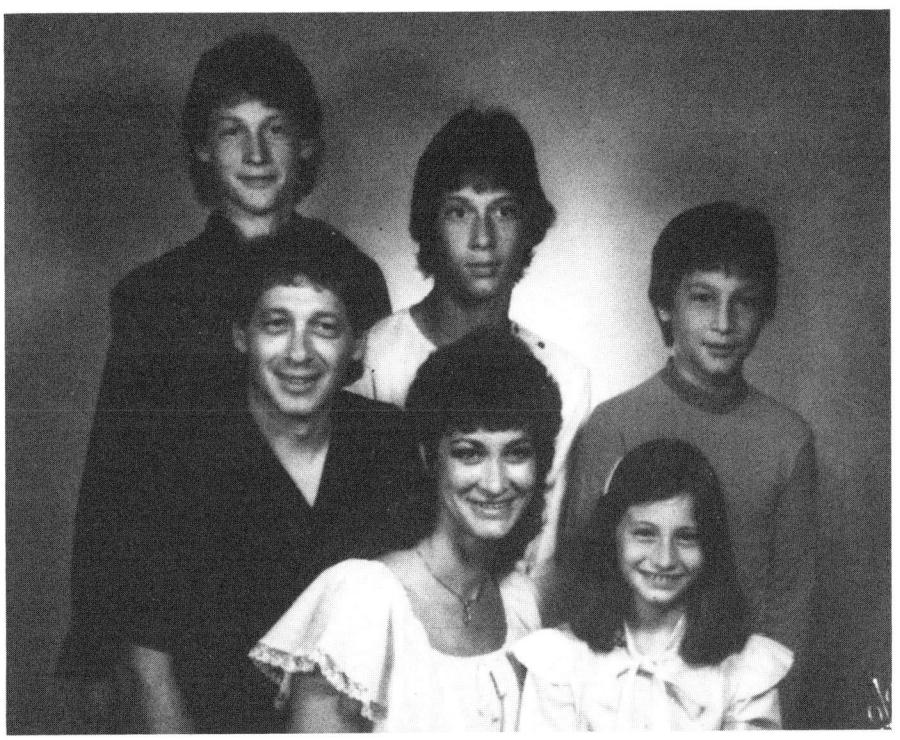

FIGURE 20:15 Patient (M.S.) with wife and four children (all normal) thirty years after surgery. Courtesy Dr. C. Walton Lillehei.

On 3 December 1954, Lillehei and his group operated on a nineteen-month-old boy, who, when admitted to hospital, was intensely cyanotic, in heart failure, and judged to be dying. The child was suffering from tetralogy of Fallot, but this time Lillehei was able to correct the defects completely. The child recovered rapidly, and when he was examined six months later he was found to have a normal heart.[45]

By February 1955 with the aid of cross circulation, Dr. Lillehei and his group had performed thirty-two open heart operations with twenty-five survivors and seven deaths. None of the deaths were attributable to the cross-circulation technique. They had occurred in the postoperative period and were usually due either to technical errors in what were radically new procedures, or to respiratory difficulties. One three-month-old infant who developed heart block momentarily, while the defect in its septum was being sutured, died suddenly twelve hours after the operation. Dr. Lillehei thought that its sudden, unexplained death might have resulted from a recurrence of the heart block.[46]

In successive operations, Lillehei and his group modified the cross-circulation method to include a reservoir of venous blood, and instead of a single catheter inserted through the jugular vein into the two venae cavae, they inserted two catheters into the superior vena cava and inferior vena cava, respectively through separate stab wounds in the right atrium. During by-pass they circulated through the patient a current of blood about two to three times the azygos flow, or 30 to 40 percent of the resting heart output. A great advantage of the lower flow of blood was the significant reduction in loss of blood from the coronary veins while the heart was open, together with a corresponding improvement in visibility of structures within the heart. The heart surgeon's goal was a dry, bloodless field in which to work within the heart. Because Lillehei and his colleagues found that occasionally as they manipulated the heart in suturing the septum, arterial blood leaked back through the aortic valve, they began routinely to place a tourniquet around the base of the aorta and to draw it tight whenever the field became bloody.

By April 1955 when Dr. Lillehei described their experience with the surgical correction of tetralogy of Fallot to a meeting of the American Surgical Association at Philadelphia, they had performed nine operations for tetralogy of Fallot with four deaths. The results among the five survivors were excellent. During the discussion of their paper at Philadelphia, Alfred Blalock commented: ". . . . I never thought I would live to see the day when this type of operative procedure could be performed." He commended the Minnesota group ". . . for their imagination, their courage and their industry."[47] Nevertheless, Blalock suggested that the ultimate answer to the support of the patient's circulation during open heart surgery would not be cross circulation but the artificial heart-lung developed by Dr. Gibbon.

At the Philadelphia meeting, Dr. Lillehei did not comment on Dr. Blalock's suggestion, but on that day he knew that at the University of Minnesota they had ready an artificial heart-lung that was more effective, safer, and far simpler than any of the elaborate machines developed by John Gibbon, Clarence Dennis, or others. Such oxygenators worked on the principle of creating a large interface between blood and oxygen by spreading out the blood into a thin film, which moved through an oxygen atmosphere. However, an enormous blood-oxygen interface could also be created in another way by bubbling oxygen through the blood. In 1950 at Antioch College in Yellow Springs, Ohio, Leland C. Clark, Jr. and two coworkers had developed a small bubble oxygenator. Previous investigators who had tried the bubble method had found it too slow, and with too great a tendency to make the blood foam. Clark and his colleagues were able to prevent foaming by passing the blood through a tube containing small glass rods or glass beads coated with *DC Antifoam A,* a compound made by the Dow-Corning Company of Midland, Michigan. With their apparatus, Clark and his group were able to maintain small dogs, while the dogs breathed an atmosphere of pure nitrogen.[48] In 1952 Clark and two colleagues described a larger all glass bubble oxygenator capable of maintaining animals of up to 20 kg. in complete heart-lung by-pass.[49]

In the fall of 1954 a young physician, Richard A. De Wall, who had graduated from the university's medical school just the year before and then taken an internship at a hospital in Chicago, came to see Dr. Lillehei to say that he wanted to do research on heart surgery. He was practicing medicine at Anoka, a small community just north of Minneapolis. Since Lillehei needed someone to supervise the pumps during open heart operations by cross circulation, he asked De Wall to take over that job and arranged his appointment as a resident. Residents in the Department of Surgery were required to apply for admission to the graduate school in order that they might pursue graduate degrees in surgery. A few weeks later Dr. Lillehei received a call to come to Dr. Wangensteen's office. When he arrived Wangensteen told him that Theodore Blegen, dean of the graduate school, had refused to admit De Wall because his grades in medical school were too low. Dr. Wangensteen added that he had not had much luck in persuading Dean Blegen to change his mind in such matters, so they would have to accept the decision. When Lillehei returned to the laboratory and told De Wall the news, De Wall suggested that Lillehei appoint him as a laboratory animal attendant. Lillehei accepted the idea, Dr. Wangensteen agreed, and De Wall became an animal attendant and went right on doing what he had been doing before. The only difference was that his pay was somewhat higher than when he was a surgical resident.

For a research project, Lillehei asked De Wall to work on the development of an oxygenator on the bubble principle. He suggested that De Wall ignore all that had been published previously on bubble oxygenators and start from first principles. The chief difficulty with bubble oxygenators was the problem of removing bubbles from the blood, and the avoidance of foaming. De Wall began by exploring the possibility that if the bubbles of oxygen were kept relatively large, they would be easier to remove from the blood, yet would still provide a large area of blood-oxygen interface for the exchange of oxygen and carbon dioxide. When they came to set up a trial bubble oxygenator, De Wall and Lillehei obtained polyvinyl plastic tubing from Mayon Plastics of Hopkins, Minnesota, a company that had been created specifically to make plastic tubing for the commercial production of mayonnaise. In the manufacture of mayonnaise, foaming had been a problem, but the Hopkins firm had overcome the difficulty by coating the interior of portions of the plastic tubing with the same silicone compound, *DC Antifoam A,* used four years earlier by Clark to prevent foaming in his bubble oxygenator at Antioch College. Unaware of Clark's work, De Wall and Lillehei thought that if *DC Antifoam A* would prevent the foaming of mayonnaise, it might also prevent the foaming of blood. It did, but although *DC Antifoam A* prevented the foaming of the blood and removed many of the bubbles, it did not remove all of them. The possibility of air embolism from remaining bubbles persisted. Because bubble-containing blood was lighter than bubble-free blood, if the oxygenated blood were held in a vertical settling tube the bubble-free blood would settle to the bottom, while the bubbles would rise to the top. The process was nevertheless slow because the hydrostatic forces tending to move the lighter blood upward were opposed by the downward movement of the heavier blood, and the viscosity of the blood hindered the convection currents by which the bubble-containing blood moved to the top of the tube. To overcome the viscosity resistance to the separation of the lighter bubble-containing blood, Richard De Wall hit upon the idea of using a spirally coiled settling tube instead of a straight one. The polyvinyl tubing could be bent easily into a spiral helix. As the oxygenated blood descended through the helical coil, the lighter blood containing bubbles of free oxygen rose to form an upper layer, while the heavier blood, free of bubbles, flowed beneath it and constantly pushed the lighter blood upwards. The hydrostatic forces created by differences in density thus acted across the short distance of the diameter of the tube instead of along the length of a straight vertical-settling tube, and the separation of bubbles could be accomplished by laminar flow as the blood descended the upper portion of the helical tube. When De Wall tried the helical settling tube, it worked beautifully, giving a rapid, dependable, and complete elimination of bubbles from the blood. During the winter of 1954–55, De Wall tested the bubble oxygenator thoroughly in experimental trials on some seventy dogs. The experience gained from open heart operations with cross circulation showed that twenty minutes of perfusion was sufficient to complete most procedures. De Wall, therefore, used a total by-pass interval of twenty-five minutes on the dogs and perfused them at various low multiples of their azygos flow. In his early trials he did not appreciate the importance of keeping the blood warm as it circulated through the oxygenator, and at the end of the perfusion, the dogs' temperatures had dropped several degrees. Later he immersed the oxygenator reservoir in a water bath kept at constant temperature. De Wall judged twenty-two of the perfusions to be failures because of the death or injury of the animal, but in each instance he was able to identify the cause of failure and later correct it. He discovered the importance of smooth connections at the junctions between all tubes and catheters in order to avoid turbulence of the blood and the resultant formation of blood clots. He found also that by arranging filters in parallel he could reduce the rate of flow through the filters sufficiently to elimi-

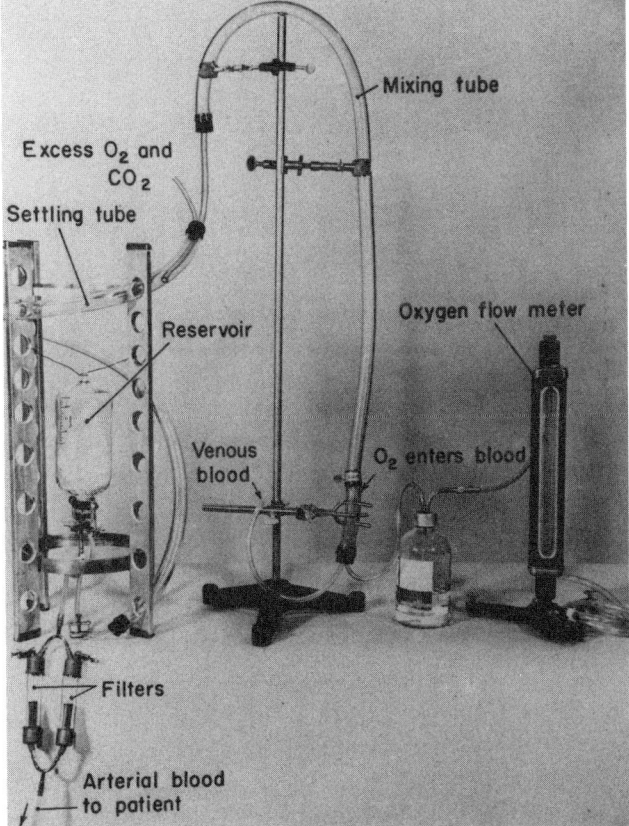

FIGURE 20:16 De Wall's Model I Bubble Oxygenator. Courtesy Dr. Richard A. De Wall.

nate clot formation.[50] By May 1955, De Wall had an oxygenator that he and Lillehei judged was ready for use with human patients.

In the Model I Oxygenator first used on patients, De Wall introduced large bubbles of oxygen through eighteen intravenous needles inserted through an ordinary rubber stopper at the bottom of a vertical plastic tube through which venous blood from the patient flowed slowly upward. The bubbles of oxygen ascended through the rising column of blood to the top of the mixing tube where the blood entered a U-shaped debubbling chamber, its interior walls coated with *DC Antifoam A*. There most of the bubbles escaped from the blood. The oxygenated blood then poured over into the helical coil of plastic tubing down which it flowed by gravity into a reservoir. As the blood descended any residual bubble-containing blood rose upward, while the bubble-free blood flowed downward along the lower surface of the tube. At the bottom of the helical settling tube, oxygenated blood, now completely free of bubbles, passed into a reservoir. From the reservoir it passed through standard blood filters before it entered the arterial system of the patient.

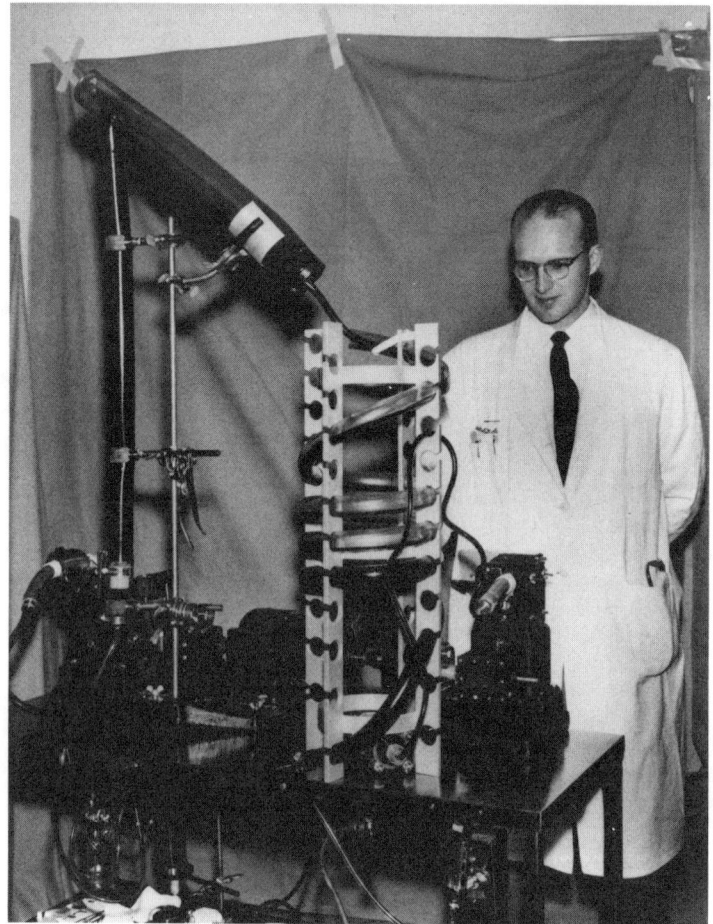

FIGURE 20:17 Richard A. De Wall with Model III Bubble Oxygenator. Courtesy Mn U Archives.

On 13 May 1955, Lillehei and his group used the De Wall oxygenator to perform open heart surgery on a three-year-old child suffering from a ventricular septal defect and pulmonary hypertension. The operation went well, but eighteen hours after the operation the child died. By 9 August 1955, Lillehei and his group had used the bubble oxygenator for seven open heart operations on children ranging in age from nineteen months to seven years with two deaths. All seven patients awakened immediately after the operation without showing any sign of damage to the nervous system, liver, or kidneys. Both deaths were explained at autopsy on an anatomic basis, and neither was related to the use of the bubble oxygenator. The five survivors were discharged from hospital as normal children, cured of their heart defects. The bubble oxygenator proved so successful that Lillehei and his group began to use it entirely in place of the human cross-circulation donor which,

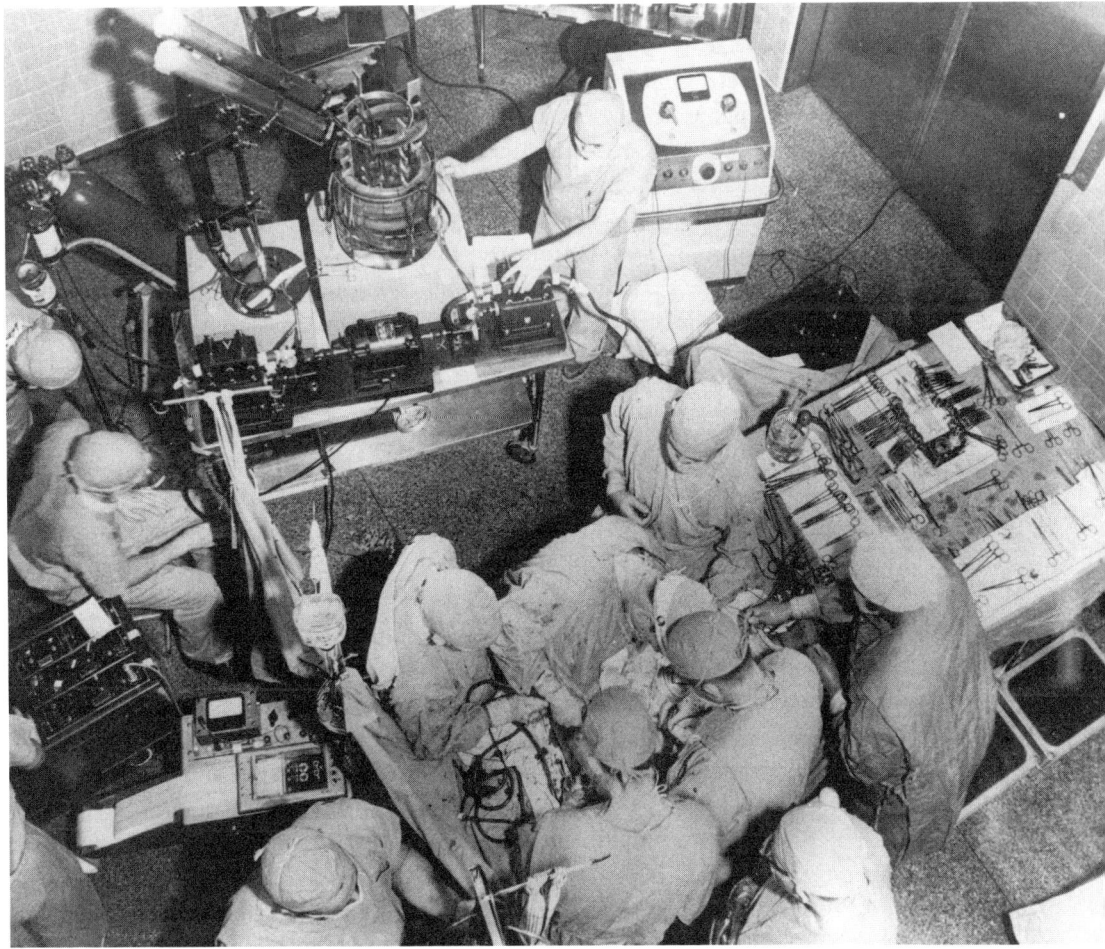

FIGURE 20:18 Open heart surgery using the bubble oxygenator.
Courtesy Mn U Archives.

they said " . . . previously had set the standards in our clinic for safety and effectiveness because of its physiologic superbness."[51]

The seventh patient, operated upon on 9 August 1955, was a seven-year-old child, who was perfused at the rate of 600 cc. per minute, the largest flow of blood yet passed through the bubble oxygenator. At that level of flow, Lillehei and his group detected a significant rise in the plasma hemoglobin indicating an increasing destruction of red blood cells. At a flow of 600 cc. per minute, the blood was driven against the connection between the mixing tube and the helix with enough force to produce a significant destruction of blood cells. Higher perfusion rates also required more oxygen, but if oxygen were admitted under greater pressure, an increased agitation of the blood would likewise damage the red blood cells.

To increase the capacity of the oxygenator while minimizing the turbulence of the blood, De Wall enlarged the debubbling chamber and added more coils to the helical settling tube, incorporating such changes in his Model II Oxygenator which was capable of oxygenating up to two liters of blood per minute. At the upper limit of capacity of the Model II, problems of turbulence again developed, this time in the central reservoir, but De Wall decided that by making the helical settling tube still longer, he could eliminate the central reservoir and have the oxygenated blood pass directly from the lower end of the helix through standard blood filters to the patient's arterial system. With this and other minor changes was born the Model III Oxygenator, which was used for open heart operations through 1956.

In contrast to the elaborate screen oxygenators, with their numerous moving parts and complex controls, the De Wall-Lillehei bubble oxygenator was elegantly simple. It had no moving parts; it was assembled from lengths of polyvinyl plastic food hose; and it could be sterilized in its entirety by autoclaving. Because it was so simple and cheap, Lillehei and his colleagues preferred to dispose of the oxygenator after each operation instead of cleaning it and reusing it. They could adapt each oxygenator to the patient for whom it was intended, making a small oxygenator for open heart surgery on an infant, or a larger model for similar surgery on an adult. Thus they did not need to use more donor blood than necessary to prime the oxygenator, and thereby reduced the chances both of hemolytic transfusion reactions and of heat loss as the blood circulated through the oxygenator. The bubble oxygenator proved remarkably free of harmful effects on the blood.

By 5 May 1956, Lillehei and his colleages had performed eighty open heart operations with the aid of the bubble oxygenator. They had also operated on forty-five patients using controlled cross circulation, on five patients with a reservoir of arterialized blood, and on fourteen with a dog lung oxygenator, a total of 144 open heart operations. They had operated on eighty-seven patients to close a defect in the interventricular septum and on thirty-three to correct tetralogy of Fallot. They had operated on nine patients suffering from a common atrioventricular canal.[52]

During the first two years after the introduction of the bubble oxygenator in 1955, more than 350 patients underwent open heart surgery with its aid at the University of Minnesota Hospital. It was simple, cheap, easily sterilized, and worked very well. Because of its preeminent virtues, Dr. Vincent Gott, a surgical resident working with Dr. Lillehei, sought to incorporate the essential features of the De Wall oxygenator in an equally effective oxygenator that could be manufactured commercially. In 1957 Gott and his colleagues announced that they had developed a plastic sheet oxygenator suitable for open heart surgery.[53]

Whereas in the original De Wall oxygenator the oxygenated blood descended the inclined plane of a helical coil, approximately ten feet in length, in the sheet oxygenator Gott and his colleagues in effect flattened the helical coil to fit between two sheets of plastic, heat-sealed together. The oxygenated blood still descended

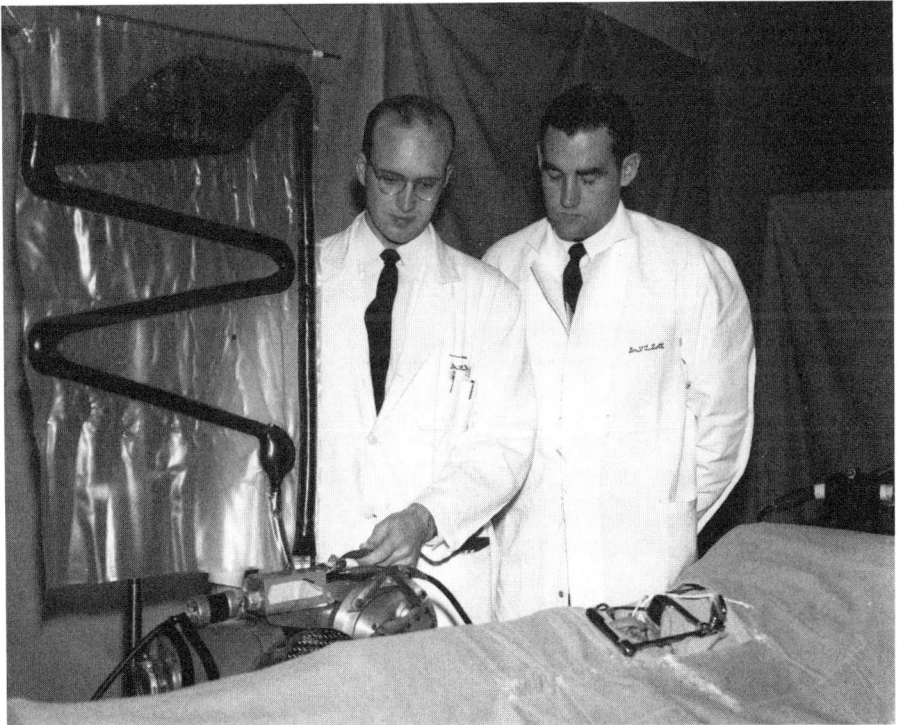

FIGURE 20:19   Richard A. De Wall and Vincent Gott (right) with a sheet bubble oxygenator. Courtesy Mn U Archives.

an inclined plane, which, although shorter than that of the helix, proved to be a dependable barrier to the transmission of bubbles. The great advantage of the plastic sheet oxygenator was that it could be manufactured easily and distributed in sealed, sterile containers to surgical operating rooms anywhere in the world.

The introduction of the bubble oxygenator thus made possible the spread of cardiac surgery from a very few centers to any modern, well-equipped hospital with surgeons trained in the special techniques of intracardiac surgery. There were estimated to be 50,000 infants born with congenital heart defects annually in the United States alone. Children's hospitals throughout the world contained large cardiac wards in which stunted, cyanotic children gasped out their brief lives. When in 1954 the possibility of complete and permanent cure for such children emerged, surgeons began to come to the University of Minnesota from all over the world — the older surgeons to watch the Lillehei team operate and to learn as much as possible of the new technique, the younger surgeons to begin residencies in the Department of Surgery. Between 1951 and 1967, Dr. Lillehei trained fifty-one residents from the United States and seventy-six residents from thirty-eight foreign countries in cardiac surgery. Before 1954 the Department of Surgery was

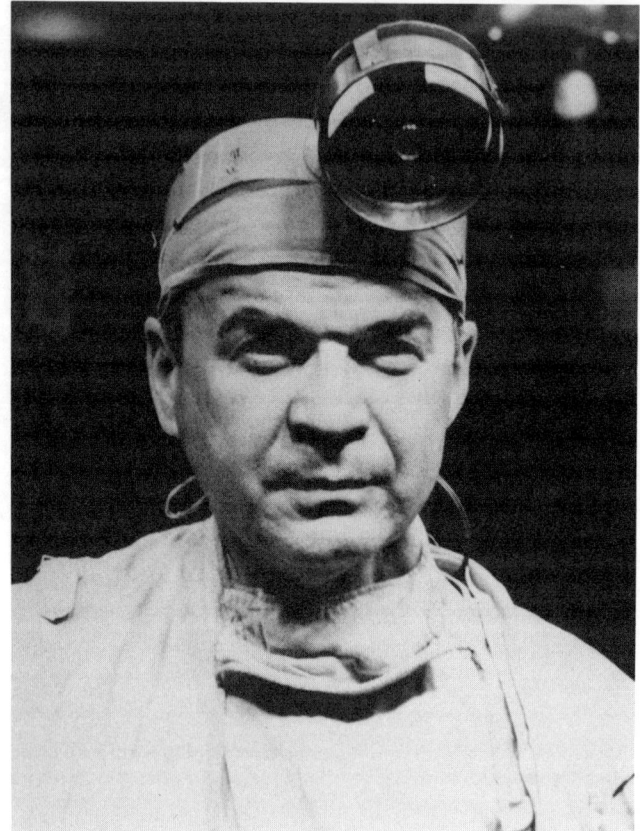

FIGURE 20:20   C. Walton Lillehei, 1958. Courtesy Mn U Archives.

already famous because of Dr. Wangensteen's numerous and immensely important contributions to surgery for intestinal obstruction and gastric surgery and for the introduction of gastrointestinal suction. Dr. Wangensteen had also been remarkably successful in the training of creative young surgeons who had taken up academic appointments at other medical centers. But with the advent of open heart surgery, Minnesota became not merely famous but the focus of world attention.

In 1957 C. Walton Lillehei reviewed the experience that he and his colleagues had gained from operations performed on 305 patients ranging in age from six weeks to sixty-six years. Two hundred and four patients survived. The initial experience gained with forty-five operations using cross circulation had demonstrated that extensive surgical repair of the hearts of even seriously ill persons was not only possible, but life saving. Once the circulation of the patient was connected to that of the donor, the patient began to receive a steady supply of warm, oxygenated blood, maintained in homeostatic balance by the donor's lungs, kidney, liver, and other organs. Nevertheless, the De Wall pump oxygenator had proven almost equally effective in maintaining the seriously ill heart patient. Dr. Lillehei mentioned one eight-week-old baby girl upon whom they had operated as an emergency at night because the cardiologist in charge of her did not think she would live until morning.[54] In operations performed in such circumstances, Lillehei and his colleagues could not always avoid failure, especially because they were often operating upon previously little known heart defects for which they had to improvise corrective procedures on the spot. In 145 operations for ventricular septal defect there were forty-five deaths, or a mortality of 29 percent, but most of the deaths were among children suffering before the operation from severe pulmonary hypertension because of the defect. The risks were also greater in operations on children under the age of two. In children two years or older with considerable, but not severe pulmonary hypertension, the risk of a corrective surgical operation was less than 7 percent. The experience with the correction of atrial septal defects and tetralogy of Fallot demonstrated the vast superiority of corrective procedures performed under direct vision in the open heart to operations performed blindly in the closed heart, or to the creation of a palliative artificial ductus arteriosus. Thus, despite the mistakes and disappointments inevitable in the pioneer exploration of new and unknown surgical territory, the results of the first three years were an immense accomplishment. By 1957 Lillehei and his group could operate on heart defects with far greater certainty of success than in 1954.

Nevertheless, serious problems remained. During or after open-heart surgery, and particularly when a defect in the interventricular septum was being closed, the ventricles sometimes went into fibrillation and the heart might stop. Heart block had occurred. In the first seven patients who developed complete heart block, Lillehei and his team attempted to overcome the heart block with drugs such as epinephrine, ephedrine, atropine, or sodium lactate. Although drug treatment sometimes restored the heartbeat temporarily, none of the seven patients survived. In 1955 they began to use a new drug, Isuprel (isoproternol), with somewhat greater success. Sixty percent of patients in whom complete heart block developed survived the immediate postoperative period.[55] Often later they died suddenly from, Dr. Lillehei suspected, a recurrence of heart block.

In 1954 at the Beth Israel Hospital at Boston, Massachusetts, Paul Zoll and his colleagues used electric stimulation to overcome ventricular fibrillation in patients suffering from Stokes-Adams attacks. They placed electrodes on the skin of the chest directly over the heart and sent periodic electrical impulses through them with a frequency corresponding to the heart rate. Their instrument, which they called a cardiac pacemaker, could restore and maintain a normal heartbeat, but the electrodes irritated the skin and patients often found the repeated electrical shocks painful. Furthermore, the apparatus, which was a modification of the electrical stimulator used in physiological laboratories, was cumbersome; it had to be kept connected to a source of electric power; and it was impractical to keep it ready for instant use in case a patient suddenly went into complete heart block.

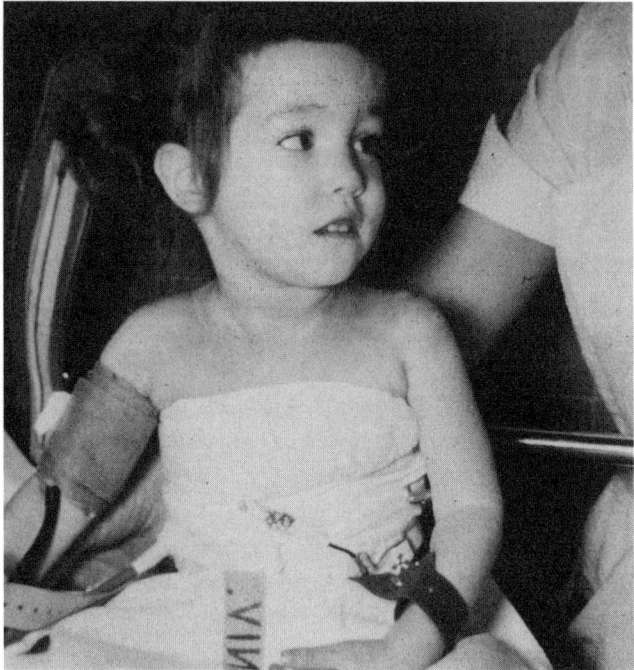

FIGURE 20:21 The first patient to have successful treatment of complete heart block by means of a myocardial electrode connected to a pulse generator, 30 January 1957. She is seen three days after surgery for closure of a ventricular septal defect. Courtesy Dr. C. Walton Lillehei.

Because the mortality among cardiac surgical patients at the University of Minnesota Hospital remained high even with the use of Isuprel, and because of the pain and burns caused by electrodes on the skin, Lillehei and his group began to experiment with dogs to see whether it might be possible in insert a wire from an electric stimulator directly into the heart muscle. They induced heart block by placing a suture in the wall of the atrium near the origin of the atrioventricular bundle, and inserted a wire attached to an electric pacemaker directly into the wall of the right ventricle. By stimulating the dogs' hearts with low voltages at the desired heart rate, the heartbeat was restored and the blood pressure rose to normal levels. The results on dogs were so successful that on 30 January 1957 Lillehei and his team for the first time used the electrical pacemaker on a human patient suffering from heart block as a result of open heart surgery. Dr. Samuel Hunter, then a resident with Dr. Lillehei, has described the early use of the pacemaker in surgery for an interventricular septal defect on a twelve-year-old boy.

> During the closing moments of the procedure we encountered a severe bradycardia [slowing of the heart] of about 30 beats per minute. Dr. William Weirich was summoned and appeared shortly with a device that resembled a large table radio. Two

stainless steel, Teflon coated wires connected to this device were immediately sutured to the right ventricle and subcutaneous tissue respectively by Dr. Lillehei. The patient's rate immediately jumped from 30 to 85 beats per minute.[56]

By early 1958 Lillehei and his group had used the pacemaker to overcome heart block in eighteen patients. They used it only until the patient's heart was able to maintain its beat spontaneously, but they were obliged to keep one patient connected to the pacemaker for twenty-one days before the heart could sustain its own beat.[57] The surgeons no longer had to watch helplessly while a patient died in heart block, and the mortality among open heart patients began to drop sharply.[58] Whenever heart block developed during open heart surgery, even momentarily, Lillehei routinely inserted an electrode in the heart muscle and left it in place when they closed the chest. Later, when the heartbeat returned to normal, they withdrew the wire from the heart and out through the chest wall. Sometimes, in patients who had shown no sign of heart block during surgery, heart block developed in the days following the operation. With the chest closed and no electrode in the heart muscle, Lillehei and his group then had to depend on Isuprel to restore the heartbeat. Since heart block did not occur often enough to justify the placement of a myocardial wire in every patient, they decided to develop a method for the insertion of a wire through the skin into the wall of the right ventricle. Such a method would also have life-saving value for nonsurgical patients who might suffer a Stokes-Adams attack.

Again Lillehei and his group turned to experiments on dogs. In a series of dogs, they first operated to create heart block by placing stitches in the wall of the right atrium. After closing the chest wall, they inserted a hollow needle through the sixth intercostal space and passed a wire through the needle until it touched the beating heart. They then inserted the wire slightly into the wall of the right ventricle. When the pacemaker was turned on, they tested its ability to overcome the heart block and to maintain a steady heartbeat and normal blood pressure. The experiments on dogs proved successful, and one of Lillehei's residents, André Thevenet, then carried out studies on cadavers to determine how a wire might be inserted through the human chest wall so as to reach the heart muscle while avoiding other organs. He found that he could pass a wire through the fourth or fifth intercostal space directly into the wall of the right ventricle without penetrating the pleural spaces.[59]

As Lillehei and his colleagues used the pacemaker, they became frustrated by the awkwardness and danger of the existing machines, which had been adapted from those used in physiological laboratories. Not only was the pacemaker large and cumbersome, but it had to be kept plugged into an electric outlet. Thus the patient could not be moved further than the length of the cord. Disconnection of the cord, or a failure of electric power, would be disastrous, and if a short circuit should occur in the machine, it would instantly electrocute the patient. Since the pacemaker delivered electrical impulses at only one or two volts, the electric currents were very small and might be supplied by a very small power source. Lillehei

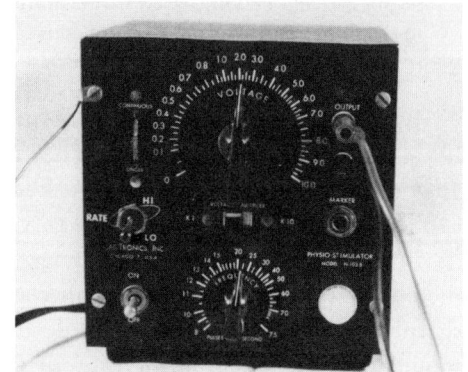

FIGURE 20:22 The pulse generator used to overcome heart block in thirty-eight patients was a Grass Physiologic Stimulator, which gave effective control of the heart rate, but limited the mobility of the patient. Courtesy Dr. C. Walton Lillehei.

thought, therefore, that it ought to be possible to make a miniature pacemaker, powered by batteries, that the patient could carry about with him. Early in 1958 he described the problem to Earl Bakken, the electrical engineer whom the surgery department was accustomed to call in when electrical equipment in the operating room failed to work. At that time Bakken, in partnership with his brother-in-law Palmer Hermundslie, operated an electrical equipment business in a garage in northeast Minneapolis. They sold medical equipment to physicians, often modifying such equipment as electrocardiographs to meet a particular physician's special needs. They also repaired television sets. Within a few weeks, Bakken returned to the university hospital with a small battery-powered pacemaker, which could be adjusted to give the desired heart rate and could be carried easily by a patient in a small holster. Such a small pacemaker was possible only because of new developments in electronics, including the transistor, improved mercury cell batteries, and other miniature components.

The new pacemaker met the need so exactly that Lillehei encouraged Bakken to make more of them. In 1958 Bakken and Hermundslie incorporated their business under the name Medtronic, Inc., to manufacture the small, portable pacemakers, and by 1960 Dr. Lillehei and his coworkers had used the Medtronic pacemaker to overcome complete heart block in sixty-six patients.[60] After two to three weeks of continued electrical stimulation, a majority of patients regained a normal heartbeat and the pacemaker was turned off. Nevertheless, an accompanying transistor monitor remained attached to the patient, and if the pulse rate slowed, the pacemaker again took over. In 1960 one patient had already been sustained on a pacemaker for fifteen months. The miniature pacemaker proved so safe, reliable, and relatively convenient that it also began to be used for nonsurgical patients suffering from heart block as a result of coronary artery disease or other causes.

About 10 percent of patients undergoing open heart surgery suffered heart block. If they survived the immediate postoperative period, three quarters of them recovered a normal sinus rhythm within four weeks. Others continued to suffer chronic complete heart block. Before 1956 none of the latter group survived very long. When in 1957 they began to use the pacemaker to overcome heart block until the heart regained its normal sinus rhythm, Lillehei and his colleagues anticipated that such recovered patients would have a normal or near normal life expectancy. They soon found that they were quite wrong. Among twenty-eight patients who recovered from heart block after surgery between 1956 and the end of 1961, seventeen died as a result of Stokes-Adams attacks, fourteen of them dying during the first year after operation. Among the eleven surviving patients, two had had Stokes-Adams attacks, and the electrocardiograms of seven revealed that they suffered from intermittent complete heart block. By 1961 Lillehei and his colleagues concluded that all patients who suffered heart block, no matter how briefly, during or soon after open-heart surgery, remained vulnerable to sudden death from a Stokes-Adams attack.[61] Such patients, therefore, ought to remain connected to a pacemaker indefinitely. Fortunately, in 1960 several medical and engineering developments combined to make long-term heart pacemaking feasible.

In 1957 when Dr. William Weirich, working with Lillehei, first inserted an electrode in a patient's heart, he used a single stainless steel wire that acted as a unipolar electrode. The single wire electrode worked well at pacing the heart for short periods, but it stimulated the formation of scar tissue that increased the electric resistance. After several weeks, in order to maintain control of the heartbeat, the voltage had to be increased to a level at which the thoracic muscles began to twitch. To overcome the difficulties of the single pole electrode, in 1959 Samuel Hunter, assistant professor in the Department of Surgery and director of cardiac research at St. Joseph's Hospital in St. Paul, worked with Norman A. Roth, chief engineer for Medtronic, Inc., to develop a bipolar stainless steel electrode that required a much smaller electric current. The bipolar electrode worked successfully to maintain the heartbeat in dogs for five to six months. Encouraged by these results, on 4 April 1959 Dr. Hunter implanted a bipolar electrode in the heart of a seventy-two-year-old man suffering from complete heart block as a result of a myocardial infarction and attached it to a Medtronic pacemaker. The patient, who had been deteriorating steadily despite medical treatment, began immediately to improve and achieved an almost complete recovery.[62] By 1961 Dr. Hunter had placed bipolar electrodes in the hearts of three patients suffering from total heart block, and after two years the first patient was still living.[63]

In 1960 at Buffalo, New York, Wilson Greatbatch, an engineer working with Dr. William Chardack, a surgeon, developed a very small, disc-shaped pacemaker designed to be implanted beneath the skin of a patient. In August 1959, Chardack and Greatbatch received from Hunter and Roth at St. Paul a preliminary report on the bipolar electrode, so they were able to use it with their implantable pacemaker when they first installed it in a sixty-five-year old man who had been suffering twenty Stokes-Adams attacks a day. The patient's attacks ceased and he became able to walk. When he died more than a month later from a myo-

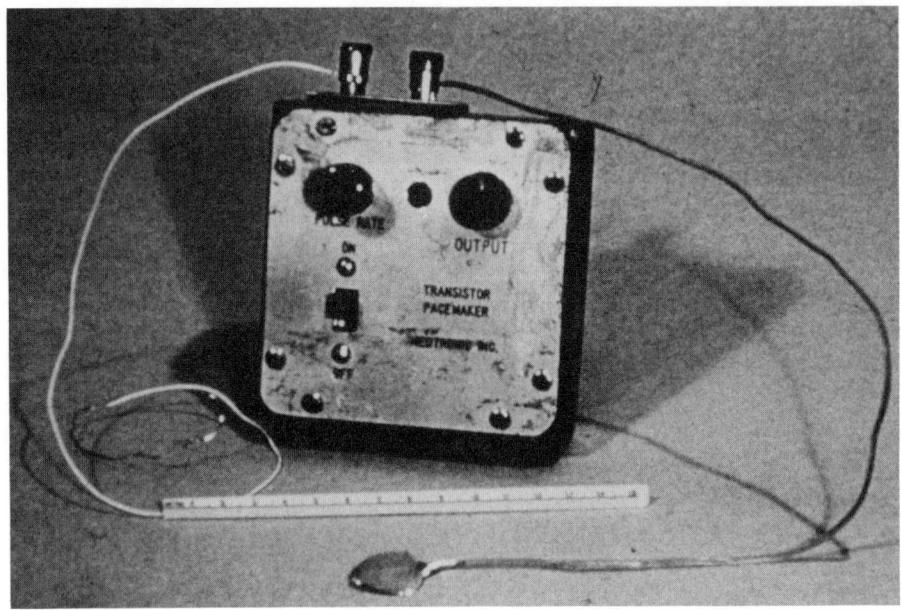

FIGURE 20:23 The first battery-operated transistor pacemaker, developed by Earl Bakken for experimental research in dogs, and used in humans beginning 14 April 1958. Courtesy Dr. C. Walton Lillehei.

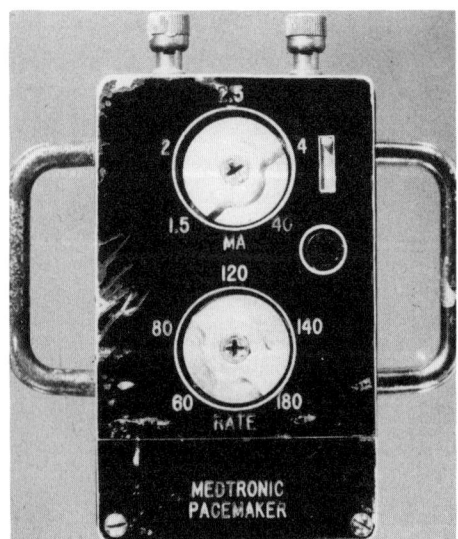

FIGURE 20:24 The first battery-operated transistor pacemaker designed specifically for clinical use in May 1958. Courtesy Dr. C. Walton Lillehei.

cardial infarction, at autopsy the tissues surrounding the electrode were found unchanged.[64] In 1960 Medtronic, Inc. concluded an agreement with Wilson Greatbatch to produce and market his implantable pacemaker.[65] The need for implantable pacemakers proved far greater than anyone anticipated at the time because the danger of heart block was not then appreciated fully. A person with mild

Stokes-Adams symptoms might die suddenly without warning. Their death would be attributable to a coronary attack, especially because, if an autopsy were performed, the coronary arteries would be found diseased. Yet the immediate cause of death might have been a Stokes-Adams attack. By 1964 Lillehei and his colleagues concluded that probably all patients suffering from complete heart block after heart surgery should receive an implantable pacemaker even though the heart block occurred only intermittently. The pacemaker should also be used in acute heart block following myocardial infarction.[66]

The succession of important contributions to heart surgery that emerged from Minnesota during the 1950s was so extraordinary as to make the medical school renowned throughout the world. Moreover, the young surgeons who trained at Minnesota as residents during that period continued to make significant contributions to heart surgery after they left to work at other medical centers, most notable being the contributions of Norman Shumway at Stanford University and Christian Barnard at Capetown, South Africa to the development of heart transplantation. Although he did not himself participate directly in the work on heart surgery, the guiding spirit, who made so many surgical successes possible at Minnesota, was Owen H. Wangensteen. From the beginning of his career, Dr. Wangensteen perceived the importance of the laboratory to surgery and especially to the training of the young surgeon. Instead of keeping the surgical resident occupied in routine clinical duties, Dr. Wangensteen required each resident to spend at least one year, and preferably longer, in experimental work in the laboratory. He required residents to do advanced work in physiology, and he attributed the development of open heart surgery at Minnesota to the cooperation of the head of physiology, Maurice Visscher, both in providing physiological training to surgical residents and in opening the facilities of his laboratory to them. A striking feature of the development of heart surgery at Minnesota was that each new procedure was worked out carefully and fully on dogs before it was attempted on human beings. As a result the mortality among even the earliest series of patients operated on for correction of heart defects, whether using hypothermia, cross circulation, or the pump oxygenator, was very low. By contrast early developments in gastric surgery and lung surgery had evolved through experimental operations on human beings with mortalities as high as 60 percent for gastrectomy and 40 percent for pneumonectomy.[67] For all their bold adventurousness, the Minnesota surgeons proceeded cautiously in the development of cardiac surgery and avoided as much as possible any unnecessary risk to human life. They could not attempt new operations without taking risks, and risk meant the possibility of disaster, but if disaster occurred they would seek to learn from it and not be dismayed by it. In any trouble they could count on Dr. Wangensteen to advise, support, and, if need be, to defend them. In that knowledge they did their utmost.

Epilogue

Dr. Lillehei kept track of the patients upon whom he and his group performed open heart operations during the early years, and in 1986 he published two studies of the long-term results, the first of the forty-five patients on whom Lillehei and his group had operated in 1954 and 1955 to correct various heart defects and the second of 106 patients on whom they had operated from 1954 through 1960 to correct tetralogy of Fallot.[68] The two groups overlapped somewhat, but in both the long-term results of surgery were excellent. Among the 106 patients who had undergone surgery to correct tetralogy of Fallot, 84 (77 percent) were still living. Following their operations performed when they were children, thirty-four patients had completed college, two had received Ph.D. degrees, two had become physicians, and one a lawyer. One patient, with advanced degrees in aeronautical engineering, headed a research division in a large aircraft manufacturing company. Another patient whose education had been limited to high school, nevertheless owned a large chain of restaurants. As a group, the former patients were leading healthy, productive lives, pursuing successfully a variety of professions and trades. They had married and many had children. In 1956, during the pioneering phase of open heart surgery, Dr. Lillehei had insisted that the operations to correct heart defects were not merely corrective, but curative, an opinion that was challenged as rash and presumptuous.[69] Rash it may have been, but by 1986 the experience of thirty years demonstrated that Lillehei's early judgment was right.

NOTES

1. Robert E. Gross and John P. Hubbard, "Surgical ligation of a patent ductus arteriosus," *J. Am. med. Ass.*, 1939, *112*, 729–731.

2. M. J. Shapiro and Ancel Keys, "Clinical and physiologic analysis of twenty-three patients with persistent patent ductus arteriosus," *New int. Clins*, 1941, *4*, 149–165.

3. Morse J. Shapiro and Ancel Keys, "The prognosis of untreated patent ductus arteriosus and the results of surgical intervention. A clinical series of 50 cases and an analysis of 139 operations," *Am. J. med. Sci.*, 1943, *206*, 174–183.

4. Ibid., p. 183. By 1947 three surgeons, Robert Gross at Boston, Clarence Crafoord at Stockholm, and Owen H. Wangensteen at Minneapolis, had performed a total of 172 sections of the ductus arteriosus with no fatalities, and Dr. Shapiro concluded that the surgery for this condition had become so safe and so effective that all children with patent ductus arteriosus should be operated upon whether or not they showed any signs of heart strain. See M. J. Shapiro, "The results of surgery in patent ductus arteriosus," *J. lab. clin. Med.*, 1947, *32*, 329–330.

5. Information about the origins of the Variety Club Heart Hospital is derived largely from Margaret Ayling Stanchfield, *A history of the Variety Club Heart Hospital of the University of Minnesota Hospitals.*

6. Alfred Blalock and Helen B. Taussig, "The surgical treatment of malformations of the heart," *J. Am. med. Ass.*, 1945, *128*, 189–209.

7. The Variety Club was a service organization made up of people in the entertainment business. From the time of its origin at Pittsburgh, Pennsylvania in 1928, the Variety Club

had been concerned with helping needy children. In keeping with their origin as entertainers, the local chapter of the Variety Club in each city was called a Tent, after a circus tent, and its presiding officer, Chief Barker, after a circus barker. During the ten years since its founding in Minneapolis in February 1934, Tent 12 of the Variety Club had sponsored, among other charities, a milk fund for needy children in Minneapolis and had given funds to Sister Kenny for the care of polio patients.

8. On 23 September 1946, at a testimonial dinner in the Coffman Memorial Union at which the radio comedian Fred Allen acted as master of ceremonies, the Variety Club of the Northwest presented the university with a check for $250,000 for the construction of the heart hospital and renewed their pledge of $25,000 annually for its support. When construction of the hospital began in November 1948, the amount raised was more than $300,000. The university had applied for federal matching funds under the Hill-Burton Construction Act, and the Variety Club had pledged itself to raise an additional $160,000 for which it was organizing a new fund drive.

9. The fourth floor was devoted to research, the third floor with forty beds to pediatric heart patients, the second floor to adult heart patients, and the first floor to outpatient heart clinics for both children and adults.

10. Morley Cohen to Leonard G. Wilson, 22 January 1987, Personal communication, deposited in Mn U Archives.

11. John H. Gibbon, Jr., "The gestation and birth of an idea," *Phila. Med.*, 1963, *59*, 913-914.

12. John H. Gibbon, Jr. "Artificial maintenance of circulation during experimental occlusion of the pulmonary artery," *Archs Surg., Chicago*, 1937, *34*, 1105-1131.

13. John H. Gibbon, Jr., "The maintenance of life during experimental occlusion of the pulmonary artery followed by survival," *Surg. Gynec. Obstet.*, 1939, *69*, 602-614.

14. Gibbon went to New York City to consult the director of research at the IBM Corporation who arranged for him to meet Thomas Watson, chairman of the board of IBM. When Gibbon explained his project and said that he did not wish to make money from the project either for himself or for IBM, but that he did need engineering assistance, Watson promised to give help and sent IBM engineers to Philadelphia to confer with Gibbon.

15. Stephen L. Johnson, *The history of cardiac surgery 1896-1955*, p. 143.

16. T. L. Stokes and J. H. Gibbon, Jr., "Experimental maintenance of life by a mechanical heart and lung during occlusion of the venae cavae followed by survival," *Surg. Gynec. Obstet.*, 1950, *91*, 138-156.

17. Karl E. Karlson et al., "Pump oxygenator to supplant the heart and lungs for brief periods. I. Evaluation of oxygenator techniques; an efficient oxygenator," *Surgery*, 1951, *29*, 678-696.

18. Clarence Dennis et al., "Pump-oxygenator to supplant the heart and lungs for brief periods. II. A method applicable to dogs," *Surgery*, 1951, *29*, 697-713.

19. Bernard J. Miller, John H. Gibbon, Jr. and Mary H. Gibbon, "Recent advances in the development of a mechanical heart and lung apparatus," *Ann. Surg.*, 1951, *134*, 694-708, p. 706.

20. W. G. Bigelow, J. C. Callaghan, and J. A. Hopps, "General hypothermia for experimental intracardiac surgery," *Ann. Surg.*, 1950, *132*, 531-539. Cf. W. G. Bigelow, *Cold hearts*, pp. 42-61.

21. C. Walton Lillehei et al., "Role of cardiovascular stress in the pathogenesis of endocarditis and glomerulonephritis," *Archs Surg. Chicago*, 1951, *63*, 421-434, pp. 432-433.

22. Ibid., p. 433. When Dr. Lillehei presented his results to a meeting of the Central Surgical Association at Chicago on 23 February 1951, Dr. Willis J. Potts of Chicago commented: " . . . . Dr. Lillehei and his coworkers sought information on heart strain by

making arteriovenous aneurysms and found endocarditis. Upon [such] serendipity depends future great advances in medicine." Ibid., p. 434.

23. M. J. Shapiro and Ancel Keys, "The prognosis of untreated patent ductus arteriosus and the results of surgical intervention . . . ," *Am. J. med. Sci.*, 1943, *206*, 174-183.

24. C. Walton Lillehei, Ivan D. Baronofsky, and Richard L. Varco, "The surgical treatment of congenital heart disease — analysis of the results in 388 cases," *Bull. Univ. Minn. Hosp. & Minn. med. Fndn*, 1952-53, *24*, 75-93, p. 87.

25. Paul D. White, *Heart disease;* B. J. Clawson, "Incidence of types of cardiac deaths in 50,730 autopsies," *J.-Lancet*, 1950, *70*, 15-17.

26. Lillehei, Baronofsky, and Varco (n. 24).

27. A. T. Andreasen and F. Watson, "Experimental cardiovascular surgery," *Br. J. Surg.*, 1952, *39*, 548-551.

28. R. C. Brock, "Pulmonary valvulotomy for the relief of congenital pulmonary stenosis," *Br. med. J.*, 1948, *i*, 1121-1126.

29. Alfred Blalock and Richard F. Kieffer, Jr., "Valvulotomy for the relief of congenital valvular pulmonic stenosis with intact ventricular septum," *Ann. Surg.*, 1950, *132*, 496-516.

30. Richard L. Varco, discussion of a paper by William H. Muller, Jr. and W. P. Longmire, Jr., "The surgical treatment of cardiac valvular stenosis," *Surgery*, 1952, *30*, 29-42, pp. 41-42.

31. Morley Cohen et al., "The tolerance of the canine heart to temporary complete vena caval occlusion," *Surg. Forum*, 1952, *3*, 172-177.

32. Morley Cohen and C. Walton Lillehei, "A quantitative study of the 'azygos factor' during vena caval occlusion in the dog," *Surg. Gynec. Obstet.*, 1954, *98*, 225-232.

33. Ibid., p. 231.

34. Morley Cohen, Herbert E. Warden, and C. Walton Lillehei, "Physiologic and metabolic changes during autogenous lobe oxygenation with total cardiac by-pass employing the azygos flow principle," *Surg. Gynec. Obstet.*, *1945*, *98*, 523-529.

35. Morley Cohen and C. Walton Lillehei, "Autogenous lung oxygenator with total cardiac by-pass for intracardiac surgery," *Surg. Forum*, 1953, *4*, 34-40.

36. F. John Lewis and Mansur Taufic, "Closure of atrial septal defects with the aid of hypothermia; experimental accomplishments and the report of one successful case," *Surgery*, 1953, *33*, 52-59.

37. F. John Lewis, Richard V. Varco, and Mansur Taufic, "Repair of atrial septal defects in man under direct vision with the aid of hypothermia," *Surgery*, 1954, *36*, 538-556.

38. Carleton B. Chapman and Robert Fraser, "Clinical and hemodynamic features of uncomplicated interatrial defect in adults," *Am. Heart J.*, 1953, *46*, 352-363.

39. A. T. Andreasen and F. Watson, "Experimental cardiovascular surgery. Discussion of results so far obtained and a report on experiments concerning a donor circulation," *Br. J. Surg.*, 1953, *41*, 195-206.

40. Herbert E. Warden et al., "Controlled cross circulation for open intracardiac surgery. Physiologic studies and results of creation and closure of ventricular septal defects," *J. thorac. Surg.*, 1954, *28*, 331-343.

41. C. Walton Lillehei et al., "The results of direct vision closure of ventricular septal defects in eight patients by means of controlled cross circulation," *Surg. Gynec. Obstet.*, 1955, *101*, 446-466, p. 460.

42. Ibid., p. 459.

43. Ibid., p. 460.

44. C. Walton Lillehei et al., "Direct vision intracardiac surgical correction of the tetralogy of Fallot, pentalogy of Fallot, and pulmonary atresia defects. Report of first ten cases," *Trans. Am. surg. Ass.*, 1955, *73*, 98-125, pp. 110-112.

45. Ibid., pp. 114–115. Cf. C. Walton Lillehei et al., "Complete anatomical corection of the tetralogy of Fallot defect," *Archs Surg., Chicago*, 1956, *73*, 526–531.

46. C. Walton Lillehei et al., "The direct-vision intracardiac correction of congenital anomalies by controlled cross circulation. Results in thirty-two patients with ventricular septal defects, tetralogy of Fallot, and atrioventricularis communis defects," *Surgery*, 1955, *38*, 11–29.

47. Lillehei et al., ". . . Surgical correction of the tetralogy of Fallot . . . ," *Trans. Am. surg. Ass.*, 1955, *73*, 98–125, p. 122.

48. Leland C. Clark, Jr., Frank Gollan, and Vishwa B. Gupta, "The oxygenation of blood by gas dispersion," *Science*, 1950, *111*, 85–87. DC Antifoam A was a compound made by the Dow-Corning Company of Midland, Michigan.

49. Leland C. Clark, Frederick Hooven and Frank Gollan, "A large capacity, all-glass dispersion oxygenator and pump," *Rev. sci. Instr.*, 1952, *23*, 748–753.

50. Richard A. De Wall et al., "The helix reservoir pump oxygenator," *Surg. Gynec. Obstet.*, 1957, *104*, 699–710. Cf. Richard A. De Wall, "The helix reservoir bubble oxygenator for use in open intracardiac surgery," M.S. thesis, University of Minnesota, 1961, pp. 32–36.

51. C. Walton Lillehei et al., "Direct vision intracardiac surgery in man using a simple, disposable artifical oxygenator," *Dis. Chest*, 1956, *29*, 1–8, p. 5.

52. Richard A. DeWall et al., "Total body perfusion for open cardiotomy utilizing the bubble oxygenator: physiologic responses in man," *J. thorac. Surg.*, 1956, *32*, 591–563.

53. Vincent L. Gott et al., "A self-contained disposable oxygenator of plastic sheet for intracardiac surgery. Experimental development and clinical application," *Thorax*, 1957, *12*, 1–9. Cf. Vincent L. Gott et al., "A disposable unitized plastic sheet oxygenator for open heart surgery," *Dis. Chest*, 1957, *32*, 615–625.

54. C. Walton Lillehei, Herbert E. Warden, Richard A. De Wall, Paul Stanley, and Richard Varco, "Cardiopulmonary by-pass in surgical treatment of congenital or acquired heart cardiac disease," *Archs Surg.*, Chicago, 1957, *75*, 928–345, p. 935.

55. C. W. Lillehei, discussion paper by John W. Kirklin et al., "Surgical correction of ventricular septal defect: anatomic and technical considerations," *J. thorac. Surg.*, 1957, *33*, 45–59, pp. 57–59. The discussion took place in May 1956 at the annual meeting of the American Association for Thoracic Surgery at Miami Beach, Florida.

56. Quoted in David Chas. Schechter, "Background of clinical cardiac electro stimulation. VII. Modern era of artificial cardiac pacemakers," *N. Y. St. J. Med.*, 1972, *72*, 1166–1191.

57. William L. Weirich, Vincent L. Gott, and C. Walton Lillehei, "The treatment of complete heart block by the combined use of a myocardial electrode and an artificial pacemaker," *Surg. Forum*, 1958, *8*, 360–363.

58. William L. Weirich et al., "Control of complete heart block by use of an artificial pacemaker and a myocardial electrode," *Circ. Res.*, 1958, *6*, 410–415.

59. André Thevenet, Paul C. Hodges, and C. Walton Lillehei, "The use of a myocardial electrode inserted percutaneously for control of complete atrioventricular block by an artificial pacemaker," *Dis. Chest*, 1958, *34*, 621–631.

60. C. Walton Lillehei et al., "Transistor pacemaker for treatment of complete atrioventricular dissociation," *J. Am. med. Ass.*, 1960, *172*, 2006–2010.

61. C. Walton Lillehei et al., "Chronic post surgical complete heart block," *J. thorac. Surg.*, 1963, *46*, 436–456.

62. Samuel W. Hunter et al., "A bipolar myocardial electrode for complete heart block," *J.-Lancet*, 1959, *79*, 506–508.

63. Samuel W. Hunter and Norman A. Roth, "The platform bipolar mycardial electrode for prolonged treatment of total heart block," *J.-Lancet*, 1961, *81*, 115–117.

64. William M. Chardack, Andrew A. Gage, and Wilson Greatbatch, "A transistorized, self-contained, implantable pacemaker for the long-term correction of complete heart block," *Surgery,* 1960, *48,* 643–654.

65. In 1984 Medtronic, Inc. reported sales of $422.7 million, and employed 5,500 people worldwide.

66. C. Walton Lillehei et al., "The use of a myocardial electrode and pacemaker in the management of acute postoperative and postinfarction complete heart block," *Surgery,* 1964, *56,* 463–472.

67. Henry Swan, "How cardiac surgery transformed surgery," *Archs Surg., Chicago,* 1963, *87,* 365–368.

68. C. W. Lillehei et al., "The first open-heart repairs of ventricular septal defect, atrio ventricular communis, and tetralogy of Fallot using extracorporeal circulation by cross-circulation: a 30-year follow-up," *Ann. thorac. Surg.,* 1986, *41,* 4–21; C. Walton Lillehei et al., "The first open heart corrections of tetraology of Fallot, a 26–31 year follow-up of 106 patients," *Ann. Surg.,* 1986, *204,* 490–502.

69. Discussion of Kirklin et al. (n.55), pp. 57–59.

CHAPTER 21

The Development of Organ Transplantation at Minnesota

During the 1960s the most exciting and rapidly developing field of surgery was that of the transplantation of organs and tissues. The failure of kidney, heart, liver, or pancreas creates serious disease, and unless the function of the failed organ can be replaced promptly, the patient will die. In 1921 Banting and Best isolated insulin from the pancreas, and thereafter diabetics were sustained by daily injections of insulin, but the functions of other organs were less easy to replace, and even pancreatic function was not replaced fully by administration of insulin. The level of blood sugar fluctuates widely in diabetics receiving insulin, and such fluctuations harm the blood vessels throughout the body. Over the longer term diabetics may become blind, acquire kidney disease, and their feet or hands may become infected, all as a result of impaired circulation. The onset of diabetes is usually gradual, its effects accumulating over years, by contrast kidney failure creates an immediate emergency that can bring death within a short time.

Shortly after 1900 at Lyons, France, Alexis Carrel developed a technique for joining blood vessels end to end with sutures, and Carrel foresaw that the techniques would permit the transplantation of organs. In 1905 at the Rockefeller Institute, he and Charles Guthrie transplanted the kidney of a dog from its normal position to the neck, where they found that in its new location the kidney secreted urine even more abundantly than before, thus demonstrating that the secretion of urine depended entirely on the circulation of the blood through the kidney and not upon its nervous connections.[1] Other investigators confirmed Carrel's results. In 1950 in England, W. J. Dempster found that when a kidney was transplanted from one dog to another, although it began to secrete urine, the secretion stopped after the fifth day. The animal became acutely ill but could be cured immediately by surgical removal of the transplanted kidney.[2] In 1944 at Oxford, England, P. B. Medawar showed from a study of skin grafts that the process by which a transplanted organ was rejected by its host occurred in two stages. First, the transplanted organ induced an immunity in the host against itself; then the immune system of the host attacked the transplant. The latter stage corresponded to the acute illness created by a transplanted kidney in dogs.

Despite the discouraging results in dogs, in the early 1950s David M. Hume and his colleagues at the Peter Bent Brigham Hospital in Boston performed several kidney transplantations in patients because they thought it important to learn how the disease that had destroyed the patient's own kidneys would affect a transplanted kidney, and whether a transplanted kidney in man would behave in the same way as in the dog. Among nine transplanted kidneys, only four became functional, but they secreted urine for 37 to 180 days, periods much longer than had been observed in dogs.[3] Such transplantations could be done only because of development in the 1940s of the artificial kidney which permitted very sick, uremic patients to be prepared for surgery and sustained them until the transplanted kidney began to function.[4] In 1954 Hume and his colleagues concluded that kidney transplantation was not yet a treatment suitable for human patients.

Nevertheless, in the fall of 1954, one of Hume's colleagues, Dr. John P. Merrill, decided to transplant a kidney into a twenty-four-year-old man suffering from kidney disease because the patient had an identical twin willing to donate a kidney. Since skin grafts between human identical twins were known to survive permanently, Merrill thought that a kidney transplant similarly should have a good chance of survival. The transplantation did prove successful and the patient recovered normal health.[5]

After their first success, Merrill and his group continued to perform transplants between identical twins, some of whom came to Boston from distant places for the surgery, and by 1958 they had performed seven such transplants.[6] In January 1959, Merrill performed a kidney transplantation between fraternal twin brothers. He was encouraged to do so because, although the brothers were not identical twins, a comparison of their blood groups showed that they had twenty-five factors in common. In an attempt to avoid an immune response, Merrill gave the recipient whole body irradiation before transplantation. The transplantation was successful, and a rejection episode eight months after the operation was overcome by a second course of irradiation together with treatment by adrenal cortical hormones. In 1962, three and a half years after transplantation, the patient was in normal health, had completed graduate school, and married.[7]

In 1958 a new possibility for prevention of the rejection of transplanted organs appeared when Robert Schwarz and his coworkers at Tufts University School of Medicine found that the drug 6-mercaptopurine could inhibit the development of an immune response in rabbits.[8] In 1960 Schwartz and Dameshek also showed that 6-mercaptopurine would prevent the rejection of homotransplanted kidneys in dogs.[9] The difficulty with 6-mercaptopurine was that it was quite toxic, especially to the bone marrow. In 1961 at the Peter Bent Brigham Hospital in Boston, Roy Calne and Joseph Murray found that another drug, Burroughs Wellcome 57–322, azathioprine (later named *Imuran*), was as powerful as 6-mercaptopurine in preventing rejection, but less toxic.[10] In 1961 at the Peter Bent Brigham Hospital, Murray and his colleagues began to use azathioprine to prevent the rejection of kidneys transplanted into patients from cadavers. At first they had difficulty in determining the correct dose, but gradually they found that if azathioprine were given steadily in small doses it could prevent rejection without excessive impairment of the patient's immunological system.[11] They learned to combat episodes of rejection by additional treatment with prednisone.

By 1962 kidney transplantation was beginning to emerge as a possible method of extending and improving the lives of patients with kidney disease, who could otherwise be kept alive only with the aid of the artificial kidney. In March 1962, Thomas Starzl and his colleagues at the University of Colorado performed their first kidney transplantation. By May 1963, they had done twelve kidney transplantations, and similar numbers had been performed at the University of California Los Angeles and the Medical College of Virginia at Richmond. A total of 194 human kidney transplantations had been performed in the United States and Europe of which 29 were between identical twins, 49 from related donors, and 57 from unrelated donors, usually from cadavers.[12]

While American surgeons concentrated their attention on immunosuppression by drugs, in 1962 at the Necker Hospital in Paris, Jean Hamburger transplanted a kidney into a thirty-seven-year-old man from a nonidentical twin brother, using total body radiation to suppress the immune system.[13] Before making the transplantation Hamburger sought the help of an immunologist, Jean Dausset, who determined that among nine serum tests of the brothers there was only one discordance, the recipient possessed one antigen lacking in the donor. Hamburger attributed the success of their first transplant from a nontwin donor in 1962 to their matching of the tissues of donor and recipient.[14] Dausset went on to study further the antigens carried on human leucocytes in an effort to identify the immunological factors that influenced compatibility between the tissues of donor and recipient. Dausset had discovered the first histocompatibility antigen in 1958, but soon others were identified. The discovery of histocompatibility antigens meant that, as transplantation surgery developed, the surgeon would be involved ever more deeply in questions of immunology. The significance of immunology for transplant surgery was reinforced in 1964 when at Edinburgh, Woodruff and Anderson found that an antilymphocytic serum could prolong the survival of skin homografts in rats.[15]

The successive stages in the development of kidney transplantation during the 1960s may be illustrated from the experience of Starzl and his colleagues in Colorado. In each case the patients upon whom they performed transplants were suffering from end stage renal disease, which meant that their kidneys had stopped functioning, and they were being kept alive by periodic dialysis with the artificial kidney—a restricted, precarious, and troublesome existence. In 1962, Starzl and his colleagues began their first series of kidney transplants, using azathioprine and prednisone to prevent rejection of the implanted kidney. The doses of azathioprine were so large that many of the patients suffered bone marrow depression, and almost complete inhibition of their immune systems. As a result they became extremely susceptible to infections. Starzl and his colleagues were faced frequently with a choice between a regime that would prevent rejection, but would permit the patient to die of infection, and one that would restore resistance to infection, but with rejection of the implanted kidney and death from loss of kidney function. Among forty-six patients in their first series, who received kidneys between November 1962 and the end of March 1964, fifteen were dead seven months after receiving the implant. On the positive side, in 1970, twenty-seven of the recipients were still alive, twenty-five of them with the original implants, six to seven-and-a-half years after operation. In 1964, Starzl and his colleagues began to do histocompatibility matching of donor with recipient, but their limited choice of donors placed a severe restriction on their efforts to achieve improved matches. In their second series of twenty-five patients who received kidneys from October 1964 through March 1966, twenty-one (84 percent) remained alive seven months after operation, but after two, three, and four years, the results were slightly worse than in their first series. Among the twenty-five recipients, thirteen remained alive in 1970, four to five and a half years after transplantation. In both series, Starzl and his colleagues found that their best results were with kidneys from living related donors.

In April 1966, Starzl and his colleagues again modified their procedure. After Woodruff's and Anderson's observation in 1964 that antilymphocytic serum could prolong the survival of skin homografts in rats, various investigators began to study the effect of antilymphocytic serum on the survival of transplanted kidneys in dogs. In 1966 Anthony Monaco and his colleagues at Harvard found that antilymphocytic serum was unusually powerful in its ability to prevent the rejection of kidney transplants in dogs.[16] Other groups at Edinburgh and in Starzl's laboratory published similar findings. Thus in their third series of patients begun in April 1966, in addition to improved histocompatibility matching, Starzl and his colleagues reduced the doses of azathioprine and prednisone and began to give antilymphocytic globulin for four months after transplantation. The result was a dramatic improvement in the survival rate of both patients and implanted kidneys. Thirty-two of thirty-four patients were still alive a year after operation, and thirty-one remained alive at the end of two years.[17]

Nevertheless, the administration of antilymphocyte globulin was not without harmful side effects and potential dangers. The antiserum was prepared by successive injections of human lymphocytes into horses so as to immunize the horses specifically against human lymphocytes. The antilymphocyte globulin, therefore, possessed the potential capacity to produce serum sickness, anaphylactic reactions, and other reactions to foreign proteins. To minimize such possible reactions, Starzl and his colleagues injected the antilymphocyte globulin intramuscularly into the patients. The injections were painful, and patients might develop hives, itching, or rashes. About 20 percent of patients suffered some form of anaphylactic reaction and almost every patient developed antibodies against horse protein. Yet the benefits of antilymphocyte globulin were so impressive as to outweigh its risks and drawbacks.[18]

At the University of Minnesota the first kidney transplant was performed on 7 June 1963, and during the next four years a total of eighty kidney transplants were carried out with forty-two deaths. With a death rate in excess of fifty percent, kidney transplantation at Minnesota was regarded as an experimental procedure, and a high risk one. Yet by the 1960s transplantation was clearly becoming an important part of surgery. Thus it was natural that as Dr. Wangensteen's retirement approached in 1967, the medical school should seek as the new chief of surgery a surgeon interested in transplant surgery and familiar with immunology. They chose Dr. John S. Najarian, a professor of surgery at the University of California medical school in San Francisco. A native Californian, Dr. Najarian graduated with distinction from the University of California-Berkeley, and then studied medicine at San Francisco. After his surgical residency there, he spent a year at the University of Pittsburgh as a special research fellow in immunopathology and two years as a senior fellow in transplantation immunology at the Scripps Clinic and Research Foundation at La Jolla. Dr. Najarian thus studied transplantation immunology during the years when transplantation was coming of age as a practicable field of surgery. In 1964 he was appointed a Markle scholar in academic medicine.

At the University of California in March 1964, Dr. Najarian began to perform kidney transplants from living related donors. Three of his first ten patients to receive transplants died, two within a month after transplantation. In an analysis of the causes of death, Dr. Najarian noted that in a number of cases there was a significant delay before the implanted kidney began to secrete urine, a fact which suggested that the kidney had undergone injury before implantation. Since Najarian and his colleagues had cooled the kidney as soon as it was removed from the donor, and they had kept the time period that it was deprived of circulating blood to about twenty minutes, well within the range considered tolerable, he decided that the kidney must have undergone some unrecognized form of injury during its removal from the donor. When he studied the records of the operations, Najarian noted that the donor's blood pressure tended to fall steeply shortly before the kidney was removed, and that as soon as dissection was begun around the renal artery, the flow of urine from the kidney dropped sharply, sometimes even stopped. In an effort to protect the donor kidney, in December 1964 Najarian began to give the donor large amounts of water, together with mannitol, before operation so as to maintain the flow of urine. On the new regimen the transplanted kidneys began to function promptly, and the number of deaths declined. Among twenty-one patients who received kidneys from December 1964 through March 1966 there were only four deaths.[19]

When he arrived at Minnesota in the summer of 1967, John Najarian established protocols for kidney transplantation designed to avoid or minimize the various risks in the procedure. By 1967 deaths from the transplantation surgery itself were rare, and most deaths among patients after transplantation were caused by infections.[20] Because patients who received transplanted organs were treated with immune suppressive agents to prevent rejection, their resistance to infection was greatly reduced. Nevertheless, transplant patients usually did not die of infections acquired casually. More than half who died of infections following transplantation had an active focus of infection at the time of transplantation, usually in the urinary tract. Dr. Najarian decided that transplantation should not be performed in the presence of infection. Instead, the patient should be maintained on dialysis until infections were eliminated. If the patient's kidneys were infected, they should be removed and the patient allowed to recover before transplantation. Dr. Najarian thought that the amount of surgical trauma to which the patient was subjected at the time of transplantation should be kept to a minimum. If the urinary bladder were infected, such infection could be removed by irrigating the bladder with antibiotic solutions. Before transplantation, the patient should be checked for other possible infections by cultures from the nose, throat, urine, stool, and hemodialysis cannula.

Since the uremia resulting from kidney failure produced pulmonary edema, kidney patients often developed pneumonia. To eliminate uremia, and with it any special susceptibility to pneumonia, patients were given hemodialysis for a period of time before transplantation. Almost a third of patients who died of infection following kidney transplantation developed leakage where the ureter of the implanted kidney joined the urinary bladder. To prevent such leakage, Dr. Najarian adopted a submucosal tunneling technique in which the bladder was closed in three layers. The technique worked so well that none of the seventy transplants that Najarian performed during his first two years at Minnesota developed urinary tract infections.

An even more serious source of infections were wound infections from the transplantation surgery itself. Dr. Najarian sought to avoid wound infections by keeping operations brief with minimal loss of blood, by irrigating the wound with sterile saline to remove dead tissue, and by closing the wound carefully.

Finally, Najarian limited the dose of azathioprine and prednisone given to overcome episodes of rejection, thinking it better to let the kidney reject, if it must, than to endanger the life of the patient by too much suppression of the immune system. If the implanted kidney functioned poorly, he restricted azathioprine even further, because if the drug were not being removed in the urine, even small doses would tend to accumulate in the body.

By such steps, no one of them by itself revolutionary, John Najarian developed a regimen that lowered the mortality among kidney transplant patients significantly. His emphasis throughout was on the prevention of infection even more than on the avoidance of rejection. The whole plan of treatment was adapted intelligently to the physiology and immunology of the patient. It proved very effective. Among the seventy transplantations that Najarian and his colleagues performed at the University of Minnesota from August 1967 through July 1969 there were only ten deaths; and two that died were desperately ill and had received pancreas transplants in addition to kidney transplants.[21] The results were better than those of other transplantation centers at the time.

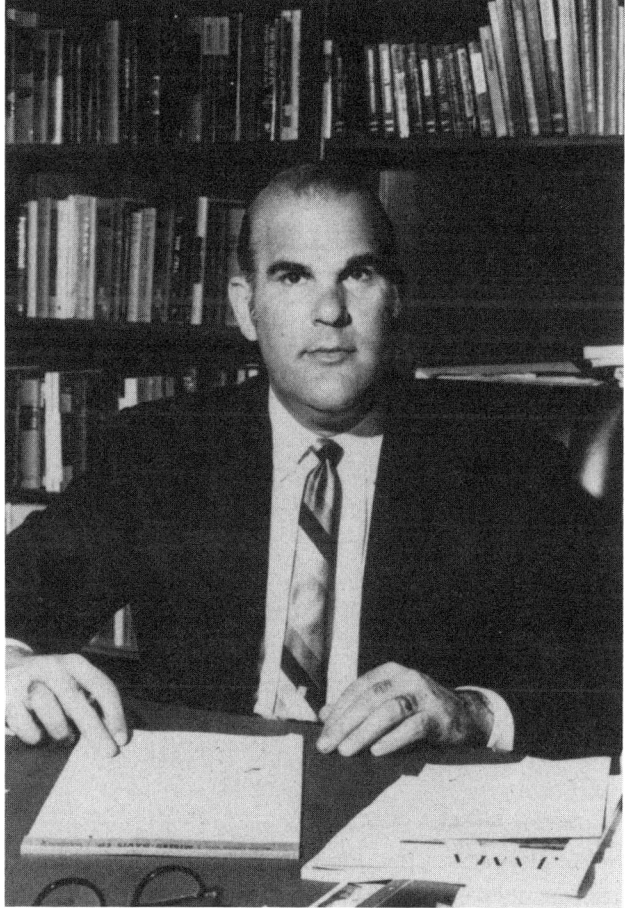

FIGURE 21:1 John Najarian, circa 1968. Courtesy Department of Surgery.

During the first two years of the new kidney program at Minnesota, Najarian and his colleagues used only azathioprine and prednisone to prevent rejection, but were keenly aware from the work of Starzl's group of the potential value of antilymphocytic globulin as an immunosuppressant. In 1968 Dr. Najarian brought Richard L. Simmons to Minnesota from Columbia University. Simmons, who had pursued postresidency training in tissue transplantation at the Massachusetts General Hospital, collaborated with Najarian and others on the preparation of antilymphocyte globulin.

In their work on antilymphocytic globulin, Najarian and Simmons obtained the collaboration of the Roswell Park Memorial Institute at Buffalo, New York, which provided lymphocytes obtained from the peripheral blood of healthy volunteers and grown in culture in 200-liter vats. The pure cultures of human lymphoblasts were shipped from Buffalo to Minneapolis where they were injected into horses at ten-day intervals. When the horses had been immunized to a sufficient antibody-titer, they were bled and continued to be bled at intervals, after repeated booster infections of lymphocytes, for a period of six months. The horse blood was filtered, and the serum subjected to repeated electrophoresis to obtain the immune globulin free of other serum proteins.[22] In its highly purified form the antilymphocyte globulin could be given to patients intravenously, thereby avoiding painful intramuscular injections, and the purified globulin tended to reduce the incidence of fever, hives, rashes, or other allergic reactions. On a trial basis, Dr. Najarian and his colleagues began to give antilymphocyte globulin to transplant recipients daily for two days before and ten days after transplantation, and then every other day for five more doses. They also gave azathioprine and prednisone. The initial results were encouraging. Among nineteen patients treated with antilymphocyte globulin, who received kidneys from living related donors during 1968 and 1969, no kidneys were lost, no patients died, and the number of rejection episodes was noticeably fewer than in earlier series.[23] Similarly improved results were obtained with kidneys transplanted from cadavers.[24]

After the introduction of purified antilymphocyte globulin the next significant immune suppressive agent to be introduced into transplantation was cyclosporin A in 1978. Nevertheless, in 1973 Gerhard Opelz and his colleagues at the University of California-Los Angeles noted that patients who had received blood transfusions before transplantation had better kidney survival rates than patients who had not had transfusions.[25] Thereafter Opelz and Paul Terasaki found that blood transfusions before transplantation improved markedly the survival of kidneys transplanted from cadavers.[26]

From 1968 through 1981, 1,295 patients received kidney transplants at the University of Minnesota, and 76 percent of them survived at least four years. Whenever possible Dr. Najarian and his group transplanted kidneys from living related donors, but 504 of their transplantations were from cadavers. The survival rates were better for patients receiving kidneys from related donors; for cadaver transplants the survival rates were about the same as those for cadaver transplants at other centers in the United States and Europe.[27]

In 1969 Dr. Najarian and his colleagues began to do kidney transplants on diabetic patients. Few transplantation centers then were willing to attempt kidney transplantation on diabetics because they were considered to have a high risk of developing infection, progressive cardiovascular disease, or other complications. Nevertheless, diabetic patients did not do well on hemodialysis; 70 percent of those who began dialysis were dead within three years. By 1975 Najarian and his colleagues had performed kidney transplants for 132 diabetic patients, 9 of whom received a second transplant. Seventy-seven patients lived at least two years after transplantation and twenty-one more than five years. In 1975, eighty-eight of the diabetics who had received kidney transplants were still living. Furthermore, whereas before transplantation, such patients were rapidly going blind, after transplantation their vision often stopped deteriorating and even improved, and they were able to lead more normal lives. Among twenty-two patients who before transplantation were unable to walk, sixteen had improvement in muscle strength and in their ability to walk.[28]

Pancreas Transplantation

The failure of the kidneys was but one consequence of a general deterioration of small arteries throughout the body of young diabetics even when their diabetes was carefully controlled by insulin and diet. Therefore, when transplantation of organs became feasible in the 1960s, surgeons began to consider the transplantation of the pancreas to cure the primary diabetes. The dual functions of the pancreas, namely, its secretion of pancreatic juice through the pancreatic duct into the duodenum as well as its internal secretion of insulin into the circulating blood, and its complex arterial and venous connections, made it extraordinarily difficult to transplant. Furthermore, in order to preserve its function of secreting pancreatic juice, the duodenum had to be transplanted together with the pancreas, because the walls of the duodenum produce a hormone, *secretin,* which stimulates the pancreas to secrete pancreatic juice. In 1966 Dr. Felix Largiader, who had come to the University of Minnesota from Zurich to work with Dr. Richard Lillehei, succeeded in transplanting the pancreas and duodenum together into dogs from whom the pancreas had previously been removed. Ten dogs survived the transplantation for periods of four to nine days, during which the transplanted pancreas secreted both pancreatic juice and insulin.[29] After Largiader and Lillehei established a workable surgical technique for transplantation of the pancreas, Yasuo Idezuki, also working with Richard Lillehei at Minnesota, carried out pancreatic transplants on a further series of dogs to learn whether rejection of the engrafted pancreas could be prevented by the administration of azathioprine and prednisone. Although many of the dogs died from one cause or another in what was highly experimental surgery, one survived more than 150 days with azathioprine treatment. Another survived 98 days without any immunosuppressive treatment. At no time after transplantation did the dogs show signs of diabetes. Idezuki and his colleagues believed the results sufficiently encouraging to justify pancreatic transplantation for selected patients with severe diabetes and its complications.[30]

Patients who developed diabetes during childhood or in adolescence were described by Richard Lillehei as "the pariahs of medicine."[31] When their kidneys failed, medicine had little to offer them. Diabetics with kidney failure were difficult to dialyse and did not survive long on dialysis. Likewise they were considered poor candidates for kidney transplantation programs. Thus, although the risks of a new and untried procedure such as pancreatic transplantation were great, they were less than the known consequences of severe diabetes that had begun in childhood.

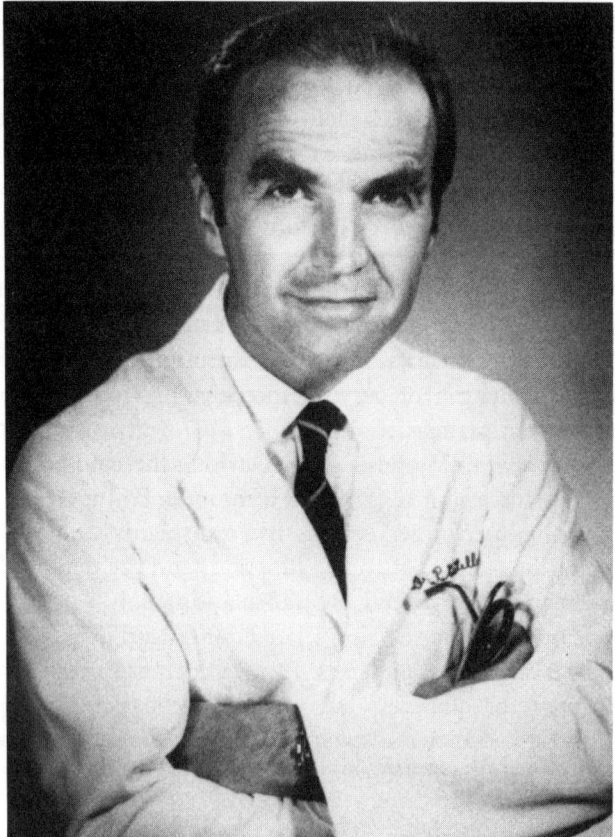

FIGURE 21:2   Richard Lillehei. Courtesy Mn U Archives.

At the university hospital on 17 December 1966, William D. Kelly and Richard Lillehei transplanted both kidney and pancreas into a twenty-eight-year-old woman who had suffered from diabetes since the age of nine, and from kidney disease since she was nineteen. In June 1966 she had begun hemodialysis but did badly, and in November she was admitted to the university hospital, requesting consideration for transplantation. The transplanted kidney did not begin to secrete urine at first, but the patient's blood sugar immediately began to fall, indicating that the transplanted pancreas was secreting insulin. Although the kidney slowly began to secrete urine, the patient developed pancreatitis; kidney and pancreas had to be removed two months after transplantation. A month later the patient died from pulmonary embolism.[32]

On 31 December 1966 Richard Lillehei performed a second pancreatic and kidney transplantation on a thirty-two-year-old woman who had suffered from diabetes since the age of eleven. She survived four and a half months after transplantation before dying from infection. Although she suffered from chronic rejection of the implanted kidney, the pancreas continued to function and appeared normal at autopsy. By 1970, Lillehei had performed eleven pancreatic transplants among whom no patient had survived transplantation longer than eleven months. Despite such discouraging results, he felt justified in continuing pancreatic transplantations because in almost every case the pancreas had functioned normally after transplantation, and the patient had not required insulin during the postoperative period. He thought that the problems leading to early death after transplantation would prove solvable.

From 1966 through June 1977, fifty-seven pancreas transplants were performed throughout the world. Only two patients survived more than a year, one of them for slightly over four years. After 1977 the number of pancreas transplants rose sharply and the length of survival increased. Among 262 patients who received pancreatic transplants after 1 July 1977, 187 were still alive in June 1983. In 1978 at the University of Minnesota, Dr. David Sutherland began a new series of pancreatic transplants using a segmental technique. By June 1983, Sutherland and his colleagues had performed seventy-five transplants. Some of the patients have had excellent long-term pancreatic function, and the deterioration of their small arteries seemed to be arrested. By transplanting only a portion of the pancreas, Sutherland was able to use living related donors and thereby to achieve better survival of the transplanted pancreas. Pancreatic transplantation will never be a general treatment for diabetes, but for diabetic patients who require immunosuppression for a kidney transplant or whose diabetic complications are severe, it may be a helpful and life-preserving treatment.[33]

Bone Marrow Transplantation

In July 1968, Dr. Jerome A. L'Heureux of Meriden, Connecticut, telephoned Dr. Robert A. Good at the University of Minnesota about a patient, a four-month-old boy, who a month before had begun to develop extensive skin infections marked by numerous draining pustules on the scalp and other areas of the body. Although such an infection normally would stimulate the production of immune globulin in the blood, the child showed a low level of gamma globulin in the serum. What made his condition particularly grave was that in his family there was a history of eleven male infants who had died before they were a year old, each overwhelmed by a similar general infection. In 1963 at the Boston Children's Hospital, a first cousin had been diagnosed before death as suffering from a deficiency of lymphocytes and gamma globulin. Since the child was clearly suffering from immunologic deficiency, Dr. L'Heureux wished to send him to the University of Minnesota for study and possibly for treatment by bone marrow transplantation.

When the child was admitted to the university hospital on 16 July, his tissues were found to match those of one of his four sisters at the HLA-locus. On 24 July

Dr. Good and his colleagues performed a bone marrow transplant from the sister to the infant boy. A week later the boy began to vomit and developed a fever. A rash appeared over his face and back. At this stage, Dr. Good realized that the lymphocytes developed from the cells in the bone marrow transplant were attacking the child's own tissues, but from his experience in mice, Good thought that the reaction would be temporary because the donor and recipient were matched at the HLA-locus. Such proved to be the case. Within three days the fever subsided and the rash disappeared. Then the child developed anemia as his new immunological system attacked his blood-forming cells, but a second bone marrow transplant provided him also with a new blood-forming system, his blood type changing from type A to that of the donor, his sister, which was type O.[34] Thereafter the little boy was healthy and grew steadily, possessing normal immunological and blood-forming systems. In 1982, fourteen years after receiving the bone marrow transplant, he was a normal, healthy adolescent boy, who resisted infection fully as well as other normal members of his family.[35]

By 1980 throughout the world, approximately fifty-five patients suffering from severe immune deficiency disease had been endowed successfully with immune systems by bone marrow transplants from a brother or a sister. At Minnesota eight bone marrow transplants had been performed with the survival of five of the patients.[36] Severe combined immunological deficiency is a very rare condition, but this tiny group of unfortunate patients had provided invaluable information about the defenses of the body against infection, against cancer, and against transplanted organs and tissues. To Dr. Good in 1968, it was particularly satisfying to be able to repay the debt he owed to the children with immune deficiencies he had studied in earlier years, without being able to help, by providing one of them with the immune system that Nature had failed to give him.[37]

Heart and Liver Transplantation

In December 1967 at Capetown, South Africa, Dr. Christian Barnard performed the first human heart transplant. In January 1968 at Stanford University, Dr. Norman Shumway, who, by extensive experimentation on dogs, had developed the methodology for heart transplantation, also transplanted a human heart. Both surgeons had taken surgical residencies at the University of Minnesota in the 1950s when open heart surgery was developing rapidly. During the next two years over 150 heart transplants were performed all over the world, but the results were so unsuccessful that heart transplantation was soon given up at most medical centers. Nevertheless, Dr. Shumway and his colleagues continued to perform heart transplants at Stanford with steadily improving results. By the late 1970s they had established heart transplantation as an accepted treatment for selected patients who would otherwise die from heart failure. In 1986 one of Dr. Shumway's students, Dr. Stuart W. Jamieson, came to Minnesota to inaugurate a program for heart-lung transplantation in the Heart-Lung Institute established by the university in 1987.

Since the 1960s surgeons at the University of Minnesota have also performed liver transplants, pioneered in March 1963 by Thomas Starzl and his colleagues at the University of Colorado. In the 1980s liver transplantation has become increasingly successful, especially for young children with biliary atresia, who would have no hope of growing to adulthood without a liver transplant.

During the more than three decades that transplantation of organs and tissues has developed into an accepted treatment for otherwise hopeless diseases, Minnesota has been continuously active in both research and surgical achievement. Occasionally a pioneer, Minnesota has responded promptly to new developments in surgery and immunology whether made at Minnesota or elsewhere. The early studies in hematology at Minnesota by Hal Downey laid a foundation for Robert Good's brilliant achievements in immunology, as early surgical research and research laboratories created a tradition and facilities within which John Najarian developed his outstandingly successful transplantation program.

NOTES

1. Alexis Carrel and C. C. Guthrie, "Functions of a transplanted kidney," *Science*, 1905, *22*, 473.

2. W. J. Dempster, "Observations on the behaviour of the transplanted kidney in dogs," *Ann. roy. Coll. Surg. Engl.*, 1950, *7*, 275–302.

3. David M. Hume et al., "Experiences with renal homotransplantation in the human: report of nine cases," *J. clin. Invest.*, 1955, *34*, 327–382.

4. An effective artificial kidney was first used clinically in Holland in 1944 by Kolff and Berk. See W. J. Kolff and H. J. J. Berk, "The artificial kidney: a dialyser with a great area," *Acta med. Scand.*, 1944, *117*, 121–134. In 1946 Nils Alwall at Lund, Sweden, and Gordon Murray and his colleagues at Toronto, Canada, each independently developed an artificial kidney. See Nils Alwall, "On the artificial kidney: Apparatus for dialysis of the blood in vivo," *Acta med. Scand.*, 1947, *128*, 317–325; Gordon Murray, Edmund Delorme, Newell Thomas, "Development of an artificial kidney. Experimental and clinical experiences," *Archs Surg., Chicago*, 1947, *55*, 505–522.

5. John P. Merrill et al., "Successful homotransplantation of the human kidney between identical twins," *J. Am. med. Ass.*, 1956, *160*, 277–282.

6. Joseph E. Murray et al., "Kidney transplantation between seven pairs of identical twins," *Ann. Surg.*, 1958, *148*, 343–359.

7. Joseph E. Murray et al., "Kidney transplantation in modified recipients," *Ann. Surg.*, 1962, *156*, 337–355, pp. 342–343.

8. Robert Schwarz et al., "Effect of 6-mercaptopurine on antibody production," *Proc. Soc. exp. Biol. Med.*, 1958, *99*, 164–167.

9. Robert Schwarz and William Dameshek, "The effects of 6-mercaptopurine on homograft reactions," *J. clin. Invest.*, 1960, *39*, 952–958; Roy York Calne, "The inhibition of renal homograft rejection in dogs by 6-mercaptopurine," *Lancet, Lond.*, 1960, *i*, 417–418.

10. Joseph E. Murray et al., "Kidney transplantation in modified recipients," *Ann. Surg.*, 1962, *156*, 339–355.

11. Joseph E. Murray et al., "Prolonged survival of human kidney homografts by immunosuppressive drug therapy," *New Engl. J. Med.*, 1963, *268*, 1315-1323.
12. Willard E. Goodwin and Donald C. Martin, "Transplantation of the kidney, spring 1963," *Urol. Surv.*, 1963, *13*, 229-248, p. 231.
13. J. Hamburger et al., "Transplantation d'un rein entre jumeaux non monozygotes après irradiation du receveur. Bon fonctionnement au quatrième mois," *Presse médicale*, 1959, *67*, 1771-1775.
14. Jean Hamburger et al., *Renal transplantation theory and practice*, p. vii.
15. M. F. A. Woodruff and N. F. Anderson, "The effect of lymphocytic depletion by thoracic duct fistula and administration of antilymphocytic serum on the survival of skin homografts in rats," *Ann. N.Y. Acad. Sci.*, 1964, *120*, 119-128.
16. Anthony P. Monaco et al., "Antiserum to lymphocytes. Prolonged survival of renal homotransplants in dogs," *Transplantation*, 1966, *4*, 628-632; Ralph T. Huntley et al., "Use of anti-lymphocyte serum to prolong dog homograft survival," *Surg. Forum*, 1966, *17*, 230-233.
17. T. E. Starzl et al., "Long-term survival after renal transplantation in humans: (with special reference to histocompatibility matching, thymectomy, homograft glomerulonephritis, heterologous ALG, and recipient malignancy)," *Ann. Surg.*, 1970, *172*, 437-472.
18. Thomas E. Starzl et al., "Heterologous antilymphocyte globulin, histoincompatibility matching, and human renal homotransplantation," *Surg. Gynec. Obstet.*, 1968, *126*, 1023-1035.
19. John S. Najarian et al., "Protection of the donor kidney during transplantation," *Ann. Surg.*, 1966, *164*, 398-417.
20. Rolla B. Hill, Jr. et al., "Death after transplantation," *Am. J. Med.*, 1967, *42*, 327-334.
21. Richard L. Simmons, Carl M. Kjellstrand, and John S. Najarian, "Sepsis following kidney transplantation," in James D. Hardy, ed., *Critical surgical illness*, pp. 559-580.
22. A. W. Moberg et al., "Forced flow electrophoretic purification of antihuman antilymphoblast globulin," *Surgery*, 1970, *68*, 862-869.
23. John S. Najarian et al., "Antihuman lymphoblast globulin," *Fed. Proc.*, 1970, *29*, 197-201.
24. Richard L. Simmons et al., "Immunosuppressive assay of antilymphoblast globulin in man. Effect of dose, histocompatibility, and serologic response to horse gamma globulin," *Surgery*, 1970, *68*, 62-68.
25. Gerhard Opelz et al., "Effect of blood transplantation on subsequent kidney transplants," *Transpl. Proc.*, 1973, *5*, 253-259.
26. Gerhard Opelz and Paul I. Terasaki, "Dominant effect of transfusions on kidney graft survival," *Transplantation*, 1980, *29*, 153-158.
27. D. E. R. Sutherland et al., "Kidney transplantation," in Shimon Slavin, ed., *Bone marrow & organ transplantation, achievements & goals*, pp. 127-318, esp. pp. 187-202.
28. John S. Najarian et al., "Kidney transplantation for the uremic diabetic patient," *Surg. Gynec. Obstet.*, 1977, *144*, 682-690.
29. Felix Largiader et al., "Orthotopic allotransplantation of the pancreas," *Am. J. Surg.*, 1967, *113*, 70-76.
30. Yasuo Idezuki et al., "Experimental pancreaticoduodenal preservation and transplantation," *Surg. Gynec. Obstet.*, 1968, *126*, 1002-1014.
31. Richard C. Lillehei and J. Octavio Ruiz, "Pancreas," in John S. Najarian and Richard L. Simmons, eds., *Transplantation*, pp. 627-645, p. 636.
32. W. D. Kelly et al., "Allotransplantation of the pancreas and duodenum along with the kidney in diabetic nephropathy," *Surgery*, 1967, *61*, 827-837.

33. D. E. R. Sutherland et al., "Pancreas and islet transplantation," Slavin, ed., *Bone marrow* (n. 27), pp. 365–410.

34. Richard A. Gatti et al., "Immunological reconstitution of sex-linked lymphopenic immunological deficiency," *Lancet, London,* 1968, *ii,* 1366–1369.

35. R. N. Pahwa and R. A. Good, "Bone marrow transplantation in primary immunodeficiency diseases," Slavin, ed., *Bone marrow* (n. 27), p. 32.

36. Robert A. Good et al., "Current approaches to the primary immunodeficiencies," in M. Fourgereau and J. Dausset, eds., *Immunology 80. Progress in immunology IV,* pp. 906–929, p. 908.

37. Robert A. Good, "Immunologic reconstitution: the achievement and its meaning," *Hosp. Pract.,* 1969, *4,* 41–47.

CHAPTER 22

Change and Expansion after 1970

In 1959 the United States Surgeon General's Consultant Group on Medical Education drew attention to a growing shortage of physicians in the United States.[1] The rapid rise in population during the postwar period combined with the greater use of medical services brought about by a rising standard of living, increased use of health insurance, and medical advances all acted to add to demands for the services of physicians. At the same time a growing number of physicians was being diverted from medical practice to research or teaching. The rapid expansion of medical specialties reduced further the number of physicians in general practice—the part of the profession that provided primary medical care to patients. In 1959 there were 249,000 physicians in the United States, or 141 per 100,000 people. Schools of medicine and osteopathy were then graduating about 7,400 physicians annually. If the United States population were to grow by 1975 to 235 million, as was projected, the nation would by then require some 330,000 physicians in order to maintain the ratio of physicians to population existing in 1959. To provide 330,000 physicians by 1975, schools of medicine and osteopathy would have to raise their annual production of physicians by about 50 percent from the 7,400 graduated in 1959 to approximately 11,000 annually by 1975. Furthermore, in order to graduate 11,000 physicians by 1975 the schools would have to be prepared by 1971 to admit approximately 12,000 students. Such a massive increase in medical students would require both the creation of new medical schools and the large-scale expansion of existing schools. Neither could be accomplished without extensive building to provide the lecture rooms, laboratories, and teaching hospitals required to accommodate the crowds of additional students.

During the 1950s American medical schools, including the university's medical school, received substantial sums of money in federal matching grants for the construction of research facilities under the Federal Research Facilities Construction Program and occasionally for the construction of hospitals under the Hill-Burton Construction Act, but there were no federal funds available for the con-

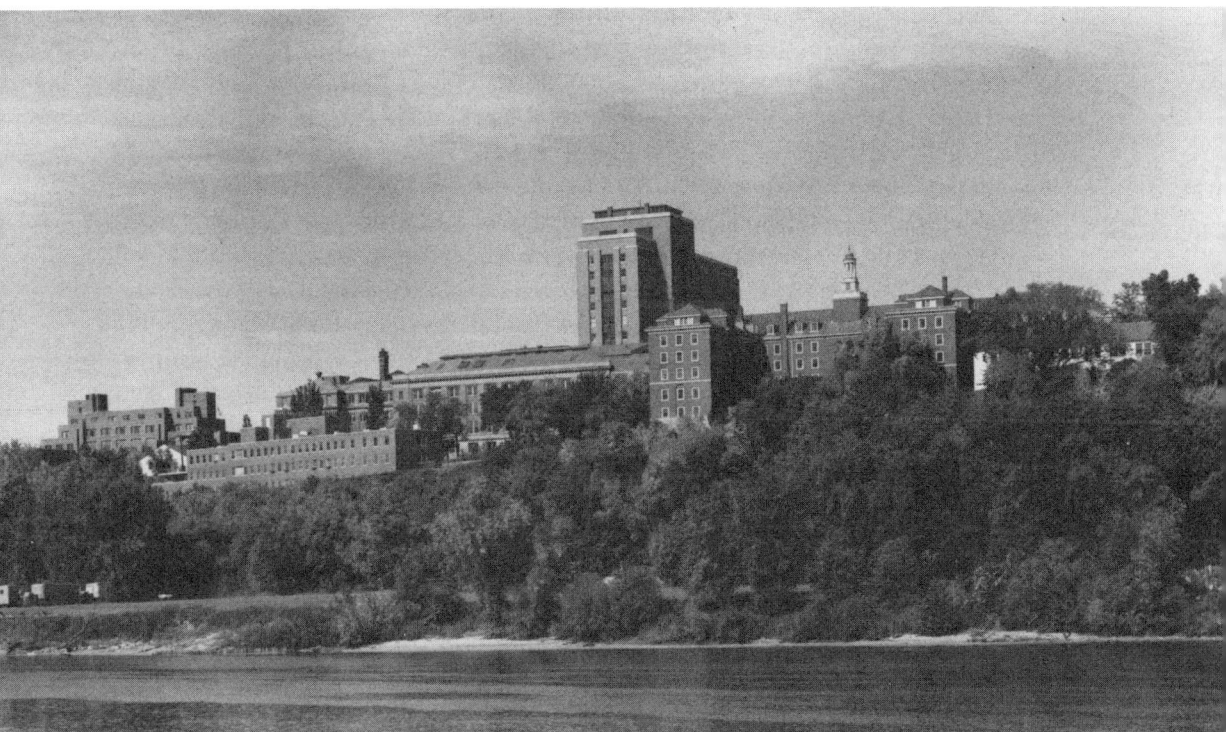

FIGURE 22:1 University of Minnesota Medical Center, 1955. From left to right: Students' Health Service, Variety Club Heart Hospital, Elliot Memorial Hospital, Mayo Memorial, Powell Hall (nurses' residence). Courtesy Mn U Archives.

truction of buildings to be used for medical teaching. As a result, the teaching facilities at most American medical schools tended to be older buildings, poorly adapted to modern needs, and severely overcrowded. From 1948 to 1958, funds for grant-supported research in medical schools had grown from $17 million to $88 million—a five fold increase. Since much research was necessarily carried on in medical school buildings that were also used for teaching, the enormous growth of research intensified the overcrowding of teaching facilities. In 1959 medical schools were, therefore, ill prepared to receive large numbers of new students. At no school was that fact more painfully true than at Minnesota.

In 1959 the Surgeon General's Consultant Group recommended that the federal government provide emergency matching funds for the construction of new medical buildings, and especially for buildings to be used for teaching.[2] In 1963 Congress responded to such urgings by passing the Health Professions Educational Assistance Act which provided matching funds for the construction of teaching facilities for medical schools on a two for one basis. Research facilities would continue to receive matching funds on a one for one basis.

The year before, in June 1962, the Minnesota State Legislature, concerned at the impending shortage of physicians and dentists, asked the university to estimate the funds that would be required for expansion of the dental and medical schools. After considering the question, the university decided that it did not know the extent of the perceived shortage of physicians and dentists and in September 1963 it recommended that a study be made of foreseeable needs for physicians, dentists, and other health professionals in Minnesota and adjoining states. At the request of the university the Hill Family Foundation of St. Paul decided in May 1964 to sponsor a regional study of the projected need for dentists and physicians in the upper Midwest. The foundation created a Health Manpower Study Commission under the direction of Professor Osler L. Peterson of Harvard University. In June 1965 Professor Peterson and Dr. Ivan J. Fahs began to collect data on the need for physicians and dentists in Minnesota, the Dakotas, and Montana. The four states formed a unified region from the standpoint of training physicians and dentists because the only schools for these professions in the four states were at the University of Minnesota, and the University of Minnesota educated many of the physicians who practiced in North and South Dakota and Montana. Peterson and Fahs found that in 1965 Minnesota had 145 physicians per 100,000 people, slightly more than the national average of 143, but that with the growth of population it would by 1975 have 200 to 300 fewer physicians than would be needed to maintain the 1965 ratio of physicians to population. Meanwhile, the passage of Medicare legislation, the growth of personal income, and the extended use of health insurance were expected to increase the demands for physicians. Even without such factors, the increasing differentiation of the medical profession into various specialties would require more physicians merely to fill present demands and needs.

To meet the predicted need for physicians, the Health Manpower Study Commission recommended that the University of Minnesota Medical School expand its entering class from 150 students to 200 students, and plan in the future to expand to 250 students. The commission noted that because all physicians took at least one year of internship after receiving the M.D. degree, and many took three years of hospital residency after the internship, there would be a delay of as long as eight years before an increase in the entering class of the medical school would bring about an increase in the number of practicing physicians. Thus an increase in the entering class in 1967 would not provide more physicians until at least 1972 and probably not until 1975.[3] The commission also recommended that the medical school accept transfer students who had completed the first two years of the medical course at the universities of North Dakota or South Dakota.

While the Hill Family Foundation's Health Manpower Study Commission was at work, the university had proceeded on the assumption that, while the exact scale and character were yet to be determined, a major expansion of the health sciences at the university must be undertaken. In October 1964 President O. Meredith Wilson appointed a Committee for the Study of Physical Facilities for the Health Sciences, with Elmer W. Learn, assistant to the president, as chairman.

After preliminary meetings the committee by March 1965 decided that before they could begin to consider the buildings that the health sciences might need, they would first need to study the role of the health sciences in the university, and the teaching and research functions they were intended to fulfill. The committee organized seven subcommittees and began an intensive examination of how the College of Medical Sciences and the School of Dentistry worked in the third quarter of the twentieth century. In October 1965 the committee completed its role and program report, which was submitted to President Wilson in 1966.

The committee's study of the medical school in 1965 occurred at a time when, after more than three decades of growth and change, the school was undergoing major changes both in its leadership and in the conditions under which it must work. Through all the vicissitudes of the Great Depression, World War II, the Korean War, the war in Viet Nam, and the enormous expansion of medical research supported by federal funding, the heads of major departments had continued either unchanged or with a continuity of philosophy despite a change in head. Owen Wangensteen had led the Department of Surgery for thirty-five years and Maurice Visscher physiology for thirty years. In the Department of Medicine, Cecil Watson had been in the department since 1932 and its head since 1942. In pediatrics, Irvine McQuarrie had retired in 1954 only to be succeeded by his former student, John A. Anderson, who continued the McQuarrie tradition uninterruptedly. When after thirty years of service Leo Rigler retired from Minnesota in 1957, he left the Department of Radiology in the hands of his former student and colleague, Harold O. Peterson. In 1965 the long continuity of leadership was drawing to a close. In 1966 Cecil Watson would retire early from the medical school. Owen Wangensteen was due to retire in 1967 and Maurice Visscher in 1968. A total of five department chairmen were due to retire within three years.

Aware of impending retirements and their possible implications for the school, the committee's Clinical Medicine Task Force under the chairmanship of Lyle A. French interviewed the chiefs of the various clinical departments. From their testimony and that of others, the task force distinguished two trends that were influencing teaching and research in clinical medicine. One was the assignment of groups of hospital beds to specific diseases, as had occurred in the creation of the Variety Club Heart Hospital and in the kidney transplantation program. The restriction of hospital beds to particular purposes, although necessary for special programs, imposed a somewhat less efficient use of hospital beds, and required, therefore, a larger number of hospital beds to achieve the same amount of clinical teaching. Thus the university hospital must expand merely to meet the needs of medical school classes at the existing level. If classes were to be enlarged, even more beds would be needed. The growth of hospital insurance and prepaid medical care was also changing the requirements of clinical teaching. Neither the patients admitted to the university hospital nor those who came to the outpatient department were any longer for the most part indigent patients. In the university hospital patients were not content to be placed in large public wards; at the outpatient department patients refused to come to cramped and dismal examining rooms. Since much of the university hospital had been built forty to fifty years before, it reflected the needs of an earlier era and required extensive renovation. Its capacity needed to be expanded by 200 to 300 beds. Similarly, the outpatient department completed in 1929 was severely inadequate. In order to attract enough outpatients to support adequate programs of clinical teaching, the medical school must develop an efficient, complete, and pleasant clinical facility.

The committee's study of the medical school and university hospital revealed various pressures and crosscurrents. Research in the medical school had grown greatly and was expected to grow further, but the growth of research in clinical departments and improvement in basic faculty salaries tended to make members of the faculty less willing to devote time to the care of patients, and therefore limited the ability of the school to provide comprehensive medical care. In his testimony before Dr. French's task force, Dr. Wangensteen noted the conflicting pressures of research and patient care when he expressed the belief that if the Department of Surgery were assigned many more beds in the university hospital, the faculty would be overwhelmed by demands for service to patients and would have insufficient time for research.[4]

To provide adequate facilities for clinical teaching, the committee thought that in addition to expansion of the university hospital, the medical school should form affiliations with various community hospitals in the Twin Cities. Such affiliations would be effective, the committee thought, if the university controlled the appointment of the clinical teaching staff in the affiliated hospital, and if the affiliated hospital were willing to provide adequate support for research as well as clinical teaching and to give medical students direct responsibility for the care of patients. Nevertheless, the university hospital, the outpatient department, and all the facilities of the medical school must be enlarged if the school were to educate large numbers of additional medical students.[5]

After the committee completed its study of the functions and programs of the health sciences in October 1965, it proceeded to compile data on the physical space that would be required to implement the educational recommendations contained in its preliminary report. In May 1966 the committee submitted its report on space needs to President Wilson and subsequently to the Board of Regents. In July the university presented the committee's space data to the Minnesota Legislative Building Commission and the following October the report was published.[6] On the assumption that in 1971 the medical school would admit 200 students, the committee projected that by 1973 the health sciences would need 1,140,000 square feet of additional space in new buildings to be constructed at an estimated cost of $47.3 million and the remodelling of 260,000 square feet of space in existing buildings at a cost of $5.4 million. The projected new buildings would about double the amount of space available to the College of Medical Sciences and the School of Dentistry.

In its projections the committee anticipated larger numbers of students in all the schools and graduate programs. The committee called for the transfer of the dental school to a new building in which there would be space to develop new programs in preventive dentistry, team teaching, and dental research. The space then occupied by the dental school in Owre Hall could be remodeled for the use of the basic science departments of the medical school. The committee's plans included a new outpatient clinic and a new university hospital. The portions of the Mayo Memorial Building and existing university hospital vacated by the transfer of their functions to the proposed new buildings could then be used for clinical teaching and laboratories. In 1965 Mr. Jay Phillips had offered the university $1.5 million to build a new surgical research laboratory to be named for himself and Dr. Owen H. Wangensteen as the Phillips-Wangensteen surgical research laboratory, and the committee included the Phillips-Wangensteen laboratory in its comprehensive plan to provide clinical research space. The new university hospital was planned to provide 276 beds and to increase the total capacity of the university hospitals to more than a thousand beds. The new hospital would contain larger areas for each of the clinic units to permit the use of modern automated equipment. The hospital pharmacy, for instance, would become an integral part of the patient care team on each nursing floor instead of being isolated in a distant corner of the hospital basement. Growth was anticipated also in other schools. By 1973 public health was expected to more than double both its staff and its need for space.

The release of the committee's report in May 1966 with its projected needs for buildings to cost more than $53 million—construction on a scale vastly exceeding all previous building plans—was followed by the appointment of a Minnesota legislative committee to investigate the need for more dentists and physicians in the state. The questions posed by the legislative committee were answered almost immediately by the publication in June of the report of the Hill Family Foundation's Health Manpower Study Commission, which recommended that the medical school should increase its entering class from 150 to 200 students, and later to 250 students, and the dental school from 110 to 150 students and later to 200 students. Because the commission's report confirmed the projections of the university's committee, and lent urgency to its findings, the Board of Regents in July 1966 accepted the committee's projections of long-range space needs. In January 1967 the university asked the legislature for $650,000 to buy the land on which to place the proposed buildings and $500,000 to prepare preliminary architectural plans for them.

The group of new health sciences buildings were to be located on two blocks south of Washington Avenue between Union and Harvard Streets. The first building planned, called temporarily Health Sciences A, was to extend along the east side of Union Street most of the length of the block from Delaware Street to Washington Avenue and was to be a seventeen-story tower above ground, with three storys below ground level. Two-thirds of the building was to house the dental school; the remainder was to contain research and teaching laboratories for the medical school and School of Public Health. On level two were to be lecture rooms for the medical school and a student lounge and cafeteria. In 1969 the Minnesota legislature appropriated $14 million for the construction of building A, the ap-

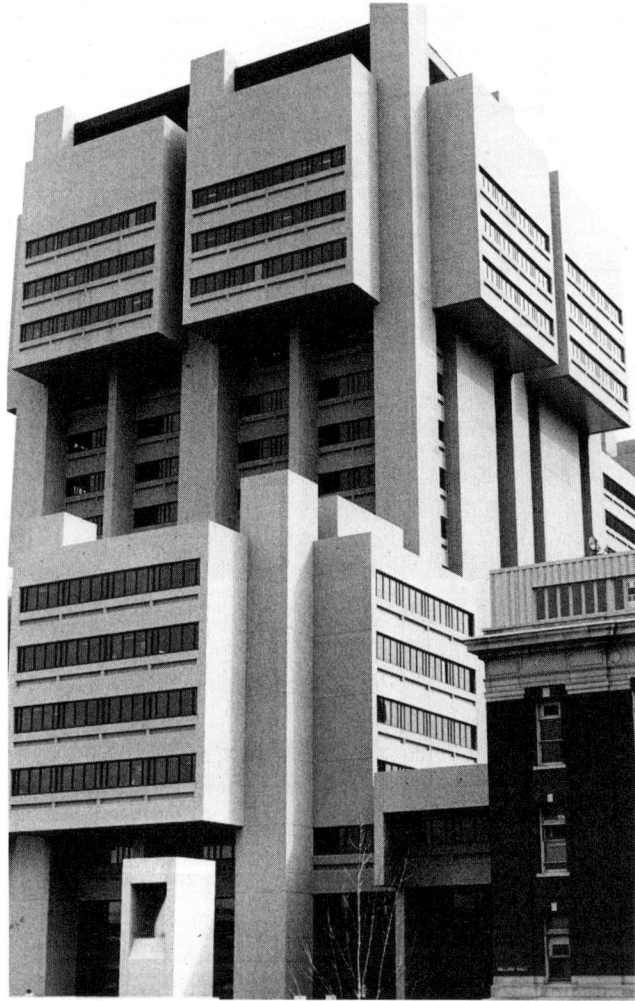

FIGURE 22:2 Malcom Moos Health Sciences Tower (Health Sciences A). Note the contrast in scale with Millard Hall on the right. Courtesy Health Sciences Public Relations.

propriation being contingent on the university's obtaining federal matching funds available under the Health Professions Educational Assistance Act of 1973. In July 1969 the university submitted a grant application and in December 1970 was awarded a grant of $22.4 million, thereby providing $36.4 million for the construction of building A.

Excavation for building A began in January 1971, the month following the award of the federal grant, and continued through the following summer. Construction proceeded over the next two years. By August 1973 the building was ready to receive its first occupants and by March 1975 it was fully occupied. On

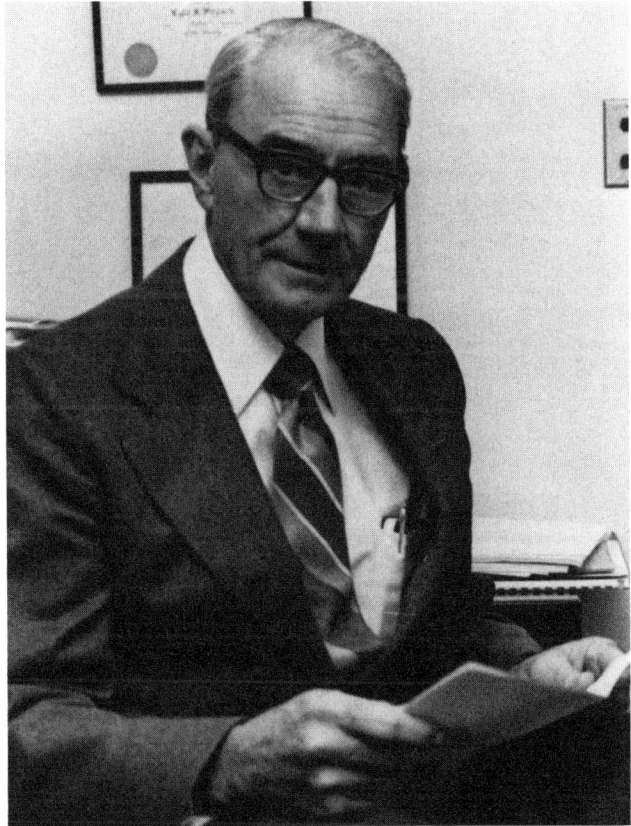

FIGURE 22:3   Lyle A. French. Courtesy Mn U Archives.

24 September 1976 building A was dedicated. In 1983 it was named in honor of former President Malcolm A. Moos as the Malcolm Moos Health Sciences Tower.

The reports of the Committee for the Study of Physical Facilities for the Health Sciences revealed such close relationships and so many interrelated needs between the College of Medical Sciences and the School of Dentistry, that the university began to consider how their administration might be coordinated. In April 1968 the Board of Regents changed the name of the Medical Center to that of the Health Sciences Center, and in March 1970 an eleven-member external committee appointed to study the organization of the health sciences at Minnesota recommended the dissolution of the College of Medical Sciences and the appointment of a chief administrative officer, or vice president, for the health sciences. The Board of Regents thereupon dissolved the College of Medical Sciences, and in July 1970 appointed Dr. Lyle A. French to be acting vice president for health sciences affairs. A year later the Board of Regents made Dr. French's appointment permanent. In 1970 Dr. Robert B. Howard, who had served since 1958 both as dean

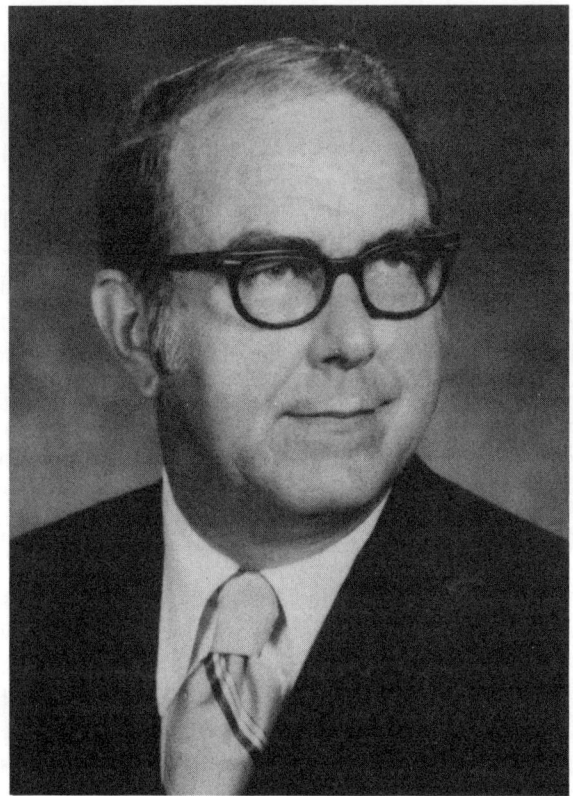

FIGURE 22:4 Neal L. Gault, Jr., 1970. Courtesy Dr. Gault.

of the College of Medical Sciences and dean of the medical school, resigned. A search committee was appointed to look for a new dean of the medical school, and in 1971 Dr. Neal L. Gault, Jr., who had left Minnesota in 1967 to go to the University of Hawaii, returned to become dean.

During the 1970s plans for new buildings to expand the health sciences continued apace. In 1973 Dr. Paul Dwan, who earlier had played an active role in the creation of the Variety Club Heart Hospital, gave $2.4 million to build a cardiovascular research and training center next to the heart hospital. The Kresge Foundation of Detroit, Michigan, contributed $750,000, the Minnesota legislature appropriated $1.7 million, and with gifts from the Variety Club of the Northwest and others, the university was able to build the K-E building for cardiovascular research at a total cost of about $9.5 million.

As the university developed plans for the second major health sciences building, referred to as health sciences B-C, the plans came under increasing criticism. The building was to contain in addition to clinical research laboratories, the new outpatient clinic. Critics of the proposed outpatient clinic suggested that instead of building a large central clinic to which patients might come from the whole metropolitan area, and indeed the whole state, the university should create a number of small community health clinics located in various poor neighborhoods of the Twin Cities. In order to build its outpatient clinic, the university had to obtain a certificate of need from the State Board of Health, a requirement that had been established to avoid unnecessary duplication of health care facilities. The State Board of Health was accustomed to issue certificates of need on the recommendation of the Metropolitan Health Board, which reviewed applications for such certificates in relation to community needs in the Twin Cities. In December 1972 the university obtained a certificate of need for the B-C building, but, because of a delay in funding, it was unable to begin construction before the certificate of need expired in December 1973. When in January 1974 the university applied to renew the certificate of need for B-C, the Metropolitan Health Board refused to recommend renewal. When the university's request then came before the State Board of Health, the board returned the request to the Metropolitan Health Board for reconsideration. At that point the university offered to reduce the number of examining rooms in the outpatient clinic from 228 to 156, to expand facilities at a community health care clinic operated by the university in south Minneapolis, and to establish a second such clinic in the Twin Cities. On 14 March 1974 the Metropolitan Health Board voted unanimously to recommend a certificate of need for B-C, a recommendation accepted promptly by the State Board of Health.

The controversy over the certificate of need for B-C reflected confusion among the public concerning health needs. It reflected also a conflict between the medical school's desire for a comprehensive, central outpatient clinic that would be most efficient for the clinical teaching of medical students and the desire of communities for small health care clinics located conveniently in their midst.

In July 1974 the university finally received $7.9 million in federal matching funds for B-C. Construction began in 1974 and the exterior shell of the building was completed in the fall, but the interior of many floors remained unfinished. The B-C building was a fifteen-story tower built at a cost of $33 million. In addition to the $7.9 million federal grant, the Minnesota legislature appropriated $15 million, and the university used university hospital funds and private gifts to make up the remainder. The B-C building was located south of building A to which it was joined by multi-level bridges and by a broad corridor that extended underground beneath what had formerly been Union Street. The underground corridor served to connect the two new health sciences buildings with each other and with Millard Hall, the Mayo Memorial, Diehl Hall, and the Masonic Hospital, thereby providing enclosed access to the whole Health Sciences Center. Union Street was converted into a broad plaza between Diehl Hall and the new health sciences towers on the east and the older buildings of the medical school and university hospital on the west.

In June 1978 the Phillips-Wangensteen Research Laboratory was dedicated in the B-C building and in 1979 the new outpatient clinics were opened. On 11 June

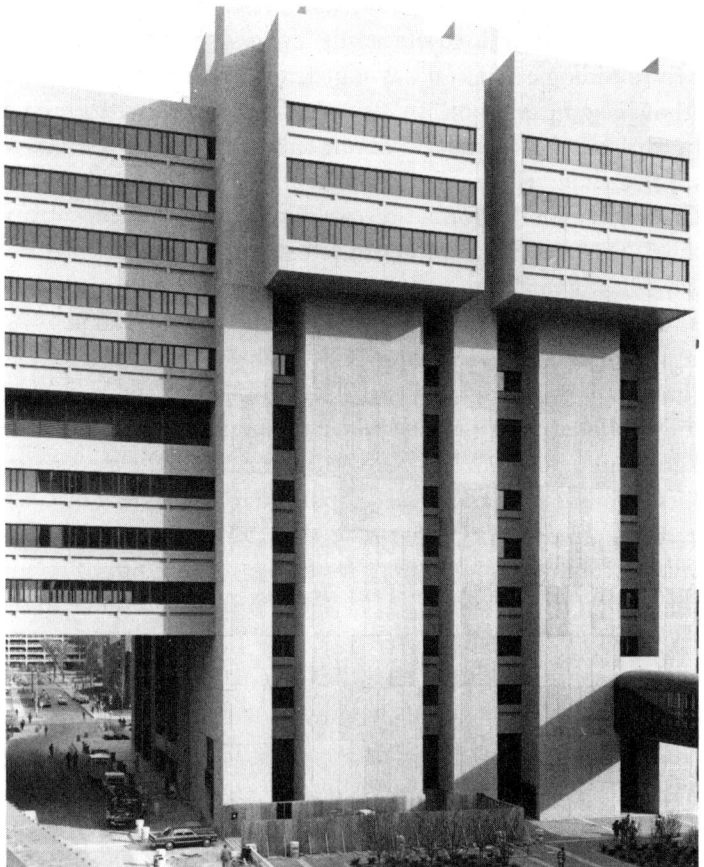

FIGURE 22:5   Phillips-Wangensteen Building (Health Sciences B - C). Courtesy Health Sciences Public Relations.

1979 the B-C building was named the Phillips-Wangensteen building in honor of Mr. Jay Phillips and Dr. Owen H. Wangensteen.

In 1977 the Minnesota legislature appropriated $13 million for a third large health sciences building, building F, for which the university obtained a federal matching grant of $8.3 million. Building F was to be an eleven story structure to the east of building A to house the pharmacy and nursing schools. Its construction began in November 1977 and was completed early in 1981.

With the completion of unit F the university had spent more than $100 million on the four large buildings for the health sciences. The cost of expansion was more than double the $47.3 million projected in 1966, but between 1967 and 1980 the United States had experienced a great currency inflation that by 1980 had reduced the purchasing power of the dollar to about a third of what it had been in 1967. The expansion transformed the Health Sciences Center, more than doubling its space, but also created the problem of remodeling the older buildings so that they might be used efficiently along with the new.

While the building expansion was in progress, the medical school was also undergoing change and expansion. In 1969 the faculty approved a revised medical curriculum, with emphasis upon a core curriculum, with time reserved for elective courses and free time. The curriculum changes were thought to be required by what was described as the "information explosion," most of the faculty being unaware that their predecessors in 1900 had felt similarly overwhelmed by the great growth of medical knowledge and medical literature at that time. In 1972 the medical school admitted 227 students in the freshman class, and in 1973, 239 students. The school also received a number of transfer students from the Dakotas so that in June 1974 the school graduated 262 seniors with the M.D. degree. Such a large number of graduates was, however, a temporary bubble; in 1975 the medical school graduated only 240 M.D.'s. During the 1970s the medical school thus expanded its enrollment in about the proportion urged upon it in 1965. The enlargement of the student body by more than 50 percent required additional faculty, and the commitment of funds for faculty salaries placed relentless pressures on the medical school budget. In 1976 the financial pressures on the medical school were relieved somewhat when Congress passed the Health Professions Educational Assistance Act, under which the federal government made annual capitation grants to medical schools based on the number of students enrolled. Through the 1970s the federal government in various ways encouraged or required medical schools to enlarge their enrollments. In 1974 the federal grant for the B-C building was made conditional upon the medical school's further expansion by 1980 of its entering class. In October 1975 the federal government announced a Health Careers Development Program intended to help minority and disadvantaged youths prepare for careers in medicine and other health professions. In 1978 the federal government began to require medical schools to admit second and third-year transfer students from foreign medical schools. Most such transfer students were Americans who had gone abroad for medical study because they were unable to gain admission to a medical school in the United States.

Nevertheless, by 1980 there was growing concern that American medical schools might be graduating too many physicians. In November 1980 a Graduate Medical Education National Advisory Committee recommended a 17 percent reduction in medical school class sizes because they projected that by 1990 there would be a surplus of 70,000 physicians in the United States.[7] At Minnesota the medical school, because of previous commitments, could not reduce its class size, but it decided not to expand to 245 students in 1981, and received permission from the United States Department of Health and Human Services to do so. In 1983 a medical school task force recommended a reduction in medical school class size to 200 students by 1988. Whether the projections in the 1980s of a surplus of physicians will be more accurate than the projections of a shortage of physicians made in 1959, only time will tell. It must be admitted that if the great expansion of new medical schools of the 1960s and 1970s had not occurred, an acute shortage of physicians would have developed in the United States.

NOTES

1. U. S. Surgeon General's Group on Medical Education, *Physicians for a growing America.*
2. Ibid., pp. 63–64.
3. Health Manpower Study Commission, *Health manpower for the upper Midwest: A study of the needs for physicians and dentists in Minnesota, North Dakota, South Dakota, and Montana,* p. 95.
4. Owen H. Wangensteen, "Report to Dean Howard's Committee . . . ," in Committee for the Study of Physical Facilities for the Health Sciences. Clinical Medicine Task Force, Minutes.
5. Committee for the Study of Physical Facilities for the Health Sciences, "Future planning for the health sciences. Part I. Preliminary Report."
6. Committee for the Study of Physical Facilities for the Health Sciences, "Future planning for the health sciences. Part II. Program, personnel and space projections."
7. U.S. Department of Health and Human Services, Graduate Medical Education National Advisory Committee, *Summary report.* This report, written in jargon, is so unclear that its conclusions are highly dubious. The evidence for the projected surplus of 70,000 physicians by 1990 is not provided in the summary report.

CHAPTER 23

New Developments in the 1980s

Although by 1981 the various schools in the Health Sciences Center possessed greatly enlarged space either in new buildings or in renovated portions of the older buildings, the university hospital remained in its existing labyrinthine quarters. The youngest part of the university hospital, the Mayo Memorial Building, had been built more than a quarter century before. Most of the rooms for patients were in still older buildings, erected between 1911 and 1929, more than half a century earlier. Because the older buildings extended around a quadrangle, both patients and staff had to traverse long corridors to get from one part of the hospital to another. The hospital was crowded; the space for laboratories and equipment was especially cramped and inconvenient. The operating rooms, designed for the simpler surgery of an earlier period, were inconveniently small for transplant surgery. As a whole, the hospital was poorly adapted for such activities as kidney dialysis and organ transplantation.

The hospital was equally inadequate for clinical teaching. It lacked conference rooms, so professors and students were obliged to gather in crowded and noisy corridors to discuss the details of patient care. Neither were there rooms in which physicians or nurses might talk privately with patients' families.[1]

The need for renewal of the university hospital became evident in the health services planning of the 1960s. When the Board of Regents dissolved the College of Medical Sciences in 1970, they made the university hospital an autonomous administrative unit responsible directly to the vice-president for health sciences affairs. In 1974 the Board of Regents established a separate board of governors for the university hospital. During the late 1970s the hospital board of governors searched for means to renew the hospital. The difficulties were formidable. The cost of a new university hospital would be greater than that of the whole of the rest of the health sciences expansion. Furthermore, there was no vacant land adjacent to the existing hospital on which to place it. The board of governors decided that the new hospital must be located on the site of Powell Hall, at the east end of Union Street. Although Powell Hall, built in 1933 for a nurses' residence, was an unusually handsome building of Georgian design, it was no longer used primarily by nurses. Instead, it operated as a low cost hotel for patients visiting the outpatient clinic or members of the families of patients in hospital. It occupied a magnificent site overlooking the Mississippi River next to the Cardiovascular Research Center and the Christian block of the university hospital.

In October 1980 the university hospital announced a plan to build on the Powell Hall site a new eleven-story hospital to cost an estimated $233 million. The university hoped to finance the building project by the sale of tax exempt bonds to be repaid over a period of thirty years from the hospital's charges for patient care. The university would seek the state's permission to issue the bonds as general obligation bonds of the state of Minnesota so that, backed by the full faith and credit of the state, the bonds would bear a lower interest rate than if the university issued them on its own credit. The new building was not intended to increase significantly the bed capacity of the hospital, but to replace obsolescent rooms and wards with a completely modern facility.[2] That fall the university applied for a certificate of need for the new hospital, which was granted in February 1981.

Nevertheless, the plans for the new university hospital aroused considerable opposition, in part because a surplus of hospital beds was developing in the Twin Cities. In presenting the case for the proposed hospital to committees of the state legislature, President C. Peter Magrath and Vice-president Lyle A. French were obliged repeatedly to argue for the special functions of the university hospital in medical teaching and research. In April 1981 the trustees of the Minnesota Medical Association questioned the size and cost of the university hospital project. Through the spring of 1981 in a series of articles in the *Minneapolis Tribune*, reporter Joe Rigert asserted that the size of the proposed hospital had been increased secretly in 1980. The director of the university hospital, John Westerman, complained to the Minnesota News Council that the *Tribune* articles were inaccurate. The plans for the hospital, Westerman said, had been presented at successive stages to meetings of the hospital board of governors, which were open to the press as were also the hearings before the various public boards concerned with the certificate of need application. Nevertheless, the charges published in the *Tribune* reflected a widespread hostility to the proposed hospital among the community hospitals and perhaps among the medical profession of the Twin Cities. The bonding request also came before the state legislature at a time when state finances were unusually tight. Despite criticism of the proposed hospital, and financial stringency, the Minnesota legislature in May 1981 passed a bonding bill to provide up to $190 million for the new university hospital. It was less than the $250 million requested, but not so much less as to cripple the project. The funds eliminated were to have paid for the remodeling of portions of the existing hospital to provide support services and a small number of beds. The new hospital would have a capacity of about 500 beds.

During the summer of 1981 Powell Hall was demolished, and in October excavation began for the new hospital. Because of extraordinarily high interest rates in 1981, the university deferred the issuance of long-term bonds to pay for the project, and instead issued $20 million in short-term notes to pay for the initial phases of construction. The unsettled conditions in financial markets created by very high interest rates caused concern whether the hospital project was financially feasible. In December 1981, the hospital board of governors proposed modifications to reduce the cost of the building by $14 million. Meanwhile, critics continued to attack the project on various grounds, most frequently because of the existing surplus of hospital beds in the Twin Cities. Critics also alleged that the high patient charges would make the university hospital so much more expensive than other hospitals that few patients would be referred to it. As a result of such criticisms, in January 1982 the Board of Regents decided to reduce the size of the hospital by eliminating the tenth floor, and with it 119 beds and four nursing stations. The reduction lowered the estimated cost of the project by $21 million to $154 million.[3] Although Vice-president French considered that the cuts were as much as could be made without endangering the effectiveness of the new hospital, on 18 January President Magrath announced that the university was to obtain an independent assessment of the financial feasibility of the hospital project by Robert Derzon of Lewin and Associates, a consulting firm in Washington, D.C. Mr. Derzon was to examine particularly the possible financial impact on the hospital of proposed changes in federal health care legislation, because President Reagan had indicated his intention to reduce federal payments under the Medicare and Medicaid programs. In March 1982 Derzon reported that although the existing facilities of the university hospital were deplorable, and the university badly needed a new hospital, the margin of financial safety in the plan to pay for it was not large enough. Current interest rates of 12 percent, said Derzon, would cost the hospital "almost $2 million a month for thirty years, or a total of $706 million for $105 million of bricks and mortar." He thought that the financial burden would be too great to be borne entirely by charges to patients. On the basis of Derzon's recommendations, the Board of Regents decided to defer the construction, which had been scheduled to begin that month, and to reexamine the size and funding of the new hospital.

Through the winter and spring of 1982 the proposed university hospital remained a great yawning hole in the ground, extending for a block and a half along the East River Road, over which ominous quiet reigned. There was no sound of men or machines at work, and no traffic to or from that gaping pit. In June the hospital administrators presented the Board of Regents with a revised plan for the new hospital that reduced its size to eight floors and 432 beds. The hospital would be primarily for acute patient care and would contain fewer offices and conference rooms. Its estimated cost was $125 million. In July 1982, the Board of Regents approved construction of one floor to house the Department of Therapeutic Radiology, which was facing a crisis, because the new linear accelerators which they needed urgently for the treatment of cancer patients and bone marrow transplant patients, could not be fitted into their existing quarters in the Mayo Memorial Building without dismantling the existing equipment and shutting down the

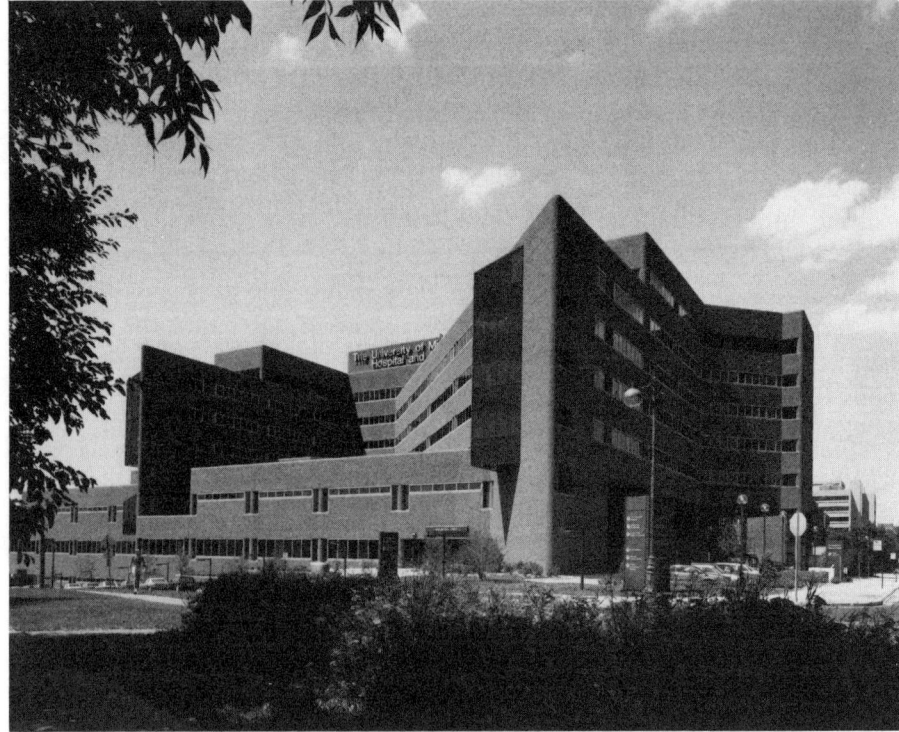

FIGURE 23:1 The new University of Minnesota Hospital, 1986. Courtesy Health Sciences Public Relations.

department for months. In October construction of the therapeutic radiology unit began. It was to be below ground level next to the Masonic Cancer Hospital.

In October 1982 the Board of Regents approved the plan to build the hospital on a reduced scale, to cost $125 million, but the university still had to decide how to finance it. That fall the construction of the therapeutic radiology unit was financed with short-term notes. Because of the financial difficulties of the state, Governor Albert Quie had imposed a moratorium on the issuance of state bonds so that the university for the time being could not use the bonding authority granted by the legislature in May 1981. In November 1982, the Board of Regents decided to finance the hospital by using its own credit to issue tax exempt thirty-year revenue bonds. The bonds would be secured by hospital revenue, rather than by the credit of the state, and would be paid off from charges to patients. In December, aided by an AA rating of its bonds by Standard & Poor's, the university succeeded in selling the whole bond issue on the New York bond market. The cost of repaying the bonds was estimated to be about $83 per patient day in the new hospital.

NEW UNIVERSITY HOSPITAL

In January 1983 the contractors began to pour footings for the new hospital, and construction proceeded swiftly. By December the steel framework of the eight-story building was complete. In contrast to university building projects of the previous forty years, the contracts for construction of the new hospital were awarded for amounts less than had been budgeted—on average about 9 percent less. When the new hospital was finished, some $11 million of the $125 million budgeted for it remained unspent and available for other purposes. As interest rates declined, the university was also able to reissue at lower interest rates the bonds used to finance the hospital, thereby lowering further the costs to be paid from patient charges.

In May 1984 the new facility for therapeutic radiology was opened to receive patients. The whole hospital, described as Unit J, was completed and opened in March 1986. On 25 April the first patients were transferred from the old hospital.

From the time of its opening the new hospital proved a remarkably successful building. As the staff became familiar with its bright rooms and corridors, their morale and efficiency rose markedly. The number of patients increased. Both staff and patients appreciated the central air conditioning that provided filtered, dust-free air—especially important for the avoidance of infection among transplant patients. Most of the patients' rooms had views of the Mississippi River. With the addition of Unit J, the university hospital possessed a total capacity of 580 beds, making it the second largest hospital in the Twin Cities. The Variety Club Children's Hospital, containing the pediatric section with 140 beds, was slightly larger than either the Minneapolis Children's or St. Paul Children's Hospitals. The whole fourth floor of Unit J was devoted to patients requiring intensive care. With the opening of Unit J the university hospital changed its official name from University of Minnesota Hospitals, which had reflected its diverse components built between 1911 and 1954, to University Hospital and Variety Club Children's Hospital to reflect the concentration of its services in the new building.

The opening of the new hospital in 1986 marked the first time in its seventy-seven year history that the hospital possessed a thoroughly modern building of adequate size in which it could provide a completely integrated hospital service. Nevertheless, the university hospital faces serious questions about its future, not the least of which is whether it can survive in an era of fierce competition among hospitals and among health maintenance organizations. The financial basis of the university hospital is payments made through Medicare, Medicaid, and private health insurance programs. The administrators of all forms of health insurance are concerned increasingly with the control of costs, but a teaching hospital such as the university hospital tends to have higher costs than community hospitals without a teaching program because of the salaries that it must pay to residents and the other costs of a teaching program. The university hospital also tends to receive patients who are acutely ill and who, therefore, require intense, prolonged, and often highly elaborate care. The care of such patients may cost more than the university is paid for them by either government or private health insurance.[4] So far the university hospital has been able to cope successfully with its financial

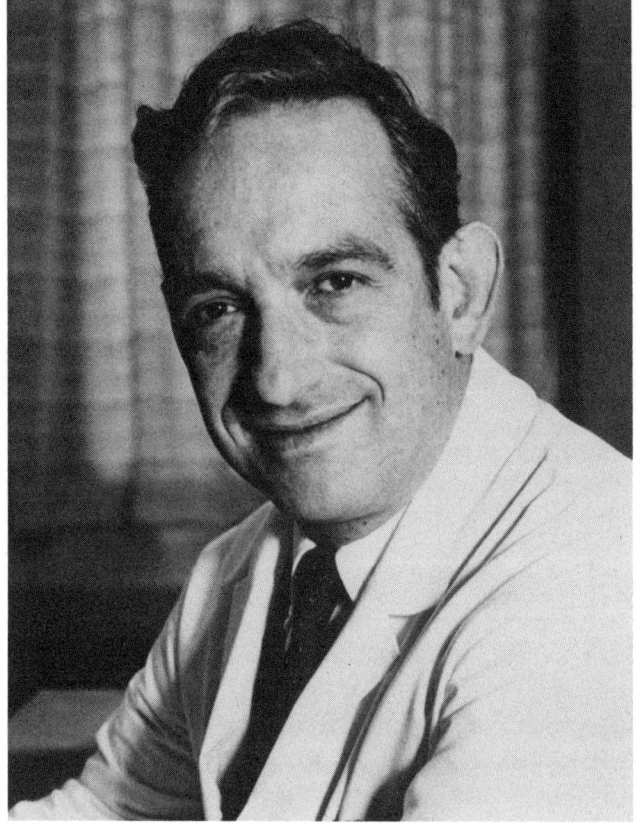

FIGURE 23:2 David M. Brown. Courtesy Medical Administration.

problems. The combination of lower building and financing costs with larger numbers of patients has kept it financially healthy.

A less tangible question posed by the new university hospital is the effect that it may have on the relations of the medical faculty with the medical profession in the Twin Cities and throughout the state. Since the reorganization of the medical school in 1913, the faculty has been separated, in greater or lesser degree, from the medical profession in the Twin Cities. Now that clinical members of the faculty possess a large, self-contained hospital in which to work, they may tend to see even less of their professional colleagues in practice, who carry on their work in the community hospitals. Unless deliberate efforts are made to overcome the resultant isolation, it could exert an impoverishing effect on the medical school.

In 1985 after fourteen years of serene and compassionate leadership through difficult times, Neal Gault resigned as dean of the medical school to be succeeded by David M. Brown, a member since 1967 of the Departments of Pediatrics and

Laboratory Medicine. Under Dean Brown's leadership the medical school enters upon its second century.

NOTES

1. Ralph Heussner, "U of M Hospitals renewal project: building for the future," *Univ. Minn. med. Bull.*, Spring 1981, pp. 1–7.
2. "U Hospitals ask $230 million to built, renovate," *Minnesota Daily,* 14 October 1980.
3. "Regents approve $21 million cut in U Hospitals project," *Minnesota Daily,* 8 January 1982.
4. Neal A. Vanselow, "Academic health centers: Can they survive?," *Issues Sci. Technol.*, 1986, *2*, 55–64.

CHAPTER 24

The Medical School in Retrospect

As the University of Minnesota Medical School enters upon its second century surrounded by many uncertainties, and perhaps real dangers, it may take both comfort and warning from its history over the first hundred years. The school has grown enormously from its beginnings in the fall of 1888 in the small buildings of the Minnesota Hospital College and St. Paul Medical College, where busy doctors took time from their practices to deliver hastily improvised lectures or to attend patients at the university dispensary. Despite its small beginnings, Perry Millard and his colleagues clearly intended that the medical school should move to stand among the leading medical schools in the United States. Within eight years they achieved three substantial buildings on the university campus, and the sciences of anatomy, chemistry, histology, embryology, and pathology were being taught by full-time medical scientists, each of whom had received advanced training in Europe. In 1908, at the end of its first twenty years, the medical school had become the sole school in the state of Minnesota, and indeed the only medical school in the vast area of the Northwest between Milwaukee to the east and Seattle to the west. The school occupied six buildings all relatively new, including two large laboratory buildings that were probably as fine and well-equipped as any in the United States. Nevertheless, the school was developing plans to move beyond the confined area of the university campus to a new medical campus in a residential area south of Washington Avenue on high ground overlooking the Mississippi River. There Dean Wesbrook and his colleagues hoped to build a new group of still larger medical science buildings in proximity to the new university hospital to be provided by the Elliot bequest. The following year the university hospital opened in several large houses on the new medical campus and the chiefs of medicine and surgery began to be paid salaries that enabled them to devote a substantial portion of their time and effort to clinical teaching. It was thus that Abraham Flexner saw the school when he visited it in May 1909 and described the medical laboratories as "excellent, exceedingly attractive, and well organized . . . ."

RETROSPECT

By 1912 the first stage of the move to the new medical campus was accomplished. The 120-bed Elliot Hospital was in operation, and the Institute of Anatomy and the new Millard Hall had both just been completed, although each had one blank wall where wings were yet to be added. The medical school had plans for additional pavilions to be added to the Elliot Hospital to enlarge its capacity ultimately to 1,000 beds. It wished to build a residence for nurses and a pathology building adjacent to the hospital. If the plans of 1912 had been carried out, the university hospital might have become by 1915 a large and complete general hospital, staffed with full-time clinical chiefs and assistants. Dean Wesbrook intended that the university hospital should serve as a consultant to the medical profession of the whole state. The university hospital would, therefore, have received charity patients and referral patients from throughout Minnesota and from adjacent states. It would have become a center of clinical research and of medical innovation.

Such plans were well within the realm of possibility in 1912; if fulfilled they would have maintained Minnesota in the leading position among American medical schools that it then occupied. Yet they were not to be. The plans of the medical faculty were cancelled by President Vincent, who instead of supporting the medical faculty, subjected it to a brutal reorganization.

The reorganization of 1913, followed by the Mayo affiliation controversies of 1915 and 1917, the disruption of the First World War, and the agricultural depression of the 1920s meant years of stagnation for the medical school. The energies of the faculty were consumed mainly by teaching; little research was done. Elsewhere throughout the United States, medical schools built large hospitals for clinical teaching and new laboratories. Minnesota slipped from its rank among the four or five leading American medical schools to a position much lower in the scale.

Renewal began in the late twenties. By 1930 the university hospital had expanded to a capacity of 600 beds—still small, but sufficient for most aspects of clinical teaching—and there were full-time chiefs of medicine, surgery, pediatrics, and radiology. The school drew strength from the vigor and intelligence of its own graduates. Despite limited budgets and inadequate facilities, success followed success through the thirties, forties, and fifties. By 1955, with the triumphant achievements of open heart surgery, Minnesota might be considered to have regained the national position which it lost after 1912.

A great source of strength to the Minnesota medical school has been its openness to students of both sexes and all races. From the beginning Minnesota admitted women to the study of medicine, and it did not exclude any ethnic group. The loyalty and generosity of all its graduates have helped to sustain the school through good times and bad.

The resilience of the medical school through successive crises—its ability to educate competent physicians despite inadequate facilities and meager budgets—has been remarkable, as has been its ability to produce research of high quality. That resilience has its historical roots in the unusual character of the physicians who settled in Minnesota when it was still a territory and in the early days of its statehood. All Minnesota physicians were then country doctors, but they were educated men who possessed a clear vision of the future of medicine. Quick to grasp the significance of antiseptic surgery in the 1880s, they rapidly exploited the even greater advantages of aseptic surgery. The most famous Minnesota surgeons were the Mayo brothers, but as very young doctors the Mayo brothers came to St. Paul and Minneapolis to learn surgery from their father's friends, Justus Ohage, Alexander Stone, and Charles Wheaton in St. Paul and James Dunn and James E. Moore in Minneapolis. Later they went to Chicago, New York, Baltimore, and Boston, but their earliest practical knowledge of the new surgery was gained in Minnesota.

Although Minnesota physicians were educated and resourceful, and although through the medical school they communicated such characteristics to their students, the power of character and training to overcome obstacles must not be exaggerated. One cannot study the history of the medical school without forming the strong impression that with more consistent and generous support, the school might have accomplished much more. Historically, even through its best periods, the school has been underfinanced. The young men who did the pioneering work in open heart surgery in the 1950s were paid so little as surgical residents that they and their families lived in near poverty. As their careers developed they were forced to depend heavily upon their income from private practice. In recent years successive retrenchments have left the clinical departments of the medical school more dependent upon income from private practice than they have been since the early days of the school. Indeed, the financial basis of the clinical departments is coming dangerously to resemble that of an old-fashioned proprietary medical school. The flow of research grants, largely from federal agencies, sustains the research activities of the school almost entirely. The concept of the full-time clinical teacher has as a result become seriously diluted with real consequences for clinical teaching and clinical investigation. The scientific departments of the medical school suffer similarly from inadequate budgets, without being able to supplement them with income from medical practice.

The reliance of clinical departments upon income from practice brings them increasingly into competition with physicians and with hospitals outside the university. The effects of such competition are not yet wholly clear, especially since the whole system of payment for health care is under obvious strain and may be about to undergo profound change. A consequence of the 1913 reorganization, and perhaps one of its occult purposes, was the separation of the medical faculty from the medical profession of the Twin Cities. That separation has persisted, and shows little sign of diminishing. The isolation of the medical school from the local medical profession may be no greater than that of other medical schools — possibly even less — but neither is it of benefit to the school, to the medical profession of Minnesota, nor to the community at large. However that may be, Minnesota medical students must continue to be trained to be competent and compassionate physicians, guided by a high sense of the dignity of the profession they are to enter.

APPENDIX I
First Faculty of the Department of Medicine, University of Minnesota

College of Medicine and Surgery Professors

Duluth	Arthur F. Ritchie, M.D.	Anatomy
Minneapolis	Richard O. Beard, M.D.	Physiology
St. Paul	H.M. Bracken, M.D., L.R.C.S.E.	Materia Medica and Therapeutics
St. Paul	Albert E. Senkler, M.D.	Theory and Practice of Medicine
Minneapolis	Charles H. Hunter, A.M., M.D.	Clinical Medicine
St. Paul	Everton J. Abbott, A.B., M.D.	Clinical Medicine
St. Paul	Charles A. Wheaton, M.D.	Principals and Practice of Surgery
Minneapolis	Frederick A. Dunsmoor, M.D.	Clinical Surgery
St. Paul	Perry H. Millard, M.D.	Clinical Surgery
St. Paul	Alexander J. Stone, M.D.	Diseases of Women
St. Paul	Parks Ritchie, MD.D	Obstetrics
St. Paul	John F. Fulton, Ph.D., M.D.	Ophthalmology and Otology
St. Paul	C. Eugene Riggs, M.D.	Nervous and Mental Disorders
St. Paul	Charles H. Boardman, M.D.	Medical Jurisprudence
St. Paul	Arthur B. Ancker, M.D.	Hygiene
Minneapolis	James H. Dunn, M.D.	Diseases of the Genito-Urinary Organs
Minneapolis	Charles L. Wells, A.M., M.D.	Diseases of Children
Minneapolis	James E. Moore, M.D.	·Orthopaedic Surgery
Minneapolis	Max P. Vanderhorck, M.D.	Diseases of the Skin

APPENDIX I

Minneapolis	W. S. Laton, M.D.	Diseases of the Throat and Nose
St. Paul	J. Clark Stewart, B.S., M.D.	Histology and Bacteriology
Minneapolis	J. W. Bell, M.D.	Physical Diagnosis and Diseases of the Chest
St. Paul	E. A. Spencer, M.D.	Surgical Anatomy

Clinical Professors

Minneapolis	Amos W. Abbott, M.D.	Diseases of Women
Minneapolis	Frank Allport, M.D.	Ophthalmology and Otology

Adjunct Professors

Minneapolis	A. B. Cates, A.M., M.D.	Obstetrics
St. Paul	A. McLaren, A.B., M.D.	Gynecology
Minneapolis	W. A. Jones, M.D.	Diseases of the Nervous System

Demonstrator

Minneapolis	Burnside Foster, M.D.	Anatomy

College of Homeopathic Medicine and Surgery

Minneapolis	William E. Leonard, A.B., M.D.	Materia Medica and Therapeutics
St. Paul	Henry Hutchinson, M.D.	Theory and Practic of Medicine
Minneapolis	George E. Ricker, A.B., M.D.	Clinical Medicine
Minneapolis	Robert D. Matchan, M.D.	Principles and Practice of Surgery
St. Paul	Warren S. Briggs, B.S., M.D.	Clinical Surgery
Fergus Falls	Henry C. Leonard, B.S., M.D.	Obstetrics
Minneapolis	Albert E. Higbee, M.D.	Gynaecology
Minneapolis	John E. Beaumont, M.D.	Ophthalmology
Minneapolis	Henry W. Brazie, M.D.	Paedology
Minneapolis	Salathiel M. Spaulding, M.D.	Mental and Nervous Diseases

APPENDIX I

St. Paul	Eugene L. Mann, A.B., M.D.	Physical Diagnosis and Laryngology
St. Paul	B. Harvie Ogden, A.M., M.D.	Genito-Urinary Diseases
Minneapolis	Henry C. Aldrich, M.D., D.D.S.	Dermatology
Duluth	D. A. Strickler, M.D.	Otology

Manuscript Sources

The largest and most essential collection of papers relating to the University of Minnesota and its various schools is the University of Minnesota Archives. The university archives contain the minutes of the Board of Regents, minutes of the faculties and their executive or administrative committees, papers of the president's office from 1911 to 1960, and the personal papers of a number of past presidents, deans, and professors. The university archives are hereafter designated Mn U Archives, and their address is:

> University of Minnesota Archives
> 10 Walter Library
> 117 Pleasant Street, S.E.
> Minneapolis, Minnesota 55455

The personnel records of deceased members of the faculty provide accurate detailed biographical information, especially concerning dates and places of birth and education, dates of appointment, salaries, and honors received. In many cases such files contain historically valuable correspondence, including letters of recommendation at the time of appointment. Personnel records are located in the:

> Academic Personnel Systems Office
> University of Minnesota
> 2 Morrill Hall
> 100 Church Street, S.E.
> Minneapolis, Minnesota 55455

For any aspect of the history of Minnesota, an indispensable source is the Minnesota Historical Society Archives which contain state records, including the papers of the State Board of Health and other institutions, together with the personal papers of many Minnesotans. They are hereafter designated MHS Archives, and their address is:

> Minnesota Historical Society Archives
> 1500 Mississippi Street
> St. Paul, Minnesota 55112

MANUSCRIPT SOURCES

The addresses of other archives are given with the papers for which they were consulted.

Administrative Services, Central Files	Administrative Services Center University of Minnesota 1919 University Avenue St. Paul, Minnesota 55104
Abbott, Amos Wilson, Papers	MHS Archives
Board of Regents, Minutes	Mn U Archives
Bracken, Henry M., Papers	MHS Archives
Cannon, Walter Bradford, Archives	Francis A. Countway Library Harvard Medical School Boston, Massachusets 02115
College of Medicine and Surgery, Executive Committee, Minutes	Mn U Archives
College of Medicine and Surgery, Executive Faculty, Minutes	Mn U Archives
College of Medicine and Surgery, Faculty, Minutes	Mn U Archives
College of Medicine and Surgery, General Faculty, Minutes	Mn U Archives
College of Medicine and Surgery, Record Book	Mn U Archives
Committee for the Study of Physical Facilities for the Health Sciences, "Future Planning for the Health Sciences"	Mn U Archives
Committee for the Study of Physical Facilities for the Health Sciences, Minutes	Mn U Archives
Cowling, Donald J., Papers	Mn U Archives
Department of Medicine, Record Book	Mn U Archives
Folwell Papers	MHS Archives
General Education Board, Papers	Rockefeller Archive Center Pocantico Hills North Tarrytown, New York 10591-1598
Gray, James, Papers	MHS Archives, Mn U Archives
Mann, Eugene Langdon, Family Papers	MHS Archives
Medical School, Papers	Mn U Archives
Medical School [papers], Affiliation with the Mayo Foundation	Mn U Archives
Medical School [papers], Miscellaneous Correspondence 1883–1948	Mn U Archives
Moore, James E., Papers	Mn U Archives
President's Office, Papers	Mn U Archives
School of Medicine, Administrative Board, Minutes	Mn U Archives
School of Medicine, Administrative Committee, Minutes	Mn U Archives

MANUSCRIPT SOURCES

School of Medicine, Executive Faculty, Minutes — Mn U Archives
School of Medicine, General Faculty, Minutes — Mn U Archives
Vaughan, Victor, Papers — Michigan Historical Collections
Bentley Historical Library
University of Michigan
Ann Arbor, Michigan 48109

Wangensteen, Owen H., Papers — Mn U Archives
Wesbrook, Frank Fairchild, Papers — University of British Columbia Archives
Library, Special Collections
1956 Main Mall
Vancouver, Canada V6T 1Y3

Abbreviations of Journals Cited

Abbreviation	Journal
Acta med. Scand.	Acta Medica Scandinavica
Am. Heart J.	American Heart Journal
Am. J. clin. Nutr.	American Journal of Clinical Nutrition
Am. J. Dis. Child.	American Journal of Diseases of Children
Am. J. Med.	American Journal of Medicine
Am. J. med. Sci.	American Journal of the Medical Sciences
Am. J. Nurs.	American Journal of Nursing
Am. J. Obstet. Gynec.	American Journal of Obstetrics and Gynecology
Am. J. Path.	American Journal of Pathology
Am. J. Physiol.	American Journal of Physiology
Am. J. pub. Hlth	American Journal of Public Health
Am. J. Roentg.	American Journal of Roentgenology
Am. J. Surg.	American Journal of Surgery
Am. Rev. Tuberc. pulm. Dis.	American Review of Tuberculosis and Pulmonary Diseases
Anat. Anz.	Anatomische Anzeiger
Anat. Rec.	Anatomical Record
Ann. intern. Med.	Annals of Internal Medicine
Ann. med. Hist.	Annals of Medical History
Ann. N.Y. Acad. Sci.	Annals of the New York Academy of Sciences
Ann. Otol. Rhin. Lar.	Annals of Otology, Rhinology, and Laryngology
Ann. roy. Coll. Surg. Engl.	Annals of the Royal College of Surgeons of England
Ann. Surg.	Annals of Surgery
Ann. thorac. Surg.	Annals of Thoracic Surgery
Annls Inst. Pasteur, Paris	Annales de l'Institut Pasteur, Paris

ABBREVIATIONS

Abbreviation	Journal
Archs Derm.	Archives of Dermatology
Archs intern. Med.	Archives of Internal Medicine
Archs Path.	Archives of Pathology
Archs Surg., Chicago	Archives of Surgery, Chicago
Ariel	Ariel
Boston med. surg. J.	Boston Medical and Surgical Journal
Brain	Brain
Br. J. Surg.	British Journal of Surgery
Br. med. J.	British Medical Journal
Bull. Am. Acad. Med.	Bulletin of the American Academy of Medicine
Bull. Hist. Med.	Bulletin of the History of Medicine
Bull. Minn. med. Fndn	Bulletin of the Minnesota Medical Foundation
Bull. Mém. Soc. méd. Hôp., Paris	Bulletin et Memoires de la Société Medicale des Hôpitaux de Paris
Bull. Univ. Minn. Hosp. & Minn. med. Fdn	Bulletin of the University of Minnesota Hospitals and Minnesota Medical Foundation
Circ. Res.	Circulation Research
Circulation	Circulation
Dis. Chest	Diseases of the Chest
Endocrinology	Endocrinology
Endokrinologie	Endokrinologie
Fed. Proc.	Federation Proceedings
Folia haemat.	Folia haematologica
Guy's Hosp. Rep.	Guy's Hospital Reports
Hoppe-Seyler's Z. physiol. Chem.	Hoppe-Seyler's Zeitschrift fur Physiologischen Chemie
Hosp. Pract.	Hospital Practice
Illinois med. J.	Illinois Medical Journal
Ind. Engng Chem. analyt. Edn	Industrial and Engineering Chemistry, Analytical Edition
Issues Sci. Technol.	Issues in Science and Technology
Johns Hopk. med. J.	Johns Hopkins Medical Journal
Johns Hopkins Hosp. Bull.	Johns Hopkins Hospital Bulletin
J. Am. diet. Ass.	Journal of the American Dietetic Association
J. Am. Hosp.	Journal of the American Hospital
J. Am. med. Ass.	Journal of the American Medical Association
J. Ass. Am. med. Coll.	Journal of the Association of American Medical Colleges [continued as The Journal of Medical Education]
J. Bacteriol.	Journal of Bacteriology

ABBREVIATIONS

Abbreviation	Journal
J. biol. Chem.	Journal of Biological Chemistry
J. Cancer Res.	Journal of Cancer Research
J. chron. Dis.	Journal of Chronic Diseases
J. clin. Invest.	Journal of Clinical Investigation
J. comp. Neurol.	Journal of Comparative Neurology
J. comp. Path. Ther.	Journal of Comparative Pathology and Therapeutics
J. dent. Res.	Journal of Dental Research
J. exp. Med.	Journal of Experimental Medicine
J. Hist. Med.	Journal of the History of Medicine and Allied Sciences
J. Immunol.	Journal of Immunology
J. infect. Dis.	Journal of Infectious Diseases
J. lab. clin. Med.	Journal of Laboratory and Clinical Medicine
J. Minn. St. med. Ass. & Northwest. Lancet	Journal of the Minnesota State Medical Association and Northwestern Lancet
J. med. Educ.	Journal of Medical Education
J. med. Res.	Journal of Medical Research
J. med. Sci., Portland, Maine	Journal of Medical Science, Portland, Maine
J. Neurosurg.	Journal of Neurosurgery
J. Nutr.	Journal of Nutrition
J. natn Cancer Inst.	Journal of the National Cancer Institute
J. natn dent. Ass.	Journal of the National Dental Association
J. Path. Bact.	Journal of Pathology and Bacteriology
J. Pediat.	Journal of Pediatrics
J. Physiol., Lond.	Journal of Physiology, London
J. thorac. Surg.	Journal of Thoracic Surgery
J.-Lancet	Journal-Lancet
Lancet, Lond.	Lancet, London
Med. Rec.	Medical Record
Mem. Univ. Calif.	Memoirs of the University of California
Metabolism	Metabolism
Mpls homeo. Mag.	Minneapolis Homeopathic Magazine
Minn. Alumni Wkly	Minnesota Alumni Weekly
Minn. Hist.	Minnesota History
Minn. med. Fdn med. Bull.	Minnesota Medical Foundation Medical Bulletin
Minn. Med.	Minnesota Medicine
Minn. med. Mthly	Minnesota Medical Monthly
Minn. Chats	Minnesota Chats
Nature	Nature
Natn. Fdn News	National Foundation News

ABBREVIATIONS

Abbreviation	Journal
New Engl. J. Med.	New England Journal of Medicine
New int. Clins	New International Clinics
N.Y. med. J.	New York Medical Journal
N.Y. St. J. Med.	New York State Journal of Medicine
Northwest. Lancet	Northwestern Lancet
Notes Rec. R. Soc. Lond.	Notes and Records. Royal Society of London
Pediat. Clin. N. Am.	Pediatric Clinics of North America
Pediatrics	Pediatrics
Phila. med. J.	Philadelphia Medical Journal
Phila. Med.	Philadelphia Medicine
Presse méd.	Presse Médicale
Proc. Ass. Res. nerv. ment. Dis.	Proceedings of the Association for Research on Nervous and Mental Diseases
Proc. Soc. exp. Biol. Med.	Proceedings of the Society for Experimental Biology and Medicine
Proc. staff Meet. Mayo Clinic	Proceedings of the Staff Meetings of the Mayo Clinic
Pub. Hlth Pap. Rep., N.Y.	Public Health Papers and Reports. American Public Health Association. New York
Pub. Hlth Rep.	Public Health Reports. United States Public Health Service
Radiology	Radiology
Rev. sci. Instr.	Review of Scientific Instruments
St. Paul med. J.	St. Paul Medical Journal
Science	Science
Surg. Forum	Surgical Forum
Surg. Gynec. Obstet.	Surgery, Gynaecology and Obstetrics
Surgery	Surgery
Thorax	Thorax
Trans. Am. surg. Ass.	Transactions of the American Surgical Association
Trans. Ass. Am. Physns	Transactions of the Association of American Physicians
Trans. Minn. St. homeo. Inst.	Transactions of the Minnesota State Homeopathic Institute
Trans. Minn. St. med. Soc.	Transactions of the Minnesota State Medical Society
Trans. natn Tuberc. Ass., N.Y.	Transactions of the National Tuberculosis Association, New York
Trans. r. Soc. trop. Med. Hyg.	Transactions of the Royal Society for Tropical Medicine and Hygiene
Transpl. Bull.	Transplantation Bulletin
Transpl. Proc.	Transplantation Proceedings

ABBREVIATIONS

Abbreviation	Journal
Transplantation	Transplantation
Univ. Minn. Hosp. staff Meet.	University of Minnesota Hospitals Staff Meeting
Univ. Minn. med. Bull.	University of Minnesota Medical Bulletin
Urol. Surv.	Urological Survey
U.S. Bureau of Animal Industry Ann. Rep.	United States Bureau of Animal Industry, Annual Reports
West. J. Surg. Obstet. Gynec.	Western Journal of Surgery, Obstetrics and Gynaecology
Wisc. med. J.	Wisconsin Medical Journal
Yale J. Biol. Med.	Yale Journal of Biology and Medicine
Z. Tiermed.	Zeitschrift für Tiermedizin
Zentbl. Bakt. Microbiol. Hyg.	Zentralblatt für Bakteriologie, Mikrobiologie, und Hygiene

Bibliography

Atwater, Isaac, ed. *History of Minneapolis, Minnesota.* 2 vols. New York: Munsell & Company, 1893.

Bell, E.T. *Diabetes Mellitus, a Clinical and Pathological Study of 2,529 Cases.* Springfield, Ill.: Charles C. Thomas, 1960.

——. *Renal Diseases.* 2nd ed. Philadelphia: Lea & Febiger, 1950.

——, ed. *A Textbook of Pathology.* Philadelphia: Lea & Febiger, 1934.

Benison, Saul; Barger, A. Clifford; and Wolfe, Elin L. *Walter B. Cannon: The Life and Times of a Young Scientist.* Cambridge, Mass. and London, Harvard University Press, Belknap Press, 1987.

Bergh, George S., and Erickson, Reuben F., eds. *A History of the Twenty-Sixth General Hospital.* Minneapolis: Bureau of Engraving, Inc., n.d.

Berglund, Hilding; Medes, Grace; Huber, G. Carl; Longcope, Warfield T.; and Richards, Alfred N., eds. *The Kidney in Health and Disease* . . . . Philadelphia: Lea & Febiger, 1935.

Bigelow, W. G. *Cold Hearts: The Story of Hypothermia and the Pacemaker in Heart Surgery.* Toronto: McClelland and Stewart, 1984.

Blegen, Theodore C. *Grass Roots History.* Minneapolis: University of Minnesota Press, 1947.

Boyden, Edward A. *Segmental Anatomy of the Lung.* New York: McGraw-Hill, 1955.

Chesney, Alan M. *The Johns Hopkins Hospital and The Johns Hopkins University School of Medicine: A Chronicle.* 3 vols. Baltimore: Johns Hopkins University Press, 1943–63.

Clapesattle, Helen. *The Doctors Mayo.* Minneapolis: University of Minnesota Press, 1941.

Cohn, Victor. *Sister Kenny: The Woman who Challenged the Doctors.* Minneapolis: University of Minnesota Press, 1975.

Corner, George W. *George Hoyt Whipple and His Friends.* Philadelphia: J.B. Lippincott Company, 1963.

——. *The Seven Ages of a Medical Scientist.* Philadelphia: University of Pennsylvania, 1981.

Cushing, Harvey. *The Life of Sir William Osler.* 2 vols. Oxford: Clarendon Press, 1925.

BIBLIOGRAPHY

Davis, Loyal. *Fellowship of Surgeons: A History of the American College of Surgeons.* Springfield, Ill.: Charles C. Thomas, 1960.

Davis, Nathan Smith. *History of the American Medical Association from its Organization Up to January 1855.* Philadelphia: Lippincott, Grambo & Company, 1855.

Downey, Hal, ed. *Handbook of Haematology.* 4 vols. New York: Paul B. Hoeber, 1938.

Ewart, William. *The Bronchi and Pulmonary Blood Vessels — Their Anatomy and Nomenclature.* London: Baillière, Tindall, and Cox, 1889.

Finland, Maxwell. *The Harvard Medical Unit at Boston City Hospital.* 2 vols. Boston: Harvard Medical School, 1982.

Flexner, Abraham. *Medical Education in the United States and Canada: A Report to the Carnegie Foundation for the Advancement of Teaching.* New York: Carnegie Foundation for the Advancement of Teaching, 1910.

Fourgereau, M. and Dausset, J., eds. *Immunology 80. Progressive Immunology IV.* London and New York: Academic Press, 1980.

Gibson, William. *Wesbrook and His University.* Vancouver, B.C.: Library of the University of British Columbia, 1973.

Gray, James. *The University of Minnesota 1851–1951.* Minneapolis: University of Minnesota Press, 1951.

Hahnemann, Samuel. *Organon of Homeopathic Medicine.* 2nd American ed. New York: W. Radde, 1843.

Hamburger, Jean, et al. *Renal Transplantation Theory and Practice.* Baltimore: Williams and Wilkins Company, 1972.

Hardy, James D., ed. *Critical surgical illness.* Philadelphia: W. B. Saunders Company, 1979.

Harris, J.A.; Jackson, C.M.; Patterson, D.J.; and Scammon, Richard E. *The Measurement of Man.* Minneapolis: University of Minnesota Press, 1930.

Health Manpower Study Commission. *Health Manpower for the Upper Midwest: A Study of the Needs for Physicians and Dentists in Minnesota, North Dakota, South Dakota, and Montana.* St. Paul: Hill Family Foundation, 1966.

Henrici, Arthur T. *Morphologic Variation and the Rate of Growth of Bacteria.* Springfield, Ill.: Charles C. Thomas, 1928.

Hirschfelder, Arthur Douglas. *Diseases of the Heart and Aorta.* Philadelphia: J. B. Lippincott Company, 1910.

Holmes, Oliver Wendell. *Homeopathy and Its Kindred Delusions.* Boston: W. D. Ticknor, 1842.

Jarchow, Merril E. *Donald J. Cowling.* Northfield, Minn.: Carleton College, 1974.

Johnson, E. Bird, ed. *Forty Years of the University of Minnesota.* Minneapolis: General Alumni Association, 1910.

Johnson, Stephen L. *The History of Cardiac Surgery 1896–1955.* Baltimore: Johns Hopkins Press, 1970.

Jordan, Philip. *The People's Health: A History of Public Health in Minnesota to 1948.* St. Paul: Minnesota Historical Society, 1953.

Kaufman, Martin. *Homeopathy in America, the Rise and Fall of a Medical Heresy.* Baltimore: Johns Hopkins Press, 1971.

BIBLIOGRAPHY

Kelly, Howard A., and Burrage, Walter L., eds. *American Medical Biographies.* New York and London: D. Appleton and Company, 1920.

Kerkhof, Arthur C., ed. *Festschrift, George E. Fahr, M.D.* Minneapolis, 1962.

Keys, Ancel. *The Biology of Human Starvation.* 2 vols. Minneapolis: University of Minnesota Press, 1950.

———. *Seven Countries: A Multivariate Analysis of Death and Coronary Heart Disease.* Cambridge, Mass.: Harvard University Press, 1980.

Lesky, Erna. *The Vienna Medical School of the 19th Century.* Translated by L. Williams and I.S. Levij. Baltimore: Johns Hopkins University Press, 1976.

Litzenberg, Jennings C. *Contributions to the Pathology of Pregnancy.* Lawrence, Kans.: University of Kansas, 1944.

Long, Joseph A. and Evans, Herbert McLean. *The Oestrous Cycle in the Rat and Its Associated Phenomena.* Berkeley: University of California, 1922.

Mayo Clinic, Rochester, Minn. *Sketch of the History of the Mayo Clinic and the Mayo Foundation.* Philadelphia and London: W. B. Saunders Company, 1926.

McClendon, Jesse F. *A Manual of Biochemistry.* New York, 1934.

———. *Advances in the Science of Nutrition.* Sendi, Japan, 1937.

———. *Iodine and the Incidence of Goiter.* Minneapolis: University of Minnesota Press, 1939.

———. *Physical Chemistry of Vital Phenomena.* Princeton: Princeton University Press, 1917.

McClendon, Jesse F., and Medes, Grace. *Physical Chemistry in Biology and Medicine.* Philadelphia and London: W. B. Saunders Company, 1925.

McQuarrie, Irvine. *The Experiments of Nature and Other Essays.* Lawrence, Kans.: University of Kansas, 1944.

Meyer, Robert. *Autobiography.* New York: Henry Schuman, 1949.

Minnesota, University. *The President's Report for 1917–18.* Minneapolis: 1918.
———. *The President's report for . . . 1918–19.* Minneapolis: 1919.
———. *The President's report for . . . 1920–21.* Minneapolis: 1921.
———. *The President's report for . . . 1922–23.* Minneapolis: 1923.
———. *The President's report for . . . 1926–27.* Minneapolis: 1927.
———. *The President's report for . . . 1928–30.* Minneapolis: 1930.

Minnesota, University. Department of Anatomy. *Contributions.* 16 vols. Minneapolis, University of Minnesota Press, 1913–40.

Moore, James E. *Orthopedic Surgery.* Philadelphia: W. B. Saunders, 1898.

Myers, Jay Arthur. *Lymanhurst, a Report of Ten Years of Activity.* Minneapolis: 1932.

———. *Masters of Medicine: An Historical Sketch of the College of Medical Science, University of Minnesota.* St. Louis: Warren H. Green, Inc., 1968.

———. *Tuberculosis among Children.* Springfield, Ill.: C. C. Thomas, 1930.

———. *Tuberculosis, a Half Century of Study and Conquest.* St. Louis: Warren H. Green, Inc., 1970.

Najarian, John S., and Simmons, Richard L., eds. *Transplantation.* Philadelphia: Lea & Febiger, 1972.

Pohl, John F. and Kenny, Elizabeth. *The Kenny Concept of Infantile Paralysis and Its Treatment.* Minneapolis: Bruce Publishing Company, 1943.

Quervain, Fritz de. *Clinical Surgical Diagnosis for Students and Practitioners.* Translated by J. Snowman. New York: W. Wood & Company, 1913.

Rasmussen, Andrew T. *Atlas of Cross Section Anatomy of the Brain. Guide to the Study of the Morphology and Fiber Tracts of the Human Brain.* Villiger-Ludwig's atlas revised and extended. Philadelphia: Blakiston Company, 1951.

Reimann, Hobart A. *The Pneumonias.* Philadelphia: W. B. Saunders Company, 1938.

Rigler, Leo G. *Outline of Roentgen Diagnosis: An Orientation in the Basic Principles of Diagnosis by the Roentgen Method.* Philadelphia: J. B. Lippincott Company, 1938.

Rosner, David. *A Once Charitable Enterprise: Hospitals and Health Care in Brooklyn and New York, 1885-1915.* Cambridge: Cambridge University Press, 1982.

Rowntree, Leonard G. *Amid Masters of Twentieth Century Medicine.* Springfield, Ill.: Charles C Thomas, 1958.

Scammon, Richard E., and Calkins, L. A.. *The Development and Growth of External Dimensions of the Human Body in the Fetal Period.* Minneapolis: University of Minnesota Press, 1929.

Shryock, Richard H. *Medical Licensing in America, 1650-1965.* Baltimore: Johns Hopkins University Press, 1967.

Slavin, Shimon, ed. *Bone Marrow & Organ Transplantation, Achievements & Goals.* Amsterdam, New York, Oxford: Elsevier, 1984.

Spink, Wesley W. *Infectious Diseases: Prevention and Treatment in the Nineteenth and Twentieth Centuries.* Minneapolis: University of Minnesota Press, 1978.

———. *The Nature of Brucellosis.* Minneapolis: University of Minnesota Press, 1956.

Stanchfield, Margaret Ayling. *A History of the Variety Club Heart Hospital of the University of Minnesota Hospitals.* Minneapolis: 1975.

Stevens, Rosemary. *American Medicine and the Public Interest.* New Haven: Yale University Press, 1971.

Tang, Jane M. "Hal Downey and the Development of Hematology in America." Ph.D. diss., University of Minnesota, 1988.

U.S. Army, Base Hospital no. 26, Allerey. *History of Base Hospital 26.* Minneapolis: 1920.

U.S. Department of Health and Human Services, Graduate Medical Education National Advisory Committee. *Summary Report.* Washington, D.C.: Government Printing Office, 1980.

U.S. Surgeon General's Group on Medical Education. *Physicians for a Growing America.* Washington, D.C.: 1959.

U.S. Surgeon General's Office. *The Medical Department of the United States Army in the World War.* 15 vols. in 17. Washington, D.C.: Government Printing Office, 1923.

———. *The Medical and Surgical History of the War of the Rebellion (1861-65).* 6 vols. Washington, D.C.: Government Printing Office, 1875.

Vincent, George Edgar. *The Social Mind and Education.* Chicago: University of Chicago Press, 1897.

Walsh, James J. *History of Medicine in New York.* 5 vols. New York: National Americana Society, 1919.

BIBLIOGRAPHY

Wangensteen, Owen H. *Owen H. Wangensteen.* Bethesda, Md.: National Library of Medicine, 1973. [Transcript of a series of tape recorded interviews between Dr. Wangensteen and Dr. Peter Olch, interviewer, as part of the National Library of Medicine Oral History Program.]

―――. *The Therapeutic Problem in Bowel Obstructions.* Springfield, Ill.: Charles C. Thomas, 1937.

―――, ed. *Elias Potter Lyon: Minnesota's Leader in Medical Education.* St. Louis: Warren H. Green, Inc., 1981.

White, Paul D. *Heart Disease.* 4th ed. New York: Macmillan, 1951.

Wintrobe, Maxwell M., ed. *Blood, Pure and Eloquent.* New York: McGraw-Hill Book Company, 1980.

Index

Abbott, Amos W., 17, 38, 92, 206(n.4), 568
Abbott, Everton J., 567
Abscess, alveolar: research by Henrici and Hartzell, 381–384
Actinomycetes: research by Henrici, 385
Adair, Fred, 284, 287
Adair, J. H., 73
Administrative Board: report of salary committee (1913), 152; search for new dean (1913), 152–154; approved Beard's control over supply budget (1913), 155; appointed Hirschfelder professor of pharmacology (1913), 155; protested loss of funds from salary and supply budgets (1913), 156; appealed for needed facilities (1914), 161–163; committee on Mayo affiliation, 167–170, 171, 173; accepted faculty resignations (1915), 190; question of private patients and per diem patients, 192–193; requested legislative funds for buildings (1916), 196–197; prepared students for military service (1917), 215; requested external review of medical alumni report (1920), 241; appointed Pirquet chief of pediatrics, 259; "practically full-time" clinical appointments, 283–284; full-time clinical appointments, 285–286; pharmacology made a department (1913), 392. *See also:* Administrative Committee; Committee on hospital and clinical development; Subcommittee on hospital extension
Administrative Committee: problem of finding a chief of surgery, 289–291, 295; appointed McQuarrie chief of pediatrics (1930), 301; approved War Department plan for mobilization (1940), 416–417; approved Masonic Hospital, 446; response to Diehl's resignation, 453. *See also:* Administrative Board (pre 1926)
Admissions standards: medical colleges (1872), 13; 1898 change, 102; 1906 change, 102–104
Agammaglobulinemia, 470–472
Aldrich, Henry C., 568
Allerey (France) Hospital Center, Mud (photo), 232; 227, 228, 231. *See also:* Base Hospital No. 26
Allison, Robert G., 298
Allport, Frank, 38, 568
Alwall, Nils, 541
Amberg, Raymond M. (port.), 438; appointed director of hospital, 325; role in securing state funds for Mayo memorial (1949), 438
Amberg, Samuel, 258
American Association of Medical Colleges, 36, 77
American Board of Internal Medicine, 448
American Cancer Society, 435, 452, 459(n.43)
American College of Surgeons, 159–160

INDEX

American Heart Association, 476
American Medical Association, 7, 36
American Public Health Association, Buffalo, N.Y., meeting (1896), Widal test demonstrated, 71; Minneapolis meeting (1899), 84–85
American Red Cross: preparation for W.W.I, 214
American Red Cross Commission to Poland, 231–232
American Surgical Association, 491, 508
Ames, Alfred Elisha, 7
Anatomical dissection (photo), 86; legalized (1872), 13
Anatomy Building (photo), 85; 83, 85–86; fire (1902), 87; fire (1908), 115; Lee on the use of, 140(n.35)
Anatomy, Department of: Lee removed as head, 143; Jackson appointed head, 151; Scammon on faculty, 305; under Jackson, 372; research (1913–41), 372–376; Lee retired (1929), 373
Anatomy, Institute of. *See:* Institute of Anatomy
Anatomy instruction (1888), 38–40, 41
Ancker, Arthur B., 567
Ancker Hospital (St. Paul), 341, 350
Anderson, Gaylord, 431
Anderson, John A., 547
Anderson, Joseph T.: research on cholesterol in diet, 410–412; controlled diet experiments, 412
Anderson, N.F., 531
Andreasen, Anthony, 493–495, 501
Anesthesia: semi-centennial observation, 76
Antiseptic surgery: antiseptic method used (1885), 4, 95, 100; carbolic acid spray first used (1882), 19; advocated by Dunn, 95;
Appendectomy: first surgical removal (1887), 4
Apprenticeship as medical training, 13
Archer, Olga, 472
Armstrong, Wallace D. (photo), 406; 486; appointed head of physiological chemistry (1946), 404; graduate study under McClendon, 404; research on radioactive isotopes in metabolic studies, 404; fluoride in prevention of tooth decay, 404–405; role in fluoridation of water supplies, 405–406
Artificial kidney, 530, 541
Asbury Hospital (Minneapolis), 46, 96
Aschoff, Ludwig, 297
Aseptic surgery: used by Moore (1890), 100
Asher, Leon, 293, 297
Atrial septal defect, 490, 499, 500, 517
Avery, Oswald, 326
Azygos flow: research on, 493–496, 503; amount of blood needed for heart-lung bypass, 508

Bacillus proteus, research by Bell and Larson, 389
Bacteria: researches on morphology by Henrici, 385–386; fresh water bacteria by Henrici, 387–388; types associated with pyorrhea and abscess, 381–384
Bacterial endocarditis, 391, 492
Bacteriology: instruction in (1894), 61; (1896), 68; curriculum (1898), 100–101; research in, 1913–41, 381–388
Bacteriology culture room (photo), 68
Bacteriology, Department of: space in Mayo Memorial Building, 442; Green appointed head (1947), 468. *See also:* Microbiology, Department of
Bacteriology Laboratory [in Laboratory of Medical Sciences building] (photo), 84
Baker, A. B., 456
Baker, Howard, 273
Bakken, Earl, 520
Baldwin, Louis B. (port.), 121; 233, 262; first superintendent of hospital (1910), 119; dedication of Elliot Memorial Hospital, 120; secured Madsen Flats (1910), 121–122; dispensary (1912), 136; purchasing agent for Base Hospital No. 26, 215–216, 217
Balfour, Donald C., 173; supported a Mayo memorial at university, 427, 429
Bang's disease, 331–332

INDEX

Barker, Lewellys F., 393
Barnard, Christian, 523, 540
Barron, Moses (photos), 219, 230; 325; role in Base Hospital No. 26, 218, 219; laboratories at Base Hospital No. 26 and Allerey Center, 222–223, 227; diphtheria epidemic at Allerey Hospital Center, 228–230
Base Hospital No. 26, (W.W.I) Bathing the wounded (photo), 226; Bishop at work (photo), 224; Captain Barron at work (photo), 230; Laboratory (photo), 229; Mud at Allerey (photo), 232; mustered at Millard Hall (photo), 220; operating room (photo), 227; unloading the wounded (photo), 224; ward (photo), 231; established, 215; personnel, 215, 216–217; medical students continued instruction, 218; description of camp, 221–222; description of facilities, 222–223, 225–226; patients at, 223, 225, 226, 228, 231; surgery at, 223, 225, 226, 231
Beard, Archie H., 219
Beard, Richard O. (port.), 40, 152; 40, 47, 87, 105, 140(n.35), 221, 567; taught physiology, 61; role in securing new Anatomy Building, 83–84; request for animal housing, 84; Historical Evening (1908), 127; appointed secretary of medical school, 143; control over supply budget (1913), 155; meeting and correspondence on Mayo affiliation, 168–169, 171, 172, 183; committee on Mayo affiliation, 167–170, 171, 173; chairman of building fund committee (1925), 267–268
Beaumont, John E., 568
Beckman, E. H.: diphtheria work at Park Rapids, 74
Bell, Charles J. (port.), 39; 39, 47, 48, 60, 66
Bell, Elexious T. (port.), 390; 151, 285, 299, 348; as head of Department of Pathology, Bacteriology and Public Health, 238, 389; medical training, 389; as teacher, 389, 391; clinical-pathological conferences, 391; researches on *Bacillus proteus*, 389; renal tumors, 389; glomerulonephritis, 389–390; renal pathology, 389, 391; diabetes mellitus, 391; valvular heart disease, 391
Bell, J. W., 568
Bell, James Ford, 430, 431, 468
Bell, William, 361
Bellevue Hospital Medical College, 17
Belsey, Ronald, 375
Bergh, George S., 366
Berglund, Hilding (photo), 319; appointed chief of medicine (1925), 297, 325, encounter with Wangensteen, 297–298; promoted research, 325; resigned (1932), 326
Berk, H. J. J., 541
Berkman, David, 129–130
Berkshire Medical Institution, 12, 28(n.14)
Bigelow, W. G., 492, 499
Billings, Frank, 241–242
Biochemistry, Department of: Armstrong appointed head (1946), 404
Bio-medical Library: space in Mayo memorial, 435, 441; need for new location, 449, 451; plan to house in Owre Hall, 450; state funds requested, (1952, 1955), 450; (1957), 451; funds raised for Diehl Hall, 450, 451, 455; opened in Diehl Hall (1961), 455. *See also:* Medical Library; Wangensteen Historical Library of Biology and Medicine
Bittner, John J. (port.), 466; research on cancer transmission in mice, 465–466, 468; appointed head of cancer biology (1942), 467
Bjork, Viking, 490
Blake, Francis, 282
Blake, Joseph A., 213
Blalock, Alfred, 483, 494, 508
Blalock-Taussig procedure, 483, 484, 493, 494, 505
Blegen, Theodore, 509
Blood-oxygenating equipment, multiple screen (photo), 491; 489–491. *See also:* Bubble oxygenator; Cross circulation in open heart surgery
Blue-babies. *See:* Blalock-Taussig procedure; Tetralogy of Fallot
Boardman, Charles H., 567

INDEX

Board of Regents: delayed establishment of medical school, 6; committee to organize College of Medicine (1882), 23–24; established College of Medicine (1883), 24–25; College of Medicine faculty selected (1883), 30(n.50); reorganization of College of Medicine (1886), 32; medical school proposed (1887), 34; appointed Millard dean (1888), 36; established Department of Medicine (1888), 36; appointed first faculty to Department of Medicine (1888), 38; approved faculty salaries (1888), 38–39; appointed C. Bell (1888), 39; homeopathic instruction part of medical department (1888), 45–46; approved change to four-year course (1891), 49, 63; approved construction of Medical Hall (1891), 49–50; accepted Millard's loan for Medical Hall, 50; established College of Pharmacy, 50; accepted private funding of dispensary, 51; advocated Minneapolis City Hospital close to campus, 55; approved construction of Medical Chemistry Building (1891), 60; approved construction of Laboratory of Medical Sciences (1895), 63–64; State Board of Health laboratories, 69; appointed Ritchie dean (1897), 82; requested funds for Anatomy Building (1898), 84; requested funds for dispensary (1898), 84; voted funds for clinical apparatus (1897), 84; appropriated money for physiology laboratory (1902), 87; contract for Hospital for Crippled Children (1897), 90, 91; accepted gift of Millard library, 92; appointed Christison, 94; appointed Sweetser, 94; appointed Wheaton, 94; approved change of titles by surgery professors (1901), 98; action on medical admissions requirement (1906), 103–104; appointed Wesbrook dean (1906), 104; Elliot estate gift rejected (1906), 109–110; accepted Elliot estate gift (1907), 111; Gilbert plan of university campus accepted (1908), 114; requested funds for anatomy building and medical sciences building (1908), 115; site for Elliot Memorial Hospital (1909), 116; houses approved as temporary hospital buildings (1909), 117, 118–119; requested funds to equip and maintain hospital (1911), 119; assigned Madsen Flats to hospital, 121–122; approved merger with Hamline medical school (1908), 127; merged College of Homeopathic Medicine and Surgery into College of Medicine and Surgery, 127–129; elected Vincent president (1910), 130; requested additional funds for medical buildings and hospital (1911), 134; effect of appropriations cut (1911), 142; Salary Committee (1910), 143; appointed committee on reorganization (1913), 147; appointed secretary for medical school, 151; control of Mayo Foundation funds, 170, 200, 204, 205–206; failure to request legislative funds for medical facilities, 171, 196–197; advised of opposition to Mayo affiliation, 180; public hearing on Mayo affiliation, 188; approved Mayo affiliation, 188–189; demanded resignation of Greene, 189; appointed Mayo staff to faculty, 191; hearing on bill to dissolve Mayo affiliation (1917), 203–204; accepted new plan of Mayo affiliation (1917), 203–206; approved Burton's building plan, 235–236; prohibited opposition to Mayo affiliation, 189–191, 239; private medical practice, 253, 277; Comprehensive Building Program money used for hospital, 255, 273, 274, 275; accepted gift for Christian Cancer Hospital, 256; on locating Minneapolis General Hospital at university, 261; funding of hospital additions (1925), 268–269, 271–272, 274–275; appointed Boynton (1935), 325; appointed Diehl dean, 325; established physiological chemistry as a department (1946), 404; architect to prepare sketches of Mayo building (1941), 428; appreciation to Cowling for work on Mayo memorial, 430; established School of Public Health (1943), 431; planning of Mayo memorial, 435, 437; requested federal funds from Hill-Burton Construction Act (1947), 436, 439; accepted Variety Club's offer to finance heart hospital, 483; action on reports of long-range space needs (1966), 549; established Health Sciences Center (1968), 551; created office of vice-president for health sciences, 551; established board of governors for hospital (1974), 557; made hospital autonomous administrative unit (1970), 557; approved construction of one floor of hospital (1982), 559; deferred hospital construction (1982), 559; issued bonds for hospital (1982), 560

Boehm, J. C., 207(n.21)
Bohr, Christian, 292
Bohr, Nils, 293
Bone marrow transplantation, 539–540
"Bowling Alley." *See:* Medical Chemistry Building
Boyd, Edith, 305
Boyden, Edward A. (port.), 376; 372; research on gall bladder, 374–375; description of lungs, 375–376
Bracken, Henry M., 65, 77, 567; typhoid fever identification, 70–72; diphtheria work at Park Rapids, 74
Bratrud, Theodore B., committee on reorganization (1913), 147
Brazie, Henry W., 46, 568
Brekkus, P. J., research on fluorine content of tooth enamel, 404–405
Briggs, Warren S., 568
Brink, William R., 473
Brock, Russell, 375, 494
Brown, David M. (port.), 562; 562–563
Brown, Edgar D., 129; appointed head of Division of Pharmacology, 391
Brown, William R., 402
Brucella abortus, 329–332
Brucella melitensis, 331–332
Brucellosis: research by Spink, 329–332
Bruton, Ogden C., 470
Bubble oxygenator, Model I (photo), 511; Model III and Richard A. De Wall (photo), 512; sheet, and Richard De Wall and Vincent Gott (photo), 515; used in open heart surgery (photo), 513; research on, 509–511; De Wall's Models I, II, and III, 511–514

Buildings planned: Medical Hall (1892), 49–50; Medical Chemistry Building (1892), 60; Laboratory of Medical Sciences (1895), 63–65; University Dispensary (1899), 82–83, 86–87; Anatomy Building (1900), 83–86; Institute of Public Health and Pathology (1904), 88–89; Elliot Memorial Hospital (1907), 109–113; Institute of Anatomy (1908), 114, Millard Hall (1908), 115; contagious disease hospital, (1914), 171; (1916), 197; Todd Memorial Clinic (1920), 251–255, 273; Christian (George Chase) Cancer Hospital (1923), 255–256, 273; Eustis Hospital (1927), 260, 274–275; outpatient department wing (1927), 274; students' health service (1927), 274; Mayo Memorial Building (1945), 428, 432, 435; Lyon Memorial Laboratory (1951), 445; Masonic Memorial Hospital (1955, 1963), 445–448; Veterans of Foreign Wars Cancer Research Institute (1956), 449; laboratory space (1956) (under Union Street), 451; Diehl Hall (1957), 452–457; Variety Club Heart Hospital (1945), 483–485; Moos (Malcolm) Health Sciences Tower (1971), 549–551; K-E building for cardiovascular research (1973), 552; Phillips-Wangensteen Building (1979), 552–554; building F (1977), 554; University Hospital (1981), 558–560

Burnham, F. W., 113
Burr, George O. (port.), 401; appointed director of Division of Physiological Chemistry (1940), 400, 404; researches on vitamin E with Evans, 400–401; fatty acids in diet, 401–403; conversion of non-drying oils to drying oils, 402; left university (1946), 404
Burr, Mildred, 400; research on fatty acids in diet, 401–403

INDEX

Burton, Marion: Comprehensive Building Program, 235; financial crisis (1920–21), 236; left university (1920), 236; attempted to raise money for hospital, 237–238; Todd gift for clinic, 251, 253; founded students' health service, 275

Butler, Pierce, 184, 188, 244

Calcium in blood: research by Gresheimer, 381
California, University, at Berkeley, research at, 292, 302, 331, 400
Calne, Roy, 530
Cameron, Angus, 326
Campbell, O.N., 307
Cancer: surgery for, 316, 319–320; treatment of gynecological, 354–356, 465; surgery for in alimentary canal, 463–465; reduced mortality, 464; "the silent interval," 464; radiation treatment, 465; "the second look," 465; university designated a training center, 465; fluorescence used to detect malignant tissue, 468–469; radioactive substances used to detect tumors, 468–469
Cancer Biology, Division of: Bittner appointed head (1942), 467
Cannon, Walter B., 151
Carbolic acid spray: first surgical use (1882), 19
Cardiac surgery: patent ductus arteriosus, 481, 494; tetralogy of Fallot, 483, 493, 494; pulmonary valvular stenosis corrected, 494. *See also:* Open heart surgery
Cardiogram: slit x-ray, 407
Carey, James B., 351
Carli, Christopher, 6
Carlson, Anton J., 393
Carpenter, Elbert L., 112, 119
Carrel, Alexis, 529
Case, J. T., 299
Cates, A. B., 109, 568
Chapman, Carleton, 410
Chardack, William, 521
Chautauqua Institution, 131
Chemistry instruction (1888), 38–40, 41
Chemistry laboratory, 1890s (photo), 62

Chemotherapy: research by Hirschfelder, 393
Chesley, Albert J., 231–232
Cholera: research by Wesbrook, 65
Cholesterol in diet, 410–412
Christian, George Chase, lecture, 465–466
Christian, Mrs. George Chase (port.), 255; (photo), 440; 255, 430
Christian, George H., 255
Christian Cancer Hospital (photo), 274; installation of radiation equipment, 273–274; Strachauer chief of (1925), 288
Christison, James T., 94
Chunn, Stanley S., 309
Churchill, Edward D., 375, 488
Citizens Aid Society, 255–256, 465, 467
City and County Hospital (St. Paul), 47, 243; first use of x-rays in surgery, 76; Hospital for Crippled Children, 90–92. *See also:* Ancker Hospital (St. Paul)
City Hospital of Minneapolis. *See:* Minneapolis City Hospital
Civil War: physicians in, 8–10, 15, 17, 30(n.45), 82; treatment of fevers, 9
Clapesattle, Helen, 429
Clark, Leland C., Jr., 509
Clarke, William, 327
Clausen, Samuel W., 303
Clawson, Benjamin J.: researches on allergic and immune responses, 391; valvular heart disease, 391
Clifford, F. W., 113
Clinical clerkships, began 1909, 117
Clinical Congress of Surgeons of North America, 159
Clinical instruction, 16–17, 20, 22, 54–55; Department of Medicine (1888), 41–43, 47; dispensary on campus (1892), 51–52, 86; university hospital advocated, 82; University Dispensary [at Seven Corners] (1900), 86–87; orthopedic surgery, 92; in surgery by Dunn (1900), 97; clinical microscopy taught by Head (1898), 101–102
Coffey, Walter C., fund-raising campaign for Mayo memorial, 431

Coffman, Lotus D. (port.), 256; 240; external Survey Committee review of medical alumni report (1921), 241–246; need to expand university hospital, 253; negotiations with Minneapolis Board of Public Welfare over city hospital, 257, 261; negotiations with Rockefeller Foundation for hospital buildings (1923), 257, 261; application for hospital funding to Rockefeller board, 263–264, 268–269, 271–273; appeal for private donations, 265, 268, 272; letter to Mayo seeking funds (1925), 267; response to alumni criticism of Lyon, 305–306; role in Wangensteen controversy, 320–323; supported screening for tuberculosis among students, 344

Cohen, Morley (port.), 496; 494–495; impressions of surgery department (1950), 487; researches on azygos flow, 495–498; cross circulation, 501–503; successful cardiac by-pass surgery on dogs, 496–497; used cardiac lobe of lung as oxygenator, 496, 500

Colby, Woodard L., 258

Cole, Wallace (port.), 359; work with polio patients, 359; interest in Sister Kenny's methods, 360–362

College of Dentistry: in Medical Hall, 86; needed more space (1907), 114; losses in fire (1909), 129

College of Homeopathic Medicine and Surgery: faculty, 40, 46–47; lecture schedule, 40; clinical instruction, 41–43, 47; curriculum, 41–42, 46–47, 56(n.28), 57(n.30); merged with College of Medicine and Surgery (1909), 127–129

College of Medical Sciences (1931–70) [administrative unit of medical school], 306, 325; abolished as an administrative unit, 551

College of Medicine: established (1883–87), 21, 23–24, 77; faculty duties, 24–27; licensing of physicians, 24, 25; purpose, 25

College of Medicine and Surgery, student body, 1889 (photo), 42; faculty, 1909 (photo), 129; faculty selection (1888), 38; tuition, 39; anxious that Elliot gift be accepted, 109; reorganized into administrative departments (1908), 124–126; student records, 125; merger with Hamline Medical School (1908), 126–127; merged with College of Homeopathic Medicine and Surgery, 127–129; reorganization by Vincent, 141, 143–150; effect of budget cut (1911), 142–143; effect of Wesbrook's resignation, 145–146; criteria for faculty selection (1913), 146–147; Beard acquired control of all supply budgets (1913), 155. *See also:* Clinical instruction; Curriculum; Executive Committee; Executive faculty; Faculty meetings

College of Pharmacy: created (1891), 50; offices in wing of Laboratory of Medical Sciences, 64

Committee for the Study of Physical Facilities for the Health Sciences, 546–549

Committee of Founders of the Mayo Memorial: created, 429–430; fund-raising campaigns (1944), 431–432; (1945), 434–435; (1947), 436; state funds requested (1945), 432–434; (1947), 435–436; (1949), 437–438; (1951), 441; national publicity about, 433, 435; building cost increases (1946), 435; (1947), 436; (1948–49), 437; (1950), 440; delays due to architect, 437, 439–441

Committee on hospital and clinical development (1913), 161–163, 191–192; promised support by Mayo, 171; recommendation not supported by regents, 174

Committee on Hospital Extension, 260; attempted to raise money for Todd Memorial Clinic, 254

Comprehensive Building Program, 235, 253 255, 268, 273, 274, 275

Congenital heart defects, 483, 484, 492, 493, 515

Continuing education courses for physicians, 247

Cook, Paul D., 207(n.21)

Copavin, 450, 459(n.43)

INDEX

Corner, George W., 302
Corser, F. G., 64
Cotton, W. E., 331
Cowling, Donald J. (port.), 430; (photo), 440; chairman of planning committee, 428; chairman, Committee of Founders of the Mayo Memorial, 429; requests to legislature (1945), 432–434; (1947), 435–436; (1951), 441; fund-raising campaigns for Mayo memorial (1944), 431–432; (1945), 434–435; appreciation by Morrill, 438; Cowling scholarships, 444; trustee of Minnesota Medical Foundation, 444; role in Masonic Memorial Hospital, 445–447; fund-raising for medical library building, 452, 455; death, 457
Crafoord, Clarence, 524(n.4)
Crawford, William H., 450
Creevy, C. Donald, 307
Crile, George, 213–214
Crippled children. *See:* Hospital for Crippled Children
Cross circulation: in dogs (diag.), 502; used in open heart surgery (diag.),504; used in first open heart surgery (photo), 505; used, second patient (photos), 506; surgical correction of tetralogy of Fallot, first patient (photos), 507; in open heart surgery, 501–504, 508
Curriculum: College of Homeopathic Medicine & Surgery (1888), 41–42, 46–47, 56(n.28), 57(n.30); College of Medicine & Surgery (1888), 41–42, 56(n.28), 57(n.30); change to eight-month program (1890), 42; change to four-year program, 49, 63, 66, 76; Wesbrook's changes in bacteriology and pathology (1898), 100–101; clinical microscopy added (1898), 101–102; change to six-year program, 102–103
Curry, Cynthia, 477
Cushing's syndrome, 349
Cutts, Rollin E., medal, 100

Dahlgren, Bror E., 137
Dale-Schuster pumps, 489

Daly, Mary, 362
Dameshek, William, 530
Daniels, Asa W., 28(n.22)
Darrach, William, 289
Dausset, Jean, 531
Davis, Arch, 435
Davis, Cushman K., 58(n.45)
Day, David, 7
DC Antifoam A, 509–510, 511
Dean, H. Trendley, 405
DeBakey roller pump, 488, 489
Delplaine, C. W., 445
Dempster, W. J., 529
Dennis, Clarence, 463, 487, 492, 497; developed a multiple screen oxygenator, 486, 489–491, 493; first open heart surgery with multiple screen oxygenator (5 April 1951), 490; and W. Harris, with multiple screen blood oxygenator (photo), 491
Dennis, Warren, 486
Denny, Floyd, 473, 474
Department of Medicine: established (1888), 36, 37–38, 77; first faculty meeting (8 June 1888), 41; first term (1888), 42; extended term to eight months, 42; cooperation with homeopathic college, 43, 77; department libraries, 43, 93; role in establishing medical library, 92–93; admissions standards raised, 102–104. *See also:* College of Dentistry; College of Homeopathic Medicine and Surgery [1888–1908]; College of Medicine and Surgery [1888–1913]; College of Pharmacy; Medicine, Department of [est. 1908]
Dermatology, Division of. *See:* Medicine, Department of
Derzon, Robert, 559
De Wall, Richard A., Model I Bubble Oxygenator (photo), 511; Model III Bubble Oxgenator (photo), 512; research on bubble oxygenators, 509–514; and Vincent Gott with sheet bubble oxygenator (photo), 515
Dewey, John Jay, 6
Diabetes, 349, 380
Diehl, Harold S. (photo), 319; (port.), 24; (photo), 440; 228; American Red

590

Cross Commission to Poland, 231–232; appointed director of students' health service, 275; appointed dean (1935), 325; screening for tuberculosis among university students, 343–344; required tuberculin test on admission to hospital (1935), 345; enabled Sister Kenny to demonstrate her treatment, 358–360, 365; efforts to raise Burr's salary, 404; role in mobilizing medical school for wartime, 416–417; appeal for Mayo memorial at university, 426–428; fund-raising campaign for Mayo memorial, 431–432; requested funds from Rockefeller Foundation for School of Public Health, 431; on low faculty salaries, 436; role in securing state funds for Mayo memorial, 438; federal funding for Mayo memorial, 439; reduced size of Mayo memorial, 441; on completion of Mayo Memorial Building, 443; role in Masonic Memorial Hospital, 445–448; need for medical library, 449–450; fund raising for library building, 450; royalties from Copavin patent, 450; state funds needed for staffing Mayo Memorial Building, 450; fund raising for laboratories (Union Street), 451; resignation as dean, 452–454

Diehl, Mrs. Harold, 454

Diehl Hall, 1961 (photo), 454; 1965 (photo), 457; architect's design, 452; building cost increases, 455–456; floors 4 and 5 finished (1964), 457

Diet: role of cholesterol, 410–412

Diphtheria bacilli: classification system devised, 73–74

Diphtheria epidemics: Owatonna (1896), 73; Park Rapids (1901), 74; Benson (1904), 75; Grand Rapids (1903), 75; university hospital (1911), 121; Allerey Hospital Center, 228–230;

Diploma law. *See:* Medical practice act, 1883

Dispensaries: homeopathic, 47; on university campus, 50–51, 82–83. *See also:* University Dispensary

Downey, Hal, 93, 137, 337, 372, 471, 541; authority on hematology, 373; description of infectious mononucleosis, 373, 374

Dunn, Halbert (photo), 319; appointed director of hospital, 318; Wangensteen controversy, 318–321; resigned (1935), 325

Dunn, James H. (port.), 96; 566, 567; life, 94–95; antiseptic surgery, 95, 100; as a teacher, 96–98; death, 96, 103; philosophy of surgical education, 97–98; made chief of surgical professors (1901), 98; entrance requirements of medical school, 103;

Dunsmoor, Frederick A. (port.), 15; 94, 195, 567; interest in medical education, 14–21; first surgery with carbolic spray (1882), 19; opposed to reorganization plan, 125; Historical Evening, 127

Dwan, Paul, 552

Earl, George, 426, 427

Eastman, Nicholson J., 352

Eaton, Burt W., 183, 267

Eczema, infantile, 402

Ehrlich, Paul, 393

Einthoven, Willem, 292–293

Eitel, George D., 456; European experience (1927–28), 295–296; and Owen H. Wangensteen (photo), 296

Eitel, George G., 20

Elliot, Adolphus F. (port.), 110; 104, 109

Elliot, Frank M., 119

Elliot, Mary Ellen Hoar, 104, 109

Elliot Memorial Hospital (photo), 120, 274; 565; funded by Elliot estate, 109; funds needed to purchase site, 112; location recommended to Board of Regents (1907), 112; long-term view of hospital complex, 112–113; administration building for future hospital, 115; architect, William Kenyon, 119; dedication (1911), 119; first patients (1911), 120; service building added, 134, 139, 156

Embolisms: research on pulmonary embolism by McCartney, 390

Epilepsy: research in control of, 346
Erdmann, Bertha, 117, 118
Erdmann, Charles A., 94, 106(n.39), 334; losses in Anatomy Building fire (1908), 115
Ericksen, Lester, 356
Eustis, William H. (port.), 270; gifts for hospital expansion, 260, 265, 270–271, 274; death, 276–277; life, 277
Eustis Endowment, 346, 348
Eustis Hospital (photo), 276; Entrance (photo), 278; 274–275, 276, 277
Evans, Alice C., 331
Evans, Herbert M., 292, 302, 400
Ewart, William, 375
Executive Committee [College of Medicine and Surgery]: on the dispensary question (1898), 82–83; on plans for Anatomy Building (1898), 83; on need for animal housing (1898), 84; requested funds to enlarge dispensary (1902), 87; requested funds to replace anatomical preparations (1902), 87; requested more laboratory space (1902), 87; established permanent committee for library development (1895), 92; appropriation for library book purchases (1899), 93; revised teaching schedule (1898), 100–101; anxious that Elliot gift be accepted, 109; expansion of campus, 110, 113; site for new anatomy building (1907), 114; reallocated laboratory space (1908), 114; appropriation request for buildings and equipment (1908), 114–115; meeting with regents on future of medical school (1908), 115; Gilbert plan of medical campus (1909), 115–116; need to coordinate teaching among departments (1906), 124; plan to reorganize the faculty, 124–125; reorganization approved (1908), 125–126. After 1908 *see:* Executive Faculty meetings
Executive Faculty meetings [College of Medicine and Surgery]: organization, 124–125; increased building costs (1911), 133–135; plan for new medical campus (1912), 133–139; needs of college discussed with Vincent (1912), 134, 148; Vincent explained reorganization (1913), 144; letter of resignation (Jan. 1913), 144–145; resolution in memory of Parks Ritchie, 147; Vincent explained lack of building funds, 148; After 1912 *see:* Administrative Board
Experiments of nature, 348, 369(n.102), 474, 477

Faculty, 1909 (photo), 129; first medical school, 38–40; first salaried, 39; College of Homeopathic Medicine and Surgery, 40, 46–47; first faculty meeting (1888), 41; concept of executive faculty, 124–125; concept of general faculty, 124–125; letter of resignation (Jan. 1913), 145; Vincent's criteria for, 146–147; suspicious of motives for Mayo affiliation, 171, 173, 177; forbidden by regents to oppose Mayo affiliation, 189–191; resignations (1915) after Mayo affiliation, 189–190; restricted by limited space (1916), 197; part-time clinical, 282–283; full-time clinical, 285–286; geographical full-time plan for clinical faculty, 289
Faculty meetings, 41, 82; Medical Hall site selection (1891), 49; on raising entrance requirements (1904), 103. *See also:* Administrative Board; Administrative Committee; Executive Committee; Executive Faculty meetings; General Faculty meetings
Faculty salaries, 38–40, 143; scale of minimum salaries recommended (1912), 134; clinical chiefs on salary (1908), 141; salaries advocated for clinical staff (1913), 152; (1916), 197; clinical salary increases diverted (1913), 154, 157(n.30); after W.W.I, 236; clinical salaries in 1920s, 284; part-time, 286, 288; part-time surgeons deprived of salaries (1930), 307; Diehl on low salaries (1947), 436
Fahr, George (port.), 294; 325, 326, 327; salary, 284; as teacher,

293–295; life; 291–293; medical training, 292–293; European trip (1927), 295; diagnosis of myxedema heart, 295
Fahs, Ivan J., 546
Fairview Hospital (Minneapolis), 343
Fatty acid deficiency disease in rats (photo), 403
Fatty acids: research by George and Mildred Burr, 401–403
Fender, F. A., 309–310
Ferris, Viola, 476
Fesler, Paul (port.), 318; 277; accomplishments, 315–316
Fevers: treatment of, 9, 22, 29(n.42)
Fiber tracts (human): research on, 372–373
Fifth Minnesota Volunteer Infantry (Civil War), 30(n.45)
Finney, John M. T., 241–242
Firor, Warfield M., 463
First Minnesota Infantry Regiment (Civil War), 8
Fischer, Hans, 326
Flandrau, Charles E., 58(n.45)
Flexner, Abraham, 237, 564; report on 1909 visit, 129, 141; negotiations for Rockefeller gift for hospital buildings, 257, 261, 268–269, 272; on relation of Mayo Clinic to medical school (1923), 262–263
Flint, Austin, 17
Fluid balance, 347–348
Fluoridation of water supplies, 405–406
Fluoride: in prevention of tooth decay, 404–405
Folin, Otto, 297
Folwell, William W., 34, 291; role in creating the College of Medicine (1883–87), 23–25
Ford, Guy S., 177, 191, 204; role in McClendon's departure, 400; supported a Mayo memorial at university, 427; view on funding of Mayo memorial, 429
Ford, Joseph H., 218, 227
Forssell, Gösta, 273, 298, 299
Foster, Burnside, 39, 568
Fowler, L. Haynes, 417
Francis, Edward, 386
Freeman, Charles D., 190, 210(n.121)

French, George F. (port.), 16; 15, 17, 28(n.26)
French, Lyle A. (port.), 551; 547, 551, 558, 559
Frey, Max von, 292
Friedell, H. L.: research on comparative heart size, 407
Friesen, Stanley R. (port.), 464; 464
Fulton, John F., 19–20, 38, 50, 567
Fungal diseases: research by Henrici, 388
Fungus: research by Henrici, 385

Gale, Benjamin, 112
Gale, Sara P. 251
Gallbladder: first surgical removal (1886), 4
Gamble, James L., 309
Gardner, E. L.: research on actinomycetes, 385
Garten, Siegfried, 293
Gasparich, Sergeant, 418
Gault, Neal L., Jr. (port.), 552; 552, 562
Gay, Frederick P., 302
General Alumni Association: on the Mayo affiliation, 177–178, 180
General Faculty: meetings, 246, 286; organization, 124–125; Vincent explained reorganization (1913), 145, 148; vote on Mayo affiliation, 172–173; meeting after regents impose gag order, 190; committee on relations of clinical chiefs to medical school, 284; Lyon's plan for more full-time faculty, 286–287
Gibbon, John, 488–489, 491, 493, 497, 508, 525(n.14)
Giere, Richard W., 456
Gilbert, Cass: plan for the medical campus (illus.), 113; revised plan for the medical campus (illus.), 116; architectural plan of campus, 113–114; plan as viewed by Vincent, 136, 445
Gilfallan, James S., 190, 210(n.121)
Gillette, Arthur J.: first patient at Hospital for Crippled Children (photo), 91; 20; established Hospital for Crippled Children, 89–92; life,

INDEX

105(n.18); appointed to chair of orthopedics, 106(n.19)
Gillette, George M., 184
Gillette, Lewis S., 113
Gillette Hospital. *See:* Hospital for Crippled Children
Glass, Ameil, 375
Glen Lake Tuberculosis Sanatorium, 483
Glomerulonephritis, 492; researches by E. T. Bell and Hartzell, 398–390; by Wannamaker, 475
Glycogen formation: research by Gresheimer, 380
Goiter: research by McClendon, 379, 400
Good, Robert A. (photo), 471; bone marrow transplant, 539–540, 541; researches on agammaglobulinemia, 470–472; on thymus, 472–473
Good Samaritan Dispensary, 29(n.41)
Goodrich, Calvin G., 28(n.23)
Gorgas, William C., 213–215
Gorham, Frederic P., 75
Gott, Vincent: developed the sheet bubble oxygenator, 514–515; and Richard A. De Wall, with sheet bubble oxygenator (photo), 515
Graduate medical education, 240, 243–244, 245, 246; under Mayo Foundation, 239
Graduate Medical Education National Advisory Committee, 555
Graduate School in Medicine, 160, 174–175, 205–206
Graham, Christopher, 166
Graham, Evarts, 298
Grande, Francisco: controlled diet experiments, 412
Granger, George W. 267
Graves' disease: research by McClendon, 379
Gray, James: description of Vincent, 140(n.37)
Greatbatch, Wilson, 521, 522
Green, Robert G. (port.), 387; researches on tularemia, 386–388; on rabbit papilloma, 467; on mouse cancer milk factor, 468; death (1947), 468

Greene, Charles L. (port.), 153; used Widal test, 71; chief of medical division in hospital, 117; dedication of Elliot Memorial Hospital, 119; committee on reorganization (1913), 147; refused deanship, 152–154; recommended Hirschfelder, 155; on the Mayo affiliation, 172, 173–174, 175–177, 178–179, 184–186; regents demanded resignation, 189; opposed 1916 plan for clinical expansion, 198–200
Greer, E. K., 341
Gresheimer, Esther M., 397(n.38); researches on glycogen formation, 380; on respiratory irregularities, 380; on blood calcium, 381
Gross, Robert E., 481, 482, 524(n.4)
Gross, Samuel D., Prize, 323
Guilford Bill, 180, 181–182, 183, 184, 187–188
Guthrie, Charles, 529

Haden, Russell L., 309
Hahnemann, Samuel C., 43–44
Hahnemann Medical Society, 30(n.45)
Haines, Samuel F., 351
Hall, Alexander R., 190
Hall, Robert A., 210(n.121)
Hall, Wendell, 476
Halsted, William S., 165
Hamburger, Jean, 531
Hamilton, Arthur S. (port.), 287; 149, 325; opposed Lyon's plan for reducing part-time faculty, 286–287;
Hamilton, Charles H., 47
Hamilton, Frank, 17
Hamline University, Department of Medicine, 15, 29(n.41); entrance requirements raised (1898), 102; merged with university medical school (1908), 126–127
Hamline University Medical School. *See:* Hamline University, Department of Medicine
Hammond, W. S., 188
Hand, Daniel W. (port.), 9; 8, 9–10, 28(n.22), 34; treatment of fevers, 9; interest in medical education, 10, 12–13

INDEX

Hankin, E. H., 75
Hansen, Arild: research on infantile eczema, 402
Hare, E. R., 207(n.21)
Harrington, Francis E. (port.), 333; commissioner of public health for Minneapolis (1920), 332–333; tuberculosis major problem, 333–335
Harris, W. and Clarence Dennis with multiple screen blood oxygenator (photo), 491
Hart, M. C.: synthesized Saligenin, 393
Hartwell, John A., 309, 312
Hartzell, Thomas B.: researches on bacteria in pyorrhea and abscesses, 381–384; on infected pulp of teeth, 384–385; on glomerulonephritis, 389–390; on valvular heart disease, 391
Harvey, Valerie, 361
Hastings, Donald, 456
Hatch, Philo L., 22
Hauge, Cecilia, 417
Hawes, George, 45
Hawley, Augustine B., 10
Head, George D. (port.), 101; 150; taught clinical microscopy, 101–102; life, 107(n.63); organized alumni support for the Elliot Memorial Hospital, 110–111; on Mayo affiliation, 177, 184; resignation, 190–191, 210(n.121); on private patients at university hospital, 195, 196; chaired medical alumni committee on the medical school (1920), 238–240; chaired Committee on Medical Education (1922), 246; diagnosed tuberculosis in J. Arthur Myers, 334
Health Careers Development Program, 555
Health Professions Educational Assistance Act, 545, 551, 555
Heart: comparative sizes, 407; effect of exercise (photo), 408
Heart block: first pulse generator (photo), 520; first patient successfully treated by myocardial electrode (photo), 518; 508, 520; experiments on dogs, 519; first implantable pacemaker used, 521; first pacemaker used in patient, 521; pacemaker used in all patients with post-operative heart block, 523
Heart disease: researches on valvular disease, 391; coronary heart disease by Keys, 409–412
Heart efficiency: research by Starling and Visscher, 393–394
Heart failure: research by Visscher and Moe, 394–395
Heart-Lung Institute, 541
Heart transplantation, 540–541
Heimbeck, Johannes, 343
Hematology: research by Downey, 373–374
Hemodialysis, 530, 534, 537
Henderson, Melvin, 358, 359
Hendricks, George A. (port.), 48; 47, 61, 66, 76, 92, 94
Hennepin County Medical Society: meeting on Mayo affiliation, 188–189; meeting on paying patients at university hospital, 193–196; relocation of Minneapolis General Hospital, 261
Henrici, Arthur T. (port.), 385; 389; appointed (1913), 381; researches on bacteria in pyorrhea and abscesses, 381–384; on infected pulp of teeth, 384–385; on actinomycetes, 385; on morphology of bacteria, 385–386; on tularemia, 386–388; on fresh water bacteria, 387–388; on fungal diseases, 388; on renal tumors, 389; death (1943), 468
Henschel, Austin F.: research on effect of vitamin supplements, 407
Hermann, Edgar T., 456
Hermundslie, Palmer, 520
Hewitt, Charles N. (port.), 11; 10, 14; role in creating the College of Medicine (1883–87), 23–24; views on medical education, 34–35; conflict with Millard, 35–36, 68–69
Hickey, P. J., 299
Higbee, Albert E., 568
Hill, Harry, 478
Hill, James J., 18, 58(n.45)
Hill, Nathan B., 28(n.22)
Hill-Burton Construction Act, 436, 525(n.8)

INDEX

Hill Family Foundation's Health Manpower Study Commission, 546
Hill-Quie Syndrome, 478
Hilleboe, Herman E., 320
Hirsch, Jean, 375
Hirschfelder, Arthur (port.), 392; 155, 158(n.34), 284; appointed head of pharmacology, 392; medical training, 392–393; research on chemotherapy, 393; synthesized Saligenin, 393
His, Wilhelm: library purchased for university, 93
Histology and Embryology Laboratory (photo), 66
Historical Evening (1908), 126–127
Hodgkin's disease, 337, 356
Hoff, Eivind O., Jr., 444
Hoff, Peder A., 190, 210(n.121)
Hoffman, Franz, 392
Hoguet, J. P., 309, 312
Hoidale, Einar, 187
Holmes, Oliver W., 44
Homeopathy: origin of, 43–44; conflict with regular medical profession, 44–45; as part of medical school, 45–47
Hooper Foundation for Medical Research, 302, 308
Hormel, Jay C., 430
Hormone, ovarian: research by McClendon, 379–380
Hospital for Crippled Children (St. Paul): first patient (photo), 91; 89–92, 359
Howard, Robert B. (port.), 453; 551; appointed dean (1958), 454
Hoyt, Wayland, 51
Huenekens, E. J., 350
Hume, David M., 530
Hunt, Reid, 151
Hunter, Charles H., 19, 20, 21, 567
Hunter, Samuel, 518, 521
Hutchinson, Henry, 568
Hynes, John E., 149, 190, 210(n.121)
Hypercapnia: research by Scott, 378
Hypothermia: refrigerating blankets for heart surgery (photo), 497; hot water bath for warming patient (photo), 498; research and use in open heart surgery, 498–500
Hypoxia: research by Scott, 378

IBM, 525(n.14)
Idezuki, Yasuo, 537
Ikeda, Kano, 299
Illinois State Board of Health, 48–49
Immune deficiency diseases, 470–473
Immune suppressive agents: 530, 531, 532, 534, 535, 537; purified antilymphocytic globulin, 535–536; Cyclosporin A, 536
Immunology: compatibility for transplant surgery, 531–532, 539–540
Infectious mononucleosis: described by Downey and McKinlay, 373, 374
Influenza epidemics, 275
Institute of Anatomy (photo), 132; 427, 435, 565; funding for, 114–115, 133, 135, 148; cornerstone laid, 120; renamed Jackson Hall (1954), 450
Institute of Public Health and Pathology (photo), 88; 88–89, 104, 148
Insulin, 529, 530
Internal Medicine, Division of: Reimann appointed head (1932), 326; research during 1930s, 326–332; Watson appointed head (1936), 327. *See also:* Medicine, Department of
Intestinal obstruction: surgical intervention, 308; dehydration in, 308–309, 312; toxic theory of, 308–309, 311–312; Wangensteen and Leven identify cause of death in, 309–312; diagnosis of, 312–313; relieved by suction, 313–316
Iodine: deficiency as a cause of goiter, 379, 400
Iowa University Hospital, 257
Irvine, Harry G., 207(n.21)
Isuprel, 517, 518

Jackson, Clarence M. (port.), 150; 286, 334, 389; appointed, 150–151
Jackson Hall: formerly Institute of Anatomy, 450
James, Herbert W., 207(n.21)
Jamieson, Stuart W., 540
Janeway, Charles A., 470
Johns Hopkins Hospital, 165
Johns Hopkins Medical School, 54, 55; full-time clinical appointments (1913), 141, 283

Johnson, John A., 111
Johnson, Clarence, 277
Johnson, Delia: research on freshwater bacteria, 388
Johnson, R. M., 349
Johnston, C. H. and Company, 437, 439
Johnston, Wyatt, 71
Jones, Fred S.: demonstrations of x-rays (1896), 75–76
Jones, W. A., 194–195, 568; chaired faculty reorganization committee (1907), 124–125; editorials, 205, 244
Judd, E. Starr, 166, 173

Kean, Jefferson R., 214
Keefer, Chester S., 329
Keith, Haddow M., 346
Kelly, William D., 538
Kendall, Edward C., 166
Kenny, Elizabeth (Sister), demonstrates her methods (photo), 361; demonstrates control of muscles (photo), 363; demonstrates therapeutic techniques (photo), 363; purpose of trip to U.S., 358; methods of treatment for polio patients, 358–360; methods receive acceptance, 360–362
Kenny Institute, Sister: established at Lymanhurst, 364
Kenyon, William M., 119
Kernkamp, Leila, 339, 340
Keys, Ancel: appointed to Department of Physiology (1937), 406; established Laboratory of Physiological Hygiene, 407; developed K rations, 407; researches on effect of vitamin supplements, 407; on slit x-ray cardigram to detect heart defects, 407; on comparative heart size, 407; on effects of starvation, 408–409; on coronary heart disease, 409–412; on cholesterol in diet, 410–412; controlled diet experiments, 412; study of patent ductus arteriosus, 482, 492
Keys, Margaret, 410–412
Kidney: researches on diseases by E. T. Bell and Hartzell, 389–390; on renal pathology, 389, 391

Kidney transplant surgery: experiments on dogs, 529; first human transplant, 530; tissue compatibility, 531; immunological compatibility, 531–532; first at university, 533; statistics 1960s, 531–532, 533, 534; 1968–81, 536; on diabetic patients, 536–537; Najarian regimen reduced mortality, 534
Kildal, J. N., 184
Kilgore, Floyd V., 418, 422
Kimball, Hannibal H., 28(n.23)
Knapp, Miland E. (photo), 364; interest in Sister Kenny's methods, 360–362; directed training program in Kenny methods, 364
Knutson, John W.: research on topical treatment of teeth, 405
Kolff, W. J., 541
Kollman, Sara, 358
Kolouch, Fred, 470
Kottke, Frederic J. (photo), 364; appointed director of physical therapy (1947), 364
Kramer, Rudolph, 375
Krehl, Rudolf, 293
Kresge Foundation, 552
Krusen, Frank H., 358

Laboratory of Medical Sciences (photo), 64; Histology and Embryology Laboratory (photo), 66; Bacteriology Culture Room (photo), 68; Bacteriology Laboratory (photo), 84; 63–65, 76
Laboratory of Physiological Hygiene (photo), 408; 407, 409, 412
Langley, John N., 377
Largiader, Felix, 537
Larson, Winford P. (port.), 382; 389; researches on contagious abortion, 331; on *Bacillus proteus,* 389; appointed (1911), 381; death (1947), 468
Laton, W. S., 568
Law, Arthur A. (port.), 216; role in Base Hospital No. 26, 214, 215, 218, 219, 225–226, 227, 231
Law, Mrs. Arthur A., 418
Learn, Elmer W., 546
Le Boutellier, C. W., 8

INDEX

Lee, Thomas G. (ports.), 51, 138; 60, 66, 305; appointment, 50; teaching, 67; role in establishing medical library, 92–93, 449; on reorganization of faculty, 125; life, 137; Vincent's opinion of, 137; on use of the Anatomy Building, 140(n.35); demoted, 143, 151; omitted from all committees, 156

Lees, H. D., 340

Leidy, Joseph, 50

Leonard, Henry C., 568

Leonard, William E., 568

Leonard, William H., 29–30(n.45), 34, 45; role in creating the College of Medicine (1883–87), 23–24

Leven, N. Logan (port.), 310; work on intestinal obstruction, 310–312; and Wangensteen's diagrams of alimentary canal (illus.), 311

Levitt, Seymour, 356

Lewin, Philip, 362

Lewis, F. John: research on hypothermia, 498–499; performed with Varco and Taufic first open heart direct vision surgery (2 Sept. 1952), 499; and Richard Varco with cooling blanket and machine (photo), 500

L'Heureux, Jerome A., 539

Libman, Emanuel, 435

Licensing of physicians: first attempt, 10–11; by College of Medicine, 24

Liggett, William M., 49, 58(n.56)

Lillehei, C. Walton (port.), 516; showed relation of congenital heart defects to bacterial endocarditis, 492; developed open heart technique to correct tetralogy of Fallot, 492–493; practiced open heart surgery on cadavers, 492–493, 505–506; researches on azygos flow, 495–498; on lung as oxygenator, 500; used cardiac lobe of lung as oxygenator, 496, 500; successful cardiac by-pass surgery on dogs, 496–497; first open heart cross circulation surgery (26 March 1954), 503; second open heart cross circulation surgery (20 April 1954), 504; surgery for tetralogy of Fallot by direct vision (31 Aug. 1954), 506–508; first used De Wall bubble oxygenator (13 May 1955), 512; training program, 515–516; report on surgeries, 1954–1957, 516–517; pacemaker used in all patients with post-operative heart block, 523

Lillehei, Richard (port.), 538; 537–539

Lind, John, 115; Historical Evening, 127

Litzenberg, Jennings C. (port.), 351; 136, 137, 246, 247; committee on plans for hospital (1913), 147, 149–150; committee on Mayo affiliation, 167–170, 177; appointed chief of obstetrics and gynecology (1913), 350; research on basal metabolism and sterility, 351–352; organized graduate program, 352

Liver, 348; research on cirrhoses by McCartney, 390

Liver transplantation, 541

Loewi, Otto, 377

Long, Joseph A., 302, 400

Long Island College Hospital, 17

Loring, Charles M., 58(n.44)

Lott, Mark E., 218

Loucks, Milo, 309

Lowry, Thomas, 18, 20

Ludwig, Carl, 392

Lung: described in detail by Boyden, 376; research on pulmonary embolism by McCartney, 390

Lymanhurst (photo), 336; founding and dedication, 333–335; routine at, 336; tuberculosis clinic for children, 336–337; records kept on all cases, 337; use of Pirquet test, 337–338, 339, 340; use of chest x-rays, 338; tuberculosis in infants, 339; tuberculosis in teenagers, 340; adult clinic opened (1933), 341; school part closed (1935), 341–342; results of long-term studies, 341–343; converted to Sister Kenny Institute, 364; rheumatic fever clinic, 482; work with congenital heart defects, 482

Lymphocytes: identification of classes T and B, 473

Lynch, Francis, 312

Lyon, Elias P. (port.), 154; 246, 377; life, 155, 158(n.31); omitted Lee from all committees (1913), 156; need for additional facilities (1914), 164; committee on Mayo affiliation, 167–170; meetings and correspondence on Mayo affiliation, 169, 171, 183, 184, 185; on Mayo affiliation, 177, 178–179, 184; sought support for Mayo affiliation, 180–181; faculty resignations (1915), 189–190; on private practice, 195, 196; hearing on bill to dissolve Mayo affiliation, 204; role in organizing medical unit in W.W.I, 215; attempt to raise money for hospital, 237–238; criticism by medical alumni (1920), 239; response to Medical Alumni Association report (1920), 239–241; response to Committee on Medical Education report (1922), 248; received money for Todd Memorial Clinic, 254; arranged Pirquet appointment, 259–260; on Pirquet's resignation, 260–261; appeal for private donations, 265; on Rockefeller board application, 271–272; plan for hospital expansion accepted (1927), 274–275; on Eustis, 276–277; plan for more full-time faculty (1924), 286–287, 289; developed Wangensteen to be chief of surgery, 291, 295; developed Rigler to be chief of radiology, 299; recommended McQuarrie as chief of pediatrics (1930), 301; defended Wangensteen, 323; retired (1936), 325, 393

Lyon, Elias P., Memorial Laboratory (photo), 446; 445

MacCallum, A. B., 377

McCartney, James S., clinical-pathological conferences, 391; researches on cirrhoses of the liver, 390; on pulmonary embolism, 390

McClendon, Jesse F. (port.), 380; 404; appointed in 1914, 379; researches on goiter and Graves' disease, 379; on nutrition, 379; on pH measurement, 379; on vitamin deficiencies, 379; on ovarian hormone, 379–380; left university (1939), 400

McCollum, C. A., 126, 127

McDaniel, Orianna, 70; diphtheria work at Owatonna, 73; head of Pasteur Institute, 89; role in brucellosis research, 329, 331

McIntire, Ross T., 434

McIver, Monroe A., 309

McKelvey, John L. (port.), 353; appointed chief of obstetrics (1938), 352; medical training, 352; work at Peking Union Medical College, 352; research on gynecological cancer, 353–356

McKinlay, C.A.: description of infectious mononucleosis, 374

McKinley, Chauncey: role in organizing 26th General Hospital, 417

McKinley, John Charnley (port.), 322; defended Wangensteen, 321; appointed chief of medicine, 326

McLaren, A., 568

Maclaren, Archibald, 125, 206(n.4)

Maclean, Lloyd D., 472

McQuarrie, Irvine (port.), 301; (photo), 319, 471; 320, 475, 547; appointed chief of pediatrics (1930), 301, 346; life, 301–302; medical training, 302–303; researches on epilepsy, 346; on fluid balance, 347–348; on protein, 347–348; on liver disease, 348; identified role of liver, 348; used term "experiments of nature," 348, 369(n.102), 474; identified role of sodium in diabetes, 349; study of patient with Cushing's syndrome, 349

Madsen, Leo J., 444

Madsen Flats, 121–122

Magrath, C. Peter, 558, 559

Malaria: treated by 26th General Hospital staff, 422, 423–424

Mall, Franklin P., 285, 292

Malta fever, 331

Mann, Arthur T., 233; assisted at first clinic at university hospital, 117

Mann, Eugene L., 568

Mantoux test, 341, 342

Marsh, Fayette, 32

Marshall, William R., 58(n.45)

Martin, Franklin, 159

Masonic Cancer Relief Committee of Minnesota, 447

Masonic Memorial Hospital (photo), 448; 445–448, 460(n.80)
Masonic professorship of oncology, 447
Massachusetts Association of Boards of Health: study of diphtheria bacilli, 75
Matchan, Robert D., 568
Matson, Leroy E., 445, 447
Mayo, Charles H., as surgeon, 166; meetings on Mayo affiliation, 183; speaker for laying of cornerstone of Eustis Hospital, 276; death, 426
Mayo, Mrs. Charles H., 427
Mayo, William J. (port.), 162; 151, 289, 296; met with Wesbrook over proposals for new buildings (1908), 114–115; dedication of Elliot Memorial Hospital, 119; Historical Evening, 127; role in reorganization (1913), 145–146; refused to meet Greene's conditions (1913), 154; as regent received appeal for needed facilities (1914), 161–163; as surgeon, 165–166; meetings on Mayo affiliation, 168–169, 183; speech at legislative hearing on anti-Mayo affiliation bill (1917), 203–204; new plan of affiliation proposed (1917), 204–206; role in organizing medical unit in W.W.I, 213–215; invited Rowntree to Mayo Clinic, 236–237, 238; invited Robertson to Mayo Clinic, 238; Survey Committee interview (1921), 241–243; response to Survey Committee Report (1921), 244–245; question of paying patients, 253–254, 255; protested limited size of classes, 254; tried to discourage Todd gift, 254; refused to donate funds to medical school, 266–267, 272; response to complaints against Wangensteen, 322–323; death, 426
Mayo, Mrs. William J., 430
Mayo, William Worrall, 165, 203
Mayo affiliation: first mentioned (1913), 159; effect on medical school, 172, 173, 175, 179, 188, 197; opposition to, 173, 175–178, 180, 184–186, 188, 194; public discussion, 174, 177, 178–179, 181, 185, 186, 188, 201–202, 203–205; advocated, 174–175, 184; terms, 168, 204–206; first exchange of students, 191; call to terminate (1917), 200; defense by foundation (1917), 200–201
Mayo Clinic: new building (photo), 163; waiting room (photo), 164; pathology laboratory (photo), 167; 176, 429, 430; new building (1914), 163–165; medical practice, 165–166; began teaching program (1912), 167; administrative board negotiated with university, 168; beneficiary of Mayo Foundation endowment, 176, 200–201, 205–206, 426–427; development as a surgical center, 182–183; personnel at Base Hospital No. 26, 215, 217
Mayo Foundation for the Promotion of Medical Education and Research: origin of, 169–170, 173; Board of Regents to control endowment, 170, 200, 204, 205–206; confusion over terms of agreement, 181, 183; defense of affiliation (1917), 200–201; rapid growth of graduate education, 239; Survey Committee interview (1921), 241–243; on the Mayo memorial, 426, 430, 432
Mayo Memorial Auditorium, 435, 443
Mayo Memorial Building (photo), 442; ground breaking (photo), 440; fitting memorial for Doctors Mayo, 427–428; plans and architectural design, 428, 432, 434–435; building cost increases (1946), 435; (1947), 436; (1948–49), 437; (1950), 440; ground-breaking ceremony, 441; reduced in size to meet funding, 441; construction bids, 441–442; completed 1954, 442; dedication, 443; state funds needed for additional staff, 450. *See also:* Committee of Founders of the Mayo Memorial
Mayo Memorial Commission, 426–429
Mayo Properties Association, 266–267, 429, 430–431, 459(n.43)
Medawar P. B., 529
Medical Alumni Association: 196, 207(n.21); response to Mayo affiliation, 167–168, 171–172, 179; report on medical school (1920), 238–240;

INDEX

critical of Dean Lyon (1920), 239; (1930), 305-306; Survey Committee Report (1921) on the alumni report, 241-246; treated Minnesota Medical Foundation, 443-444
Medical Center, 1955 (photo), 545
Medical Chemistry Building (photo), 62; Chemistry laboratory (photo), 62; 60-61
Medical colleges: 1870s, 13, 14-16; 1880s, 16-17; in Minneapolis and St. Paul, 20-22; 19th century American, 23-24
Medical education: 1850s, 8; 1860s, 10; 1870s, 12-16, 23; apprenticeships, 13; qualifications for students, 13; effect of medical practice act (1887), 33-34; subject of Osler's dedicatory speech, 52-54. *See also*: Clinical instruction; Curriculum
Medical Hall (photo), 53; construction (1892), 49-50; dedication (4 Oct. 1892), 51-54; name changed to Millard Hall, 105. *See also:* Millard Hall
Medical library: gifts from faculty, 92, 94; established (1895), 92-93; Millard gift, 92-93; His library acquired, 93; size of collections, 93; losses in fire (1909), 129. *See also:* Bio-medical Library
Medical practice act (1883), 32-33; (1887), 33-34
Medical school: staff involved in W.W.I, 213-214, 233; inability to keep clinical teachers (1920s), 282, 288, 295; tuberculosis among students, 341, 343-345; need for expansion in 1960s, 546; enrollment changes in 1970s, 555. *See also:* College of Medicine and Surgery [1888-1913]
Medical societies, 7-8, 10-11
Medicine, Department of: Rowntree appointed head (1916), 191; resignations over Mayo affiliation (1916), 191; Blake leaves, 236; White appointed head (1920), 238, 283, 284; Fahr appointed (1921), 293; Berglund appointed chief, 297; McKinley appointed chief (1932), 326; Watson appointed chief (1942), 547. *See also:* Internal Medicine, Division of
Medtronic, Inc., 520, 521, 522
Merriam, William R., 51, 58(n.45)
Merrill, B. J., 25
Merrill, John P., 530
Mesobiliviolin, 327
Metabolic studies, use of radioactive isotopes, 404
Metabolism, basal, 351-352, 380
Meyer, Karl F., 302, 331
Meyer, Robert (port.), 354; 352, 353-355
Michelson, Henry E., 325
Microbiology, Department of: Syverton appointed head (1948), 468. *See also*: Bacteriology, Department of
Millard, Caroline Swain, 36
Millard, George S., 92
Millard, John Jay, 92
Millard, Perry H. (ports.), 37, 78; 100, 564, 567; role in creating the College of Medicine (1883-87), 23-24; drafted medical practice act, 1887, 32-34; role in establishing the medical school, 34-36; conflict with Hewitt, 35; appointed dean of medical school, 36, 77; European experience, 36, 65; life, 36-37, 56(n.18), 76-78; role in construction of Medical Hall, 49-50; funding of dispensary, 50-51; appointed professor of surgery, 63; role in management changes in State Board of Health, 68-69; used x-rays in surgery, 76; final illness, 77-78; funeral, 78-79; gave personal library to university, 92-93; Medical Hall renamed Millard Hall, 105
Millard Hall (old), formerly Medical Hall, 105; fire (1909), 129
Millard Hall (photo), 133; 427, 435, 565; cornerstone laid, 120; increased cost to build, 133, 135; remodeled (1955), 450
Millet, Melvin C., 166
Millikan, Robert A., 292
Minneapolis Board of Public Welfare: new city hospital contemplated, 256-257, 261, 267-268; application for funds to Rockefeller board,

263–264, 271; Harrington as commissioner, 332–335; tuberculosis health problem, 333; converted Lymanhurst into the Sister Kenny Institute, 364
Minneapolis City Hospital, 47, 55, 96, 197. *See also:* Minneapolis General Hospital
Minneapolis Civic and Commerce Association, 192, 193, 196
Minneapolis College of Physicians and Surgeons, 21, 126, 127
Minneapolis Free Homeopathic Dispensary, 47
Minneapolis General Hospital, 243, 245, 333, 350, 359, 474; new hospital contemplated, 256–257, 259, 267–268; application for funds to Rockefeller board, 263–264, 271; Fahr at, 294–295, 303; ward for polio patients, 360–361; clinical-pathological conferences, 391. *See also:* Minneapolis City Hospital
Minneapolis Homeopathic Hospital, 22, 29(n.42), 58(n.44)
Minneapolis Surgical Society: paper on use of suction following abdominal surgery (1932), 316
Minnesota Academy of Medicine: results of Widal test presented (1896), 71
Minnesota Cancer Society, 445
Minnesota College Hospital (photo), 19; 17–20, 21
Minnesota Experiment (photo), 409; 408–409
Minnesota Homeopathic Medical College, 22, 35, 45, 58(n.44)
Minnesota Hospital College (photo), 21; 35, 50, 127, 564; organized, 20–21
Minnesota Medical Association, 558
Minnesota Medical Foundation, 431, 443–445, 455
Minnesota Medical Society, 7, 10, 38
Minnesota State Board of Health, 35, 38, 45; created (1872), 13–14, 28(n.22); offices in Laboratory of Medical Sciences, 63–65; appointed Wesbrook, 68; management changes, 68–69; testing kit designed for Widal test, 71–72; typhoid fever epidemics, 72; diphtheria epidemics, 73–75; Pasteur Institute for rabies treatment, 89. *See also:* Minnesota State Department of Health
Minnesota State Board of Medical Examiners, 22, 38, 77
Minnesota State Department of Health: role in brucellosis research, 329, 331
Minnesota State Homeopathic Institute, 22, 45
Minnesota State Insane Examining Board, 45
Minnesota State Medical Association, 36, 163, 196, 260; joint meeting with Medical Alumni Association (1920), 238–240; Committee on Medical Education report (1922), 246
Minnesota State Medical Society, 10–11, 45; advocated regulation of medical practice, 13–14
Minnesota State Legislature: buildings appropriation (1891), 50; appropriation for Laboratory of Medical Sciences (1895), 64, 68; appropriation for Institute of Public Health and Pathology (1903), 88; bill to fund care of crippled children (1897), 89–90; visit to Hospital for Crippled Children, 91–92; Elliot Memorial Hospital Bill (1907), 111; appropriation for anatomy building and medical science building, 115; appropriation for land for Gilbert Plan (1909), 115; cut in university appropriation (1911), 142; Guilford Bill, 181–182, 183, 184; hearing on bill to dissolve Mayo affiliation (1917), 203–204; approved Burton's building plan, 236; emergency appropriation (1921), 236; created Committee of Founders of the Mayo Memorial, 429; state funds requested for Mayo memorial, (1945), 432–434; (1947), 435–436; (1949), 437–438; (1951), 441; funds requested for bio-medical library, (1952, 1955), 450; (1957), 451; appropriation for Health Sciences A, 549–550; appropriation for Health Sciences B-C, 553; appropriation for Health Sciences F, 554; passed bonding bill for hospital (1981), 558

INDEX

Minnesota State Public Health School for Dependent and Neglected Children, Owatonna: diphtheria outbreaks, 73–74
Minnesota Territorial Legislature: established university (1851), 6
Minnesota Territory: early physicians, 6–7
Minot, Charles S., 137
Minot, George, 328
Moe, Gordon K.: research on heart failure, 395
Monaco, Anthony, 532
Moore, George E. (photo), 469; research on fluorescence in malignant tissue, 468–469; on radioactive substances to detect tumors, 468–469
Moore, James E. (ports.), 99, 130; 92, 94, 566, 567; expressed need for a university hospital, 82; role in university dispensary, 82–83; work with crippled children, 90; appointed professor of surgery, 98, 106(n.19); life, 98–100; appointed professor of orthopedic surgery, 99–100; antiseptic and aseptic surgery, 100; as teacher, 100; Elliot Hospital site committee, 112; effect of Anatomy Building fire (1908), 115; first clinic at university hospital, 117; chief of surgery division in hospital, 117; dedication of Elliot Hospital, 119; injured at Millard Hall (1910), 129–130; committee on reorganization (1913), 147; advocated graduate program in surgery (1914), 159, 160; met with Regent Mayo on building needs (1914), 163; committee on Mayo affiliation, 167–170; death, 233
Moore, James T., Historical Evening, 127
Moos (Malcolm) Health Sciences Tower (Health Sciences A) (photo), 550
Morrill, James L. (photo), 440; (port.), 439; appointed president (1945), 434; appreciation of Cowling's work, 438; role in securing state funds for Mayo memorial, 438–439; role in building fund for medical library, 450
Morton, John J., 311–312

Mueller, August, 472
Mueller, Friedrich, 326
Mullin, Gerald T., 444
Multiple screen oxygenator (photo), 491
Murphy, John B., 181
Murphy, John Henry, 7
Murray, George R., 52
Murray, Gordon, 541
Murray, John G., 430
Murray, Joseph, 530
Mussey, Robert D., 219, 351
Myers, A. W., 181
Myers, Jay Arthur (port.), 335; ill with tuberculosis, 334–335; medical education, 334–335; medical director at Lymanhurst, 335; research on tuberculosis at Lymanhurst, 336–343; screening for tuberculosis among university students, 340, 343–344; research on tuberculosis among medical personnel, 341–346; evicted from Lymanhurst (1942), 364; role in Variety Club Heart Hospital, 483

Najarian, John (port.), 535; appointed chief of surgery (1967), 533; medical training, 533; transplant regimen reduced mortality, 533–534; production of purified antilymphocytic globulin, 535–536; kidney transplantation on diabetics, 536–537
National Cancer Institute, 460(n.56), 465
National Foundation for Infantile Paralysis, 357, 358, 360, 361, 362
National Heart Institute, 445, 460(n.46)
National Institutes of Health: construction funds available, 451, 455
Nelson, Benjamin F., 115
Nelson, E.: research on actinomycetes, 385
Nelson, Russell M., 490
Nervous and Mental Diseases, Division of. *See:* Medicine, Department of
Newton, Francis, 289
Northrop, Cyrus O., 49, 51, 77; role in establishing the medical school, 34, 38; Millard memorial service, 79; admissions standards of medical school,

103; testimonial banquet for Ritchie, 105; Historical Evening 127
Nunn, William L., 461(n.80)
Nurses: Erdmann as superintendent, 117, 118; Powell as superintendent, 118; need for residence, 122, 161–162
Nursing school: hindered by Mayo affiliation, 173; tuberculosis among students, 341, 343–346
Nutrition: fatty acid deficiency disease (photo), 403; research by McClendon, 379; fatty acids, 402

O'Brien, Alice, 456
Obstetrics and Gynecology, Department of: Litzenberg appointed chief (1913), 350; research 1910s to 1930s, 351–356; McKelvey appointed chief (1938), 352
O'Connor, Basil, 358, 360
Offerdahl, Serena, 121
Ogden, B. Harvie, 568
Ohage, Justus, 4, 566
Opelz, Gerhard, 536
Open heart surgery: using cross circulation (diag.), 504; first successful (photo), 505; second patient (photos), 506; using bubble oxygenator (photo), 513; blood flow from Thebesian veins, 490; used multiple screen oxygenator (5 April 1951), 490; methods worked out on dogs, 490, 491, 492, 494–497, 498–500, 501–503, 510, 518, 519, 523; Lillehei tried procedures on cadavers, 492–493; significance of rate of azygos flow, 495–497; first performed under direct vision (2 Sept. 1952), 499; to correct atrial septal defect, 499; ventricular fibrillation as cause of death, 499; heart block as cause of death, 499, 508; cross circulation used, 503–504, 506, 508; for ventricular septal defects, 503–504, 506, 512; research on bubble oxygenator, 509; used Model I Oxygenator, 511–513; cross circulation abandoned, 512; used Model III Oxygenator, 514; mortality, 516–517, 523; treatment of heart block during or after, 517, 519, 521, 523
Ophthalmology: graduate program proposed, 160
Orr, Thomas G., 309
Orthopedic surgery: clinical instruction at Hospital for Crippled Children, 90, 92
O'Shaughnessy, Ignatius A., 430, 451, 452, 455
Osler, William: dedication of Medical Hall (1892), 50, 52–54, 65; attended Millard in illness, 77–78
Ospedale Militare Lorenzo Bonomo, Bari, Italy (photo), 423
Otology, graduate program proposed (1914), 160
Owen, Sidney M., 115
Owens, Jay, 19
Owre, Alfred, 129

Pacemaker: first pulse generator (photo), 520; first battery-operated transistor designed for clinical use (photo), 522; first battery-operated transistor model (photo), 522; 517; tested on dogs, 518, 519; small, battery powered, 520; bipolar used, 521; first implantable used, 521; used in all patients with postoperative heart block, 523
Paine, John R., 316, 494
Pancreas transplantation: research at university, 537; in human subjects, 538–539; statistics, 539
Papermaster, Ben, 473
Paratyphoid epidemic, 275
Park, Edwards A., 302
Partridge, George H., 264
Pasteur Institute. *See:* Minnesota State Board of Health, Pasteur Institute
Patent ductus arteriosus: surgery for, 481, 482, 492, 517
Pathology: revised curriculum (1898), 100–101
Pathology, Department of, 275; Robertson moved to Mayo Clinic, 238; E. T. Bell appointed head (1921), 238, 389; Robertson appointed head

(1913), 381; research in, 1913–41, 389–391
Pearce, Richard M., 237–238, 261
Pediatrics, Department of, 275; Sedgwick chief of, 257–258; Pirquet appointed chief (1923), 259–260; Schlutz appointed chief (1924), 285; McQuarrie appointed chief (1930), 301, 346; research in 1930s, 346–350; interdepartmental cooperation, 350; Anderson appointed chief (1954), 547
Peeler, D. B., 346
Peking Union Medical College, 297, 326, 352
Penicillin: used in streptococcal infections, 474; tested at university (1942), 476; antibiotic-resistant strains of staphylococci, 476–477
Perry, Mabel: research on fluorine content of tooth enamel, 405
Peters, Howard, 394
Peterson, Harold O., 465, 547
Peterson, Osler L., 546
Pettijohn, John J., 245, 246
Peyton, William T. (port.), 467; 307, 467, 469; research on fiber tracts, 372–373
pH measurement: research by McClendon, 379
Pharmacology, Department of: losses in fire (1909), 129; research in, 1913–41, 391–393; appointed Hirschfelder head (1913), 392
Pharmacology, Division of: appointed Brown (1907), 391
Philadelphia Academy of Surgery, Gross Prize, 323
Phillips, Elisabeth, 345
Phillips, Jay, 456, 549
Phillips-Wangensteen Building (Health Sciences B-C) (photo), 554
Phillips-Wangensteen Research Laboratory, 549
Physical Therapy, Division of: Knapp appointed director (1939), 359; Kottke appointed director (1947), 364
Physiological Chemistry, Department of: Armstrong appointed head (1946), 404

Physiological Chemistry, Division of: Burr appointed director (1940), 400, 404
Physiology: instruction in (1888), 38–40, 41; (1893), 61
Physiology, cardiac: research in, 1913–41, 393–395
Physiology, Department of: research in, 1913–41, 377–381; under Lyon and Scott, 377, 378; Visscher appointed head (1936), 393; Keys appointed (1937), 406. *See also:* Cancer Biology, Division of
Pierce, Howard, 475
Pierce, J.C., 472
Pillsbury, Alfred F., 93
Pillsbury, Charles C., 93
Pillsbury, Frederick C., 58(n.44)
Pillsbury, John S., 49, 51, 63, 93; family contributions to Elliot Hospital site committee, 112
Pillsbury, John Sargent, gift for rare medical books, 455
Pirquet, Clemens von: pediatric work 258–259; accepted appointment at Minnesota, 259–260; resignation, 260–261, 262
Pirquet test, 258–259, 337–338, 339, 340–341, 343; administered to university freshmen (1928), 340, 343–344
Pituitary gland: research on, 372–373
Platou, Erling S., 444
Plummer, Henry, 164, 166, 173
Pohl, John, 360, 371(n.132)
Poliomyelitis: traditional treatment, 358, 359; Sister Kenny method of treatment, 358–360; Kenny method adopted by National Foundation, 362; teaching program established for Kenny method, 362–364
Porphyria: research by Watson, 327–328
Potts, Thomas Reid, 7
Potts, Willis J., 525(n.22)
Powell, Louise M. (port.), 118; appointed superintendent of nurses (1910), 118; on need for nurses' residence, 122; life, 123(n.27)
Powell Hall, 558
Powers, Grover F., 302
Preventive Medicine and Public Health,

Department of, 247. *See also:* School of Public Health
Private practice controversy, 193–196, 198, 253, 284–285; Columbia University's experience, 289
Protein, serum, 347–348
Public health: vital statistics required, 13; board of health created (1872), 13–14. *See also:* Minnesota State Board of Public Health
Pulmonary artery: stenosis of, 506
Pulmonary hypertension, 481–482, 517
Pulmonary valvular stenosis, 494
Pyorrhea: research by Henrici and Hartzell, 381–384

Quervain, Fritz de, 296
Quie, Albert, 560
Quie, Paul: appointed to pediatrics (1958), 477; researches on defenses against staphylococcal infection, 477; on fungal septicemia associated with intravenous catheterization, 477–478; on staphylococcal cell wall, 478; Hill-Quie Syndrome, 478

Rabies: distribution in Minnesota (illus.), 69; in Minnesota (1906), 89; Pasteur Institute at Minnesota State Board of Health, 89
Radiation therapy: for gynecological cancer, 354–356; 465
Radioactive isotopes: use of in metabolic studies, 404
Radiology, Department of: Peterson appointed, 465
Radiology, Division of: Rigler named chief, 273–274, 299; changes in (1920s), 298–300; development under Rigler, 300–301; research in 1930s, 356–357
Rammelkamp, Charles H., 474
Ramsey, Alexander, 8, 58(n.45)
Ramsey, Walter, 350
Ramsey County Medical Society: on the Mayo affiliation, 177
Rasmussen, Andrew T. (port.), 373; 349, 372, 395(n.2); researches on fiber tracts, 372–373; on pituitary gland, 372–373
Rea, Charles, 487
Red Lake Indian Reservation, 474–475
Reed, Charles A., 50, 58(n.58)
Rees, Soren P., 195–196
Reid, Mont R., 288, 290
Reid, Whitelaw, 435
Reimann, Hobart A., 326, 327
Reiner, Joel K., 36
Remington, W. P. (photo), 224; 217, 231
Respiratory irregularities: research by Gresheimer, 380
Rheumatic fever, 391, 473–476, 482
Rheumatic heart disease, 391, 475, 482, 483
Rice, Edmund, 58(n.45)
Richardson, Senator, 426, 429
Richdorf, Lawrence, 261
Ricker, George E., 568
Rigert, Joe, 558
Riggs, C. Eugene, 125, 567
Rigler, Leo (port.), 300; 326, 375, 486, 547; appointed director of radiology (1927), 273–274; medical training, 298–299; European experience, 299; interest in radiology, 299; reorganization of radiology, 300–301; use of x-ray to detect pleural effusion, 356; research in diagnostic radiology, 356–357; role in organizing 26th General Hospital, 417
Ritchie, Arthur F., 38, 39, 47, 567
Ritchie, Harry P.: used Widal test, 71
Ritchie, Parks (port.), 83; 567; appointed dean of College of Medicine and Surgery, 82; admissions standards of medical school, 103; faculty opposition, 103–104; resignation as dean, 103–104; accomplishments as dean, 104; testimonial banquet (1906), 105; chief of obstetrics division in hospital, 117; on reorganization of faculty, 125; Historical Evening, 127; letter of resignation (1913), 147; death, 147
Robertson, Harold E., 233, 238, 389; appointed head of pathology (1913), 381
Rockefeller General Education Board, 237–238, 431; funds sought for

hospital buildings, 257, 261, 268, 271; response to request for funds (1923), 263–264
Rockne, A. J., 433
Roswell Park Memorial Institute, 535
Roth, Norman A., 521
Rothrock, John L., 70
Rowntree, Leonard G. (port.), 192; appointed chief of Department of Medicine, 191; on need for larger hospital and faculty, 193–194, 283; reasons for move to Mayo Clinic, 236–237, 238, 248(n.6), 262, 282; salary, 284
Ruge, Carl, 352

St. Barnabas Hospital (Minneapolis), 20
St. Joseph's Hospital (St. Paul), 10, 13, 47
St. Mary's Hospital (Minneapolis) (photo), 97; 96, 97
St. Paul Children's Hospital, 359, 482
St. Paul City and County Hospital. *See:* City and County Hospital (St. Paul)
St. Paul Medical College, 35, 50, 82, 127, 564; organized (1878), 14–16, 22
Saint Paul Salvation Army Home, 350
St. Paul School for Medical Instruction, 13, 14
Sauerbruch, Ferdinand, 297
Scammon, Richard E. (port.), 306; 372; as teacher, 305; appointed dean of College of Medical Sciences (1931), 306; Wangensteen controversy, 318; resigned as dean, 324–325; research on human growth, 373
Scarlet fever, 474
Schauta, Friedrich, 352
Schlutz, Frederic W. M.: appointed chief of pediatrics, 285; resigned (1930), 301
Schmid, Rudi, 327
Schmidt, Garden & Erickson, 435
School of Public Health: received endowment from Mayo Properties Association, 430–431; Rockefeller funding requested, 431; established (1943), 431; to have space in Mayo memorial, 435, 442
Schroeder, E. C., 331

Schwartz, Samuel P., 327
Schwarz, Robert, 530
Scott, Frederick H. (port.), 378; 393; researches on secretory function of neurons, 377; on effects of hypercapnia and hypoxia, 378
Sedgwick, Julius P. (port.), 258; 149, 233, 350; practice and chief of pediatrics, 257–258; identified Bang's disease in children, 331
Senkler, Albert E. (port.), 95; 94, 567; life, 106(n.40)
Shapiro, Morse J. (port.), 484; 362; research on rheumatic heart disease, 482; study of patent ductus arteriosus, 482, 492; role in Variety Club Heart Hospital, 483
Shaw, E. B., 331
Shimonek, Anton, 4
Shimp, Byron W., 431–432, 435, 436, 458(n.25), 459(n.37)
Shipley, Arthur E., 65
Shriners' Hospital for Crippled Children (Minneapolis), 350, 359
Shumway, Norman, 523, 540
Simmons, Richard L., 535–536
Simpson, *Sir* James Y., 28(n.15)
Sivertsen, Ivar, 343
Slater, Sidney A., 338
Smallpox epidemic (1924–25), 275
Smith, Philip E., 302
Smith, Vespasian, 28(n.22)
Snyder, Fred P., 183, 190, 203–204, 253, 265
Spaulding, Salathiel M., 568
Speckman, E. V., 319
Spencer, E. A., 568
Spencer, Edward C., 18
Spink, Wesley W. (port.), 330; 486; appointed to Department of Medicine (1937), 328; researches on trichinosis, 329; on brucellosis, 329–332; used isolation unit to control staphylococcal infections in hospital, 477
Staehalin, Rudolph, 293
Staley, John S., 231
Stanford, Edward B., 451
Staphylococcal infections: antibiotic-resistant strains, 476–477; controlled by isolation units, 477; role of cell wall, 478

INDEX

Staples, Franklin, 13
Starling, Ernest, 377, 393, 399(n.77)
Starvation: research by Keys, 408–409
Starzl, Thomas, 531–532, 541
Stassen, Harold E., 426, 429, 468
State Hospital for the Crippled and Deformed (St. Paul), 202
Steffes, Al W., 483
Stem, Allen H., 58(n.58)
Stenstrom, Annette, 273–274
Stenstrom, Karl Wilhelm (port.), 355; 273–274, 465, 486; radiation therapy in gynecological cancer, 354–356; treatment of Hodgkin's disease, 356
Sterility: caused by low basal metabolism, 351–352
Stewart, Chester (photo), 319; 335
Stewart, J. Clark (port.), 49; 47, 48, 50, 63, 568; role in bringing Wesbrook to Minnesota, 65; made professor of the principles of surgery (1900), 98
Stewart, Jacob H. (port.), 10; 8, 9–10; interest in medical education, 10, 12–13
Stinchfield, Augustus W., 166
Stokes-Adams attacks, 517, 519, 521, 523
Stone, Alexander J. (port.), 12; 4–5, 38, 566, 567; interest in medical education, 12–13, 14, 22; on reorganization of faculty, 125; Historical Evening, 127
Stone, Royal A. and Olive W., 444
Storer, Horatio R., 15
Strachauer, Arthur C. (port.), 288; 285, 286; chief of surgery, 282, 291, 295; resignation, 282, 288; defended Wangensteen, 323
Streptococcal infections, 473–476
Streptococcus viridans, cause of pyorrhea, 382–384
Strickler, D. A., 568
Students' Health Service (photo), 276; 275–276, 325; screening for tuberculosis, 340, 343–344
Subcommittee on hospital extension: report on need for larger hospital (1916), 197–198
Sundwall, John, 275, 343
Surgery: first gallbladderectomy (1886), 4; first appendectomy (1887), 4; antiseptic method used (1885), 4, 95; carbolic acid spray first used (1882), 19; early use of x-rays, 76; first at university hospital (1909), 117–118; graduate program proposed, 159
Surgery, Department of: Strauchauer chief of surgery, 282, 291, 295; problem of finding a new chief (1926), 289–291, 295; Wangensteen appointed chief, 295, 297; research during 1930s, 307–316, 323–324; residency program, 486–487; weekly surgical review conferences, 487; cardiac training center, 515–516; Najarian appointed chief, 533
Survey Committee on Medical Alumni Association report (1921), 241–246
Sutherland, David, 539
Swain, Caroline E. *See:* Millard, Caroline Swain
Sweeney, Arthur, 184
Sweetser, H. B., 94, 188
Swenson, Oscar, 433
Szlapka, Thaddeus L., 223

Taufic, Mansur: research on hypothermia, 498–499; performed with Lewis and Varco first open heart direct vision surgery (2 Sept. 1952), 499
Taussig, Helen B., 483
Terasaki, Paul, 536
Tetanus: Wesbrook's study of, 65
Tetralogy of Fallot: first patient with surgical correction (photos), 507; 483, 493, 494, 505–508, 517
Therapeutic Radiology, Department of, 559–560, 561
Thevenet, André, 519
Thomas, Gilbert J., 223
Thomas, Lewis, 474
Thompson, D'Arcy, 385–386
Thompson, Willis H., 347
Thye, Edward J., 431, 433, 434, 436, 451
Thymus: role of, 472–473
Todd, Frank C. (port.), 252; 87; Elliot Memorial Hospital committee, 113; advised sale of University Dispensary; 138–139; advocated graduate pro-

INDEX

gram in ophthalmalogy and otology (1914), 160; death, 233

Todd, Mrs. Frank C., 251, 253, 254

Todd Memorial Clinic (photo), 274; self-supporting through private patients, 252; Todd and Gale gifts received, 254; fund-raising efforts, 254–255, 273; Todd amphitheater, 273

Tooth decay: preventive role of fluoride, 404–405

Tooth infections: research by Henrici and Hartzell, 381–385

Trask, Walter, 109

Traxler, C. J., 188

Tuberculosis: as cause for crippled children (photos), 91; as cause for crippled children, 89–90; among medical profession, 94, 341, 343, 345–346; among medical students, 94, 341, 343, 345; screening among students, 276, 340, 343–344; in Minneapolis among children, 333–335; long-term study, 334, 341–343; role of Lymanhurst in treating infected children, 336–342; detection by x-rays, 338, 342, 344–345, 356–357; course of infection in children, 338–339, 341; in infants, 339; in teenagers, 340; treatment for children, 342; effect of reinfection, 342–343, 345; effect of sanatoria, 342–343; identification of first-infection cases, 344–345; treatment for medical students, 344–345; isolation techniques needed to protect personnel, 345–346; research on blood calcium levels, 381

Tularemia: research by Henrici and Green, 386–388

Tuohy, Edward L., 207(n.21), 460(n.55); committee on reorganization (1913), 147; on Guilford Bill, 182

26th General Hospital, Assi Ameur, North Africa (photo), 419; looking southeast (photo), 420; Nurses' laundry (photo), 421; 26th General Hospital at Assi Ameur, North Africa (photo), 423; 486; organized, 417; called to active duty, 417; farewell banquet, 418; at Fort Sill for training, 418; arrived in North Africa, 419; built hospital at Assi Ameur, 419–420; patients at Assi Ameur, 420–421; medical cases, 421–424; mortality rates, 422, 423; moved to Bari, Italy, 422; patients at Bari, 422–424; received Meritorious Unit Service Plaque, 424; staff returned home, 424

Typhoid fever, 22, 29(n.42); standardized test for, 70–72; in Minneapolis (1897), 72; (1887), 96; medical students infected, 93–94

Ulrich, Henry L., 299, 349

Undulant fever, 332

United States Public Health Service, 460(n.56), 460(n.80)

United States Surgeon General's Consultant Group on Medical Education, 544

University Dispensary [Seven Corners] (photo), 87; need to enlarge, 87–88, 149, 161, 202; visited by Vincent (1912), 136

University Free Homeopathic Dispensary, 47

University of Minnesota: founded, 6; enrollment increase, 1911–1919, 235, 236

University of Minnesota Hospital, ca. 1930 (photo), 317; staff (photo), 319; 1986 (photo), 560; need for medical school, 82; Elliot bequest, 104; free medical care (1907), 111, 112, 239; opened in temporary quarters (1909), 117; Baldwin first superintendent (1910), 119; need for clinical facilities for nervous and mental diseases (1912), 134–135; (1914), 171; need for clinical facilities for children's diseases (1912), 134–135; (1914), 171; need for additional facilities (1914), 161–162; private fund raising, 192; per diem patients, 192–196, 197–200, 253, 277; need to enlarge (1916), 193–196; private patients, 193–196, 198, 253, 277, 353; Burton's attempt to enlarge hospital, 237–238; committee for building funds (1925), 267–268; Christian Cancer Hospital, 273; Todd Memorial Clinic, 273; Todd amphitheater, 273; Eustis Hospital, 274; students' health service (1927), 274–275; outpatient department (1927), 274–275; increased census (1929), 277–278; Dunn director (1932-35), 318, 325; tuberculin test required on admission (1935), 345; isolation techniques developed for tuberculous patients, 345–346; ward for polio patients, 361; staphylococcal infections controlled by isolation unit, 477; need for renovation in 1960s, 547–548; made autonomous administrative unit (1970), 557; inadequacy for 1980s medicine and teaching, 557; board of governors established (1974), 557; first patients transferred (25 April 1986), 561. *See also:* Elliot Memorial Hospital

University of Minnesota Medical Center, 1955 (photo), 545

Vanderburgh, Charles E., 18
Vanderhorck, Max P., 567
Vannier, Marion L., 233
Varco, Richard, responsible for patent ductus and Blalock-Taussig procedures, 494; performed with Lewis and Taufic first open heart direct vision surgery (2 Sept. 1952), 499; and F. John Lewis, with cooling blanket and machine (photo), 500
Variety Club Children's Hospital, 561
Variety Club Heart Hospital (photo), 485; 364, 443, 474, 525(n.8), 525(n.9)
Variety Club of the Northwest, 524–525(n.7), 552
Variety Club, Tent 12, 483–485, 525(n.8)
Vaughan, Victor C., 173, 180–181, 241–242
Ventricular fibrillation, 499, 503, 517
Ventricular septal defect, 503–504, 506, 512, 517

Veterans of Foreign Wars Cancer Research Institute, 449
Vice-president for health sciences affairs, 551, 557
Vincent, George E. (port.), 131; 292, 565; dedication of Elliot Memorial Hospital, 119; life, 130–132; inauguration as president, 132–133; responses to plan for new medical campus, 133–139; executive faculty presented needs of college (1912), 134; opinion of Gilbert plan of campus, 136, 445; opinion of Lee, 137; description by Gray, 140(n.37), reorganization of College of Medicine and Surgery, 141, 143–150; took control of school away from Wesbrook (1913), 143–144; criteria for faculty, 146–147; on funding for medical school buildings, 148; on Wesbrook's resignation, 149; refused to meet Greene's conditions (1913), 154; role in the Mayo affiliation, 167–168, 169, 180, 190, 203; committee on Mayo affiliation, 167–170; meetings on Mayo affiliation, 169, 172, 183; effect of his administration, 235; as president of Rockefeller Foundation visited medical school, 237–238; negotiations for Rockefeller gift for hospital buildings, 257, 261, 272–273; letter to Mayo seeking funds (1924-25), 266
Vincent, Mrs. George E., 131–132
Visscher, Maurice B. (port.), 394; 453, 486, 547; appointed head of physiology (1936), 393; medical training, 393–394; researches on efficiency of the heart, 393–394; on heart failure, 394–395; on mouse cancer milk factor, 467–468; physiology-surgery conference, 395, 487; role in surgical residency program, 395, 487, 523; role in McClendon's departure, 400; efforts to raise Burr's salary, 404
Vital statistics, registration required (1871), 13
Vitamin deficiencies, research by McClendon, 379
Vitamins: research on supplemental vitamins by Keys and Henschel, 407

Wade, E. M., research on tularemia, 387
Walsh, Ellard A., 418
Wangensteen, Owen H. (port.), 290; (photo), 319; "the chief" (port.), 488; 289, 335, 375, 449, 453, 486, 509, 516, 547; appointed to Department of Surgery, 290; life, 291; medical training, 293–294; taught by Fahr, 293–295; appointed chief of surgery, 295, 297; European experience (1927–28), 295–297; encounter with Berglund, 297–298; research developed (1930), 307; vision of surgery department (1930), 307; part-time faculty deprived of salaries, 307; surgery for cancer, 316, 319–320; controversy with Dunn and Scammon, 318–323; offered to resign (1933), 321, 323; receipt of Gross Prize, 323; research on intestinal obstruction, 308–316, 323–324; benefits of suction tube in abdominal surgery, 323–324; physiology-surgery conference, 395, 487; role in organizing 26th General Hospital, 417; president of Minnesota Medical Foundation, 444; fund raising for laboratories (Union Street), 451; funds received from I. A. O'Shaughnessy, 451, 452, 455; requested assistance of Cowling for library building funds, 452, 455, 461(n.90); fund raising for medical library, 455, 456; illness (1962), 456; developed technique of aseptic anastomosis, 463; surgery for cancer of alimentary canal, 463–465; advocated "the second look," 465; surgery for patent ductus arteriosus, 481, 482, 524(n.4); philosophy for training surgeons, 486–487, 516, 523; weekly surgical review conferences, 487; Phillips-Wangensteen Research Laboratory, 549; and George D. Eitel (photo), 296
Wangensteen, Owen H., Historical Library of Biology and Medicine, 462(n.121)
"Wangensteen alleys," 486

Wangensteen suction apparatus (illus.), 314
Wangensteen suction sets, 421, 486
Wangensteen suction tube in use (photo), 315
Wangensteen's and Leven's diagrams of alimentary canal (illus.), 311
Wannamaker, Lewis (port.), 475; researches on streptococcal infections, 473–476; on rheumatic fever, 473–476; on acute nephritis associated with streptococcal infections, 474–475; on antistaphylokinase with Paul Quie, 477; identified type 49 streptococcus, 475; appointed career investigator of American Heart Association, 476
Warden, Herbert (port.), 501; researches on cardiac by-pass surgery on dogs, 498; on cross circulation, 501–503
Washburn, William D., 58(n.44)
Watson, Cecil (port.), 328; 453, 486, 547; medical training, 326–327; research on bile pigments and porphyrins, 326–328; appointed head of Division of Internal Medicine (1936), 327; appointed chief of medicine (1942), 547
Watson, Frank, 493–495, 501
Webber, C. C., 362
Weber, Adolph, 293
Weirich, William, 518, 521
Welch, William H., 55; on the quality of laboratories at Minnesota, 84–85
Wells, Charles L., 94, 567
Wells, *Sir* Thomas Spencer, 28(n.15)
Wesbrook, Frank F. (ports.), 67, 142; 129, 381, 564, 565; cholera and tetanus work at Cambridge, 65; appointed to faculty, 65, 69; teaching duties (1896), 67–68; appointed to State Board of Health, 68–69; rabies identification in Minnesota, 69–70; typhoid fever identification, 70–72; diphtheria bacilli identification, 73–75; diphtheria epidemics investigations, 74–75; anthrax bacillus work, 75; additional laboratory equipment (1899), 84; European trip (1904), 88; planned Institute of Pub-

lic Health and Pathology, 88; revised curriculum for bacteriology and pathology (1898), 100–101; appointed dean, 104; need for a university hospital, 105; need for expanded medical campus, 109–110; Elliot Hospital site committee, 112; conferred with Mayo on proposal for new buildings (1908), 114–115; dedication of Elliot Memorial Hospital, 119; cornerstone laid for new Millard Hall, 120; reorganization of College of Medicine and Surgery into administrative departments (1908), 124–126; Historical Evening, 126–127; merger with Hamline medical school (1908), 126–127; response to Vincent's reorganization, 141; budget cut (1911), 142–143; resignation, 144, 145; committee on reorganization (1913), 147; death, 230–231

Wesbrook Hall. *See:* Laboratory of Medical Sciences

Westerman, John, 558

Wheaton, Charles A., 19, 63, 100, 566, 567; interest in medical education, 22; appointed professor of surgery, 94

Whipple, George H., 302, 308–309, 311, 365(n.7)

White, J. C., 309–310

White, S. Marx (port.), 217; 150, 152, 286, 325, 418; on reorganization by Vincent, 143; on regents' gag order, 190; on need for larger hospital, 194; subcommittee on hospital extension, 197–200; role in Base Hospital No. 26, 216, 218, 219, 223, 231; appointed chief of Department of Medicine (1920), 238; interest in Todd Memorial Clinic, 253, 254; resignation, 282, 297; on limited private practice, 283

Widal, Fernand: diagnostic test for typhoid fever, 71

Wilkie, David, 297

Williamson, Alonzo P., 46

Williamson, George, 359

Wilson, Louis B., 137; study of kidney tissues, 61; rabies research for State Board of Health, 69–70; typhoid fever identification, 70–71; designed testing kit for Widal test, 72; diphtheria research, 75; committee on reorganization (1913), 147; developed pathology collection at Mayo Clinic, 166; on Mayo affiliation, 178, 182, 184, 185–186; opposition to medical alumni report on medical school (1920), 240

Wilson, O. Meredith, 546, 548

Winch, George D., 28(n.22)

Winslow House, 16, 18, 20

Witzel, Oscar, 308, 313

Woodruff, M. F. A., 531

World War I: American volunteers, 213; medical school staff involved, 213–214, 233; medical personnel who served, 213–234, 293, 384, 482; contributions to war effort, 215, 216. *See also:* Base Hospital No. 26

World War II: medical school continued training, 416; medical personnel who served, 494. *See also:* 26th General Hospital

Wright, Charles B., 287

Wright, Franklin R., 287

Wulling, Frederick J., 50

X-ray therapy, used in gynecological cancer, 354–356

X-rays: demonstrated to physicians (1896), 75–76; diagnostic use in intestinal obstruction, 312–313; for tuberculosis, 338, 342, 344–345, 356

Youngdahl, Luther W., 436, 437

Ziegler, Edward, 129–130

Ziegler, Mildred R., 258, 346, 347, 349

Zimmerman, Harry B., 219

Zoll, Paul, 517

Zondek, Bernard, 295